Essentials of Dental Surgery and Pathology

R. A. Cawson MD BDS FDS RCPS Glas FRCPath

Emeritus Professor of Oral Medicine and Pathology,
University of London and
Visiting Professor in Oral Pathology,
Baylor Dental College, Dallas, Texas.

FIFTH EDITION

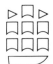

CHURCHILL LIVINGSTONE
EDINBURGH LONDON MELBOURNE NEW YORK AND TOKYO 1991

CHURCHILL LIVINGSTONE
Medical Division of Longman Group UK Limited

Distributed in the United States of America by Churchill
Livingstone Inc., 650 Avenue of the Americas, New York,
N.Y. 10011, and by associated companies, branches and
representatives throughout the world.

First edition 1962
Second edition 1968
Third edition 1978
Fourth edition 1984
Fifth edition 1991

ISBN 0-443-04042-7

British Library Cataloguing in Publication Data
CIP catalogue record for this book is available from the
British Library.

Library of Congress Cataloging in Publication Data
CIP catalog record for this book is available from the Library
of Congress.

Produced by Longman Singapore Publishers (Pte) Ltd.
Printed in Singapore

Preface

This edition has been extensively rewritten. A good deal has been added and much has been deleted in the attempt to reflect some of the changes in dentistry.

The profession seems to feel that dentistry is currently in something of a state of transition. Dental caries—once the main area of dental work—has declined strikingly. This applies to children particularly, but this change may spread to adults, and the dental health of the nation seems gradually to be improving. There have also been considerable developments in dental restorative materials and (by a strange coincidence) concern about mercury-containing amalgams.

Another change is that the increasing demand for safety in virtually every conceivable object or activity now directly involves dentistry. Not unreasonably, some feel that dentistry is about as safe to both dentist and patient as any activity can be. However, a vociferous minority of the general public have quite unrealistic ideas about the absolute necessity for total safety in *everything*. It is almost as if they wish to be in glowing health, like Aztec sacrifices, before offering themselves to be killed or maimed, as they are in their hundreds of thousands on the roads each year.

Dentistry has therefore come under the eagle eye of the Health and Safety Executive. Legally enforceable safety standards are now applied to such matters as radiography and cross-infection control, and the conduct of anaesthesia and sedation have been greatly circumscribed. It may seem therefore to the future dentist that it is becoming necessary to be as knowledgeable about legislation that may enmesh him as about dentistry itself. However, if concern shifts from the safety of the dental pulp—for so many years the obsession of examiners—to the safety of the patient, the change can only be healthy.

As a consequence, a chapter on occupational hazards in dentistry has been added, and this will give some indication of some of the legal problems that may have to be faced. Increased emphasis has also been given to radiation protection and the legal requirements involved.

A chapter on investigation of oral disease has been added partly because the multiplicity of investigations currently available must be bewildering. They are often overused, but failure to investigate a patient adequately, can itself be a source of medicolegal claims.

With regard to the rest of this text it might have been desirable to add many more illustrations. However, this would have added considerably to the cost, and there are plenty of other books available (as indicated in the lists of suggested further reading) to make up for any deficiency. Nevertheless, despite my having sought advice from as many experts as possible, reviewers will no doubt suggest that either too much or too little has been included. Whatever its limitations, therefore, the aim of this book still remains to provide an adequate background to clinical practice and to help the student with the degree examination. For that matter it could considerably help postgraduates with the Fellowship. During many years as a Fellowship examiner, it was a continual surprise that so few of the candidates knew enough of the contents of this student text to give a presentable performance.

Once again I should like to express my gratitude to many colleagues for their much-needed help and encouragement. In particular I should like to thank Dr David Brown, Dr J. W. Eveson,

Miss Rhona Hickman, Dr Richard Palmer, who has extensively revised the chapter on periodontal disease, Miss Pat Reynolds, Professor Crispian Scully, Mr Ray Shaw, Miss Meg Skelly, and Mr Eric Whaites. I especially wish to thank Professor Norman Waters for so generously providing facilities to do the necessary writing and Dr Martyn Sherriff for his invaluable help with my computer (and its many whims) also to Mr Sidney Luck for his indefatigable help with references and to Miss Phyllis Gale and the staff of the Wills and Warner Libraries for their expert and generous assistance.

London 1991

R. A. C.

Contents

1. Investigation of oral disease

The purpose of any investigation is to make as precise a diagnosis as possible, to help the clinician decide the best form of treatment and gain some idea of the prognosis. A typical example is that of deciding whether or not an ulcer or swelling is a malignant tumour. It is also essential to establish whether there is anything, particularly in the patient's history, to suggest that there may be some underlying complaint. This has become particularly important now that AIDS has become widespread. Systemic disease may be the cause of the lesion under investigation, or it may affect the management of the patient, or both.

Innumerable types of investigation are possible, and it may be difficult to refrain from asking for every conceivable investigation in the anxiety not to miss some unsuspected trouble and to avoid possible medicolegal complications. Though it may be tempting to look into every possibility, however remote, this approach may prove counterproductive in that it can produce innumerable reports that may confuse rather than inform. In addition, laboratory staff soon become aware of, and become less than helpful towards, those who overburden them. Particular investiga-

tions should only be requested when specifically indicated.

The main lines of investigation include:

1. Clinical investigation—particularly, careful history taking
2. Radiography and other imaging techniques
3. Biopsy and histopathology. In special circumstances, frozen sections, immunocytochemistry, electron microscopy or other techniques may be required
4. Other laboratory investigations, particularly haematology or biochemistry for underlying systemic disorders.

CLINICAL INVESTIGATION

The dental history

The duration of the history and the clinical features of individual lesions must be evaluated. The symptoms and rate of progress of the complaint alone may strongly suggest (for example) whether that patient has a tumour and, if so, whether it is benign or malignant. Some diseases, such as cancer, mainly affect the elderly, whilst others, such as the autoimmune diseases, more frequently affect females. An elderly woman with a swollen parotid gland due to lymphocytic infiltration is likely to have Sjögren's syndrome (Ch. 17), but, in a young man, a histologically similar lesion is far more likely to be a feature of AIDS (Ch. 8). Other diseases, particularly those which result from sex-linked recessive traits, such as haemophilia, are seen only in males. Knowledge of the age and sex of the patient may therefore contribute greatly to making a diagnosis.

The medical history

The great majority of dental patients are ambulant, and routine dental treatment presents no threat to their health. However, unsuspected diseases can sometimes affect their management (particularly now that sedation is so widely used) or be the cause of some complaint in the mouth. This is obviously important in relation to HIV infection. To ensure that nothing significant is forgotten, a simple questionnaire can be prepared for patients to complete, and this is valuable also in helping to avoid medicolegal problems. As a minimum, the following 12 questions should be asked:

1. **A**naemia or **A**llergies?
2. **B**leeding tendencies?
3. **C**ardiorespiratory complaints?
4. **D**rug treatment?
5. **E**ndocrine disorders?
6. **F**its?
7. **G**astrointestinal complaints?
8. **H**ospital admission or attendance?
9. **I**nfections?
10. **J**aundice or other liver disease?
11. **K**idney disease?
12. **L**ikelihood of, or existing, pregnancy?

The questionnaire can be modified as much as the user wishes but, even if it asks only the minimal amount of information as suggested above, it saves a good deal of time and provides a written record that the patient's medical background has been taken into consideration.

It is, however, also worthwhile to leave a final section open for patients to supply any other information that they think might be relevant. In the writer's experience, one apparently healthy and

conventional-looking young man admitted, in this open section, to an impressive list of sexually transmitted diseases and that he was currently under investigation for AIDS.

As well as considering the possibility of any systemic disease, the details of drugs being taken should be emphasised. For example, in a woman complaining of dryness of the mouth, a history of rheumatoid arthritis strongly suggests that she has Sjögren's syndrome (Ch. 17). By contrast, if the patient has a history of depression and is taking a drug such as amitriptyline, that alone will cause severe xerostomia. Drugs can also cause mucosal lesions which can mimic other diseases such as lichen planus, whilst other drugs, particularly long-term corticosteroid treatment, can significantly affect the management of the patient.

Patients should also be asked if they carry a *medical card*. This may indicate that the patient is, for example, a haemophiliac or is on long-term corticosteroid therapy with obvious implications.

Clinical examination

Oral examination

Only too often teeth have been filled and periodontal disease has been ignored. Dental examination should be thorough both for the patient's sake and because successful claims have been made against dentists who have failed to recognise or treat caries or periodontal disease, sometimes as a consequence of not taking the necessary radiographs.

Even though only routine dental care is required, it is important also to inspect the rest of the mouth systematically. Early carcinomas, for example, can be painless red areas, unnoticed by the patient. The reality of such a possibility is driven home by the fact that examination of *dentists* at meetings of the American Dental Association revealed, in some, malignant tumours, as well as a significant amount of oral and perioral disease. Nevertheless dentists are sometimes the first to notice abnormalities such as these in their patients.

It is also important to palpate the cervical lymph nodes. Lymphadenopathy is the most common manifestation of infection by the AIDS virus, and the cervical lymph nodes are often first affected by lymphomas.

Medical examination

It is essential to *look* at patients and not simply focus on their teeth. Anaemia, thyroid disease, long-term corticosteroid treatment, parotid swellings, or significantly enlarged cervical nodes are only a few of the conditions that can affect the facial appearance. If the history suggests, or examination reveals, any condition not already under treatment, referral for medical examination may be necessary. Examples are unexplained cervical lymphadenopathy or an abnormal blood picture indicating (for example) anaemia—a surprisingly common cause of mouth complaints.

IMAGING TECHNIQUES

The main examples include:

- Radiography and computerised tomography (CT)
- Magnetic resonance imaging (MRI)
- Ultrasound.

Radiography is in everyday use in dentistry because of the ready recognition of hard tissue lesions affecting the teeth or jaws. Radiographs are usually essential for the assessment of dental caries and periodontal disease. Some other lesions such as cysts of the jaws can usually be recognised with almost complete certainty by radiography alone, though histological confirmation is also necessary to exclude rare cystic tumours.

Computerised tomography (CT) scans also use X-rays but show, in much greater detail, normal and abnormal structures of both hard and soft tissues in any chosen plane. They are valuable, for example, for determining the extent of a tumour involving the maxilla. The disadvantages of these methods is the increasing anxiety about the dangers of X-rays (Ch. 22). CT scanning is also expensive and not universally available.

Sialography, in which radiopaque material is injected into the duct of a salivary gland can show abnormalities of the duct structure or distortion of their normal pattern by a tumour or radiolucent stone.

Magnetic resonance imaging (MRI) is a different technique which does not use X-rays. Though very expensive it is invaluable for showing lesions in the soft tissues, in remarkable detail. Even the grey matter of the brain can be readily distinguished from the white matter, but hard tissues appear as blank areas. MRI will also provide an image of any chosen plane of the body and is frequently useful for indicating the extent of a soft-tissue tumour, but may not show whether it has started to invade bone.

Ultrasound is little used in dentistry but may occasionally be useful to give some idea of the extent of a tumour when CT or MRI equipment is not available. It is quick, safe and inexpensive, and capable of showing to the expert even minute soft-tissue lesions, such as vegetations on the heart in infective endocarditis (Ch. 8).

HISTOPATHOLOGY AND RELATED METHODS

Conventional histopathology using paraffin-embedded sections is still the most widely used laboratory technique in dentistry for the investigation of anything other than dental caries and periodontal disease. The diagnosis of the latter diseases is made on their clinical features supplemented by radiographs.

Biopsy

The specimens for histopathology should usually be taken, before treatment, by *biopsy*—this term encompasses both removal of a part or the whole of a lesion, and its examination by microscopy. In the case, particularly, of cysts of the jaws or parotid gland tumours, microscopic examination is usually made postoperatively, on the whole specimen. This is because, as mentioned earlier, cysts are usually reliably recognisable by their clinical and radiographic features, but microscopy is necessary particularly to ensure that a cystic tumour has not been mistaken for a simple cyst. Though anxiety has been expressed about the risk of spreading tumour cells when a biopsy incision has been carried out, there is little evidence otherwise that this happens. Moreover, such a risk, if it exists, must be taken to ensure that an accurate preoperative diagnosis is made. Parotid gland tumours are an important exception, because the most common type, the pleomorphic adenoma, has an unusual tendency to seed its cells and recur in the incision wound. Such tumours should therefore be examined microscopically only *after* excision.

Some of the more important requirements of biopsies are as follows.

1. The specimen is of adequate size and (wherever possible) at least 1 cm long.
2. The specimen is not crushed by forceps, distorted by the local anaesthetic injection or otherwise damaged, during removal.
3. The specimen is put immediately into fixative, usually buffered formal-saline (NOT *normal* saline). Fixation is essential to preserve the microscopic detail of the tissue. Delay in putting the specimen in fixative leads to drying and autolysis, so that the specimen quickly becomes useless for diagnosis. A variety of other fixative agents may be used for special purposes such as electron microscopy. Some of these fixatives change the microscopic appearances of the cells appreciably.
4. The patient's name and (usually) an identifying number is put on the specimen bottle—only too easily and disastrously forgotten.
5. The request form should also identify the patient, the clinician and supply as much clinical detail as possible. The purpose of this exercise is to ensure as accurate a diagnosis as possible and not (as some clinicians seem to think) some sort of a competition with the pathologist as to who can make the better guess.

Clinical information is particularly important as it is sometimes impossible to make a definitive diagnosis on the microscopic features alone, and it is important to appreciate the limitations of histopathology as discussed later. In the case of recurrent aphthae (Ch. 15), for example, the microscopic features are non-specific, and the history of repeated recurrences is more informative.

However, in the case of a major aphtha which may clinically resemble a carcinoma, microscopy will show whether or not the ulcer is due to a tumour.

Tissue processing

Complete fixation usually takes about 12 hours or longer for large specimens. The tissue is then processed to dehydrate it (by immersion in a series of solvents) and to enable it to be impregnated with, and embedded in, paraffin wax (or other, special-purpose embedding media). These processes are usually carried out overnight in a tissue-processing machine so that the section should be ready for sectioning on the following day. The block can then be mounted on a microtome. Sections are usually cut at about 5 μm thickness, then persuaded onto microscope slides, 'de-paraffined' with solvent and stained to provide visual differentiation of the various tissues present.

It usually takes 24–48 hours to process, section and stain a specimen before the pathologist can report on it.

Some common stains used for microscopy

Stained paraffin-mounted microscopy sections provide an artefactual, two-dimensional picture of a lesion, but the use of histopathology over more than a century, supplemented by other methods of investigation such as electron microscopy, has resulted in the accumulation of so vast a body of knowledge for interpreting the appearances that may be seen, that most lesions can be reliably recognised by this means.

Haematoxylin and eosin (H & E) are the routine stains. Haematoxylin stains chromatin (nucleic acids bound to protein) blue-black and can show nuclear abnormalities which may be important in the diagnosis of cancer (Ch. 16). Eosin stains the cytoplasm of most cells varying shades of pink, and the configuration of the tissue is usually clearly displayed in these contrasting colours. Typical staining of important tissues or cell products is shown in Table 1.1. Substances which stain with eosin are sometimes termed acidophilic, whilst haematoxylin staining may be termed basophilic.

Table 1.1 Examples of haematoxylin and eosin staining of various tissues

Eosin (acidic)	Haematoxylin (basic)
Cytoplasm of most cells*	Nuclei (DNA & RNA)
Keratin	Mucopolysaccharide-rich ground substance
Muscle	
Bone (decalcified)	Bone (undecalcified)
Collagen	Reversal lines in bone

* The cytoplasm of some cells (as in some salivary gland tumours) is intensely eosinophilic. In others such as plasma cells it is basophilic or intermediate (amphophilic).

In this relatively simple way, therefore, microscopy can, among many other things, usually confirm whether or not a tumour is malignant, partly on the basis of nuclear abnormalities but, more important, by showing invasion of the adjacent tissues. In addition the degree of differentiation of the tumour cells may give some indication of how aggressive it is likely to be.

Some of the great variety of tissue patterns used to identify the many lesions that can affect the mouth can be seen in the illustrations in the subsequent text, where the great majority of the sections were stained with H & E.

Other, more complex stains such as picro-Mallory are much prettier than boring old H & E but rarely contribute significantly more information.

Connective-tissue and other special stains

Periodic acid Shiff (PAS) reagent is taken up by a variety of carbohydrates and mucinous substances which stain pink. This may be useful in helping to identify a mucoepidermoid carcinoma (for example) when there is little mucin visible with H & E. Other, uncommon tumours contain glycogen which stains positively with PAS but is removed by diastase. Candidal hyphae (Ch. 15) also stain strongly with PAS, and this is useful for demonstrating hyphae invading epithelium since they are frequently invisible in H & E-stained specimens.

Silver stains will, for example, demonstrate reticulin. This may be helpful in distinguishing follicular lymphomas (Ch. 16) from diffuse types which are usually more malignant, or for outlining blood vessels in uncommon tumours such as haemangiopericytomas where the vessel lumens are not apparent. Similarly the remains of the elastic lamina of arterioles which have been destroyed as a result of arteritis (Ch. 20) can be demonstrated. Van Gieson's stain can be modified as in the Verhoff–van Gieson stain and also shows elastic tissue (black). Fungi in the tissues usually also stain well with silver stains.

Stains for microorganisms. Bacteria and fungi in direct smears are usually quickly and satisfactorily stained by Gram's method. All fungi are strongly Gram-positive but, since the bacteria of ulcerative gingivitis are Gram-negative, another stain such as Becker's shows up the fuso-spirochaetal complex more clearly.

Special stains usually have to be used to demonstrate microbes in the tissues. Many fungi such as aspergillus species or *Candida albicans* in the tissues may be difficult to discern with H & E staining but take up silver stains strongly and also stain well with PAS as mentioned earlier.

Decalcified and hard (undecalcified) sections

For routine purposes teeth and some jaw tumours need to be decalcified before they can be sectioned. This may delay the diagnosis by days or weeks according to the size of the specimen. Another disadvantage of decalcification (though rarely important) is that the enamel, having little organic matrix, is usually lost. When it is essential to visualise abnormalities of the enamel or other hard tissues, the section can be cut with diamond or other abrasive-impregnated mechanical saws, but such methods are largely for research purposes.

Frozen sections

Frozen sections can usually provide an answer within 10 minutes of taking the specimen but show some microscopic features slightly less well than paraffin sections. Incorrect diagnoses are therefore occasionally possible. Frozen sections are only indicated under such circumstances as the following:

1. To establish, at operation, whether or not the tumour is malignant and whether, as a consequence, the excision needs to be extended
2. To confirm that the excision margins are free of tumour at the time of operation
3. For immunofluorescence microscopy or for immunocytochemistry.

Frozen sections for tumours are usually only justifiable if the definitive operation is to be carried out immediately. Fixed, paraffin-blocked sections are always preferable for light microscopy if the elective operation is going to be carried out some days later and, in any case, are always prepared later for confirmation.

Tissues must be quickly frozen, preferably to about $-70°C$ by, for example, immersion in liquid nitrogen. Delay in freezing leads to autolysis, while slow freezing (in a domestic deepfreeze at $-10°C$ or warmer, for example) results in the growth of damaging intracellular ice crystals and grossly distorted microscopic appearances. In many cases, a cryostat (a refrigerated microtome) is kept in a side room of the theatre, and the specimen can then be prepared for sectioning almost immediately. The frozen section is slid onto a slide, briefly immersed in a dehydrating fixative agent then stained with haematoxylin and eosin. If the tissue has to be taken to a separate laboratory it can be carried in liquid nitrogen in a Thermos flask or surrounded by solid CO_2.

With reasonable precautions and facilities, frozen sections for tumour diagnosis provide a rapid and, usually, a reliable answer but will not of course deal with hard tissues.

Limitations of histopathology

Microscopy will solve many but by no means all diagnostic problems. There are several reasons for its limitations as follows.

1. Specimens may be inadequate, unrepresentative, or otherwise unsatisfactory. They may be too small to be useful, may have missed some crucial area in the lesion or may have been sent unfixed or have been otherwise damaged.
2. Sections are frequently only cut in one plane, and some critical feature may not be present in that plane.
3. A few diseases, such as recurrent aphthae in particular, do not have sufficiently specific microscopic appearances to make a definitive diagnosis possible. In other lesions, such as the granulomas typical of tuberculosis, there are many other possible causes (Ch. 20) and diagnosis depends on other investigations such as bacteriology.
4. There are some diagnostic catches which can occasionally cause difficulties. Examples of these diagnostic hazards include the following.
   a. It can be difficult to decide the nature of a poorly differentiated tumour. In the past it was sometimes impossible to decide whether one was a carcinoma or a lymphoma. However, in many cases, the advent of immunocytochemistry, as discussed below, has simplified this problem.
   b. By contrast, other tumours can be well differentiated and cytologically benign, but nevertheless malignant in behaviour. It may only be possible to recognise this if the specimen includes an area of invasion. Acinic cell and muco-epidermoid carcinomas of salivary glands are an example of tumours whose behaviour is unpredictable from their usually benign microscopic appearance. Pleomorphic adenomas can also present difficulties as they are one of the few benign tumours that can undergo malignant change, but the carcinomatous area can be very small and may be missed. In the case of chondromas and some neurofibromas the borderline between the benign and malignant is ill-defined and malignancy only established later by the tumour's behaviour.
   c. Nuclear changes characteristic of malignancy may be seen but there may be no signs of invasion. It is then difficult or impossible to decide whether malignancy

is likely to develop at some time in the future or whether it has already happened in some other part of the lesion. In many such cases, the problem may be settled by more extensive examination of the specimen. However, this is only possible if the specimen is large enough. A related problem is that the assessment of degrees of cellular dysplasia (Ch. 16) can only be subjective. Hence it is virtually impossible to predict reliably the likelihood of malignant change in some mucosal white lesions.

Fibro-osseous bone lesions form another area where behaviour of the lesion may be unpredictable. In other cases, inflammation may mask the essential features or, in the case of ameloblastomas, cyst formation may compress the tumour cells so that they can resemble those of a simple cyst.

Another, but fortunately uncommon, area of difficulty is that of distinguishing malignant lymphomas from non-neoplastic lymphoproliferative diseases.

These are only a few examples but it is important to appreciate that microscopy can occasionally either produce the wrong answer or no useful answer at all. In some cases the microscopic diagnosis may differ or be at variance with the clinical picture or history. In such cases there should be no hesitation in repeating the biopsy and discussing the problem with the pathologist.

Immunofluorescence microscopy and immunocytochemistry

Immunofluorescence depends on the binding of an antibody, tagged with a fluorescent dye, to an antigen in the tissues. Surplus reagent is washed off and a positive antigen–antibody reaction is visible by its fluorescence in an ultraviolet light microscope. As mentioned earlier, frozen sections are required, as the antigens will not withstand the processing necessary for production of paraffin blocks. A typical use of immunofluorescence is for detection of autoantibodies (immunoglobulins) attached to the intercellular substance in pemphigus vulgaris (Ch. 15) or for the diagnosis of other vesiculobullous diseases. It should be noted that the precise nature of the autoantibodies is not detected in this way. Only the class of immunoglobulin (of which the autoantibody consists) is recognised as an antigen and binds the anti-immunoglobulin/stain complex, to produce the fluorescence in positive cases.

Immunocytochemistry

This depends on the preparation of antibodies (often now monoclonal) which react with specific cell or cell membrane antigenic components. The basis of the technique is the same in principle as that of immunofluorescence but the antibodies for immunostaining are conjugated with a tracer (such as horseradish peroxidase) and the process is often sensitive enough to allow the use of paraffin-embedded sections. The amount of tracer-conjugated antibody binding to a minute amount of tissue antigen, and hence the sensitivity of the test, can be increased by using an indirect, two-stage reaction. By means of a chemical reaction with the peroxidase bound to them, positively reacting cells stain brown and, for better differentiation, the tissue can be counterstained with haematoxylin.

One of the simplest applications is to examine immunoglobulin (or, more strictly, lambda or kappa light chain) production in lymphoproliferative lesions. If this immunoglobulin is monoclonal, then it is the product of a single clone of lymphocytes. This indicates that the lymphocytes are neoplastic and a malignant lymphoma is present.

Other monoclonal antibodies react with specific cell products, such as hormones, to enable a poorly differentiated endocrine tumour to be identified.

Another application is that of identifying membrane markers of lymphocytes. This may enable different subsets of lymphocytes to be recognised and, for example, T helper to be differentiated from T suppressor cells. This may suggest their activity in a lesion. Monoclonal antibodies can also be used to differentiate lymphomas of B cell origin from those of T cell origin. T cell lymphomas are uncommon and have only been recognised with certainty in recent years by means of such markers.

Intermediate filaments. Yet other types of monoclonal antibodies react with intermediate filaments (components of the cytoskeleton), including keratins (in epithelial cells), vimentin (in mesenchymal tissues), or desmin (in muscle). This often enables an undifferentiated tumour to be categorised with more certainty. Unfortunately, many quite different types of cell share antigenically similar components (epitopes), and, for example, a few mesenchymal cells stain with epithelial markers. S100 protein was thought to be neurone-specific but in practice will stain a variety of cells, including melanoma cells. As a result, the overall microscopic appearances have to be taken into account and a panel of monoclonal antibodies may have to be used before a reasonably firm diagnosis can be made.

In addition to the sharing of markers by cells of different origin, neoplastic cells may lose specific markers. The techniques must also be meticulously carried out, are time-consuming and require adequate controls to ensure that both false-positive and false-negative results are avoided.

Lectin histochemistry is being increasingly used. Lectins are glycoproteins, and the technique depends on the fact that different lectins bind, non-immunologically, to carbohydrates (in glycoproteins, glycolipids, or polysaccharides) on cell surfaces and, when used with a marker such as horseradish peroxidase or fluorescein, can be used as an alternative to monoclonal antibodies. Endothelial cells, for example, can be identified by means of a monoclonal antibody that binds to factor VIII, or alternatively with a lectin which binds to this factor's specific glycoprotein.

Lectins are, incidentally, ubiquitous in nature. In the body they mediate many cell-to-cell interactions and play a critical role in many normal and pathological processes. One of the first of these to be recognised was the mechanism by which the influenza virus binds to and agglutinates erythrocytes by means of a lectin. In the mouth, lectins help several streptococcus and actinomyces species to adhere to tooth surfaces (Ch. 3).

Exfoliative cytology

Exfoliative cytology is the examination of cells obtained by scraping a superficial lesion or, less frequently, by aspiration of cells shed into a cyst cavity. It is quick, easy and does not require the use of a local anaesthetic.

Smears of exfoliated cells from the mouth are usually stained with haematoxylin and eosin. Some of the uses of cytology are to show virally-damaged cells in herpetic infections or acantholytic cells of pemphigus (Ch. 15). As with sections, immunostaining can also be applied (such as fluorescent antibodies for herpes simplex antigens or anti-immunoglobulins for the examples just given) and will improve diagnostic specificity.

However, cytology is not a reliable method of diagnosing cancer, because false-positive or false-negative results can be obtained. Biopsy is always more reliable and, since it can be so readily carried out in the mouth, is mandatory when cancer is suspected.

Other laboratory investigations

Haematology

Blood investigations are clearly essential for the diagnosis of diseases such as leukaemias, myelomas, or leukopenias which have oral manifestations, or for identifying defects of haemostasis which can greatly affect management. A preoperative blood picture is also desirable to detect unsuspected disease—particularly anaemia, which increases the risk of hypoxia during anaesthesia and can be dangerous if there is any substantial blood loss. Blood investigations are also helpful in the diagnosis of other conditions such as HIV infection (lymphopenia), and sore tongues or recurrent aphthae which are sometimes associated with anaemia.

There are many different types of haematological examinations, and the request form must give the haematologist enough clinical information to decide what investigations are necessary. A routine blood picture provides automated measurement of the haemoglobin level, many red cell indices such as their number, size (to indicate whether micro- or macrocytosis is present) and haemoglobin content, and a differential white cell count. It is essential to put the blood into the appropriate tube, such as an EDTA (anti-coagulant) tube, for routine indices. However, the latter will provide little direct information about haemorrhagic disorders unless there is an obvious deficiency of platelets. Many tests of coagulation function require citrated blood, and a haematologist will *not* be impressed with a request for assessment clotting function on a specimen of coagulated blood.

The erythrocyte sedimentation rate (ESR) is raised in all inflammatory diseases. This is sometimes informative but especially so in cranial (giant cell) arteritis (Ch. 20). If treatment of this disease is stopped before the ESR has returned to normal, blindness can result from the still active but otherwise asymptomatic disease.

Microbiology

Despite the fact that most oral disease is infective in nature, microbiology is surprisingly rarely of practical diagnostic value in dentistry. Direct Gram-stained smears will quickly confirm the diagnosis of thrush, and H & E-stained smears can show the distorted, virally infected epithelial cells in herpetic infections. However, even in the case of ulcerative gingivitis the clinical picture is so distinctive that metronidazole is usually given without further investigation other than, perhaps, a direct smear. Nevertheless the causative organisms of osteomyelitis, cellulitis, acute parotitis, deep mycoses (frequently mistaken for tumours), or other severe infections need to be identified if appropriate antimicrobial treatment is to be given. However, such treatment has usually to be started without this information, and none of these diseases is common in Britain. Further, particularly in the case of fungal infections (in AIDS, for example), the possibility may not have been suspected clinically and the diagnosis may have to be made on the biopsy appearances. Special stains as mentioned earlier may then be helpful.

Despite hopes to the contrary, intensive study of the bacteriology of periodontal disease has not yielded any species of bacteria that is a reliable marker of disease activity. In the case of dental caries, diagnosis and treatment are carried out without consideration of the bacteriology.

Serology

Some infections, particularly syphilis, and, theoretically at least, others such as herpes or mumps, HIV infection and infectious mononucleosis (Paul Bunnell test) require serological confirmation. More important perhaps is to detect whether a patient is a hepatitis B antigen carrier.

Chemistry

Examples are blood sugar levels for the diagnosis of diabetes mellitus or blood calcium, phosphate or phosphatase levels for the diagnosis of a variety of bone diseases such as hyperparathyroidism, Paget's disease, or prostatic metastases.

Immunological tests

Autoantibody studies and other immunological tests are discussed in Chapter 20. However, it should be emphasised that there are no tests which will enable a positive diagnosis of immunologically mediated disease to be made, and autoantibody studies must be interpreted in relation to the clinical and other findings.

SUGGESTED FURTHER READING

Frable W J 1989 Needle aspiration biopsy: past, present and future. Hum Pathol 20: 504–517

Goltry R R, Ayer W A 1986 Head neck and oral abnormalities in dentists participating in the health assessment program. JADA 112: 338–341

Heyderman E, Warren P J, Haines A M R 1989 Immunocytochemistry today—problems and practice. Histopathology 15: 653–658

Huang H K 1990 Advances in medical imaging. Ann Intern Med 112: 203–220

Jacobson H G (ed) 1988 Council on Scientific Affairs. Magnetic resonance imaging of the head and neck region. J Am Med Assoc 260: 3313–3326

Lam E W N, Hannam A G, Wood W W et al 1989 Imaging orofacial tissues by magnetic resonance. Oral Surg, Oral Med, Oral Pathol 68: 2–8

Morgan P R, Shirlaw P J, Johnson N W et al 1987 Potential applications of anti-keratin antibodies in oral diagnosis. J Oral Pathol 16: 212–222

Rode J 1989 Fine needle cytology versus histology.
Histopathology 15: 435–439
Rodu B 1990 The polymerase chain reaction. Am J Med Sci
210: 210–216
Sawady J, Berner J J, Siegler E E 1988 Accuracy of and
reasons for frozen sections: a correlative, retrospective
study. Hum Pathol 19: 1019–1023

Schmitt F C, Bacchi C E 1989 S-100 protein: is it useful as
a tumour marker in diagnostic immunocytochemistry?
Histopathology 15: 281–288
Swanson P E 1988 Foundations of immunohistochemistry. A
practical review. Am J Clin Pathol 90: 333–339

2. Disorders of development of the teeth and related tissues

Abnormalities in the number of teeth
Isolated hypodontia or anodontia
Hypodontia or anodontia associated with systemic defects
Other conditions associated with hypodontia
Additional teeth: hyperdontia
Disorders of eruption
Delayed eruption associated with skeletal disorders
Changes affecting buried teeth
Defects of structure: hypoplasia and hypocalcification
Deciduous teeth
Permanent teeth
Amelogenesis imperfecta
Dentinogenesis (odontogenesis) imperfecta
Shell teeth
Dentinal dysplasia ('rootless' teeth)

Regional odontodysplasia (ghost teeth)
Hypophosphatasia
Ehlers Danlos (floppy joint) syndromes
Infection—congenital syphilis
Severe disturbances of nutrition and metabolism
Tetracycline pigmentation
Other acquired developmental anomalies
Dental fluorosis—mottled enamel
Treatment of hypoplastic defects
Odontomas
Genetic disorders of the soft tissues and jaws
Epidermolysis bullosa
Prognathism
Clefts of the lip and palate
Other genetic diseases relevant to dentistry

The development of an ideal dentition, depends on

1. Formation of full complement of teeth
2. Normal structural development of the dental tissues
3. Eruption of each group of teeth at the appropriate time into an adequate space and into the correct relationship with their opposite numbers.

In view of the complexity of the organisation of the development of the teeth, serious defects of structure are remarkably uncommon. By contrast, disorders of occlusion due to irregularities of the teeth in the arch or abnormal relationship of the arches to each other are so common that their treatment has become a specialty in its own right.

The main groups of disorders affecting development of the dentition may be summarised as follows.

1. Abnormalities in the number of teeth
   —Anodontia or hypodontia
   —Anodontia or hypodontia associated with systemic disorders
   —Additional teeth (hyperdontia)
2. Disorders of eruption of the teeth
   —Local obstructions to eruption
   —General disorders of eruption
3. Defects of structure of the teeth
   —Disorders of development of the enamel
   —Disorders of development of the dentine
4. Developmental anomalies of several dental tissues
   —Odontomas.

ABNORMALITIES IN THE NUMBER OF TEETH

These disorders are usually very minor, affect the dentition alone and are without any apparent systemic abnormality.

Usually only one or two teeth are missing or there may be an additional tooth.

11

Isolated hypodontia or anodontia

Failure of development of one or two teeth is relatively common and often hereditary. The teeth most frequently missing are third molars, second premolars, or maxillary second incisors.

Absence of third molars can be a disadvantage if first or second molars, or both, have been lost. The absence of lower premolars increases the severity of malocclusion if there is already disparity in size between an underdeveloped mandible and a normal upper arch. Otherwise absence of these teeth may have little or no noticeable effect.

Absence of lateral incisors can sometimes be conspicuous because the large, pointed canines come into position in the front of the mouth beside the central incisors. It is usually impossible to prevent the canine from erupting into this empty space, even if the patient is seen early. It is also very difficult to make room between the centrals and canines by orthodontic means to replace the laterals. An attempt has often therefore to be made to disguise the shape of the canines.

Total failure of development of a complete dentition (anodontia) is exceedingly rare. If the permanent dentition fails to form, the deciduous dentition is retained for many years, but when these deciduous teeth become excessively worn or too much damaged by caries then they must be replaced by dentures.

Hypodontia or anodontia associated with systemic defects

Anhidrotic (hereditary) ectodermal dysplasia. This disorder of ectodermal development is usually transmitted as a sex-linked or, less often, as a simple recessive trait. Males are therefore usually affected and the main manifestations are (1) hypodontia, (2) hypotrichosis and (3) hypohidrosis. In extreme cases there may be complete failure of development of the dental lamina so that no teeth form. More often, many or all the deciduous teeth form but there are few or no permanent teeth. The teeth are usually peg-shaped or of simple conical form.

Where there is anodontia, the alveolar process, without teeth to support, fails to develop. The profile then resembles that of an elderly person because of the gross loss of vertical dimension.

In most cases the hair is fine and sparse but, even when the hair appears normal, there is typically a thin or almost bald area in the tonsural region. In more severe cases the hair is little more than a thin downy fluff, while the skin is smooth and shiny, and dry due to absence of sweat glands. Heat is therefore poorly tolerated. The finger nails are usually also defective.

All that can be done to improve the patient's appearance and mastication is to fit dentures, which are usually well tolerated by children.

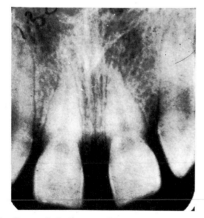

Fig. 2.1 Congenital absence of lateral incisors with spacing of the anterior teeth.

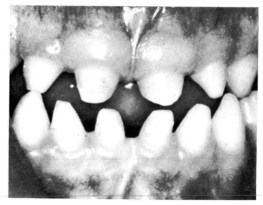

Fig. 2.2 Ectodermal dysplasia. The teeth are deficient in number and of simple conical form. Defects of the hair and nails were associated.

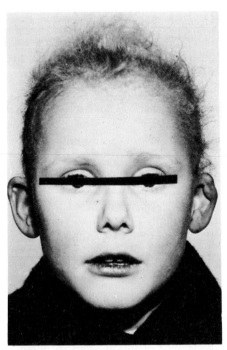

Fig. 2.3   Anhidrotic ectodermal dysplasia. This shows the typical fine and scanty hair. There is also scaling of the lower lip.

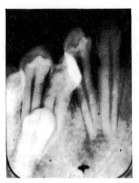

Fig. 2.4   Additional teeth; there are two additional premolars. One has erupted partially; the other remains embedded within the jaw.

Other conditions associated with hypodontia

There are many rare syndromes where hypodontia is a feature, but the only common one is Down's syndrome (Mongolism). In this condition there seems to be no defined pattern of hypodontia. One or more third molars are absent in over 90% of these patients, while absence of individual teeth scattered about the arch is also common. Anodontia has also been reported, but is rare.

Palatal clefts are another developmental disorder associated with hypodontia.

Additional teeth: hyperdontia

Additional teeth are relatively common. They are usually of simple conical shape (*supernumerary teeth*) but may resemble teeth of the normal series (*supplemental teeth*). These are the result of excessive but organised growth of the dental lamina of unknown cause.

Additional (supplemental teeth). Occasionally a supplemental maxillary incisor or premolar and, rarely, a fourth molar develops.

Supernumerary teeth. Conical or more severely malformed additional teeth are more common than supplemental teeth and are usually in the maxillary incisor region. Occasionally they form in the midline (mesiodens), particularly of the maxilla, or, even more rarely, in the mandible.

Effects and treatment. Additional teeth usually erupt in an abnormal position labial or buccal to the arch, creating a stagnation area leading to caries or periodontal disease. In other cases a supernumerary tooth may prevent a normal tooth from erupting. In most cases these additional teeth should be extracted.

Syndromes associated with hyperdontia

These syndromes are all rare but probably the best known is cleidocranial dysplasia (Ch. 12) where there is development of many supernumerary teeth. These may be so crowded as to become distorted (Fig. 12.4). In addition there is a widespread failure of eruption, with the consequence that most of these teeth remain buried in the jaw, producing *pseudoanodontia*.

DISORDERS OF ERUPTION

Eruption of deciduous teeth starts at about 6 months, usually with the appearance of the lower incisors, and is complete by about 2½ years. The

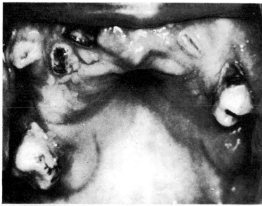
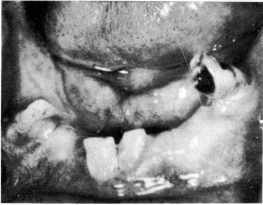

Fig. 2.5 Cleidocranial dysplasia. The upper and lower jaws of a patient of forty-one. Most of the missing teeth are still embedded in the jaws as shown in the radiographs in Chapter 12.

Table 2.1 Chronology of tooth development

Tooth	Calcification begins	Appearance in mouth
Deciduous		
Incisors	4 months (fetal life)	6–9 months
Canines	5 months (fetal life)	16–18 months
1st molars	6 months (fetal life)	12–14 months
2nd molars	6 months (fetal life)	20–30 months
Permanent		
Incisors	3–4 months (upper lateral incisor 10–12 months)	Lower 6–8 years Upper 9–7 years
Canines	4–5 months	Lower 9–10 years Upper 11–12 years
Premolars	$1\frac{1}{2}$–$2\frac{1}{2}$ years	10–12 years
1st molars	Birth	6–7 years
2nd molars	$2\frac{1}{2}$–3 years	11–13 years
3rd molars	7–10 years	17–21 years

eruption of many teeth or of the whole dentition may be delayed or fail altogether but only very rarely. More often a single tooth is prevented from erupting by local obstruction. In the case of the permanent dentition, delay in eruption of a tooth or, more commonly, too early loss of a deciduous predecessor tends to cause irregularities because movement of adjacent teeth closes the available space.

The times at which the deciduous teeth should appear are shown in Table 2.1, but there is considerable individual variation; a delay of 6 months or even longer is not unusual.

Delayed eruption associated with skeletal disorders

Delayed eruption of the teeth is associated with metabolic diseases affecting the skeleton, particularly *cretinism* and *rickets*. Though these diseases are now uncommon, they are the main causes of delayed eruption of many teeth. Treatment of these diseases usually restores the eruption rate to normal.

In the rare disease *cleidocranial dysplasia*, as mentioned earlier, eruption of most of the permanent teeth usually fails, or is long delayed.

In severe *hereditary gingival fibromatosis* eruption may apparently fail merely because the teeth, although normally erupted, are buried in the excessive fibrous gingival tissue and only their tips show in the mouth.

In cherubism (Ch. 12) several teeth may be displaced by the proliferating connective tissue masses containing giant cells and are prevented from erupting. The number of teeth affected in this way depends on the severity of the disease.

Local factors affecting eruption of deciduous teeth

Having no predecessors, the deciduous teeth are not often prevented from erupting. Occasionally an eruption cyst may overlie a tooth but is unlikely to block eruption.

Local factors affecting eruption of permanent teeth

A permanent tooth may be prevented from coming into position by such causes as the following.

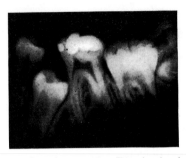

Fig. 2.6 Impaction of a premolar. Eruption has been prevented by closure of the space between first premolar and molar, following early loss of the deciduous molar.

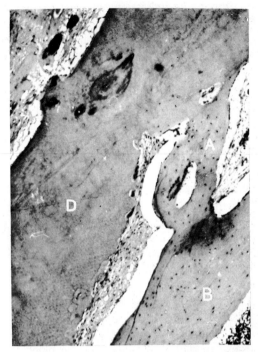

Fig. 2.7 Ankylosis of a deciduous tooth. Resorption is an intermittent process: periods of osteoclastic activity are followed by partial repair. Occasionally, excessive repair tissue (A) may form, uniting the dentine (D) to the bone (B) of the jaw. Below the point of ankylosis, osteoclasts are actively resorbing the dentine.

1. *Loss of space.* Early loss of deciduous teeth may allow adjacent teeth to drift together. The lower second premolars are the teeth most frequently displaced by this cause.
2. *Abnormal position of the crypt.* The lower third molar and the upper canine are most often misplaced and fail to erupt.
3. *Overcrowding.* Inadequate space in the alveolar ridge is a common cause of delayed eruption, especially of lower third molars.
4. *Supernumerary and supplemental teeth.* One of these may erupt before, and occupy the space of a normal tooth.
5. *Dentigerous cysts.* The tooth involved in the cyst is displaced deeply, and is prevented from erupting.
6. *Retention of a deciduous tooth.* A deciduous tooth occasionally becomes ankylosed to the bone. Resorption may very rarely be delayed by periapical infection, but infected teeth are usually shed normally.

Treatment depends on the circumstances, but room has usually to be made for the unerupted tooth by orthodontic means or extractions.

When a deciduous tooth is retained, radiographs should be taken to make sure that there is a permanent successor before extracting the deciduous tooth.

If the buried tooth partially erupts and becomes infected, it may have to be removed; mandibular third molars are the main source of trouble of this sort (Ch. 9).

Changes affecting buried teeth

Teeth may occasionally remain buried in the jaws for many years without complications. The roots of these teeth may undergo hypercementosis or they may become resorbed. Enamel usually resists resorption and if the crown of the buried tooth comes into contact with the roots of an adjacent tooth, the roots are resorbed and the enamel remains undamaged. Similar changes may affect a tooth in a dentigerous cyst. Occasionally the crown becomes resorbed during the course of many years (see Ch. 5).

DEFECTS OF STRUCTURE: HYPOPLASIA AND HYPOCALCIFICATION

Minor structural defects of the teeth, such as pitting or discolouration, or, occasionally, more serious defects may be seen. These changes may be of interest as indications of past disease, but only on rare occasions is the disease still active.

Hypoplasia of the teeth is not an important contributory cause of dental caries; indeed, hypoplasia due to fluorosis is associated with increased resistance. The main clinical problem is usually how best to improve the appearance of hypoplastic teeth.

Deciduous teeth

Calcification of the deciduous teeth begins about the fourth month of intra-uterine life. Disturbances of metabolism, or infections that affect the fetus at this early stage without causing abortion, are rare. Defective structure of the deciduous teeth is therefore uncommon, but, in a few places, such as parts of India, where the fluoride content of the water is excessively high, the deciduous teeth may be mottled.

The deciduous teeth may be discoloured by abnormal pigments circulating in the blood. Severe neonatal jaundice may cause the teeth to become yellow, or there may be bands of greenish discolouration. In congenital porphyria, a rare disorder of haemoglobin metabolism, the teeth are red or purple. Tetracycline given during dental development is probably, even now, the main cause of permanent discolouration.

Permanent teeth

The permanent teeth may be affected by local influences and by systemic diseases. Though permanent teeth are more frequently hypoplastic than are deciduous teeth, the incidence of serious structural defects is small.

Local causes

Infection. Local periodontitis of a deciduous tooth, especially a molar, may damage the underlying permanent successor. This tooth may be malformed to a greater or lesser degree. The enamel is commonly pitted, and sometimes the affected part of the crown may be much smaller than the rest (Turner teeth).

Systemic disorders

The main causes are as follows.

1. Genetic
   a. Amelogenesis imperfecta
      —Hereditary enamel hypoplasia
      —Hereditary enamel hypocalcification
   b. Dentinogenesis imperfecta
   c. Multisystem disorders with associated dental defects
2. Infection—congenital syphilis
3. Severe disturbances of metabolism—fevers and other childhood infections, rickets and hypoparathyroidism
4. Tetracycline pigmentation
5. Other acquired developmental anomalies
   —Fetal alcohol syndrome
   —Cytotoxic chemotherapy
6. Fluorosis

Amelogenesis imperfecta

There are several genetically determined disorders of enamel formation. Genetic factors act more or less severely throughout the whole duration of amelogenesis. Characteristically, therefore, all the teeth may be affected and defects involve a large part of, or are randomly distributed throughout, the enamel. In contrast, exogenous factors affecting enamel formation (with the important exception of fluorosis) tend to act only for a short time and leave a pattern of defects only in that part

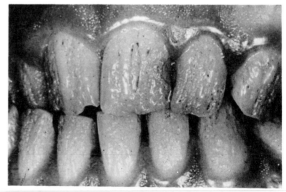

Fig. 2.8 Amelogenesis imperfecta—hypoplastic, sex-linked dominant type. This shows the vertically ridged enamel in a female.

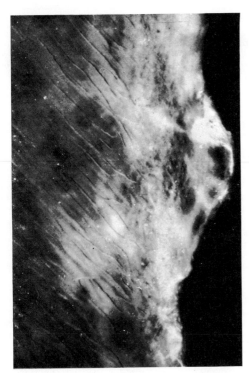

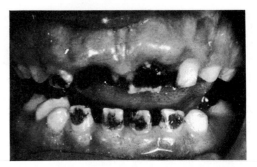

Fig. 2.10 Enamel hypoplasia. A patient with a similar defect to that in the previous picture. The darkening of the incisors is partly due to staining and partly to silver nitrate applied to prevent decay.

Fig. 2.9 Sex-linked dominant type enamel hypoplasia. This and the three subsequent pictures show the defect as it affects males. The exceedingly thin enamel lacks any prismatic structure.

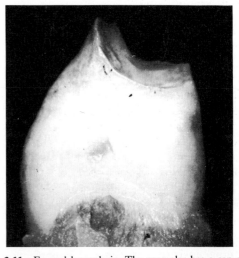

Fig. 2.11 Enamel hypoplasia. The premolar has a cap of enamel so thin that the shape of the tooth is virtually that of the dentine core.

of the enamel formed during the course of the disease.

Amelogenesis imperfecta can be divided into two main groups. *Hereditary enamel hypoplasia* is characterised by defective matrix formation but normal calcification of the enamel, whilst in *hereditary enamel hypocalcification* a normal matrix forms but is poorly calcified. Inheritance of these enamel defects follows several different patterns, but it is rarely possible to obtain a clear family history because dental defects in other members of the family have not been noticed or have been confused with caries ('the teeth came through decayed').

Hereditary enamel hypoplasia

The main defect is in the formation of the matrix. The enamel is randomly pitted, grooved or very thin, but is hard and translucent. The defects tend to become stained, but the teeth are not especially prone to caries unless the enamel is very thin and easily damaged. In these cases the enamel may lack the normal prismatic structure and appear lamellated or glassy.

There are three main patterns of inheritance. There are autosomal dominant and recessive forms and in addition—a genetic rarity—a sex-linked dominant type. The latter is characterised by almost complete failure of enamel formation in the males, while in females the tissue is vertically ridged (see Figs. 2.8–2.12).

In the USA it has been estimated that the frequency of heritable enamel hypoplasias is about 1 in 16 000.

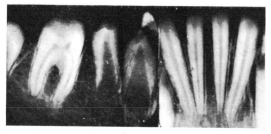

Fig. 2.12 Enamel hypoplasia. Radiographs of the same patient showing the deficiency of enamel.

Hereditary enamel hypocalcification

Enamel matrix is formed in normal quantity and, when newly erupted, the enamel is normal in thickness and form but weak and opaque or chalky in appearance.

The enamel is soon chipped away and becomes stained, usually a yellowish colour. The teeth tend to be relatively rapidly worn away and the upper incisors develop a characteristic shouldered form due to the chipping away of the thin, soft enamel of the incisal edge.

As with the hypoplastic type of amelogenesis imperfecta, autosomal dominant and recessive patterns of inheritance have been described.

In the USA the hypocalcified type of amelogenesis imperfecta is apparently more common than the hypoplastic type.

Dentinogenesis (odontogenesis) imperfecta

This is an uncommon hereditary disease, also

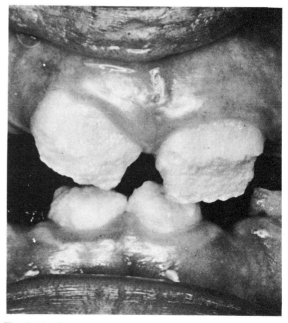

Fig. 2.14 Enamel hypocalcification. The soft, chalky enamel was virtually of normal thickness and form but has chipped away during mastication.

known as hereditary opalescent dentine, transmitted as an autosomal (simple) dominant. The gene is closely related to that of osteogenesis imperfecta and is most commonly present in Type IV of that disease. In osteogenesis imperfecta, bone formation is inadequate because of an underlying defect of collagen formation, and the fragile bones fracture repeatedly under stress (Ch. 12).

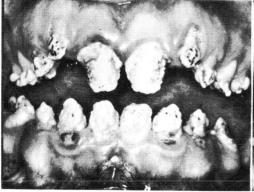
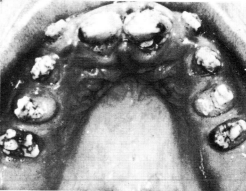

Fig. 2.13 Severe enamel hypoplasia. The enamel consists only of small irregular nodules but is hard and glossy. The pits are stained but the teeth are not carious.

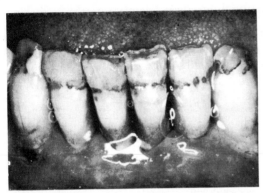

Fig. 2.15 Hypoplasia due to metabolic upset. Unlike the hereditary types of amelogenesis imperfecta the defects are linear and thought to correspond to a short period of amelogenesis disturbed by a concurrent severe illness.

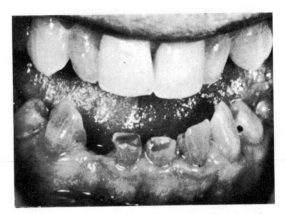

Fig. 2.17 Dentinogenesis imperfecta. The affected teeth are brownish and translucent, but of normal form. The enamel is hard but poorly attached and has chipped off, especially from the lower central incisors. The upper centrals appear unaffected.

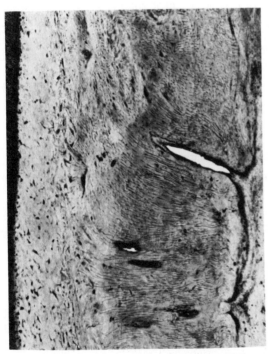

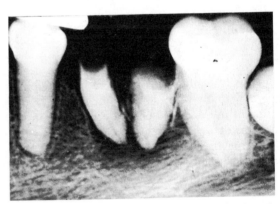

Fig. 2.18 Dentinogenesis imperfecta. Radiographs show the characteristic bulbous crowns, short roots and obliterated pulp chambers.

Fig. 2.16 Dentinogenesis imperfecta. Normal tubulated dentine can be seen along the left-hand margin. The pulp chamber has become filled with dentine containing scanty irregular tubules and more amorphous calcified tissue with many cellular inclusions.

Histological features

The dentine is soft and has an abnormally high water content. The earliest formed dentine under the amelodentinal junction usually appears nor-mal. The deeper tissue is more defective, tubules become few, calcification is incomplete and the matrix is imperfectly formed. The pulp chamber becomes obliterated early, and odontoblasts degenerate, but cellular inclusions in the dentine are common. Scalloping of the amelodentinal junction is sometimes absent, and the enamel tends to split from the dentine. The enamel is normal in typical cases.

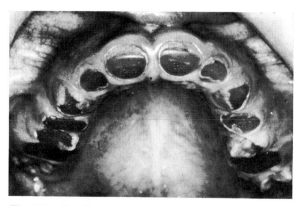

Fig. 2.19 Dentinogenesis imperfecta. A boy of fourteen with complete destruction of the crowns of the teeth by attrition due to progressive chipping away of the enamel and wearing away of the relatively soft dentine. Obliteration of the pulps has prevented their exposure.

Clinical features

The enamel appears normal but the tooth is of a uniform brownish or purplish colour and abnormally translucent. The form of the teeth is essentially normal, but the crowns of the molars tend to be bulbous and the roots are usually short. The enamel tends to chip away from the dentine abnormally easily until in severe cases the teeth become rapidly worn down to the gum. The early fitting of full dentures becomes inevitable in such cases, as the relatively soft dentine and short roots make crowning impractical.

In some patients only a few teeth are severely affected, while the remainder appear normal.

Radiographically the main features are obliterated pulp chambers and stunted roots.

Shell teeth

This rare anomaly is so called because only a thin shell of hard dental tissue surrounds overlarge pulp chambers. Shell teeth appear to be a variant of dentinogenesis imperfecta in that there is normal, but thin, mantle dentine which covers irregular dentine. The pulp lacks a normal odontoblast layer and consists of coarse connective tissue which becomes incorporated into the deep surface of the dentine.

Dentinal dysplasia ('rootless' teeth)

In dentinal dysplasia, the roots are very short and conical. The pulp chambers are obliterated by multiple nodules of poorly organised dentine containing sheaves of tubules. Not surprisingly, these teeth tend to be lost early in life.

Regional odontodysplasia (ghost teeth)

In this localised disorder of development, a group of teeth is affected. They are both malformed and poorly calcified.

The enamel is thin, grossly hypoplastic and hypomineralised; it is surrounded by irregular calcifications formed in the reduced enamel epithelium. The dentine is thin and has a disproportionately thick zone of predentine, and the pulp chamber is correspondingly large.

In radiographs, ghost teeth have a characteristic crumpled appearance and are abnormally radiolucent.

The function of ghost teeth is poor as the defects are too severe to repair, and early loss is inevitable.

Hypophosphatasia

Hypophosphatasia is a rare genetic disorder in which (among other effects) there may be failure of formation of cementum leading to premature exfoliation of the teeth (Ch. 6).

Ehlers Danlos (floppy joint) syndromes

This group of disorders of collagen formation is characterised (in varying degree) by hypermobile joints (Ch. 14), loose hyperextensible skin, fragile oral mucosa (Ch. 20) and (in type VIII) juvenile periodontitis (Ch. 6).

The main dental abnormalities are small teeth with short roots and multiple pulp stones.

Gardner's syndrome (familial adenomatous polyposis)

Gardner's syndrome is characterised by multiple osteomas, especially of the jaws, colonic polyps and skin tumours. In addition the majority of patients have dental abnormalities. These include impacted teeth other than third molars, supernumerary or missing teeth and abnormal root formation. The colonic polyps in these patients have an almost 100% frequency of malignant change, and the mortality is high. The dental abnormalities can be detected in childhood or adolescence and recognition of this syndrome may be life-saving by suggesting the need for colectomy.

Infection—congenital syphilis

Prenatal syphilis, the result of maternal infection, may give rise to a characteristic deformity of the teeth, described by Hutchinson in 1858. The effects are due to direct action of the *Treponema pallidum* within the dental follicle and it has been suggested that the organisms provoke a typical chronic inflammatory reaction and fibrosis of the tooth sac. This was thought to cause hypoplasia by compressing the developing tooth and distorting the ameloblast layer. It has also been shown that *Treponema pallidum* causes proliferation of the odontogenic epithelium which bulges into the dentine papilla causing the characteristic central notch.

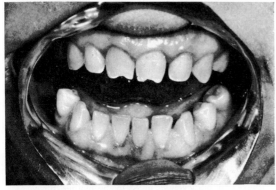

Fig. 2.20 Congenital syphilis; Hutchinson's teeth. The characteristics are the notched incisal edge and the peg shape, tapering from neck to tip.

Clinical features

If the fetus becomes infected at a very early stage, abortion follows. Infants born with stigmata of congenital syphilis are the result of later infection of the fetus, and the permanent teeth are affected. The characteristic signs are seen most often in the upper central incisors, less frequently in the first molars and sometimes in the canines and lateral incisors.

The incisors (Hutchinson's incisors) are small, barrel-shaped, and taper towards the tip. The incisal edge sometimes shows a crescentic notch or deep fissure which forms before eruption and can be seen radiographically. An anterior open bite is also characteristic.

The first molars may be dome-shaped (Moon's molars) or may have a rough, pitted occlusal surface with compressed nodules instead of cusps (mulberry molars).

This defect is now exceedingly rare.

Severe disturbances of nutrition and metabolism

General disturbances of metabolism affecting the development of the teeth may be caused by the childhood fevers and by infantile gastro-enteritis if sufficiently severe.

Unlike inherited forms of hypoplasia, only a restricted area of enamel is defective, corresponding to the state of development at the time of the metabolic disturbance. Measles with severe secondary bacterial infection was perhaps the most common cause of this limited type of dental defect. This seems to have become uncommon, presumably due to more effective treatment (Fig. 2.15).

Clinically, the most common type of defect is one or more rows of horizontally disposed pits or grooves across the crown of the incisors. These are usually in the incisal third, suggesting that the disorder had its effect during the first year or two of life, at a time when such infections are most dangerous.

Rickets can cause hypocalcification of the teeth, as shown in Figure 2.21 but has to be unusually severe for the effects to be apparent.

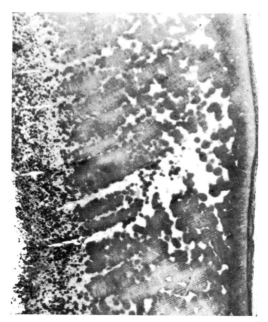

Fig. 2.21 Rickets. In this case of renal rickets, defective calcification has left a wide band of predentine and many interglobular spaces (×45).

Idiopathic hypoparathyroidism of early onset is rare but causes (for unknown reasons) ectodermal effects. The teeth may therefore be hypoplastic, the nails may be defective and there may be complete absence of hair. Patients with early onset idiopathic hypoparathyroidism may later develop other endocrine deficiencies (polyendocrinopathy syndrome).

Tetracycline pigmentation

Tetracycline is taken up by calcifying tissues, and the band of tetracycline-stained bone or tooth substance fluoresces bright yellow under ultraviolet light.

The teeth become stained only when tetracycline is given during their development, and it can cross the placenta to stain the developing teeth of the fetus. More often, permanent teeth are stained by tetracycline given during infancy.

Tetracycline is deposited along the incremental lines of the dentine and, to lesser extent, of the enamel. The more prolonged the course of treatment the broader the band of stain, and the deeper the discolouration. It has been suggested that very heavy dosage of tetracycline may cause hypoplasia, but usually the teeth are of normal form.

The teeth are at first bright yellow, but become a dirty brown or grey. The stain is permanent, and when the permanent incisors are affected the ugly appearance can only be disguised.

When the history is vague the brownish colour of tetracycline-stained teeth must be distinguished from dentinogenesis imperfecta. In dentinogenesis imperfecta the teeth are obviously more translucent than normal and, in many cases, chipping of the enamel from the dentine can be seen. In the tetracycline-induced defect the teeth show no structural defect. In very severe cases, intact teeth may fluoresce under ultraviolet light. Otherwise the diagnosis can only be confirmed after a tooth has been extracted. In an undecalcified section the brilliant yellow fluorescence of the tetracycline deposited along the incremental lines can be easily seen. Needless to say, teeth should not be extracted merely for diagnostic purposes.

It is no longer necessary to give tetracycline during the period of dental development, as there

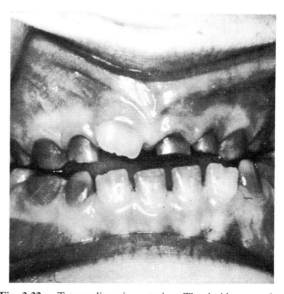

Fig. 2.22a Tetracycline pigmentation. The deciduous teeth, all affected by tetracyclines given to the mother during pregnancy, have acquired the typical greyish brown discolouration. The permanent teeth stained by tetracyclines given during infancy are still yellow but will gradually become brown or greyish.

are equally effective alternatives. Nevertheless tetracycline pigmentation is still seen. The period when tetracycline must be avoided is when the crowns of the permanent anterior teeth are calcifying (from approximately the 4th month to at least the 6th year of childhood).

Other acquired developmental anomalies

Fetal alcohol syndrome

Infants of mothers who have consumed excessive amounts of alcohol may have developmental

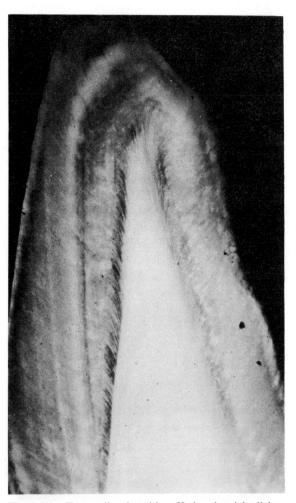

Fig. 2.22b Tetracycline deposition. Under ultraviolet light the whole of the dentine is intensely fluorescent, while the incremental lines of the enamel are well demarcated in this undecalcified section of a heavily pigmented incisor.

defects. The eyes typically slant downwards laterally, the lower half of the face is elongated and there is mental deficiency. In addition, dental development may be delayed and there may be enamel defects such as mottled opacities of the enamel near the incisal margins but, elsewhere, increased enamel translucency.

Cytotoxic chemotherapy

Increasing numbers of children are surviving malignant disease, particularly acute leukaemia, as a result of chemotherapy with drugs such as vincristine and others.

Among the survivors, teeth developing during treatment may have short roots, hypoplasia of the crowns and enamel hypoplasia. Microscopically there may be increased prominence of incremental lines corresponding with the timing of the chemotherapy.

In extreme cases, teeth forming at this time may fail to develop.

Dental fluorosis—mottled enamel

Mottling of the enamel is the most frequently seen and most reliable sign of excessive fluoride in the drinking water. There are important features of mottling that distinguish it from other forms of hypoplasia of the teeth, as follows.

1. Mottling is endemic to areas where fluorides in the drinking water exceed about 2 parts per million; mottling therefore has a geographical distribution.
2. Neighbouring communities with a different (fluoride-free) water supply do not suffer from the disorder.
3. Only those who have lived in a high-fluoride area during the period of development of the teeth show mottling. The defect is not acquired by older visitors to the area.
4. The permanent teeth are affected; mottling of deciduous teeth is rare.
5. Mottled teeth are less susceptible to caries than normal teeth from low-fluoride areas.
6. The brown stain seen in severe mottling is acquired after eruption of the teeth.

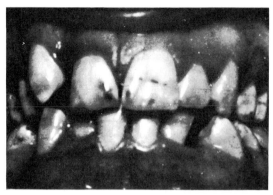

Fig. 2.23 Fluorosis. Moderately severe mottling in a patient from Maldon (Essex). All the teeth show irregular opaque white areas and some brown staining. The enamel surface is intact.

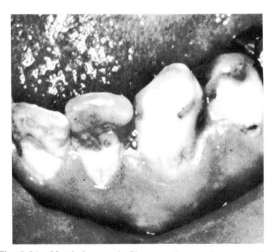

Fig. 2.24 Mottled enamel. Close-up view to show extensive paper-white areas due to hypomineralisation beneath the surface and brown staining associated with minute defects in the surface.

Clinically, mottling ranges from paper-white patches to opaque, brown, pitted and brittle enamel. It is sometimes difficult to distinguish fluorotic defects from amelogenesis imperfecta (hereditary or idiopathic) clinically when the degree of exposure of the patient to fluoride is unknown.

Pathology

Fluoride combines to form calcium fluorapatite in place of part of the normal hydroxy-apatite in the enamel. Damage to ameloblasts, leading to defective matrix formation, is seen only when the concentrations of fluorides are exceptionally high. At intermediate levels (2 to 6 ppm) the matrix is normal in structure and quantity; the form of the tooth is unaffected, but there are patches of incomplete calcification beneath the surface layer. The enamel is opaque in these areas because of high organic and water content, but is resistant to caries. Where there are high concentrations of fluorides (over 6 ppm) the enamel is pitted and brittle, with severe and widespread staining.

Clinical features

There is considerable individual variation in the effects of fluorides. A few patients may have mild mottling after exposure to relatively low concentrations of fluorides, while others exposed to relatively high concentrations may escape their effect.

Changes due to mottling are graded as follows.

- *Very mild.* Small paper-white areas on the tooth involve less than 25% of the surface.
- *Mild.* Opaque areas involve up to 50% of the surface.
- *Moderate.* The whole of the enamel surface may be affected with chalky white areas or

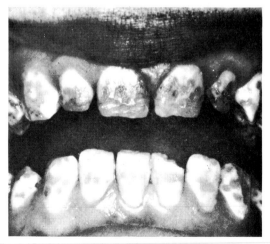

Fig. 2.25 Severe mottling. The entire enamel is opaque or brown and severely pitted; the increased brittleness has caused the incisal edges to be chipped. The patient is from Naples.

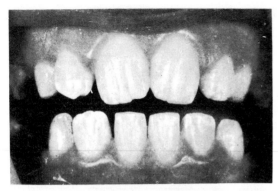

Fig. 2.26 Non-fluoride defects. The opaque flecks are distributed uniformly over the surface of the enamel.

yellowish or brown staining. Surfaces subjected to attrition become worn.

• *Severe.* The enamel is grossly defective, opaque, pitted, stained brown and brittle, and may have a corroded appearance.

With severe mottling of the enamel, other effects of excessive intake of fluorides, especially sclerosis of the skeleton may develop. Radiological evidence of increased density of the skeleton may be seen in areas where the fluoride content of the water exceeds 8 ppm, but is not harmful. Toxic effects of fluorides are discussed in Chapter 7.

Table 2.2 Fluoride concentration and its effects

Fluoride concentration	Effects	
Less than 0.5 ppm	Up to 6% of patients show 'very mild' or 'mild' defects.	Inconspicuous
0.5 to 1.5 ppm	At the upper limit of this range 22% show 'very mild' defects.	
2.5 ppm	Over 50% show 'very mild' or 'mild' defects; nearly 10% show 'moderate' or 'severe' defects.	Apparent
4.5 ppm	Nearly all patients affected in some degree; 46% have 'moderate' and 18% 'severe' defects.	Disfiguring
6.0 ppm and more	All patients affected. 50% severely.	

The milder degrees of mottling are not easily distinguished from non-specific or hereditary defects in the enamel. There is also evidence that non-specific defects are more common in low-fluoride areas where the water contains less than 1 ppm of fluorine.

Treatment of hypoplastic defects

If teeth are defectively formed there is no remedy, but when necessary the defects can be disguised. In most cases this can be done by such means as porcelain veneers. In some cases, however, it may be necessary to prepare jacket crowns. This should be delayed until adult life. In younger patients the large pulp is easily damaged during the preparation of the tooth, and injuries to the teeth are also more frequent than in older patients.

Odontomas

Odontomas are produced by aberrant development of the dental lamina. The most minor examples, though they are not usually called odontomas, are slight malformations such as an exaggerated cingulum or extra roots or cusps on otherwise normal teeth. All gradations exist between these and composite odontomas where the dental tissues have developed in a completely irregular and haphazard manner bearing no resemblance to a tooth and occasionally forming a large mass (Ch. 11).

GENETIC DISORDERS OF THE SOFT TISSUES AND JAWS

Major groups of these disorders are as follows.

1. *The gingivae and periodontium.* The main examples are:
   a. *Hereditary gingival fibromatosis*
   b. *Ehlers Danlos syndrome (type VIII)*
   These are discussed in Chapter 6.
2. *The oral mucosa.* Important examples, which are mainly discussed in Chapter 16, include:
   a. *White sponge naevus*
   b. *Epidermolysis bullosa*
   c. *Ehlers Danlos syndrome*
3. *The jaws.* Important examples include:
   a. *Hereditary prognathism*

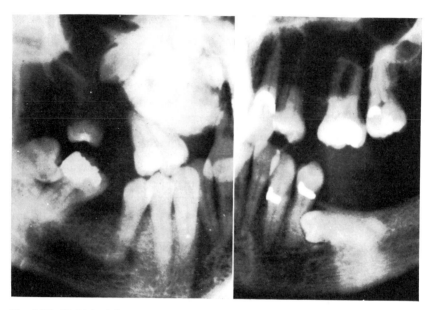

Fig. 2.27 Multiple defects of dental development. On the left in the upper jaw, there is a large composite odontoma, above and behind which is the canine. In the lower jaw on the left the third molar is impacted in a mesioangular position behind the second molar. On the right, the second molar lies horizontally, embedded in the jaw and has caused resorption of the root of the tooth in front of it.

b. *Clefts of the palate and/or lip*
c. *Craniofacial anomalies*
d. *Cleidocranial dysplasia* (Ch. 12)
e. *Cherubism* (familial fibrous dysplasia) (Ch. 12)
f. *Gorlin Goltz syndrome* (multiple jaw cysts, skeletal anomalies and basal cell naevi) (Ch. 10)
g. *Gardner's syndrome* (multiple osteomas, especially of the jaws, and sometimes odontomas or other dental anomalies, colonic polyps and skin tumours)
h. *Osteogenesis imperfecta* (brittle bone syndromes) (Ch. 12).

Epidermolysis bullosa

Epidermolysis bullosa is a blistering disease of the skin and sometimes of the oral mucosa. Four main types are distinguished on the basis of whether bulla formation is intra-epithelial or subepithelial; all are genetic except type IV, but there are several patterns of inheritance.

The hereditary types of epidermolysis bullosa have their onset at or within a few weeks of birth.

Oral mucosal involvement is rare in type I (intra-epidermal) and seen in a variable proportion of types II and III. Oral bullae and ulceration are most common and severe in the type III, autosomal recessive, scarring subtype. In this latter disease the bullae form below the PAS positive basement membrane and there is blistering and scarring of the skin so severe as to cause contractional deformities of the hands with destruction of the fingers and nails in some cases. There may also be pitting hypoplasia of the enamel and oral mucosal scarring and contracture due to minor trauma such as toothbrushing. This can lead to tongue-tie, obliteration of the sulci and limited opening. Dental treatment is difficult because of the ease with which the mucosa can be damaged, but retention of the teeth is essential as dentures cannot be tolerated or even retained. Fluoride and chlorhexidine rinses, and avoidance of sweet sticky foods, may lessen caries activity and limit plaque formation and are important ancillary measures.

Dental defects in epidermolysis bullosa

A variety of abnormalities have been reported.

They include fine or coarse pitting defects, or thin and uneven enamel. The latter may also lack prismatic structure. The amelodentinal junction may also be smooth. Dental defects vary in the different subtypes of the disease but are most frequent in the autosomal recessive scarring type of epidermolysis bullosa in which there may be delayed, or failure of, eruption.

Prognathism

For historical reasons hereditary prognathism is the best known of these defects in that the Spanish branch of the Hapsburg royal family showed the defect in striking form as is obvious from contemporary portraits. The disease has been traced through nine generations of this family, beginning with Ernst in the 14th century and ending with Karl II in the 17th century.

Clefts of the lip and palate

Clefts can form in the lip or palate alone or in both. The aetiology is unknown but there is a genetic component in approximately 40% of cases. The risk of having such defects is greatly increased if one, and particularly if both, of the parents are affected.

Cleft lip (with or without a palatal cleft) is more common in males, while cleft palate alone is approximately twice as common in females. The incidence of cleft lip is about 1 per 1000 live births, while that of isolated palatal clefts is about 1 per 2000 live births. In terms of relative frequencies, cleft lips form about 22%, combined defects of lip and palate form about 58% and isolated palatal clefts form about 20% of this group of defects.

The reasons for the variations in the sites of clefts is that the lip and anterior palate (the primary palate) develop before the hard and soft palates (the secondary palate). Fusion of the secondary palate is from behind forwards.

Isolated cleft lip is therefore the result of an early developmental disorder, while isolated cleft palate results from influences acting later, after the primary palate has closed. By contrast, a prolonged disorder of development can prevent both primary and secondary palates from closing and leaves a severe combined defect.

Developmental disorders associated with clefting

In Down's syndrome, cleft lip or palate is present in approximately 1 in 200 patients (see also Ch. 23). In the less common trisomy 13 (Patau's syndrome) cleft lip or palate or both is present in up to 70% of cases. However, multiple defects of the brain and other organs lead to early death. Clefts are also a feature of many other genetic craniofacial syndromes.

Classification

The main types of cleft lip are as follows:

1. Unilateral (usually on the left side), with or without an anterior alveolar ridge cleft
2. Bilateral, with or without alveolar ridge clefts—either can be complete or incomplete.

Palatal clefts can be of the following degrees of severity:

1. Bifid uvula
2. Soft palate only
3. Both hard and soft palate.

The main types of combined lip and palatal defects are:

1. Unilateral, complete or incomplete
2. Cleft palate with bilateral cleft lip, complete or incomplete. In the worst cases there is complete separation of the anterior palate, which projects forward with the centre section of the lip and is attached above only by the nasal septum.

Associated defects

1. *Local*. Teeth in the region of the defect are typically absent or malformed.
2. *Systemic*. Major congenital abnormalities such as heart disease, limb defects, spina bifida or mental defects are associated in about 50% of cases and can seriously affect the management of these patients. This is

particularly so in the case of Down's syndrome.

Management

Important considerations include:

1. Provision for feeding in infancy when palatal clefts are severe
2. Prevention of collapse of the two halves of the maxilla
3. Measures to counteract speech defects
4. Cosmetic repair of cleft lips.

Repair of these clefts has, for long, been carried out at 15 to 18 months after birth. However, early operation can severely inhibit growth both by damaging the delicate growing tissues and, particularly, by subsequent scar tissue formation. Severe malocclusion can result, and operation may be necessary to lessen the effect of the reduced growth.

More recently, observation of untreated clefts has shown that, contrary to earlier beliefs, the growth potential of these tissues is virtually normal. In some centres, therefore, a soft palate cleft is repaired early but repair of a hard palate cleft is delayed until 8 or 9 years after temporary closure with an obturator. The results are good facial growth and occlusion, but speech may be impaired to some degree.

Early operation is still frequently carried out, but great experience and expertise are needed to avoid damage to the developing tissues and to minimise scarring.

Submucous cleft palate

Submucous clefts are an abnormality of the attachment of the muscles of the soft palate beneath an intact mucosa. They are present in approximately 1 in 1200 births but frequently missed.

The chief effects are slowness in feeding and nasal regurgitation. Middle ear infections and speech defects result from the defective muscle attachments as frequently as in those with overt clefts, and only 10% of cases may have no symptoms.

Clinically, a submucous cleft is visible as a translucent area along the midline of the soft palate and frequently a bifid uvula. On palpation, a notched posterior nasal spine may be felt, but the diagnosis can be confirmed by imaging techniques, such as videofluoroscopy.

Operation to repair the muscle attachments is usually delayed for about $2\frac{1}{2}$ years, to enable the degree of the defect to be assessed.

Other genetic diseases relevant to dentistry

There are many rare hereditary disorders which can affect the mouth or jaws, but from the practical clinical viewpoint haemophilia is the most important (Ch. 20).

SUGGESTED FURTHER READING

Asher-McDade C, Shaw W C 1990 Current cleft lip and palate management in the United Kingdom. Br J Plastic Surg 43: 318–321

Battagel J M, Levinkind M 1988 Dentinogenesis imperfecta: an interdisciplinary approach. Br Dent J 165: 329–331

Berkovitz B K B 1990 How teeth erupt. Dental Update 17: 206–209

Carl W, Sullivan M A 1989 Dental abnormalities and bone lesions associated with familial adenomatous polyposis: report of cases. JADA 119: 137–139

Cawson R A 1987 Oral pathology—colour aids in dentistry. Churchill Livingstone, Edinburgh

Cawson R A, Eveson J W 1987 Oral pathology and diagnosis. William Heinemann Medical Books, London and Gower Medical Publishing, London

Crawford P J M, Aldred M J 1989 Regional odontodysplasia: a bibliography. J Oral Pathol Med 18: 251–263

Dahllof G, Ussisoo-Joandi R, Ideberg M, Modeer T 1989 Caries, gingivitis and dental abnormalities in preschool children with cleft lip and/or cleft palate. Cleft Palate J 26: 233–238

Desai S N 1990 Cleft lip repair in newborn babies. Ann R Coll Surg 72: 101–103

Fridrich K L, Fridrich H H, Kempf K K, Moline D O 1990 Dental implications in Ehlers-Danlos syndrome. Oral Surg, Oral Med, Oral Pathol 69: 431–435

Grossmann P 1988 An integrated treatment approach to severe hypodontia. Dental Update 15: 208–211

Jackson I T, Hussain K 1990 Craniofacial and oral manifestations of fetal alcohol syndrome. Plastic Reconstr Surg 85: 505–512

Kinirons M J, O'Brien, Gregg T A 1988 Regional odontodysplasia: an evaluation of three cases based on clinical, microradiographic and histopathological findings. Br Dent J 165: 136–139

Macfarlane J D, Swart J G N 1989 Dental aspects of hypophosphatasia: a case report, family study and literature review. Oral Surg, Oral Med, Oral Pathol 67: 521–526

Macleod R I, Welbury R R, Soames J V 1987 Effects of cytotoxic chemotherapy on dental development. J R Soc Med 80: 207–209

Maguire A, Craft A W, Evans R G B et al 1987 The long-term effects of treatment on the dental condition of children surviving malignant disease. Cancer 60: 2570–2575

Maguire A, Murray J J, Craft A W et al 1987 Radiological features of the long term effects from treatment of malignant disease in childhood. Br Dent J 162: 99–102

Milosevic A, Slade P D 1989 The orodental status of anorexics and bulimics. Br Dent J 167: 66–70

Mitchell L 1989 Supernumerary teeth. Dental Update 16: 65–70

Moss A L H, Piggott R W, Jones K J 1988 Submucous cleft palate. Br Med J 297: 85–86

Owens J R, Jones J W, Harris F 1985 Epidemiology of facial clefting. Arch Dis Child 60: 521–524

Rintala A E, Ranta R 1989 Periosteal flaps and grafts in primary cleft repair: a follow-up study. Plastic Reconst Surg 83: 17–24

Welbury R R 1990 A simple technique for removal of mottling, opacities and pigmentation from enamel. Dental Update 17: 161–163

3. Dental caries

For sweetness and decay are of one root and sweetness ever riots to decay*

The reader will have to accept that the details of what is involved in the process of dental caries may be inexpressibly tedious to read. Even worse is the endless flood of so-called literature on the minutiae of this subject; this is often opaque, conflicting, or difficult to relate either to the clinical problem or to other work in the same field. It may become apparent that the present writer has failed to overcome this problem.

Unfortunately it is tempting to take the easy way out and argue that since caries is mostly dealt with by mechanical means (restoration or extractions), there is little need to know much about the nature of the disease. Cobblers, after all, do not need to know about diseases of the feet, but even within the dental profession the extent of knowledge about caries often seems to be limited to the idea that it is 'caused by refined carbohydrates'. Quite apart from the fact that this is inaccurate (or at best a naive oversimplification) this level of knowledge suggests an almost total lack of interest in dental caries as a disease and an essentially technical and somewhat primitive view of dentistry. This in turn suggests that most of dentistry might be equally well—probably better—done by auxiliaries.

Some consideration of the details of the aetiology and pathology of dental caries is not necessarily

*Author, regrettably, unknown.

31

the waste of time that it may seem. It provides a rational basis for the management of the disease and its effects, and for ways in which it may be prevented.

Whether you like it or not, a major part of your working life is likely to be spent in remedying or preventing the effects of decay. Might it not be worthwhile therefore to try to give the subject some thought?

Introduction

Dental caries can be defined as progressive, largely irreversible bacterial damage to teeth exposed to the oral environment. Caries is one of the most common of all diseases and is still a major cause of loss of teeth.

The ultimate effect of caries is to break down enamel and dentine and to open a path for bacteria to reach the underlying tissues. This causes infection and inflammation of the pulp and, later, of the periapical tissues. Acute pulpitis and periodontitis caused in this way are the most common causes of toothache. Infection can spread from the periapical region to the jaw and beyond. Though this is rare in Britain, people in other countries— even America—occasionally die from this cause.

Enamel and dentine are not cellular, have no blood supply, and there is no natural repair of decayed tissues apart from secondary dentine formation. Established caries rarely stops spontaneously, and once a cavity of significant size has formed the only practical way of dealing with the damage and arresting the process is by excising the infected tissue and restoring it by use of artificial materials. These must prevent the disease from becoming re-established and this is the essential requirement of cavity preparation and restorative treatment.

Aetiology of dental caries

Background

Many bacteria ferment sugars to produce acid or secrete enzymes that digest proteins. In 1890, W. D. Miller showed that lesions similar to dental caries could be produced by incubating teeth in saliva when carbohydrates were added. Miller concluded that caries could result from decalcification caused by bacterial acid production followed by invasion and destruction of any remaining tissue. Though he took a laudably cautious view as to how these findings should be interpreted, Miller's basic hypothesis has been upheld even though nearly a century had to pass before the infective nature of the disease could be established.

Prerequisites for the development of dental caries

Dental caries develops in the presence of three interacting variables. These are:

1. *Bacterial plaque containing cariogenic bacteria*
2. *Bacterial substrate, especially sugar*
3. *Susceptible tooth surfaces.*

MICROBIOLOGICAL ASPECTS

Simple clinical observation of the limited sites where dental caries is active shows that the bacteria responsible are not those floating free in the saliva. Dental caries is not the result of a reaction at the interface between tooth surface and saliva but at the interface between tooth surface and dental plaque in stagnation areas.

To a great extent, the formation and properties of dental plaque depend on the microorganisms and their products which form its substance. Bacteria and bacterial plaque are therefore for all practical purposes inseparable in consideration of the processes leading to dental caries. Nevertheless, it appears that certain kinds of bacteria must be present for plaque to be cariogenic.

Though it had been suggested much earlier that dental caries might be caused by microorganisms, this belief did not become firmly established until Miller's experiments in the 19th century. These findings were of course far from conclusive, and evidence that dental caries was a bacterial disease remained circumstantial until 1954 when Orland and his associates in the USA showed that caries did not develop in germfree animals.

Germfree and gnotobiotic studies

Animals can be reared free from bacteria. This

depends on delivery of an initial pair by Caesarean section under conditions of strict asepsis and the maintenance of these animals in isolators. Food has to be delivered into and excreta removed from these isolators using a meticulous aseptic technique.

To all intents and purposes, microorganisms are absent from the bodies of germfree animals. They do not develop dental caries when they are fed a sugar-rich diet which causes caries in animals having a normal oral flora.

It is not of course possible to confirm these experiments in man, but indirect evidence of various different kinds makes it virtually certain that human caries is a microbial disease.

It is possible to show which bacteria are capable of causing caries by inoculating single, known strains into the mouths of germfree animals. Animals where the bacterial flora is thus precisely known or controlled are called *gnotobiotes*.

Experiments using gnotobiotes have shown that the most potent mediators of dental caries are strains of acid-producing streptococci. Only a few strains of these organisms are able to cause caries even with the help of a sugar-rich diet. Other bacteria such as a few strains of lactobacilli, enterococci and actinomyces have been shown to be capable of causing caries under special conditions, but are less virulent.

Transmissibility of caries in animals

Many strains of rats and hamsters remain free from caries irrespective of diet. If, by contrast, caries-susceptible animals are given penicillin, the resulting change in the oral flora renders them insusceptible to caries. Unexpectedly, this is a persistent state but caries becomes active again if these animals are caged with, or fed, faecal material from animals with active caries.

These experiments suggest that caries is dependent on a narrow range of microorganisms and that these organisms are transmissible between animals. Caries must therefore be regarded as a bacterial infection and, while it is still not yet certain that it is an entirely specific infection, the organisms responsible have specific properties not widely shared by members of the oral flora.

Cariogenic bacteria

As discussed later, carious destruction of teeth is largely mediated by acid. However, acid must be concentrated at the sites of attack if it is to cause deep, localised lesions. This localised attack depends on the formation of *bacterial plaque* which, among other properties, enables concentrations of bacteria to adhere to the teeth and prevents dilution or effective buffering of bacterial acids by saliva.

Essential features of cariogenic bacteria therefore include the following capabilities:

1. To form acid from any appropriate substrates, i.e. to be acidogenic
2. To produce a pH sufficiently low (usually lower than pH 5) to decalcify tooth substance
3. To survive and continue to produce acid at low levels of pH, i.e. to be aciduric
4. To have attachment mechanisms for firm adhesion to smooth tooth surfaces
5. To produce abundant polysaccharides for the formation of bacterial plaque matrix
6. To produce insoluble polysaccharides that resist dissolution by saliva or dietary fluids.

Streptococci

The bulk of evidence suggests that streptococci are important if not essential for the development of caries, particularly of smooth (interstitial) surfaces.

Viridans streptococci are among the most numerous bacteria that can be isolated from the mouth. They are so termed because they are a heterogeneous group which produce variable degrees of haemolysis on blood agar. This group includes *Streptococcus mutans*, *S. salivarius*, *S. mitior* and *S. sanguis*. *S. mutans* is so-called because its morphology varies with the pH of its environment.

These viridans streptococci vary among themselves in their ability to attach to different types of tissues, in their biochemical characteristics (particularly in their ability to ferment sugars and the concentrations of acid thus produced), and in the different types of polysaccharides that they form.

In addition there are considerable differences

in the properties of the various strains even of *S. mutans*, some of which are, as a consequence, strongly cariogenic while others are not. The role of *S. mutans* in experimental and human caries is discussed later but its cariogenic properties depend largely on its attachment mechanisms, its ability to make an essential contribution to plaque formation and its acidogenic and aciduric properties.

These bacteria have been intensively studied for their ability to cause dental caries in animals and their association with caries in humans. They can be categorised in various ways: by their bacteriological characteristics, biochemical activities and serological characteristics. There are also many strains of the individual members of the viridans streptococci group and different strains even of *S. mutans* vary widely in their ability to cause caries.

S. mutans is strongly acidogenic and, under favourable conditions (at low pH and with freely available sugar), also stores an intracellular, glycogen-like reserve polysaccharide. When substrate is not freely available, this reserve is used and acid production continues for a time.

Drastic reduction in dietary sugar intake is followed by virtual elimination of *S. mutans* from plaque and reduces or abolishes caries activity. The effect is transient and *S. mutans* rapidly recolonises the plaque once sugar is freely available again.

The role of *Streptococcus mutans* in experimental dental caries

The differing ability of streptococci to cause dental caries has been investigated by inoculating various strains into the mouths of gnotobiotes and maintaining them on a high sugar diet.

Hamsters which are normally caries-free have an oral microflora which does not include the pathogens capable of initiating the disease. *S. mutans* has proved to be able to cause rampant caries in these animals, while other streptococci and lactobacilli have proved ineffective. In gnotobiotic rats, by contrast, several streptococci and some lactobacilli can cause pit and fissure caries, but only *S. mutans* causes smooth surface caries. One of the reasons for this difference is that organisms impact in pits and fissures, and these sites provide an environment favourable to the development of caries. The teeth of hamsters are not, however, characterised by deep fissures, so that caries, when it develops, affects only smooth surfaces. The ability of *S. mutans* to cause smooth surface caries in hamsters, rats and man appears to be related to its ability to adhere to enamel surfaces and to form large amounts of adhesive polysaccharide.

Bacterial polysaccharides

The ability of *S. mutans* to initiate smooth surface caries in animals and to form large amounts of adherent plaque appears to be related to its ability to polymerise sucrose into high-molecular-weight (long-chain) dextran-like polysaccharides. These polysaccharides are glucans. Glucans help these streptococci to adhere to one another and to the tooth surface. Minute quantities of high-molecular-weight glucans also cause suspensions of *S. mutans* to aggregate; this suggests that these streptococci may have specific surface receptor sites to which glucans can attach, but which other streptococci lack. Similarly, *S. mutans* can be stimulated to adhere to the surfaces of extracted teeth which have been treated with minute quantities of glucan. These interactions between *S. mutans* and glucans suggest that the latter may be important in initiating the attachment of these organisms to the teeth as well as playing a major role in the building up of larger masses of plaque. Glucans do not account for the attachment of other microorganisms, notably filamentous types to the tooth surface.

The sticky, insoluble, extracellular glucan produced by some strains of *S. mutans* is closely associated with their cariogenicity.

Streptococcus mutans in human caries

S. mutans has been found in human mouths, particularly in plaque in persons having a high dietary sucrose intake and with high caries activity. *S. mutans* isolated from such mouths have been shown to be virulently cariogenic in animal experiments of the type already described. Conversely, when sugar intake is reduced and caries activity diminished, it becomes more difficult to isolate *S. mutans* from caries-susceptible sites.

It must be emphasised that *S. mutans* is not a single organism and that, quite apart from the number of strains, it is difficult to characterise these organisms with consistency and precision. It is not always certain, therefore, that, in spite of its name, the same organism is being discussed in different reports.

Research has nevertheless to a large degree concentrated on *S. mutans* and aspects of its behaviour and metabolism relevant to dental caries. It is widely accepted that strains of this organism are the most important causative organisms of the disease.

Lactobacilli

Among W. D. Miller's later findings were the isolation of '*Bacterium acid lactici*' from carious teeth and that lactic acid was produced by the breakdown of dietary carbohydrates by bacteria from the saliva. Despite the antiquity of this discovery, the importance of lactic acid in the pathogenesis of caries has been fully confirmed only in relatively recent years, as discussed later.

Lactobacilli have been extensively investigated over the years. They were at one time regarded as the main cause of dental caries because they were present in large numbers in the saliva and could be isolated from carious cavities. They are also acidogenic.

There are many strains of lactobacilli, but *Lactobacillus acidophilus*, which was isolated from carious teeth at pH 3.5, is representative of the homofermentive (lactic acid producing) group, though *L. casei* is present in larger numbers in plaque.

Lactobacilli are present only in relatively small numbers in dental plaque though they may be present in large numbers in the saliva. It has also been shown that the number of lactobacilli in plaque increases only after caries has developed.

In gnotobiotes the lactobacilli that have been tested are not potently cariogenic but some can produce fissure caries. In general there is little evidence that lactobacilli are clinically important in dental caries. Under favourable conditions lactobacilli may be able to cause or maintain tooth destruction. However, there is little evidence that they have the necessary properties for initiating caries on smooth surfaces in humans and are mainly found in the depths of established cavities. Their role in plaque formation is also small.

The *lactobacillus count* has been used as an index of caries activity. Though low caries activity and low-sugar diets are usually associated with low lactobacillus counts, this is certainly not true of every individual. Quite apart from the lack of evidence implicating lactobacilli in the initiation of caries, there is little evidence that the numbers of lactobacilli in the saliva bear any relationship to their numbers in, or the activities of, plaque in stagnation areas. The proliferation of lactobacilli in mouths where caries is active is probably a secondary phenomenon, the growth of lactobacilli being favoured by the acid conditions associated with the development of caries.

Other plaque bacteria

Many other microorganisms can also be found in plaque. The role of the filamentous forms present in enormous numbers is not known. Strains of actinomyces are also found, particularly when caries is rampant, but have not been shown to be cariogenic in germfree animals except for root surface lesions.

Pit and fissure caries

Plaque seems to be of crucial importance in the development of smooth-surface (approximal and cervical) caries. It is less certain that it is essential for the development of pit and fissure caries.

The morphology of pits and fissures is such that bacteria and sugars can impact in their depths undisturbed and the formation of an adherent plaque appears not to be necessary. Diffusion from the depths of the fissure is also limited. There is a little evidence that the microflora in pits and fissures differs from that in the interstitial areas. Certainly there is no way by which the pit and fissure environment can be changed. Fibrous foods are sometimes forced past the contact-

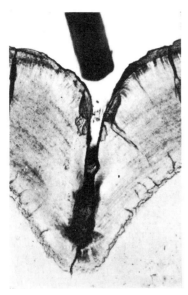

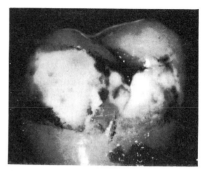

Fig. 3.2 An artificial stagnation area. Chalking of the enamel has developed under a clasp where foodstuffs and bacteria lodged undisturbed.

Fig. 3.1 A stagnation area in an occlusal pit. A ground section of a molar showing the size of the stagnation area in comparison with a toothbrush bristle placed above it. The complete inaccessibility of the stagnation area to cleansing is obvious.

points, and flossing of the interdental areas is carried out by a fanatical few. Both of these disturb interstitial plaque, but their effect is transient.

No comparable disturbance can affect pits and fissures and, in theory at least, a quite different ecosystem could develop. *S. mutans* has been isolated from occlusal pits but nevertheless may not play so essential a role there as in smooth-surface caries.

The sheer technical difficulty of studying this confined area has meant that little is known of the microbiology and ecology of pit and fissure caries. It has not been possible therefore to establish whether plaque is present in, or essential for caries to develop in, these sites.

In gnotobiotes, organisms of low cariogenicity have been shown to be able to induce caries in pits and fissures. These organisms include *S. sanguis* and lactobacilli which, though they produce some polysaccharide, are unable to produce those plaque polysaccharides essential for smooth-surface caries to develop.

These findings strongly suggest that plaque is less essential or may perhaps be unnecessary for pit and fissure caries.

BACTERIAL PLAQUE

Plaque is a tenaciously adherent deposit that forms on tooth surfaces. It consists of an organic matrix containing a dense concentration of bacteria.

Bacteria exist in the mouth either freely in saliva (the fluid phase) or in an adherent mass on surfaces such as the teeth (the solid phase, or bacterial plaque). Bacterial plaque is in micro-biological terms a *biofilm*. Biofilms, of which dental plaque is an example, consist of a hydrated viscous phase formed from bacteria, together with their extracellular polysaccharide matrices. In such a film, molecules and ions exist in concentrations that may be widely different from those of the surrounding fluid phase (saliva). Further, bacteria in biofilms can exhibit cooperative activity and behave differently from the same species in isolation in a culture medium. As a consequence, a biofilm, even when it consists of a single species of bacterium, can be resistant to antimicrobials or to immunological defences to which the individual bacteria are normally sensitive.

It is important to appreciate therefore that bac-terial plaque must, ideally, be investigated as a living entity not as individual bacteria. Con-sequently, valid information about its behaviour, such as its response to anti-plaque agents, can only be obtained by experiments in vivo.

It may be noted that many of the special pro-perties of dental plaque, such as its ability to concentrate and retain acid, were recognised long before the peculiarities of biofilms were dis-covered. However, other properties of biofilms are

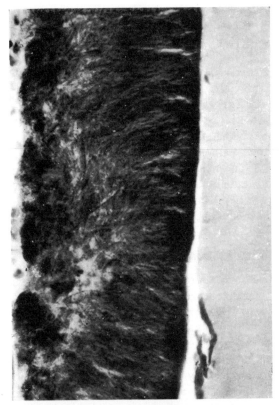

Fig. 3.3 Bacterial plaque. A decalcified section showing darkly staining plaque with enamel prisms just discernible beneath. The plaque has remained intact and adherent to the enamel throughout the processes to which the specimen was subjected in preparation for sectioning. It can also be seen that plaque consists of an almost solid mass of microorganisms predominantly filamentous in type (× 500).

more recent discoveries. For example it is possible that the effects of experimental vaccines, acting on individual species of bacteria such as *Streptococcus mutans*, may not have the same effect on dental plaque in the mouth.

Clinically, bacterial plaque is a tenaciously adherent deposit on the teeth. Its adherence is such as to resist the friction of food during mastication, and plaque can only be readily removed by toothbrushing. However, neither toothbrushing nor fibrous foods will remove plaque from inaccessible surfaces or pits (stagnation areas).

Plaque becomes visible, particularly on the labial surfaces of the incisors, when toothbrushing is

stopped for 12–24 hours. It appears as a translucent film with a matt or ground glass surface that dulls the otherwise smooth and shiny enamel. It can readily be picked up as a creamy mass with the tip of a probe and is made grossly obvious when stained with disclosing agents.

Some plaque forms even under conditions of starvation, but it forms most rapidly and abundantly on a high-sugar diet.

Bacterial plaque forms thick deposits in stagnation areas where it is undisturbed. The thickness of this deposit appears to be a crucial factor in its cariogenicity.

Supragingival and subgingival plaque. The bacterial plaque responsible for the production of periodontal disease (Ch. 6) is another example of a biofilm. However, its effects are strikingly different from the biofilm causing dental caries. Though cariogenic and periodontopathic plaque together form a continuous deposit on the teeth, their bacterial populations differ considerably. It is largely for this reason that plaque in interstitial areas and pits can induce caries under favourable conditions, while plaque on the gingival margins and subgingival tissues is a crucial factor in the production of periodontal disease.

Despite the presence of plaque in both caries and periodontal disease, it is rare for both diseases to be active in the same sites. The main exception is when plaque forms thickly at the gingival margin in neglected mouths. This can result in both cervical caries and gingivitis. However, caries of the cementum or dentine *within* periodontal pockets is exceedingly rarely seen despite the fact that *S. mutans* is numerous in subgingival plaque.

The main factor which probably affects the nature of the disease produced by plaque on different sites on the teeth may therefore be the types of substrate most freely available in each site.

It may be worth noting that viridans streptococci from the mouth can cause a totally different type of disease as a result of their ability to adhere to the endocardium, where they can give rise to the disease infective endocarditis (Ch. 8). The special properties of these biofilms are well exemplified by the difficulties in overcoming these infections despite the apparent sensitivity, in laboratory tests, of the component bacteria to antibiotics.

Bacterial adhesion to tissues

Adhesion of microbes to tissues, from which they would otherwise be washed away by the flow of fluid such as saliva, is an essential prerequisite for the formation of dental plaque and for the colonisation and infection of many other tissues. The study of bacterial mechanisms in the mouth since 1970, particularly by van Houte and Gibbons, has made a major contribution to knowledge of the mechanisms of establishment of many infectious diseases. Typical examples are the attachment mechanisms of gonococci to urinary tract epithelia and of cholera vibrios to the gut wall.

In the case of the mouth there are both soft and hard tissues, each of which have different characteristics. However, bacteria show remarkable selectivity in the surfaces to which they can attach. *S. salivarius*, for example, mainly colonises the keratinised surface of the tongue. *S. mitis* appears to be able to attach to either buccal mucosa or tooth surfaces. By contrast, *S. mutans* and *S. sanguis*, among others, do not merely colonise tooth surfaces but appear to have an absolute requirement for them. These bacteria are not found in the mouths of infants before teeth erupt.

Mechanisms of bacterial attachment to teeth

Knowledge about this difficult subject is still incomplete. However, it is known that many bacteria form 'adhesins' which bind specifically to complementary molecules ('receptors') on tissue surfaces. In the case of the teeth, components of the acquired pellicle appear to serve as receptors for *S. mutans* whereas absorbed glucans and/or glucosyltransferase appear to mediate attachment of *S. sobrinus* (formerly regarded as a serotype of *S. mutans*). Both of these streptococci are potentially cariogenic.

Components of the pellicle, important in acting as adhesion receptors, include a group of *proline-rich proteins (PRPs)* from the saliva. These PRPs have features in common with collagen. *Fibronectin*, a glycoprotein which forms part of connective tissue matrices, is also present, in its soluble form, in saliva. Among other functions, fibronectin on the surface of pharyngeal epithelium mediates ad-

hesion of *S. pyogenes* and appears to be involved in the binding of *S. sanguis*. However, there is little information as yet of the role of fibronectin in dental plaque formation.

Actinomyces species which can contribute to dental caries, particularly of root surfaces, are dependent on *lectin* formation for attachment to teeth. Lectins are glycoproteins which also mediate cell-to-cell interactions in many normal pathological body processes. In the case of *A. naeslundi* and *A. viscosus*, their lectins bind either to galactose residues on epithelial surfaces or on the surface of other bacteria such as *S. sanguis*.

Stages of formation of bacterial plaque

If teeth are thoroughly cleaned by polishing with an abrasive, plaque quickly reforms. The first stage is the deposition of a structureless cell-free pellicle. This starts almost immediately; it does not appear to be due to bacterial action. This cell-free pellicle will form in germfree animals and seems to be derived by deposition of salivary mucinous substances such as glycoproteins. Further deposition of this pellicle is probably enhanced by bacterial action precipitating these proteins.

Within 24 hours this cell-free layer becomes colonised by microorganisms, mainly streptococci and particularly sanguis and mutans strains. After 48 hours these streptococci comprise some 70% of the cultivable flora. As the plaque matures, filamentous organisms proliferate and form the second largest group after the streptococci. In addition a wide variety of other bacteria join the plaque population and include lactobacilli, actinomyces, diphtheroids and various Gram-negative anaerobes. This last group are probably important in the pathogenesis of periodontal disease.

Plaque polysaccharides

These substances, synthesised by bacteria, play an essential role in the pathogenesis of dental caries. The bacterial polysaccharides are both intracellular and extracellular. The proportions of the different types of polysaccharide, and the overall amounts formed, depend both on the kinds of bacteria present and the different dietary sugars available.

On a sucrose-rich diet the main extracellular polysaccharides are glucans. Fructans formed from fructose are produced in smaller amounts; they are also more soluble and less important in caries. The cariogenic properties of *S. mutans* seem to depend as much on its ability to form extracellular glucans in large amounts as on its ability to produce acid. Acid-producing microorganisms that do not produce suitable polysaccharides do not appear to be able to cause caries of smooth surfaces. Even mutant strains of *S. mutans* which produce a more soluble polysaccharide seem not to be cariogenic.

Polysaccharides thus contribute to the adhesiveness, bulk and resistance to solution of plaque.

Effect of plaque thickness

Even in the presence of suitable organisms and substrate, plaque needs to form in a certain critical thickness for caries to develop. Plaque forms on all tooth surfaces. Though continually removed from accessible surfaces by conscientious tooth-

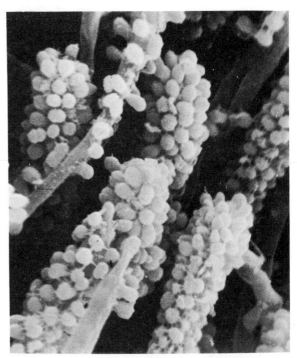

Fig. 3.5 This scanning electron micrograph at higher power shows cocci attached to filamentous organisms to produce the corn cob type of arrangement sometimes seen in plaque. (Original magnification × 6500. Figs. 3.4 and 3.5 kindly lent by Dr Sheila J. Jones.)

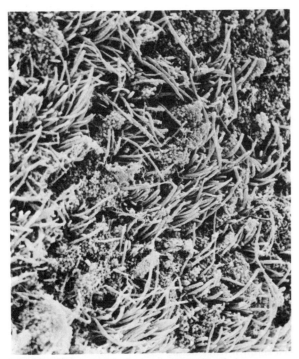

Fig. 3.4 This scanning electron micrograph of plaque shows the large number of filamentous organisms as in the previous picture and, in addition, many cocci clustered among them. (Original magnification × 2000.)

brushing in many patients it can be found on labial and lingual smooth surfaces. Caries does not, however, develop in these areas even in the most neglectful patients. In such patients, however, sufficiently thick plaque can accumulate at the necks of teeth in the angle between the gingival margin and the tooth. Caries can then develop to produce cervical caries.

A critical thickness of plaque is therefore necessary to maintain the concentration of acid at the tooth surface, to resist salivary buffering and to form reserve carbohydrate stores if caries is to develop.

Plaque minerals

In addition to bacteria and their products, particularly polysaccharides, salivary components also contribute to the plaque matrix.

Of the inorganic components, calcium, phosphorus and, often, fluorides are present in significant amounts. There is some evidence of an inverse relationship between calcium and phosphate levels in plaque and caries activity or sugar intake.

The level of fluoride in plaque may be high, ranging from 15 to 75 ppm or more, and is largely dependent on the fluoride level in the drinking water and diet, though there is wide individual variation. This fluoride is probably mostly bound to organic material in the plaque, and, at normal pH levels, little seems to be available in ionic form.

Acid production in plaque

Sugars can diffuse rapidly into plaque, and acid production quickly follows. These changes have been measured directly in the human mouth using microelectrodes in direct contact with plaque. It has been shown by this means that, after rinsing the mouth with a 10% glucose solution, the pH falls within 2 to 5 minutes often to a level sufficient to decalcify enamel.

Even when no more sugar is then taken and the surplus is washed away by the saliva, the pH level does not equally quickly return to normal but remains at a low level for about 15 to 20 minutes; it returns only gradually to the resting level after about an hour. These changes are shown in Figure 3.6. The clinical effects of the ingestion of sugars are discussed in a subsequent section.

The rapidity with which the pH falls is a reflection of the speed with which sugar can diffuse into plaque and the activity of the concentration of enzymes produced by the great numbers of bacteria in the plaque.

The slow rate of recovery to the resting pH—a critical factor in caries production—probably depends mainly on the following:

1. Rapid production of a high concentration of acid within the plaque, temporarily overcoming local buffer substances

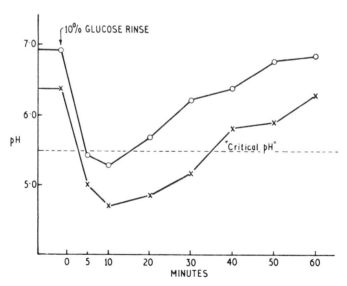

Fig. 3.6 Stephan curves. This is the usual form of curves obtained when changes in reaction in bacterial plaque are measured directly. When the pH falls below the critical level enamel may become demineralised. Patients with active caries tend to show a lower fall in pH, as in the lower curve. The most noteworthy features are the very rapid fall in pH, and the slow recovery to the normal level in spite of the very short time the sugar is in the mouth. Carbohydrates which are retained on the teeth will have a more prolonged effect still.

2. Diffusion of acid outwards into the saliva, delayed by the diffusion-limiting properties of plaque and its thickness*
3. Diffusion of salivary buffers into plaque delayed by the diffusion-limiting properties of plaque and its thickness
4. Continued sugar production from intra-cellular polysaccharides.

It is generally accepted that acid production is responsible for the carious attack and that lactic acid is probably mainly responsible. Indeed when plaque is sampled after exposure to sucrose, lactic acid is quantitatively by far the most important acid during plaque activity, particularly during the trough of the Stephan curve. In the resting state, by contrast, volatile acid radicals, particularly acetate and propionate, may be dominant. It should also be noted that since lactic acid has a lower pK constant it causes a greater fall in pH than when equimolar solutions of acetic or propionic acids are added to plaque.

SUGAR AS A PLAQUE SUBSTRATE

It is generally accepted within the dental profession that, in the matter of dental caries, sugar is the arch enemy. To prove that this is the case has been and remains a major problem. Much of the evidence is based on laboratory experiments. However, it is not justifiable to extrapolate the results from in vitro or animal experiments and assume that they apply equally strongly to humans. The only way to solve this problem is to test the cariogenicity of sugar on humans, but this presents enormous problems as discussed later.

However, even if it is accepted that sugar plays a major role in dental caries, it is still necessary to establish the nature of the biochemical mechanisms by which sugar contributes to the pathogenesis of the disease.

Despite all these considerations, a considerable

amount of evidence indicates that in the absence of sugar, caries fails to develop or, at worst, is at a very low level of activity. Nevertheless, it is foolish to believe (as some seem to) that sugar (in however small amounts or in any form) *always* damages the teeth.

If it becomes overwhelmingly boring to continue to read in such detail about something so 'obvious' as the evidence for sugar's role in dental caries, it may help to point out that the professions and the public still seem to need to be convinced of this proposition. Thus, exactly a *century* after Miller made the fundamental findings, it still seems to be necessary for a national committee (Committee on Medical Aspects of Food Policy: COMA) to reiterate these facts.

The importance of sucrose as a substrate and as a major contributory cause of dental caries depends on the following main types of studies, some of which overlap in varying degree.

1. Epidemiological studies:
   a. Caries prevalence in populations with high or low sugar intakes
   b. Archaeological evidence of caries prevalence in earlier eras
   c. The effects of sugar shortages in wartime Europe
   d. Caries prevalence in disorders of sugar metabolism (hereditary fructose intolerance).
2. Experimental animal and in vitro studies:
   a. The effects of route, quantity, timing and texture of sugar consumption in animals
   b. The effects of sugar on plaque pH
   c. The effects of sugar intake on plaque polysaccharide production.
3. Experimental studies in humans:
   a. The effects of additional intake of sugar in different forms
   b. The effects of substituting artificial sweeteners for sugar.

* If plaque behaves as a membrane which conforms with Fick's laws of diffusion for small molecules, its diffusion-limiting properties will vary with the square of its thickness. However, specific interactions between the molecules moving through plaque and the plaque components are likely to complicate the process considerably.

Epidemiological studies

Caries prevalence in populations with high and with low sugar intakes

Though it has shown a recent decline, dental

caries has been most prevalent in well-nourished, Westernised communities, such as Britain, the USA and others with similar lifestyles where large amounts of sugar, particularly in the form of sweets or snack bars are eaten.

In the past particularly, there have been many studies of poor communities living on traditional diets with little or no sugar content. A low prevalence of caries has been shown (for example) in parts of China and of Africa, the Seychelles, Tristan da Cunha, Alaska and Greenland.

Though an obvious criticism of early work such as this, is that it used unsophisticated or insensitive methods of diagnosis, comparisons between different populations by the same worker are of reasonable validity and at the very least give an indication of the varying prevalence of gross caries.

Many studies were carried out on Eskimo races who were frequently virtually or entirely caries-free when consuming their traditional diet of seal or whale meat, and fish. In all studies on these populations, caries prevalence increased at least ten-fold when a modern diet became available. Similarly in Bantu races, despite a high-starch carbohydrate diet, caries was found in fewer than 9% of those examined, but greatly increased when there was access to a modern diet. Even in Europe, in the 1930s and 1940s there were isolated communities such as the Outer Hebrides or the Lotschental in Switzerland, where dental caries prevalence increased twenty-fold or more when sugar and sweets became widely consumed.

In such studies no association has been found between malnutrition and caries. Generally the reverse is true, and, when nutrition is poor, caries is infrequent. These diets also vary widely in content, from rice as the staple in China or coarsely ground cereals in Africa to a mainly meat and fish diet among Eskimos. The common feature of these diets, and one differentiating them sharply from Westernised diets, is low or negligible consumption of sugar.

Britain is an example of a country where consumption of sugar is exceptionally high, and where the rest of the diet is more than adequate. Figures vary according to the area examined, but it is obvious that the deciduous teeth are attacked soon after eruption and the disease spreads rapidly. A survey in England and Wales in 1973 showed, for example, that (in spite of the benefits of a National Health Service) 78% of 8-year-old children had active decay, to say nothing of teeth which had been filled or lost from this cause. A survey in 1978 showed that dentate adults had on average only 13 sound and unfilled teeth.

In Britain and other countries, the incidence of caries has run roughly parallel with increasing consumption of sugar. The incidence of caries has risen in spite of the much greater consumption of so-called 'protective' foods, namely dairy products, meat and fruit, in recent years. As a consequence of this more varied diet, carbohydrates overall have formed a smaller proportion of the diet. Nevertheless, sugar forms a higher proportion of the carbohydrate component.

Effects of changes in dietary patterns of sugar intake. Where there has been a change from simple natural diets to a Westernised diet, as in Alaska, caries has increased sharply, and Eskimo children now have a caries incidence at least as high as other American children. A similar state of affairs is starting to develop in Africa as sweet eating and sweet between-meals 'snacks' have become popular. In Nigeria many of the older adults are still totally caries-free but the prevalence of dental caries among children and young people who have picked up sweet-eating habits is rising rapidly.

This effect has been strikingly well documented in the population of Tristan da Cunha who, up to the late 1930s, lived on a simple meat, fish and vegetable diet with a minimal sugar content and had a very low caries prevalence. With the adoption of westernised diet, the caries prevalence had increased up to eight-fold in some age groups by the mid-1960s.

Effect of wartime sugar shortages

The effect of reducing sugar consumption has been shown on a vast scale.

Those countries which suffered food shortages during the 1939–45 war had severe restrictions, mainly of meat, fats and sugar. In occupied Norway, where shortages were particularly severe, the pattern of dental caries during and after the war has been carefully followed. The disease declined rapidly after the start of rationing in spite of greatly increased overall consumption of starchy carbohydrates. As sugar became more plentiful at the end of the war the disease progressively increased (Fig. 3.7).

In Japan also, increased caries prevalence has been associated with increased sugar consumption. Near the end of the Second World War sugar consumption and caries levels were very low. However, in more recent years, Japan is one of the few countries where sugar consumption has substantially increased from 16.5 kg per head in 1961 to reach a peak at 29 kg per head in 1970, and caries prevalence has increased in parallel. Unlike most other countries, this picture has not been significantly masked by increasing use of fluoride toothpastes. In Britain, the market share of fluoride toothpastes is 95%, but in Japan it is only 15%.

Archaeological evidence of caries prevalence in earlier eras

Caries is not a modern disease but has become epidemic only in relatively recent years.

Britain has shown a pattern of sugar consumption and of caries prevalence that is informative since there was a sudden change in the level of sugar consumption in the middle of the 19th century. This resulted both from the decreasing cost of production and, in 1861, the sudden lifting of a tax on sugar. Sugar then ceased to be a luxury for the relatively rich and consumption in the population as a whole increased rapidly. Archaeological evidence from exhumed skulls confirms the low prevalence of caries before sugar became widely available and the steady increase in prevalence thereafter.

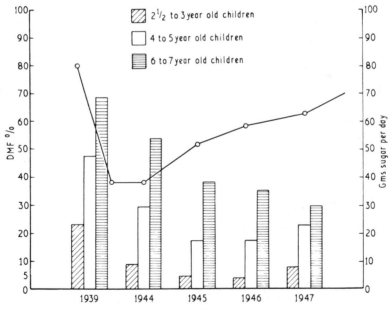

Fig. 3.7 The wartime restrictions on diet, and caries in Norway. The continuous line (above) shows an estimate of the individual daily sugar comsumption during and after the war. The heights of the columns show the incidence of caries in children of various ages. Rationing of sugar started in 1938 but it is apparent that the incidence of caries declined slowly and continued for a short time after sugar became freely available. The greatest reduction in caries was in the youngest group of children whose teeth were exposed to the wartime diet for the shortest periods; the mothers of these children on the other hand had been exposed to the wartime diet throughout pregnancy and for a long period before this. (Mainly after Toverud G 1949 Journal of the American Dental Association 39: 127.)

'Whole food' fanatics may suggest that the increased consumption of sugar in the 19th century would have been of less importance than (for example) reduced consumption of 'natural foods', particularly of whole wheat flour. However, the production of cheap white, highly-refined flour started, and white bread became a staple food even of the poor, many years before sugar became cheap.

Experimental studies

Caries activity in relation to sugar intake in animals

Production of caries in animals is dependent on a significant proportion of sugar in the diet. Conversely, dental caries fails to develop in animals, even when cariogenic bacteria are present and the animals are genetically susceptible, unless a critical, minimum quantity of sugar is added to the diet.

Experimental aspects of dietary carbohydrates—local effects. In susceptible animals, caries becomes active when a high sucrose diet is given. That this effect is a local one has been shown by feeding one group of animals a high sugar diet in the ordinary way, while another otherwise similar group was fed the same diet directly into the stomach through a tube. Those fed in the normal way developed caries, while those fed by stomach-tube remained free from the disease.

Consistency and texture of the diet. A carbohydrate which clings to the teeth and is only slowly washed away by the saliva remains accessible to the oral bacteria for a longer period and can have a greater local effect. Solutions of sugars are quickly cleared from the mouth, and after half an hour little is detectable in the saliva. Other sugary foods dissolve slowly, and high concentrations of sugar may persist in the saliva. A food which does not itself cause caries may have the effect of causing a more active agent (sugar) to adhere to the teeth and, by preventing it from being cleared away by the saliva, cause it to be retained in the mouth.

This effect has also been confirmed in man in the Vipeholm study described later.

In general, therefore, sugar in freely soluble form or in liquid diets is much less cariogenic than when in a dry diet.

Clearance of carbohydrate from around the teeth also depends on salivary function. Where salivary flow is much reduced, caries activity tends to increase. Conversely, high salivary flow rates tend to be associated with lower caries activity though, as discussed later, other factors than a mechanical cleansing effect may also be involved.

Effects of sugar on acid production in plaque.

Direct measurement of pH changes in the mouth shows that there is intermittent acid production on the surface of the teeth and this follows the expected pattern as shown earlier in the Stephan curves. The ingestion of sugar leads to a burst of activity in the plaque; the pH falls to a level low enough in some cases to attack enamel, then slowly returns to the resting level. These findings suggest that the frequency with which substrate is made available to the plaque is important.

If sugar in solution is taken, any surplus (beyond the capacity of the organisms in the plaque to metabolise—or store—at the time) is washed away. If sugary solutions are taken repeatedly at (say) half-hourly intervals, the supply of substrate to the bacteria may be sufficiently frequently renewed to cause acid in the plaque to remain persistently at a destructive level. A similar effect may be caused by carbohydrate in sticky form, such as a caramel, which clings to the teeth and is slowly dissolved, releasing substrate over a long period.

The effects of maintaining plaque activity by repeated administration of sugar have been demonstrated by the use of animal feeding devices to dispense metered quantities of sugar in diets at fixed intervals—thus emulating some of the features of the cariogenic diets of the Vipeholm study discussed below. In this way it can be shown that a given amount of sugar is more cariogenic when fed in small increments but at intervals to maintain maximal plaque activity than the same amount fed on a single occasion.

Effects of sugar on plaque polysaccharide production

As discussed earlier, the cariogenicity of plaque depends to a large degree on its ability to adhere to the teeth, to resist dissolution by saliva and its protection of bacterial acids from salivary buffering. These properties depend on the formation of insoluble polysaccharides produced particularly by cariogenic strains of *S. mutans*.

The importance of sucrose in this activity depends on the high energy of its glucose–fructose bond which allows the synthesis of polysaccharides by the enzyme dextransucrase without any other source of energy. Sucrose is thus the main substrate for such polysaccharides; other sugars are, to a variable degree, less cariogenic (in the absence of pre-formed plaque), partly because they are less readily formed into cariogenic glucans.

Effects of sugar on the oral microbial flora

The establishment of cariogenic bacteria, especially *S. mutans*, is highly dependent on the sugar content of the diet. In the absence of sugar, *S. mutans* cannot usually be made to colonise the mouths of experimental animals. In humans the plaque counts of *S. mutans* also appear to depend on the sugar content of the diet. Severe reduction in the latter appears to cause the *S. mutans* to decline in numbers or disappear from plaque.

Experimental studies on humans

As suggested earlier, the only way to establish unequivocally the role of sugar in human dental caries is to test the hypothesis in experiments on humans.

Unfortunately there is wide individual susceptibility to the disease so that huge numbers of subjects for the experimental and control groups are required. These subjects then need to be kept under concentration camp-like conditions to maintain close supervision of the quantity of sugar ingested, and when and how it is consumed. This process has to be prolonged sufficiently to enable the effects of the diet on the teeth to be assessed. Moreover the experimental groups have to accept the amount of tooth destruction that is likely to have resulted. Quite apart from the cost of so vast an experiment, it is clearly ethically unacceptable now to subject people to such treatment. Some of the difficulties of trying to impose experimental diets on a largish group of people (in the Vipeholm study) are discussed later, but even within this

closed institution it was not possible fully to ensure that the different experimental diets were eaten as required. Human experimental data in this field are therefore limited.

As a result, sceptics can argue that the essential role of sugar as a cause of human dental caries is unproven. Furthermore, there has been a significant decline in caries prevalence, particularly in children, despite the absence of a comparable decline in sugar consumption. This appears, as discussed later, to result mainly from the protective effect of fluoridised toothpastes.

The Vipeholm study

In this study, over 400 adult patients divided into seven groups received a basic low-carbohydrate diet for a period to establish a baseline of caries activity for each group. The groups were then allocated diets as follows.

1. A control group received the basic diet made up to an adequate calorie intake with margarine.
2. Two groups received supplements of sugar at mealtimes, either in solution or as sweetened bread.
3. The four remaining groups received sweets (toffees, caramels, or chocolate) which were eaten between meals.

The aim was to compare the effects of sugar in different quantities and of different degrees of adhesiveness, and of eating sugar at different times. The duration of the study was nearly 5 years.

Caries activity was greatly increased by the eating, between meals, of sweets of a kind that were retained on the teeth, namely toffees and caramels. The effect of chocolate was less severe. Sugar in either form at mealtimes only, had little effect. The incidence of caries fell to its original low level when the toffees or caramels were no longer given, and caries activity was very slight in the control group having the low-carbohydrate diet.

Criticisms of the Vipeholm study. This classical study was virtually unique in that it was possible directly to supervise the diet in a closed institution. It was therefore an interventional study. The great majority of other dietary studies have

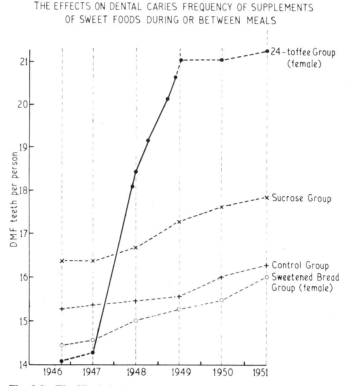

THE EFFECTS ON DENTAL CARIES FREQUENCY OF SUPPLEMENTS
OF SWEET FOODS DURING OR BETWEEN MEALS

Fig. 3.8 The Vipeholm Dental Caries Study. A simplified diagram showing the results in some of the groups of patients and in particular the striking effect on caries activity of sticky sweets eaten between meals when compared with the eating of sweetstuffs at meal times. The broken lines indicate those who consumed sugar only at meals, the continuous line shows those who consumed sugar both at and between meals. (After Gustafsson et al 1954 Acta Odontologica Scandinavica 11:232.)

been uncontrolled and based on patient's diet history. Nevertheless the Vipeholm study had inevitable limitations including the following.

1. Approximately 20% of patients, even on the most cariogenic diet (frequent eating of sweets between meals), did not develop any new carious lesions.
2. In the 8 toffee and caramel groups, caries increased not merely when the sweets were eaten between meals but also when they were given immediately after meals.
3. Caries continued to develop even in those where sugar was restricted as completely as possible.
4. Despite close supervision of the patients,

they were not forced to eat extra sweets. Some did not eat their ration, and others (contrary to instructions) swallowed the sweets whole without chewing them. It has also been suggested that some of those on sugar-limited diets were obtaining sweets illicitly.

5. Some groups had been given fluoride preparations before the experiments.

Despite these and many other criticisms that have been made of the Vipeholm study, it remains one of the most valuable pieces of evidence confirming the cariogenic effect of sucrose-containing foods when eaten between meals at relatively frequent intervals.

The Turku xylitol study

In another large-scale clinical experiment in Finland an experimental group was allowed a wide range of foods sweetened with xylitol (a sugar alcohol) but no sucrose. The control group was allowed sugar (sucrose)-containing foods as desired. After 2 years the experimental group showed 90% less caries than those who had been allowed sugar.

Caries in patients with hereditary fructose intolerance

Patients unable to metabolise fructose as a result of an enzyme deficiency cannot tolerate fructose-containing foods, including disaccharides such as sucrose where fructose forms part of the molecule. These children therefore learn to avoid all sugar-containing foods and have an unusually low incidence of caries.

Recent evidence for the cariogenicity of sugar

Overall, human evidence from epidemiological and experimental studies, as well as animal studies as discussed earlier, confirms that frequent intake of sucrose-containing foods between meals is highly cariogenic.

By contrast, more recent studies have produced less clear cut or even contradictory results for reasons such as the following.

1. It is no longer ethically acceptable to carry out interventional experiments which rot the teeth of a captive population by means of a highly cariogenic experimental diet.
2. Dietary studies have therefore to depend on the subjects' diet histories. Human memory being as unreliable as it is, there is inevitably, therefore, uncertainty about the precise amounts of sugar and the times when it has been consumed.
3. Recent diet histories have to be correlated with caries prevalence *at that time*. They can take no account of the level of caries that develops later as a result of the diet allegedly consumed. In practice, it is virtually impossible to carry out sufficiently extensive *prospective* studies, where sugar consumption for a given period is correlated with the incidence of caries that may only become detectable months later.
4. The almost universal use of fluorides, if only as dentifrices, appears to have raised the resistance of teeth to such a degree that high sugar consumption (within limits) does not always induce dental caries.

That current caries prevalence in many areas bears little relation to the level of sugar intake (for reasons just given) has been used by those with a vested interest in the subject to argue that sugar consumption has little importance in the aetiology of dental caries.

Mechanisms of cariogenicity of sucrose

The cariogenicity of sucrose depends on the fact that it is (i) an effective substrate for acidogenic bacteria and (ii) a major substrate for plaque formation. As discussed earlier, dental caries results from the interaction of plaque with the tooth surface and not between bacteria and substrates free in the saliva.

The potency of the cariogenic properties of sucrose depend on factors which include the following.

1. Sucrose promotes the formation of large volumes of plaque.
2. A major component of plaque is an insoluble polysaccharide rich in 1–3 glucose linkages. Strains of S. mutans which have lost the ability to form this polymer become non-cariogenic.
3. The polysaccharide extracellular matrix of plaque, *in itself*, contributes to cariogenicity of S. mutans. Plaque containing excessive amounts of extracellular polysaccharide but relatively few bacteria has been shown to demineralise enamel to a greater degree than greater numbers of bacteria with higher acid-producing potential, but lacking this extracellular matrix.
4. S. mutans in combination with sucrose is able to colonise both hydrophilic and hydrophobic surfaces.
5. Glucosyltransferase (GTF) catalyses the conversion of sucrose to the polymer, 1–3 linked glucan. The latter is a rigid molecule;

its rigidity facilitates the linking of such chains to one another to form a coherent mass of extracellular matrix.

6. Some evidence shows that adhesion of some cariogenic streptococci (particularly *S. sobrinus* as mentioned earlier), to tooth surfaces depends less on glucan itself than on GTF released into the environment by the bacteria. GTF molecules are highly adhesive; they adsorb onto solid surfaces, where they can produce more glucan from sucrose, and adsorb to other bacteria to bind them into the plaque matrix. These interactions between cariogenic streptococci, the glucosyltransferase that they produce, and sucrose (the specific substrate of this enzyme) have the effect that adhesion and build-up of plaque is sucrose-dependent.

Also suggestive of the role of GTF in plaque formation and adhesion is that antiplaque agents, particularly chlorhexidine and stannous fluoride, inhibit GTF.

Effects of high concentrations of sugar on acid production

The ability of bacteria to demineralise enamel depends on their ability (i) to produce acid of a sufficiently low dissociation constant (pK)—lactic acid, which has a pK of 3.8, is the main example, and (ii) their ability not merely to survive but to continue acid production at low pH, i.e. they need to be aciduric.

However, streptococci and lactobacilli do not produce lactic acid when the sugar concentration is low. The reason is that the lactic dehydrogenase that they contain is indirectly dependent on the local sugar concentration (on which the intracellular pool of fructose 1,6 biphosphate depends) and is only activated when this is high.

The ability of the bacteria to extrude protons (hydrogen ions) tends to be blocked by the re-entry of undissociated acids. With acids such as acetic or propionic acid which have a pK value of 4.8, protons re-enter the cell at a higher pH than in the case of lactic acid. Lactic acid producers should therefore be able to release protons to achieve a 10 times higher concentration than in the case of other bacteria unable to produce acids of sufficiently low pK level.

Cariogenicity of other carbohydrates

Quantitatively, sucrose (cane and beet sugar) forms by far the greatest proportion of the sugar in the diet, though semi-synthetic glucose and fructose are being increasingly used in foods and beverages.

Mono and disaccharides are more readily fermented to acid than polysaccharides by oral bacteria. Salivary amylase converts some starch into sugar but the time for which the starch is present in the mouth is limited.

Animal experiments, however, show that the cariogenicity of starchy carbohydrates is very slight in comparison with sucrose.

Epidemiological evidence also suggests that starchy carbohydrates (polysaccharides) are less important than sugars as mediators of caries. Poor, rural communities living on high-starch, low-sugar diets have little caries. Similarly, the wartime experience in many European countries was that caries declined sharply after sugar became scarce, in spite of greatly increased consumption of starchy foods, particularly bread and potatoes. Moreover in the Turku study (p. 47) substitution of sugar by xylitol reduced caries prevalence by 90% even though there was no control over the intake of other (starchy) carbohydrates in this group. Similarly caries activity remained low in the high-starch/low-sugar groups in the Vipeholm study.

Glucose and fructose are more cariogenic than starches but have been shown to be up to 30% less cariogenic than sucrose in animal diets.

Though glucose and fructose can be fermented to produce acid, sucrose is more readily built up into the glucans important in plaque structure and function. It is probable that the lesser cariogenicity of glucose and fructose under experimental conditions has been due to the fact that, having never had sucrose, these animals have failed to develop a sufficiently cariogenic plaque. In everyday life, however, most people take more than sufficient sucrose to keep the plaque active.

'Refined carbohydrates'

Apart from vegetables, eaten as such, most carbohydrates eaten today are processed or refined to some extent. White flour, for example, represents less than 75% of whole wheat. Animal feeding experiments and the findings in human studies discussed above show that starchy polysaccharides are not fermented in the mouth to any significant degree, and white bread (though highly 'refined') or unsweetened biscuits, for instance, therefore make little direct contribution to caries.

Unrefined carbohydrate such as wholemeal bread is not particularly cariogenic but is also not protective. It has also been found that rats fed on wholemeal bread had a consistently *higher* caries score than those fed on white bread. The amount of caries caused by these different breads alone was very small compared with sweet foods, but the reasons for this unexpected finding are not known.

Another unrefined carbohydrate is honey, which is a concentrated mixture of sugars. In spite of being 'unrefined' and rich in vitamins and trace elements, honey is at least as cariogenic as sucrose under comparable experimental conditions. Food cranks believe that honey has (among other effects) youth-giving properties. Those who want to take advantage of this desirable effect may also have to accept that a fair proportion of their prolonged youth will have to be spent having dental treatment or in an edentulous state.

The term 'refined carbohydrates' is therefore vague in that it encompasses a wide range of foods of widely differing cariogenicity. It shows fundamental misunderstanding of the evidence available to speak of 'refined carbohydrates' as being the main factor in the production of caries. It is also unhelpful to talk of the role of 'refined carbohydrates' when giving dental health instruction, as few patients (reasonably enough) understand what these are or will be misled into thinking that white bread is just as cariogenic as candy or toffee.

It is less pretentious and more accurate to speak of *sugar* (sucrose) as the main foodstuff causing dental decay. As a simple and sufficiently accurate generalisation, sweet (sugar-containing) foods cause caries while unsweetened carbohydrates have very little effect. The degree to which either is 'refined' is irrelevant.

SUSCEPTIBILITY OF THE TEETH TO CARIES

It seems reasonable to assume that the teeth themselves can be, to a variable degree, resistant to decay, because of factors affecting the structure of the tooth during formation.

If caries develops, then the teeth are clearly caries-susceptible. If, on the other hand, caries does not develop it cannot be assumed that the teeth are caries-resistant.

Even if a cariogenic (sugar-rich) diet is given and the teeth remain caries-free it still cannot be taken as proof that the teeth themselves are resistant. Many variables in the oral environment *may* affect caries activity. Examples of such variables are the salivary flow rate and buffering power, immune responses, or differences in the plaque flora or mineral content.

The essential problem is therefore to distinguish effects due to inherent properties of the teeth from factors affecting their environment.

Vitamin D deficiency and hypocalcification

There have been few controlled experiments to test the variation among individuals in their resistance to caries in response to the same highly cariogenic diet. This was done (in effect) in the Vipeholm study but (as mentioned earlier) not all those who had the most highly cariogenic regimen developed severe caries. However, it seems clear that not all individuals followed the instructions exactly. They were not, after all, *forced* under supervision completely to chew toffees several times a day, and it is likely that some, for example, simply bolted them so that they had little local effect. Thus those who were little affected by the cariogenic diet may have had more resistant teeth but it is equally possible that (like so many of the human race) they were simply not following instructions about what they had to eat and how they were to eat it.

Hypocalcification. Serious efforts were made in the past to establish that dental caries was due to hypocalcification of the teeth and was essentially a vitamin deficiency disease. This simplistic view ignored of course the extensive epidemiological findings that the best-nourished populations had the worst record for dental disease while poverty-stricken communities on deficient diets had a low caries prevalence as discussed earlier.

However, newly erupted teeth are generally caries susceptible, apparently because of a hypo-mineralised enamel structure which is made progressively less vulnerable by deposition of materials from saliva.

Hereditary hypoplasia or hypocalcification of the teeth which are characterised by severe disturbances of structure are also not particularly susceptible to caries.

In spite of the fact that the idea still clings on (even among *dentists*) that patients with rampant caries have 'poorly calcified' teeth, there is no evidence that the degree of calcification of the teeth affects their resistance to caries.

Effects of fluorides

Fluorides when present in drinking water and some foods are taken up by calcifying tissues during development. When the fluoride content of the water is 1 ppm or more the incidence of caries is substantially reduced. Fluoride may affect caries activity by a variety of mechanisms (as discussed later). Nevertheless the fact that fluoride has its greatest and most persistent effect in those exposed to fluorides throughout the period of dental development strongly suggests that it affects the structure of the developing teeth. Fluoride is the only nutrient which has been proved to have this action.

Despite the difficulties in distinguishing the degree of resistance of the teeth from the virulence of their cariogenic environment, it has become clear that fluorides have had a major impact on caries prevalence. As mentioned elsewhere there has been a significant decline in the prevalence of dental caries in several countries where the drinking water has been fluoridated. In Britain, as a result of widespread use of fluoridised dentifrices, there has also been so great a decrease in the disease as significantly to affect the nature of dental

practice. These changes cannot be related to any comparable decline in sugar consumption.

Other trace elements

There is some evidence to suggest that molybdenum and perhaps other trace elements, alone or in combination with fluorides, improve resistance to caries. Other elements such as selenium can apparently make teeth more susceptible. It seems likely that such trace elements can also affect tooth structure for better or worse.

The present position can be summarised by saying that, although many factors might influence the resistance of the teeth to caries, there is in most cases doubt whether they affect the structure of the developing tooth or the oral environment. Only fluorides have been shown incontrovertibly to improve resistance to caries.

SALIVA AND DENTAL CARIES

The immediate environment of the teeth is the bacterial plaque, but saliva is the medium in which plaque develops and works. Saliva may be expected to have effects upon the teeth by influencing the plaque and its metabolism. Though saliva inevitably plays some part in the process of caries, it is a complex secretion whose rates of flow, composition and properties are not easy to determine.

Effects of desalivation

The flow of saliva is of great importance in clearing cariogenic foods from the mouth. In animals, removal or inactivation of major salivary glands leads to increased caries activity roughly in proportion to the reduction in saliva production. In humans also, xerostomia due to salivary gland disease (Ch. 18) is associated with stasis of foodstuffs round the teeth and, usually, a greatly increased caries rate.

However, whether in animals or humans, caries activity under conditions of xerostomia is only increased if the diet is also cariogenic.

These considerations do not of course apply to a normal population, but during sleep salivary secretion is greatly reduced, so that food residues left on the teeth may be expected to have their most destructive effect at this time. Bedtime sweet snacks or failure to brush the teeth thoroughly then are likely to be particularly harmful.

Rate of flow, reaction and buffering power

The reaction of the saliva varies more widely than that of the blood, and the range, based on a large number of determinations, is stated to be between pH 5.6 and 7.6, with an average of pH 6.75; but estimates vary according to the way in which the pH is measured. The reaction varies during the course of the day and the pH rises as a result of increased salivary activity, especially during eating. No simple relationship exists between the reaction of the saliva and caries activity.

The buffering power of saliva depends mainly on its bicarbonate content and this is increased at high rates of flow. There is evidence that the buffering power of the saliva affects the buffering power of dental plaque and helps to prevent the pH from falling to very low levels. A rapid rate of flow, with the increased buffering power that is associated, appears to be important in this respect, and in several investigations a high buffering power has been found to be associated with a low incidence of caries.

In Down's syndrome (Mongolism) caries activity is low in spite of gross accumulation of plaque and immunodeficiencies. It is suggested that a factor may be the high rate of salivation with greater buffering power and high pH.

Whilst a rapid flow of saliva of low viscosity assists clearance of foodstuffs from the mouth, other physical properties of different salivas have not been shown to have a significant relationship to caries activity.

Other factors

Inorganic components and enamel maturation

Of the many inorganic ions in saliva, calcium, phosphorus and fluoride have been most intensively investigated. Fluoride can be adsorbed onto the enamel surface. It also appears, from use of radioactive isotopes, that there is some exchange of calcium and phosphate ions between enamel surface and saliva. Although it is suggested that the calcium and phosphate content of saliva affect susceptibility to caries, the evidence that these ions exert an important effect is not strong.

Investigations have also shown that enamel undergoes post-eruptive changes. Clinical observations suggest that newly erupted teeth are more prone to caries than teeth that have been present in the mouth for some time.

The exact nature of this post-eruptive change is unknown, but studies with radioactive tracers show that newly erupted teeth can incorporate 10 to 20 times as much inorganic material in ionic form as adult teeth.

Enzymic activity

Salivary amylase breaks down polysaccharides such as starch. This contribution to digestion is small, and the main value of this action may be to make food residues on the teeth more soluble to assist their clearance. The breakdown of polysaccharides leads to production of sugars, but the amounts and their contribution to caries are small and are only likely to be seen with experimental sugar-deficient diets. In most cases the amount of sugar usually present in the diet is far greater than that produced by amylase activity. In general, therefore, amylase activity and caries prevalence do not appear to be closely related.

Antibacterial activities

Saliva contains thiocyanates, a lysozyme-like substance and other theoretically antibacterial substances. Nevertheless the mouth teems with bacteria, and there is no evidence that non-specific antibacterial substances in saliva have any significant effect on caries activity.

Immunological defences

The contribution of salivary IgA. The main immunoglobulin in saliva is secretory IgA. Increased flow rates are associated with lower concentrations of IgA, but, overall, the increase in quantity of saliva entering the mouth may raise the amount of IgA reaching it.

Investigation of the relation of IgA to caries activity has yielded conflicting findings. In some studies, raised salivary IgA levels have been related to low caries activity. However, much depends on whether IgA levels are related to signs of active caries or related to past disease, as shown by restored or missing teeth. In the latter case, caries activity may appear to be low merely because most of the susceptible surfaces have been removed or restored.

Similar considerations apply to findings that high serum IgA and IgG levels are associated with high DMF rates.

However such findings are interpreted, the many individuals who are naturally IgA deficient (estimated at 1 in 600 of the population) are not noteworthy for rampant dental caries. This *may* result from compensatory IgG secretion, but this does not seem to have been established.

IgG and IgM normally enter the mouth via gingival exudate but in amounts so small as to be difficult to measure. The amounts entering the mouth are roughly proportional to the severity of gingival inflammation but, at most, only trace amounts reach the mouth. Any effect of these immunoglobulins is likely to be restricted to the immediate vicinity of the gingival crevice. However, this may explain the better protection of interproximal sites obtained in animals that have been vaccinated against caries.

Dental caries in immunodeficiencies

Despite a plausible case being made for the development of adoptive immunity to dental caries, there is little evidence that caries activity is increased in immunodeficiency states. The apparent lack of effect of IgA deficiency on caries activity has been discussed. In addition, in Down's syndrome (Ch. 24) there are natural defects of antibody production and susceptibility to infections. There is also massive plaque accumulation. Nevertheless caries activity is at a remarkably low level.

It is also noteworthy that dental caries is possibly the only infectious disease that does *not* become rampant as a direct consequence of the severe immunodeficiency characteristic of AIDS (Ch. 8)

Salivary minerals

Minerals and other substances from the saliva, as mentioned earlier, complete the maturation of newly erupted teeth and lessen their susceptibility to caries.

Fluoride can enter plaque from the saliva and affect caries activity. However, in this, saliva is no more than a vehicle for this important element.

Effects of saliva on plaque activity

While components of saliva contribute to plaque formation, and substances carried in saliva, particularly sugars, are taken up by plaque, it is uncertain to what degree other salivary activities influence those of plaque. The dense, insoluble matrix of the latter presents a formidable barrier, and it is hardly surprising that it is difficult significantly to affect acid production there.

Saliva and caries—summary

The main features of the saliva that appear to affect caries activity are therefore as follows.

1. Gross reduction in the amount of saliva

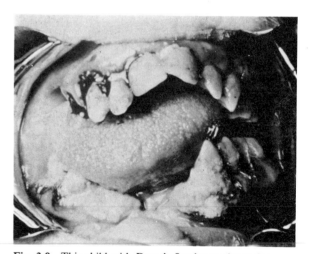

Fig. 3.9 This child with Down's Syndrome shows the typical gross accumulations of plaque but little or no caries. (Picture kindly lent by Dr Crispian Scully.)

secreted leads to an increase in caries when a cariogenic diet is eaten.

2. During sleep, salivary secretion is greatly reduced, and this is likely to make the teeth especially vulnerable at this period.

3. The buffering power of saliva appears to assist neutralisation of acid formed in the plaque, and in caries-resistant patients it may prevent acid production from reaching a destructively high level.

4. The buffering power of saliva is related to the rate of secretion and high secretion rates seem to be associated with lower caries activity.

5. Immunoglobulins, particularly IgA, are present in saliva but findings relating their concentrations to caries activity are conflicting.

AETIOLOGY OF CARIES: SUMMARY

I. Microbiological aspects

1. Dental caries is a bacterial disease and the organism mainly responsible appears to be specific strains of *Streptococcus mutans*.

2. The cariogenicity of *S. mutans* has been shown experimentally by inoculation into the mouths of otherwise germfree animals (gnotobiotes).

3. There is an association between the presence of *S. mutans* and caries activity in the human mouth, though there is as yet no conclusive evidence that it is the sole cause of human caries.

4. Other microorganisms including lactobacilli and other related strains of streptococci are only weakly cariogenic or are non-cariogenic, even though they may be effective acid producers.

5. The cariogenicity of *S. mutans* depends not merely on its ability to produce acid by fermentation of sugars, like many other organisms, but particularly also upon its ability to polymerise sugars into long-chain polysaccharides (glucans).

6. Initiation of plaque formation depends on bacterial mechanisms of adhesion to tooth substance. Bacterial polysaccharides (glucans) cause plaque to adhere firmly to the tooth, and the bacteria to adhere to one another and the tooth surface.

7. Plaque consists mainly of bacteria within this adhesive gelatinous polysaccharide matrix which is itself largely a bacterial product.

8. Plaque is cariogenic only in stagnation areas where it can form sufficiently thickly and act undisturbed for a relatively long period.

9. Plaque resists removal by the normal functional activities of the mouth but is removable from accessible areas by mechanical means such as toothbrushing.

10. The physiochemical properties of plaque matrix allow rapid diffusion of sugars into its substance but resist the escape of acids and the buffering by saliva.

11. Acid production by the bacteria of plaque is by fermentation of sugars.

12. Direct pH measurements in the human mouth show that a brief rinse with a sugar solution is followed by a fall of pH in plaque within 2 to 5 minutes but resting pH is not regained for approximately 45 minutes.

13. The slow return to resting pH probably depends both on the physiochemical properties of plaque and on continued acid production by bacteria from storage polysaccharides.

II. Dietary aspects

1. Epidemiological evidence shows that a steady increase in caries prevalence in the Western World has accompanied the progressive improvement in the level of nutrition but has been associated with a parallel increase in sugar consumption.

2. A low intake of sugar, whether because of poverty or wartime shortages, is accompanied by a low prevalence of caries.

3. Malnutrition is not a factor in dental caries, and inadequate diets of negligible sugar content are non-cariogenic.

4. Starchy carbohydrates, even when refined as in white bread, are not significantly cariogenic.

5. Direct measurement of pH changes in plaque show that frequent ingestion of sugary foods, particularly those such as caramels which stick to the teeth, usually has the most severe cariogenic effect. This has been confirmed clinically in the Vipeholm study.

6. Eating sugar or sugary foods infrequently, such as at mealtimes only, causes considerably less caries activity.

7. Sucrose is the most important foodstuff serving as bacterial substrate
   a. because of its metabolism by *S. mutans* to the glucans necessary for plaque formation and function
   b. because it is readily metabolised to form acid, and
   c. because it is eaten in greater quantity than any other sugar.

8. Glucose and fructose are only slightly less cariogenic, and unrefined sugars such as those in honey are as cariogenic as refined sugars.

9. Fluoride ingested during the calcification of the teeth is associated with a greatly decreased incidence of caries and probably increases the resistance of the tooth itself.

10. The main roles of saliva in caries are:
    a. to assist clearance of sticky carbohydrates
    b. as a buffer against acid production in the more superficial part of plaque, and
    c. as a vehicle for immune globulins.

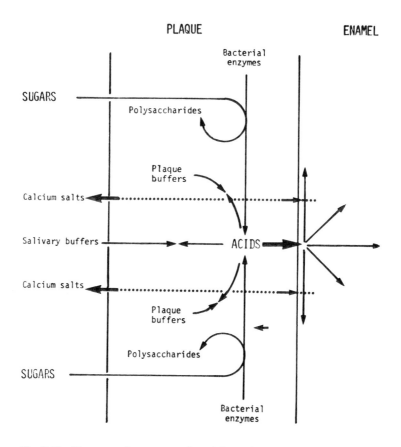

Fig. 3.10 Diagrammatic representation of the main biochemical events in dental plaque, initiating caries. (From McCracken A W, Cawson A A 1983 Clinical and Oral Microbiology. McGraw-Hill.)

PATHOLOGY OF ENAMEL CARIES

Enamel is the usual site of the initial lesion unless dentine or cementum becomes exposed by gingival recession. Enamel is the main barrier to invasion and, once breached, infection of dentine can spread with relatively little obstruction. Preventive measures must therefore be aimed primarily at stopping the attack or at making the enamel more resistant.

Routes of attack

The essential nature of the carious attack on enamel is the permeation of acid into its substance.

Part of the organic matrix of enamel is keratin-like and acid soluble but the belief that attack was initiated by dissolution of this component has not been substantiated by the microradiographic findings.

However, the organic matrix, which envelops the apatite crystals, has a relatively high water content and is permeable to hydrogen ions. By contrast, the crystalline lattice of calcium apatite crystals is relatively impermeable.

The pattern of the early attack on enamel seems likely therefore to be the result of highly mobile hydrogen ions permeating the organic matrix and then attacking the surfaces of apatite crystals. As a result further pathways are opened up. Micro-radiography suggests that a major pathway thus formed is by preferential destruction of the prism cores. The prism cores can also be seen by electron microscopy to be preferentially destroyed when enamel is etched with acid.

Once acid has started to permeate the enamel a series of submicroscopic changes take place. However, the process of enamel caries is a dynamic one and, initially at least, consists of alternating phases of demineralisation and remineralisation, rather than a continuous process of dissolution.

Microscopic changes

Enamel caries develops in four main phases:

1. The early lesion
2. Phase of enamel destruction
3. Bacterial invasion of enamel
4. Secondary enamel caries.

These stages of enamel caries are distinguishable microscopically and are also of clinical significance. In particular the early (white spot) lesion is potentially reversible, while secondary enamel caries is responsible for collapse of the enamel

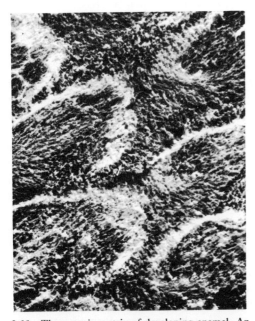

Fig. 3.11 The organic matrix of developing enamel. An electron photomicrograph of a section across the lines of the prisms before calcification showing the matrix to be more dense in the region of the prism sheaths than in the prism cores or interprismatic substance ($\times$ 5000). (From a photograph kindly lent by Dr K. Little.)

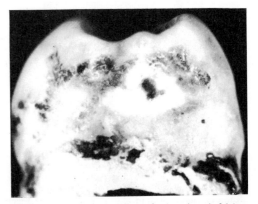

Fig. 13.12 Interstitial (smooth-surface) caries. A fairly early lesion with chalking of the enamel and a stained central area. Macroscopically the surface is intact.

and demands more or less extensive restorative procedures.

The early lesion

This term is used for the first visible changes. Clinically they are seen beneath the earliest visible sign of caries, namely the white opaque spot that forms just adjacent to a contact point. Despite the chalky appearance the enamel is hard and smooth to the probe.

The microscopic changes under this early white spot lesion are seen in undecalcified sections. They are not always clearly visible by ordinary light microscopy and are more readily visualised when polarised light is used. Microradiography provides additional information about the degree of demineralisation seen in the different zones.

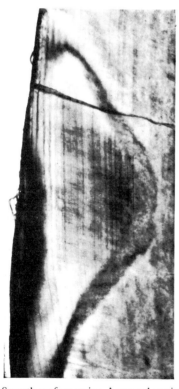

Fig. 3.13 Smooth-surface caries. A ground section of enamel at an early stage in the disease. The surface is intact but beneath it is a conical lesion in which the striae of Retzius are enhanced. Round the main body of the lesion there is a dark zone surrounded in turn by a translucent zone marking the edge of the lesion. The enamel, though altered, is intact (× 50).

This initial lesion is conical in shape with its apex towards the enamel, and a series of four zones of differing translucency can be discerned.

Working back from the advancing edge of the lesion, these zones consist first of an outer *translucent zone*; immediately within this is a second *dark zone*; the third consists of the *body of the lesion* and the fourth consists of the *surface zone*. It must be emphasised that these initial changes are not due to bacterial invasion, but are the effects of the bacterial products, namely lactic or other acids, upon the enamel. Though these changes are visible in the enamel, they are not produced by actual destruction of the tissue, even at microscopic level, but are submicroscopic.

*1. **The translucent zone.*** The translucent zone is the first observable change and is best seen when the section is mounted in quinoline which has the same refractive index as enamel.

The appearance of the translucent zone is the result of the formation of submicroscopic spaces or pores apparently located at prism boundaries and other junctional sites such as the striae of Retzius. These pores account for about 1% of the enamel volume. As a result when the tissue is mounted in quinoline, the latter fills the pores, and since it has the same refractive index as enamel the normal structural features disappear.

Precise microradiographic techniques confirm that the changes in the translucent zone are due to demineralisation. Further microdissection suggests that there is preferential removal of magnesium and carbonate-rich salts.

*2. **The dark zone.*** The dark zone is just within the translucent zone and therefore fractionally more superficial. Polarised light microscopy shows that the volume of the pores in this zone has increased to 2–4% of the enamel volume.

This increased amount of space in the tissue is due mainly to the formation of small pores in addition to the larger pores formed in the translucent zone. Two different-size pores thus coexist in the dark zone, and the small are so minute that the molecules of quinoline are unable to enter, and the tissue has become transformed into a molecular sieve. The small pores therefore remain filled with air, and this appears to be the cause for the dark appearance of this zone.

Microradiographs confirm that the dark zone

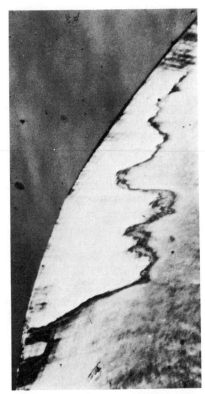

Fig.3.14 Early interproximal caries. Ground section viewed by polarised light. The specimen is in quinoline which has filled the larger pores causing most of the fine detail in the body of the lesion to disappear, but the dark zone, with its smaller pores, to be accentuated. (Original magnification × 75.)

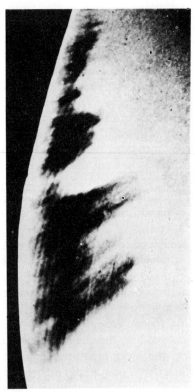

Fig. 3.15 Early interproximal caries. A microradiograph of the same section as in Fig. 3.14, showing radiolucency following the same pattern, the intact surface zone and accentuation of the striae of Retzius. (Original magnification × 75. Figs 3.14 and 3.15 kindly lent by Prof. A. I. Darling.)

has suffered a greater degree of demineralisation. However, when the lesion is exposed to saliva or synthetic calcifying solutions in vitro, the dark zone actually extends further. This may indicate that the formation of the dark zone may be due not merely to the creation of new porosities but possibly also to remineralisation of the large pores of the translucent zone so that they become micropores impermeable to quinoline. It is widely believed therefore that these changes in the dark zone are evidence of remineralisation, as discussed later.

3. The body of the lesion The body of the lesion forms the bulk of the lesion and extends from just beneath the surface zone to the dark zone. By transmitted light the body of the lesion is comparatively translucent compared with normal enamel and is sharply demarcated from the dark zone. Within the body of the lesion the striae of Retzius are well demarcated and appear enhanced, particularly when mounted in quinoline and viewed under polarised light. Polarised light examination also shows that the pore volume is 5% at the periphery but increases to at least 25% in the centre.

Microradiography, which will detect demineralisation in excess of 5%, shows that the area of radiolucency corresponds closely with the size and shape of the body of the lesion, in contrast to the surface zone which appears relatively radiopaque. Alternating radiopaque and radiolucent lines, about 30 μm apart can also be seen passing obliquely through the subsurface region. The radiolucent lines show an apparently preferential demineralisation and are thought to represent the striae of Retzius. At higher magnifications, still finer lines running at right angles to the enamel surface, and others parallel to the surface, may be discerned. These lines may represent the preferential demineralisation along the junctional sites mentioned earlier, and represent the prism boundaries and the cross striations, respectively.

4. The surface zone. The surface zone represents one of the most important changes in enamel caries that is relevant to the prevention and management of the disease. It shows the paradoxical feature that it has not merely remained intact during this stage of the attack but remains more heavily mineralised and radiopaque than the deeper zones and has a pore volume of only 1%.

The relative lack of damage to the surface zone has been attributed to its higher initial mineral and fluoride, but lower soluble protein content. For this reason therefore it was proposed that it was particularly important to protect this more resistant zone from damage during cavity preparation of an adjacent tooth. However, when the surface zone is removed and the enamel is exposed to an acid buffer, the more highly mineralised surface zone reappears over the deeper changes described earlier. This finding implies that the appearance of the surface zone is not due to specific properties of the natural enamel surface but rather that the surface zone forms partly by remineralisation. The remineralising salts may come either from those concentrated in the plaque or from precipitation of calcium and phosphate ions diffusing outwards as the deeper zones are demineralised.

Dissolution of the enamel crystals

Since all but a minute proportion of the structure of enamel consists of crystals of calcium apatite, destruction of these crystals is the essential feature of enamel caries. However, electron microscopic study of the stages of the carious destruction of enamel crystals is technically so difficult that knowledge of details of this process is limited.

In the early stages, formation of channels along the peripheries of the prisms has been reported, and the initiation of the attack may be along the prism boundaries as mentioned earlier. Later, the central core of the prisms may also dissolve to produce the appearance shown in Figure 3.18.

The attack on the apatite crystals appears mainly to consist in the removal of mineral from their surface so that they become progressively smaller in size.

This has been confirmed by microdissection of the translucent zone, which has shown that the apatite crystals have become smaller as a result of decalcification and have decreased in diameter from the normal of 35–40 nm to 25–30 nm and in the body of the lesion to 10–30 nm. In the dark zone, by contrast, enamel crystals appeared to have grown to 50–100 nm and in the surface zone to 35–40 nm. These findings also suggest that demineralisation and remineralisation are alternating processes. However, as the lesion progresses and cavitation develops, demineralisation comes to dominate the process.

Enamel destruction

There are clearly many further stages in the carious attack between the formation of submicroscopic pores in the initial enamel lesion to the stage of clinical cavity formation. However, the details of these intermediate stages are controversial, and it is not clear whether or not the different components of enamel prism structure are destroyed selectively.

Nevertheless, in broad general terms, the enamel crystallites are progressively dissolved leading to disintegration, visible microscopically. Defects eventually become large enough to allow the entry of bacteria. As shown earlier there is evidence of preferential destruction of the prism cores, and, by light microscopy, bacteria may sometimes be seen—apparently within the remnants of the enamel prisms (Fig. 3.19).

Whatever the precise nature of these changes it seems that physical penetration of enamel by bacteria is relatively unimportant until the later stages of the disease, namely secondary enamel caries and dentine caries.

Secondary enamel caries

The term 'secondary enamel caries' is used here in the histological sense, but 'secondary caries' is also used clinically to refer to recurrence of caries, particularly at the margins of restorations.

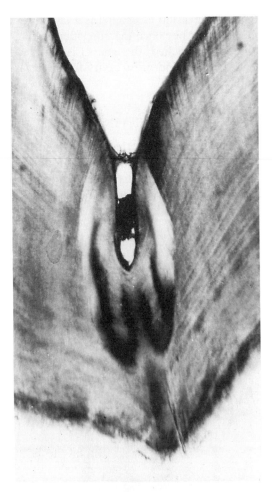

Fig. 3.16 Undecalcified section showing preinvasive acid damage to dentine surrounding and deep to an occlusal pit.

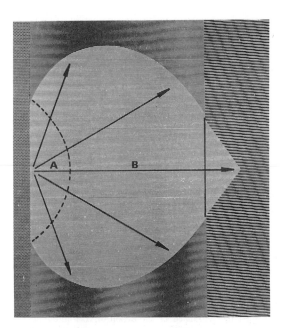

Fig. 3.17 Diagram summarising the main features of the pre-invasive phase of enamel caries. As indicated here, in this final stage of acid attack on enamel before bacterial invasion, decalcification of dentine has begun. The area (A) would be radiolucent in a bite-wing film but the area (B) could be visualised only in a section by polarised light microscopy or microradiography (see also Fig. 3.22). Clinically, the enamel would appear solid and intact but the surface would be marked by an opaque white spot over the area (A) as in Fig. 3.12 (From McCracken A W, Cawson R A 1983 Clinical and Oral Microbiology. McGraw Hill).

Once bacteria have penetrated the enamel, they reach the amelodentinal junction and can spread laterally along this zone to undermine the enamel. This has two major effects. First, the enamel becomes detached from the supporting dentine and therefore greatly weakened. Second, it is attacked from beneath.

The precise route by which bacteria spread laterally along the amelodentinal junction is unclear but this process has important clinical effects. The primary enamel lesions provide the bridgehead for the attack on enamel, but secondary enamel caries determines the gross extent (though not the depth) of a cavity. Clinically this is frequently evident when there is no more than a pinhole lesion in an occlusal pit, but cutting away the surrounding enamel shows it to be widely undermined.

As secondary enamel caries progresses, it undermines the enamel until the latter starts to collapse under the stress of mastication and to fragment around the edge of the (clinically obvious) cavity. By this stage also, bacterial acids are attacking the dentine and invading the dentinal tubules.

Pit and fissure caries

The initial lesion has been considerably more extensively investigated in smooth-surface caries. In pits the initial lesion appears to spread laterally outwards, so that, in sections, the initial changes resemble the initial lesion of smooth-surface caries on either side of the fissure. This of course is a two-dimensional view of a process which surrounds the fissure (Fig. 3.16).

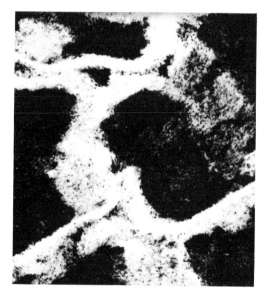

Fig. 3.18   Chalky enamel. An electron photomicrograph of chalky enamel produced by the action of very dilute acid. The crystallites of calcium salts remain intact in the prism sheaths, while the prism cores and some of the interprismatic substance have been destroyed. The same appearance is seen in chalky enamel caused by early caries (× 7500). (From a picture kindly lent by Dr K. Little.)

Enamel caries—summary

1. The earliest detectable stages of enamel caries are submicroscopic and seen as a series of changes in translucency more clearly visible by polarised light.
2. The changes in translucency of the different zones of the initial carious lesion are caused by the formation of submicroscopic pores in the enamel.
3. Microradiography confirms that these changes represent areas of increasing radiolucency and demineralisation.
4. The surface zone remains intact during the initial phases. It is less heavily demineralised than the deeper zones, and this results from remineralisation. There may also be some remineralisation of the dark zone, and the process overall may be of alternating demineralisation and remineralisation.
5. The route by which bacterial acid enters the enamel and attacks the enamel crystals appears to be via the organic matrix, which is permeable to hydrogen ions.

6. Bacterial invasion of enamel is a late stage in the process, but once the amelodentinal junction is reached, the enamel is attacked from beneath and gross cavity formation is initiated.

PATHOLOGY OF DENTINE CARIES

As in enamel the initial changes are nonbacterial and caused by the diffusion of acid into the tissue. However, once enamel has been penetrated by bacteria the dentine is open to direct bacterial attack for which the dentinal tubules form an open pathway.

The initial (nonbacterial) lesion

The initial dentine lesion forms deep to carious, but still largely intact, enamel.

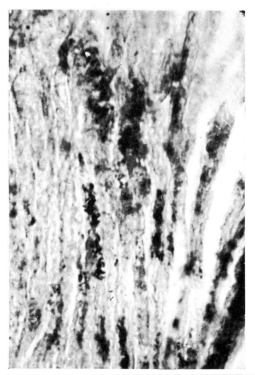

Fig. 3.19   Bacterial invasion of the enamel. A photomicrograph of a decalcified specimen showing bacteria advancing through the enamel apparently within the prisms themselves (× 800).

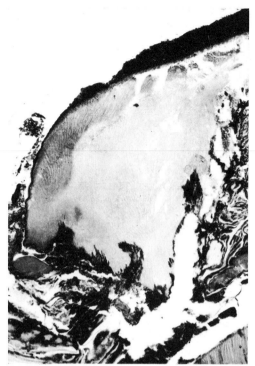

Fig. 3.20 Secondary enamel caries. Bacterial plaque forms the darkly stained layer on the enamel surface. Heavy masses of bacteria have spread beneath the enamel and are spreading through it along the general line of the prisms. Much of the enamel has already been destroyed ($\times$ 100).

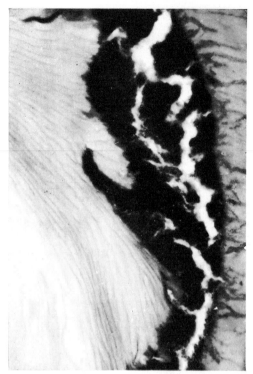

Fig. 3.21 Secondary enamel caries. Infection is spreading along the amelodentinal junction and invading the deep surface of the enamel. The terminations of the dentinal tubules are also infected but destruction, at this stage, is at the expense of the enamel ($\times$ 470).

Bacteria and the acids they produce spread laterally along the amelodentinal junction and attack the dentine over a wide area. The lesion is therefore conical with its apex towards the pulp.

Three components of this lesion, some of which are reactive, may be distinguishable. *1.* the body of the lesion is demineralised and related odontoblasts are killed. This is associated with deposition of calcified material which blocks the dentinal end of the tubule to form *dead tracts*. *2.* round the periphery of the body of the lesion, there is sclerosis of the dentine, with the formation of a narrow *translucent zone*. *3.* beyond the apex of the lesion there is a pulpal response, and reactionary dentine may be laid down across the pulpal end of the affected tubules. These reactionary changes start to develop early but may progress too slowly when caries is acute to have any great protective effect.

The infected lesion

Dentine becomes infected after bacterial invasion of the enamel and formation of a cavity. The dentinal tubules form a ready path for invasion by bacteria and there are in effect, two waves of invasion. Pioneer bacteria at the forefront are acidogenic and demineralise the dentine matrix but leave it otherwise intact and not visibly changed microscopically. Subsequently there is bacterial proteolysis of the remaining dentine matrix.

Microbial aspects

Although streptococci play a major part in the initiation of dental caries, lactobacilli are at least as numerous in dentine caries, and there is some evidence that they are the pioneer bacteria in

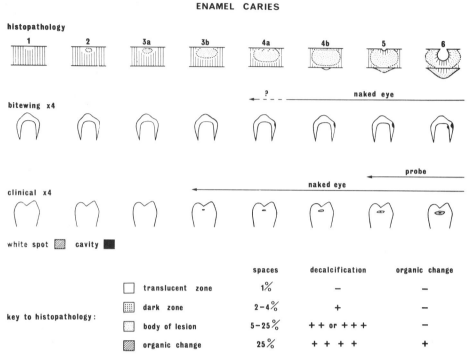

Fig. 3.22 This diagram summarises the sequential changes in enamel from the stage of the initial lesion to early cavity formation and relates the different stages in the development of the lesion with the radiographic appearances and clinical findings. (Diagram kindly lent by Prof. A. I. Darling and reproduced by courtesy of the Editor of the British Dental Journal (1959) 107: 27–302.)

dentine invasion. As the lesion progresses, the bacterial population becomes increasingly mixed and it becomes increasingly difficult to discern their relative contributions to demineralisation and proteolysis.

Histological changes

The deepest zone which is decalcified retains for a time the normal morphology of dentine, and no bacteria can be seen. More superficially, in the infected zone the tubules contain at first a few bacteria but soon become filled with them. As the softened matrix is unable to support these heavily infected tubules they become distended into a spindle shape by the expanding masses of bacteria and their products. As a result adjacent less heavily infected tubules become bent. Later still the intervening tubule walls are destroyed and collections of bacteria in adjacent tubules coalesce

to form irregular *liquefaction foci*. These in turn coalesce to form progressively more widespread tissue destruction.

In some areas bacteria also spread laterally, and, occasionally, large bacteria-filled clefts form at right angles to the general direction of the tubules. Clinically this lateral spread may explain why carious dentine can be excavated in flakes in a plane parallel to the surface.

Reactions of dentine and pulp under caries

The reactions in dentine are mainly due to the activity of the odontoblasts, so that dentine and pulp should be considered as one tissue. Their reactions are not specific, since they may be provoked by other irritants than dental caries. They comprise the following:

1. Dead tracts

2. Translucent zones
3. Reactionary dentine
4. Inflammation of the pulp.

Though these processes are reactionary in nature, they start at the time of the onset of dentine caries and precede bacterial invasion, as described earlier.

Dead tracts

Dead tracts are found under most carious cavities unless the lesion has developed exceptionally slowly. The dead tract is caused by the death of odontoblasts, followed by deposition of acellular calcific material blocking the pulpal end of the affected tubule. Dead tracts appear dark by transmitted light in ground sections because of a change of refractive index consequent upon the changes in the dentinal tubule.

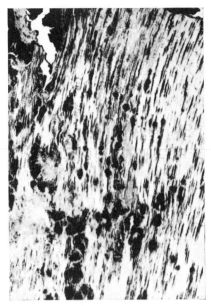

Fig. 3.24 Caries of dentine. The tubules, filled with heavily stained bacteria, are visible as dark streaks. Masses of bacteria expand tubules in the softened dentine producing globular or fusiform varicosities. As destruction progresses, these swellings coalesce to form liquefaction foci of which there are many in the lower part of the picture ($\times$ 80).

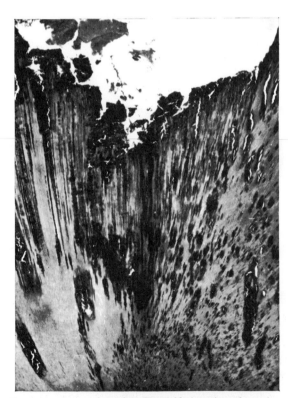

Fig. 3.23 Caries of dentine. Decalcified section of a carious lesion. The dark streaks and larger areas are due to bacteria spreading along the tubules and bursting through their walls as the dentine is destroyed. Although the dentine has been decalcified much of its structure remains intact ($\times$ 40).

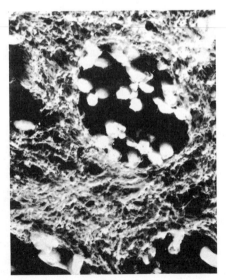

Fig. 3.25 Infection of the dentinal tubules. This electron photomicrograph shows bacteria in the lumen of the tubules. Between the tubules is the collagenous matrix of the dentine ($\times$ 7500). (From a picture kindly lent by Dr K. Little.)

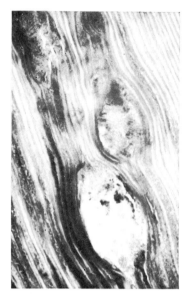

Fig. 3.26 Caries of dentine. A specimen showing infected tubules and fusiform masses of bacteria which have expanded into the softened tissue. Adjacent tubules in the demineralised dentine have been bent and pushed aside by these masses (× 360).

Translucent zones

A translucent zone is produced by mild stimulation of the odontoblast process, whereby mineral is laid down as a progressively thicker lining of the dentinal tubule (*peritubular dentine*). It is also a characteristic feature of age changes in dentine, and this response to caries may be regarded as an acceleration of a normal process. The reaction may be one of progressive withdrawal of the odontoblast process with obliteration of the tubule behind it. Alternatively calcium salts may be deposited on the tubule walls. Obliteration of the tubules by this progressive calcification presents a partial barrier to the advance of caries.

In acute caries, as in the deciduous teeth, translucent zones may not form.

Reactionary dentine

The character of reactionary dentine varies according to the severity of the stimulus. When the lesion

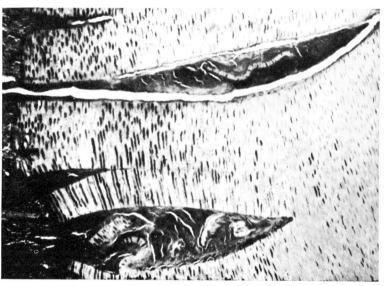

Fig. 3.27 Clefts in carious dentine. The main body of the lesion is to the left. Infection is tracking along the tubules but in this case has also spread across the tubules, forming heavily-infected clefts. Within the clefts, strips of dentine split from the rest of the tissue are lying in the mass of organisms. Further clefts are starting to form from the left-hand edge of the lesion, and the appearances suggest that there are lines of weakness in the dentine, along which infection spreads easily (× 120).

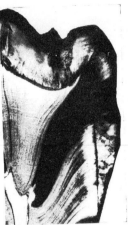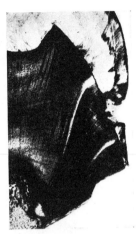

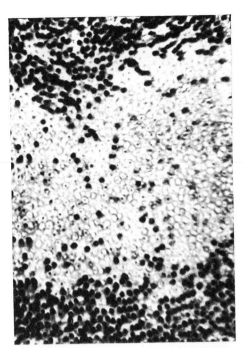

Fig. 3.28 (left) A dead tract. The empty tubules have been filled with stain to which they are permeable from the cavity, so that the whole zone appears black. At the proximal end of the tubules, the dead tract has been sealed off by a layer of impermeable calcified tissue beyond which the stain cannot penetrate; the pulp is thus protected from irritants from the cavity.

Fig. 3.29 (right) Translucent zones. These are seen on either side of a dead tract and formed by calcification and obliteration of the tubules. This is a slow process and rarely seen beneath a carious cavity, but may develop on either side of a dead tract as a result of low-grade irritation reaching the odontoblast processes by way of their lateral branches.

Fig. 3.30 A translucent zone. The dentinal tubules are seen in cross section. Those in the centre of the picture have become obliterated by calcification of their contents; only the original outline of the tubule remains visible, and the zone appears translucent to transmitted light. On either side are patent tubules filled with stain. (The three illustrations above were kindly lent by Dr G. C. Blake, and reproduced by courtesy of Honorary Editors (1958) Proceedings of the Royal Society of Medicine 51: 678.)

is advancing slowly, regular secondary dentine is formed, the tubules are almost normal in number and distribution, but the junction with the primary dentine is often marked by a darkly staining line or by a relatively abrupt change in the direction of the tubules.

Under rapidly advancing caries, there are varying degrees of damage to the odontoblasts, leading to increased malformation of any reactionary dentine. The tubules are few, irregular, or absent.

Pulpitis

Pulpitis follows penetration of dentine by bacteria or their metabolites and represents the breakdown of the protective hard dental tissues and opens the soft tissues to infection.

Clinical aspects of reactions to caries

The reactive changes described render the dentine immediately under a carious cavity more or less impermeable unless caries is advancing very rapidly. In this restricted area, therefore, the cutting of dentine in cavity preparation has little effect on the pulp. Adequate preparation of the cavity may, however, necessitate cutting dentine beyond the margins of the original cavity, and this opens up healthy, permeable tubules in direct communication with the pulp. Damage to the pulp by way of these tubules must be avoided. It is necessary therefore to use a coolant while cutting the cavity to avoid irritation by heat and to use non-irritant linings under the restoration to insulate the pulp from thermal or chemical stimuli (Ch. 4).

The formation of reactionary dentine is important in that it prevents early exposure of the pulp and often allows large cavities to be satisfactorily restored well beyond the limits of the original dentine.

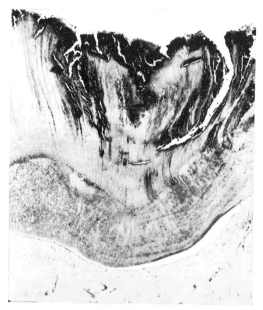

Fig. 3.31 Chronic caries and reactionary dentine formation. Infection has penetrated the full thickness of the crown but the slowness of this process has allowed time for the formation of a substantial thickness of secondary dentine. The pulp has therefore remained healthy, and deep cavity preparation is feasible.

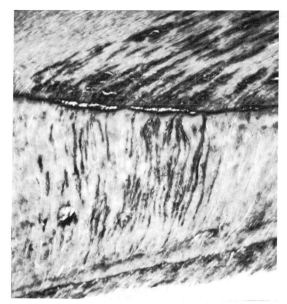

Fig. 3.32 Secondary (reactionary) dentine and caries. Regular, tubular, secondary dentine has formed under a carious cavity. A line marks the junction of the primary and secondary dentine where the tubules change direction. Caries spreading down the tubules of the primary tissue has extended along the junction and into the tubules of the reactionary dentine (× 120).

Caries of cementum

When the neck of the tooth becomes exposed by recession of the gingival margin in later life a stagnation area may be formed and the cementum attacked. Cementum is readily decalcified and presents little barrier to infection in comparison with enamel. The cementum therefore softens beneath the plaque over a wide area, producing a saucer-shaped cavity, and the underlying dentine is soon involved. Cementum appears to be invaded along the direction of Sharpey's fibres. Infection spreads between the lamellae along the incremental lines, with the result that the dentine becomes split up and progressively destroyed by a combination of demineralisation and proteolysis.

The further progress of caries in the underlying dentine is essentially similar to that in other parts of the tooth.

CLINICAL IMPLICATIONS

Prevention of dental caries depends on an under-

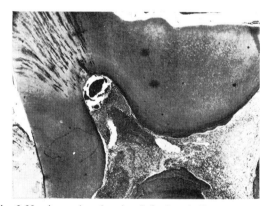

Fig. 3.33 Acute dental caries. Infection, indicated by the dark streaks in the dentine, has penetrated to the pulp too rapidly for reactionary dentine to form, causing widespread pulpitis and abscess formation.

standing of its aetiology; the practical application of this knowledge is discussed in Chapter 7.

The diagnosis and management of caries also depends on an understanding of the pathology of this disease and of the reaction to it by the pulp.

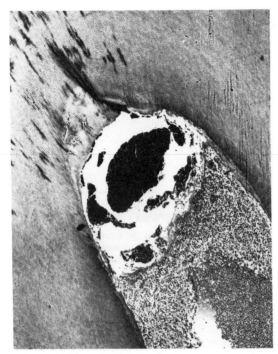

Fig. 3.34 Higher power view showing penetration of the dentine by bacteria with destruction of a cornu of the pulp, which now contains a bead of pus.

Diagnosis

By the time that a cavity has becomes obvious to the naked eye the pulp may already be infected. This is especially the case in children, where the process is rapid and there is little reactionary dentine formation. Caries must therefore be detected at an early stage, and diagnosis then depends on early evidence of decalcification.

For this purpose sharp probes, a good light and a warmed mirror are needed, but for early interstitial caries radiographs are also required. Each of the surfaces of the teeth must be examined systematically, but particular attention must obviously be paid to the stagnation areas.

Pit and fissure caries

A sharp probe will not normally 'stick' in an occlusal fissure as it cannot reach into the acutely angled depths. Early decalcification of the walls of a fissure allows a sharp probe to impact, and a sticky fissure is a reliable sign of early attack.

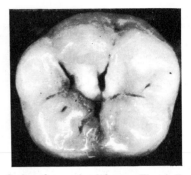

Fig. 3.35 Caries of an occlusal fissure. The chalky appearance of the enamel indicates that there is well-advanced secondary enamel caries and widespread involvement of the dentine beneath the apparently intact surface.

However, forceful use of a probe may damage the surrounding enamel and convert a lesion from being potentially arrestable into a progressive one. Later there is a small but distinct hole which allows the probe to reach softened dentine. Round the hole, secondary enamel caries causes the enamel to appear chalky and opaque, though the surface is still intact. Later still, the undermined enamel collapses under the force of mastication, and an obvious cavity appears.

Interstitial caries

An early lesion can only be seen directly if the adjacent tooth is extracted. It appears as a chalky white opacity a millimetre or two in diameter in

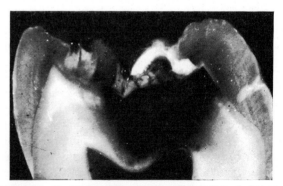

Fig. 3.36 Occlusal caries. A vertical section through the same tooth shows the spread of caries along the amelodentinal junction, extensive destruction of enamel from beneath and deep involvement of the dentine.

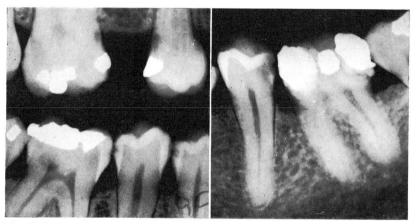

Fig. 3.37 Interstitial caries. Enlarged radiographs showing radiolucency of the enamel due to early interstitial caries in the lower premolars on the left, and a more advanced lesion affecting enamel and dentine on the distal aspect of the premolar on the right.

the region of the contact point. Such early lesions can only be reliably found radiographically, using standard bite-wing films, and are seen as small radiolucent areas just deep to the contact point. Later, especially if the embrasure is wide, a fine probe can reach sufficiently near to the contact point to allow the margin of the lesion to be felt as a roughening of the surface. Later still the cavity may become visible as a darkening or greyish discolouration of the tooth substance beneath the marginal ridge.

Remineralisation

The essential feature of active dental caries is removal of minerals from the enamel. However, this change is not entirely irreversible, and under favourable conditions the outward movement of calcium salts can be reversed and early lesions can remineralise. As mentioned earlier, re-formation of the surface layer, after its removal, can be demonstrated. Use of fluorides and consumption of a less cariogenic diet may cause a surface lesion in enamel to heal entirely. Even under natural conditions, approximately 50% of interproximal enamel lesions may show no radiographic evidence of progression for 3 years. Similarly, in some patients, secondary caries may not necessarily develop at the margins of restorations overhanging the enamel.

Principles of management

Once a tooth has been attacked, caries is usually progressive, though the rate of progress is very variable. If neglected, infection is likely to reach the pulp or eventually destroy the crown of the tooth. Effective treatment of established caries necessitates removal of infected tissue and its replacement with a resistant material to obliterate the cavity and restore the natural form of the tooth.

Cavity preparation and restoration must be carried out with the pathology of the disease in mind, and avoiding injury to other tissues, especially the pulp. It is important to bear in mind the way in which caries spreads within the tooth.

G. V. Black laid down the essential requirements for cavity preparation but Black's principles have been considerably modified in the light of more recent findings and technical developments, and in particular to reduce the amount of tissue destruction needed to produce 'classical' Black's cavities. The classes of cavity are numbered according to the frequency with which they are found; class 1 being the most common. Though these traditional principles are still widely applied, it is also suggested that, in the case of early lesions, as mentioned earlier, preventive measures should be applied to arrest the disease and, if possible, promote remineralisation, rather than resorting immediately to cavity preparation. In the case of lesions involving dentine, only carious tissue should be cut out, and Black's principle of 'extension for prevention' and conventional outline forms should in effect be abandoned. The need to retain as much healthy tooth tissue as possible has been justified by the finding that some amalgams have a useful life of no more than about 18 months before replacement becomes necessary. If, therefore, neither preventive measures can be implemented nor the restorative technique improved, the result is placement of increasingly large restorations until the tooth becomes excessively weakened. However, sceptics may question whether the amorphous restorations or newer materials now proposed will be ultimately proved to prolong the useful life of teeth. However, the main principles remain, as follows.

The pathological principles underlying conservative treatment of the teeth are to stop existing disease, to prevent its recurrence and to preserve a healthy pulp:

1. Removal of decayed enamel and dentine
2. Removal of unsupported enamel
3. Protection of the pulp
4. The placing of a watertight restoration
5. Restoration of the original form of the tooth.

Caries of the deciduous teeth

The short life of the deciduous teeth does not mean that their preservation is any less important. Early loss of deciduous teeth may prevent full growth of the alveolus and jaw, or space for the permanent successor may be lost by the drifting together of teeth on either side of the gap. Uncontrolled caries leads to death of the pulp, apical periodontitis and possible damage to an underlying permanent tooth.

Effective, durable restorations should be made in deciduous teeth, and the same general principles apply to the restoration of both permanent and deciduous teeth.

A serious problem in the treatment of deciduous teeth is the rapid progress of caries; the pulp is often involved long before the tooth is due to be shed. In these cases pulp capping, pulpotomy, or even root canal treatment may be called for to save the tooth until its successor is due to erupt.

SUGGESTED FURTHER READING

Attwood D, Blinkhorn A S 1988 Trends in dental health of ten-year old schoolchildren in South-west Scotland after cessation of water fluoridation. Lancet 333: 266–267

Attwood D, Blinkhorn A S 1989 A reassessment of the dental health of urban Scottish schoolchildren following the cessation of water fluoridation. Community Dental Health 6: 207–214

Burke F J T 1988 Restoration of the minimal carious lesion using composite resin. Dental Update 15: 232–235

Carlsson J 1989 Microbial aspects of frequent intake of products with high sugar concentrations. Scand J Dent Res 97: 110–114

Cawson R A, Eveson J W 1987 Oral pathology and diagnosis. William Heinemann Medical Books, London and Gower Medical Publishing, London

Costerton J W et al 1987 Bacterial biofilms in nature and disease. Ann Rev Microbiol 41: 435–464

Department of Health 1990 Report on Health and Social Subjects No 37, Dietary Sugars and Human Disease, Report of the Panel on Dietary Sugars, Committee on Medical Aspects of Food Policy. HMSO, London

Dummer P M H et al 1990 Factors influencing the caries experience of a group of children at the ages of 11–12 and 15–16 years: results from an ongoing study. J Dent 18: 37–48

Frank M J 1990 Structural events in the caries process in enamel, cementum and dentine. J Dent Res 69 (Spec Iss): 559–566

Gibbons R J 1989 Bacterial adhesion to oral tissues: a model for infectious diseases. J Dent Res 68: 750–760

Howe L C 1989 Minimal tooth preparation techniques for restorations with adhesive materials. Dental Update 16: 418–425

Kidd E A M 1989 Root caries. Dental Update 16: 93–101

Kishimoto D, Hay D I, Gibbons R J 1989 A human salivary protein which promotes adhesion of *Streptococcus mutans* serotype c strains to hydroxyapatite. Infect and Immun 57: 3702–3707

Levine R S 1989 Saliva: 1. The nature of saliva. Dental Update 16: 102–107

Levine R S 1989 Saliva: 2. Saliva and dental caries. Dental Update 16: 158–165

Liang L, Drake D, Doyle R J 1989 Stability of the glucan-binding lectin of oral streptococci. J Dent Res 68 (Spec Iss): 1677

Mergenhagen S E et al 1987 Molecular basis of bacterial adhesion in the oral cavity. Rev Infect Dis 9 (Suppl 5): S467–475

Moller H, Schroder U 1986 Early natural subsurface caries. A SEM study of the enamel surface before and after remineralisation. Caries Res 20: 97–102

Newbrun E 1989 Frequent sugar intake—then and now: interpretation of the main results. Scand J Dent Res 97: 103–109

Roberts M W, Li S-H 1987 Oral findings in anorexia nervosa and bulimia nervosa: a study of 47 cases. JADA 115: 407–410

Rugg-Gunn A J, Hackett A F, Appleton D R 1987 Relative cariogenicity of starch and sugars in a 2-year longitudinal study of 405 English schoolchildren. Caries Res 21: 464–473

Seaman S, Thomas F D, Walker W A 1989 Differences between caries levels in 5 year old children from fluoridated Anglesea and non-fluoridated mainland Gwynedd in 1987. Community Dental Health 6: 215–221

Shaw J H 1987 Causes and control of dental caries. New Eng J Med 317: 996–1003

Shellis R P, Dibdin G H 1988 Analysis of the buffer systems in dental plaque. J Dent Res 67: 438–446

Tabak L A, Bowen W H 1989 Role of saliva (pellicle), diet and nutrition on plaque formation. J Dent Res 68 (Spec Iss): 1560–1566

4. Diseases of the dental pulp

Pulpitis is the most common cause of dental pain and loss of teeth in young people and is usually caused by caries penetrating dentine. Pulpitis, if untreated, is followed by death of the pulp and spread of infection through the apical foramina into the periapical tissues. This in turn causes periapical periodontitis.

The main causes are as follows.

1. *Dental caries.* Caries is by far the most common cause and is usually obvious unless it has extended beneath the edge of a restoration.
2. *Traumatic exposure.* Exposure during cavity preparation allows the entry of microorganisms, and there is usually also mechanical damage to the pulp.
3. *Fracture of the crown.* Fracture may either open the pulp chamber or leave so thin a covering of dentine that bacteria can enter.
4. *Cracked tooth syndrome.* A tooth, particularly a premolar, may split, usually under masticatory stress. These minute cracks are often invisible, but may allow organisms to get into the pulp chamber.
5. *Thermal damage.* Over-rapid cavity cutting, especially of deep cavities, can cause immediate damage to the pulp. Large unlined metal restorations can also cause continuous low-grade thermal stimuli which may damage the pulp over a longer period.
6. *Chemical irritation.* Some restorations,

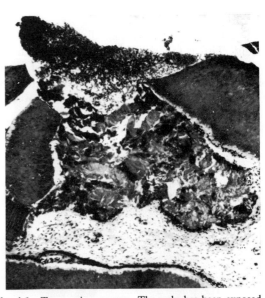

Fig. 4.1 Traumatic exposure. The pulp has been exposed during cavity preparation. Dentine chippings and larger fragments have been driven into the pulp, there is bleeding from the exposure. The tooth was extracted before an inflammatory reaction developed but it is clear that traumatic exposure causes severe injury to the pulp, and many bacteria will be introduced with the debris forced into the pulp (× 60).

particularly, in the past, silicates without a protective lining, were sufficiently irritant to kill the pulp.

When pulpitis is not a consequence of caries or of exposure, it is often the result of a combination of irritants, as described above, acting over a long period.

Pathology

The kinds of bacteria causing pulpitis are not well categorised, but in general it is likely to be a mixed infection from the mouth entering via a carious cavity or other means.

All grades of inflammation can be seen, from acute, subacute to chronic and can be localised or extend through the whole pulp. However, these changes are of variable severity and relate only to the moment when the tooth was extracted and examined. The extent of the inflammation cannot therefore be reliably correlated with symptoms.

Acute closed pulpitis

This initially consists, histologically, of hyperaemia limited to the area immediately beneath the irritant. This is followed by infiltration of the area by inflammatory cells and destruction of odontoblasts and adjacent mesenchyme. A limited area of necrosis may thus result in formation of a

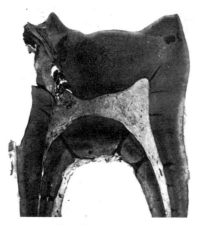

Fig. 4.2   Acute pulpitis. The dark streaks in the dentine show where bacteria have penetrated from an interstitial cavity into the pulp. Acute pulpitis has led to suppuration, and a bead of darkly stained pus fills the affected cornu (× 6).

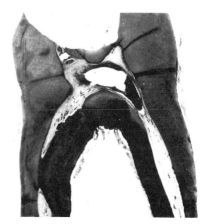

Fig. 4.3   Acute pulpitis. In this more advanced lesion, there is an exposure of the left cornu and destruction of the main body of the pulp, which has been replaced by an abscess filling the pulp chamber (× 6).

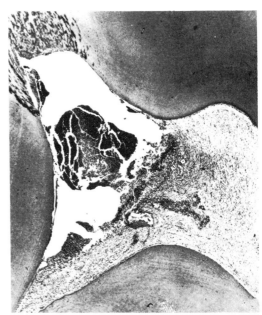

Fig. 4.4   Acute caries and pulpitis. Infection has penetrated to the pulp before any reactionary dentine has formed. Part of the pulp has been destroyed, and an abscess has formed containing a bead of pus. This is a relatively early stage and destruction is not yet widespread (× 18).

minute abscess, localised by granulation tissue formation. However, sooner or later, inflammation spreads, either with increasingly extensive necrosis or with the normal pulp obliterated by dilated blood vessels and widespread acute inflammatory infiltrate.

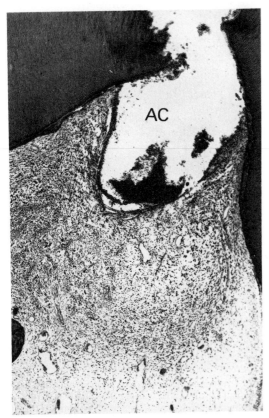

Fig. 4.5 Acute pulpitis. There is a carious exposure, destruction of a cornu of the pulp with formation of an abscess cavity (AC) and an extending inflammatory reaction. Nevertheless, immediately beyond (bottom of the picture), virtually normal pulpal tissue remains.

Chronic closed pulpitis

This is characterised by a predominantly mononuclear cell infiltrate and a more vigorous connective tissue reaction. There may be a small area of pulpal necrosis and pus formation, but localised by a well defined wall of granulation tissue, and an abscess may thus form. The remainder of the pulp may then appear normal.

Rarely, inflammation may be so well localised beneath an exposure that a partial calcific barrier forms beneath the dentine, or considerable amounts of reactionary dentine continue to form round the opening (Figs 4.8 and 4.15). Such changes are particularly likely to follow pulp capping. Calcific barriers (seen radiographically as 'dentine bridge') are frequently poorly formed, and inflammation progresses beneath them. How-

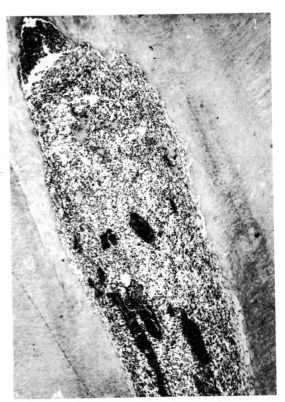

Fig. 4.6 Acute spreading pulpitis. At the coronal tip of the pulp is a bead of pus while the rest of the pulp chamber is filled with polymorphonuclear leucocytes and oedema. In the lower part of the picture are greatly dilated vessels stuffed with blood cells ($\times$ 42).

ever, in more successful cases formation of a complete barrier of tubular reactionary dentine may allow preservation of the remainder of the pulp.

Progress

The chief factor limiting pulpal responses is their enclosure within the rigid walls of the pulp chamber and, in fully formed teeth, the limited aperture for the apical vessels. In acute inflammation, the latter can readily be compressed by inflammatory oedema and thrombose. The blood supply of the pulp is thus cut off and dies. This may be rapid in the case of acute pulpitis, or delayed in chronic lesions. The relatively prolonged survival of chronically inflamed pulps is shown by the persistence of symptoms over a long period. However, pulp death is the end result.

Clinical aspects

Acute pulpitis

In the early stages the tooth is hypersensitive. Very cold or hot food causes a stab of pain but this stops as soon as the irritant is removed. As inflammation progresses, pain becomes more persistent and there may be a prolonged attack of toothache. The pain may come on spontaneously, often when the patient is trying to get to sleep.

The pain is partly due to the pressure on the irritated nerve endings by inflammatory infiltrate within the rigid pulp chamber and partly due to release of pain-producing substances from the damaged tissue. The pain at its worst is excruciatingly severe, sharp and stabbing in character. It is little affected by analgesics.

Chronic pulpitis

This may cause no symptoms. Many pulps under large carious cavities die painlessly. The first indication is then development of periapical periodontitis, either with pain or seen by chance in a radiograph. In other cases there are bouts of dull pain, brought on by hot or cold stimuli or coming on spontaneously. There are often prolonged remissions.

The pain of pulpitis is poorly localised and may be felt in any of the teeth of the upper or lower jaw of the affected side. This is because the pulps of the individual teeth are not precisely represented in the sensory cortex. Rarely, pain may be referred to a more distant site such as the ear. The pain of pulpitis is not brought on by pressure on the tooth. The patient can chew in comfort unless there is a large open cavity which allows fragments of food to press on the pulp through the softened dentine.

Diagnosis

Pulpitis is so common a cause of pain that it must be looked for in any patient complaining of pain in the region of the jaws. Pulpitis can usually be recognised from the symptoms; but to find the affected tooth is often a problem.

In practical terms:

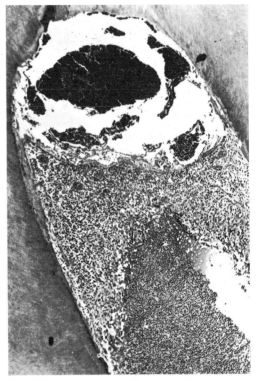

Fig. 4.7 Advanced acute pulpitis. The outline of an abscess wall is still visible beneath the collection of pus, but infection and inflammation have spread beyond; no trace of pulp structure can be seen, and the pulp chamber is filled with inflammatory cells and exudate ($\times$ 65).

1. Frequently a carious cavity indicates the source of the pain
2. Application of hot, cold, or electrical stimuli to the affected tooth should elicit pain.
3. The affected tooth may be difficult to find if there are many fillings and caries has extended under one of them.
4. Pain may be so poorly localised that it should not be assumed that the most carious or heavily restored tooth is the source.
5. When there are many heavily restored teeth, all on the affected side, including apparently sound teeth, may need to be tested.
6. Toothache following restorative treatment is likely to be the result of an exposure.
7. With fugitive pulp pain, responses to testing

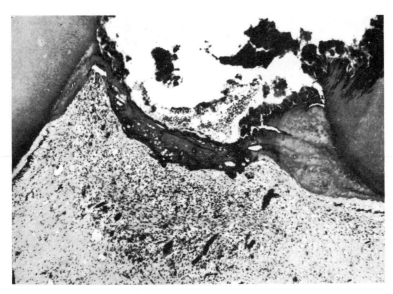

Fig. 4.8 Chronic pulpitis. Successive layers of secondary dentine have been formed and destroyed in turn; their remains are seen at the right-hand edge of the cavity. A barrier of irregular calcified tissue covers the pulp, and beneath this a localised chronic pulpitis has developed. In spite of the prolonged and massive infection there is only local inflammation, and a fibrous reaction can be seen (× 40).

    may be absent if pulp survives in only one root of a molar.

8. Cracked teeth can be particularly difficult to identify, as discussed below.
9. Tenderness to percussion or mastication may be the result of terminal pulpitis with spread of inflammation to the periapical region, but is unusual.
10. Trigeminal herpes zoster (Chapter 15) is the only extra-oral cause of pain indistinguishable from pulpitis by the patient.

Cracked tooth syndrome

Premolars, especially, may split under the force of mastication. Even an invisible hairline crack can admit bacteria and lead to pulpitis.

    The affected tooth may sometimes be identified by applying pressure to the occlusal fissure with a ball-ended burnisher to open up the crack. Pulp pain usually then results.

    Alternatively the crack may be made visible with oblique transillumination or, possibly more easily, if a source of ultraviolet light is available,

by wetting the crown of the tooth with a dye such as fluorescein.

Open pulpitis

Occasionally the pulp survives beneath a wide exposure, despite the heavy infection, and the

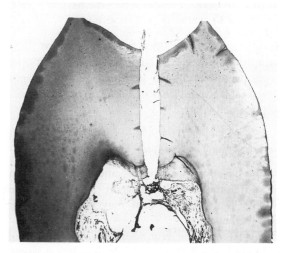

Fig. 4.9 Cracked tooth syndrome. The pulp has died beneath this crack which was undetected clinically.

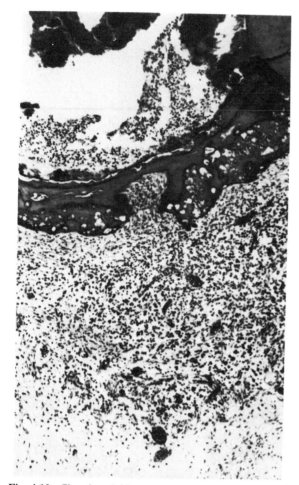

Fig. 4.10 Chronic pulpitis. This higher power view shows the calcific barrier in more detail; in particular its irregular structure and failure to hold back the infection.

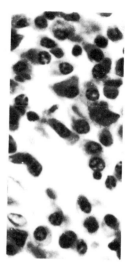

Fig. 4.11 Plasma cells. The characteristic eccentric nucleus, with irregularly arranged chromatin, and darkly staining cytoplasm can be seen. These cells are important in antibody production and are often the predominant cell in pulpitis and other dental infections ($\times$ 700).

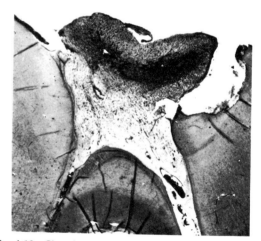

Fig. 4.12 Chronic open pulpitis. A hyperplastic nodule of granulation tissue is growing out through a wide exposure of the pulp. The masses of inflammatory cells and the many new vessels are characteristic of granulation tissue ($\times$ 9).

condition of chronic open pulpitis develops. This is traditionally believed to be associated with open apices which allow an adequate blood supply. However, open pulpitis is also seen in teeth with fully formed roots.

Chronic hyperplastic pulpitis (pulp polyp)

Rarely, despite wide exposure and heavy infection, the pulp not merely survives but proliferates through the opening. This may even happen in fully formed teeth.

In this condition few odontoblasts survive and the pulp becomes replaced by granulation tissue. As this mass grows out into the cavity in the tooth it can become epithelialised and covered by a layer of well-formed stratified squamous epithelium. This protects the mass and allows inflammation under it to subside and fibrous tissue to replace the granulation tissue.

Clinically, a pulp polyp appears as a dusky red or pinkish soft nodule protruding into the cavity.

It is painless but may be tender and bleed on probing. It should be distinguished from proliferating gingival tissue (a gingival polyp; Fig. 16.26) extending over the edge of the cavity, by tracing its attachment.

Treatment. Open pulpitis is usually associated with gross cavity formation and it is rarely possible to save the tooth, despite the vitality of the pulp.

Management

Because of the poor chances of survival of the pulp the main lines of treatment are:

1. Extraction.
2. Extirpation of the pulp and root canal filling.
3. Pulp capping

The simplest, quickest, most certain (but most destructive) way of dealing with painful pulpitis is to extract the tooth. Extraction may be the best form of treatment for reasons considered later (Ch. 9).

Pulpectomy and root canal treatment

When necessary the pulp can be extirpated and, provided that all necrotic tissue is removed and the root canal effectively sealed, the tooth remains

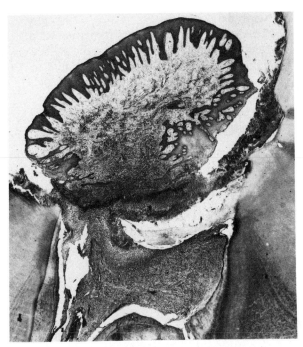

Fig. 4.14 Pulp polyp. A higher power view shows the fibrous nodule, its epithelial covering and its connection with the inflamed pulp beneath.

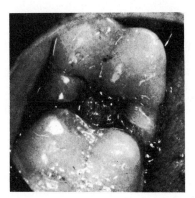

Fig. 4.15 Polyp of the pulp. A pink nodule of soft tissue fills the large carious cavity.

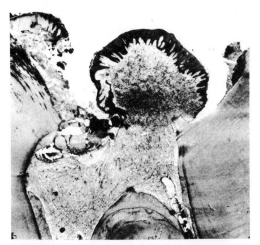

Fig. 4.13 Polyp of the pulp. A section showing the pulpal tissue proliferating through a wide carious exposure. The connective tissue has acquired a covering of stratified squamous epithelium, and the chronic inflammatory changes are less severe than in the raw granulation tissue of Fig. 4.12 ($\times$ 14).

attached by living cementum. A devitalised tooth can thus remain functional for the rest of the life of the dentition or the patient.

Provided that the periodontal condition justifies it, endodontic treatment is indicated for

1. Exposure of the pulp
2. Pulpitis or death of the pulp from any other cause

3. Apical periodontitis
4. Prevention of apical abscess formation on a deciduous molar and damage to the successor.
5. Maintenance of an intact arch in a child to allow space for the permanent teeth
6. To avoid extractions in a haemophiliac. However, great care must be taken not to damage the apical vessels.

Since apical periodontitis is usually secondary to infection in the root canal, effective débridement and sealing of the latter allows apical infection to resolve. Acute periodontitis can frequently be treated by opening the root canal through the crown and allowing exudate to drain. When the acute inflammation has subsided, the root canal can be filled.

Contraindications

Root canal treatment is unlikely to be worthwhile in the following circumstances

1. The mouth is generally neglected and the functional life of the dentition is likely to be short
2. Advanced periodontitis with deep pocketing
3. Roots so deformed or blocked by calcification that instrumentation is impossible.

Root canal treatment is also made difficult or may be unsuccessful if

1. Access is poor, i.e. posterior molars when opening of the mouth is limited
2. The tooth is incompletely formed and the apices are still open. In this case, preservation of the pulp by capping may allow development to continue until the apices have closed
3. Some types of fractures of the teeth (Ch. 5).

Principles of root canal treatment

Successful root canal treatment depends on

1. Aseptic technique
2. Complete mechanical débridement of infected pulp tissue and reaming away infected dentine. Access must therefore be adequate,

and the reamers must be able to cope with any curvature of the canal
3. Completely watertight filling and sealing of the canal
4. Avoidance of damage to the periapical tissues by overextension of the root canal filling material or use of irritant antiseptics in the preparation.

Though it was at one time believed that antiseptics or antibiotic preparations were important in the preparation of the root canal for filling, they are of no value if mechanical preparation is inadequate. Successful filling of curved root canals depends on the use of flexible instruments that will mechanically remove the infected tissue.

Complications of root canal treatment

If teeth are properly selected, root canal treatment, in competent hands, should be successful in over 80% of cases. Nevertheless the chief complication of root canal treatment is apical periodontitis (acute or chronic) due to

1. Poor preparation or sealing of the canal
2. Bacteria or irritant chemicals such as paraformaldehyde, forced through the apex
3. Extension of the filling through the apex
4. Inaccessible branches of the root canal or an apical delta
5. An instrument irretrievably broken in the canal.

In some of these cases, it may be possible to save the tooth by apicectomy (Ch. 5).

The usual practice after preparation of the root canal is to obtund the canal with a point of gutta-percha or other material in a dressing paste to fill any voids. The composition of these pastes ranges from zinc oxide in engenol to complex mixtures containing antibiotics or corticosteroids or both, or may consist of a plastic (2 hydroxyethyl methacrylate) which expands on polymerisation. The varied nature of these preparations suggests that no fully satisfactory one has been formulated or that they are used in an attempt to make up for faulty technique.

Discolouration of the crown. Discolouration of the crown can result from death of the pulp and breakdown of blood products which have leaked into the tubules. However, it may not appear until after the root has been filled. It may be possible to bleach away this stain, or it may be necessary to disguise it with a veneer.

Pulp capping

An exposed vital pulp can sometimes be preserved by capping when conventional endodontic treatment is impractical and the main indications are similar: namely, to preserve

1. A deciduous tooth to maintain the space long enough for the successor to erupt
2. 1st and 2nd permanent molars in a child to enable normal development of the jaw and occlusion
3. Deciduous molars to forestall apical abscess formation and damage to successors
4. Anterior teeth with open apices to allow normal development of the root. Conventional endodontic treatment can, if necessary, be carried out after the apices have fully formed.
5. Teeth and to avoid extractions in a haemophiliac child
6. Occasionally in an adult if preservation of the tooth is vital but endodontic treatment is impractical.

Success in pulp capping depends particularly on

1. The exposure being little more than pinpoint in size
2. Minimal trauma to, and infection of, the pulp, i.e. absence of symptoms. In the case of a potential carious exposure, indirect capping is preferable
3. Aseptic technique
4. The age of the patient—the younger the patient the greater the chance of success
5. A pulp dressing that will promote healing. Calcium hydroxide preparations are usually the most satisfactory.

An acutely inflamed pulp can be capped with a corticosteroid–antibiotic-containing pulp dressing. This usually gives rapid relief from pain but the pulp usually dies as a result of corticosteroid-induced ischaemia.

Indirect pulp capping

This refers to the placing of rapidly hardening protective dressing, usually a calcium hydroxide preparation, in the depths of a carious cavity instead of removing all softened dentine and exposing the pulp. This procedure is justified because, as pointed out in the previous chapter, decalcification precedes infection of the dentine. Calcium hydroxide appears to promote recalcification of the underlying dentine. However, experimentally, the chances of survival of the pulp depend more on the amount of existing or introduced infection than on the nature of the dressing.

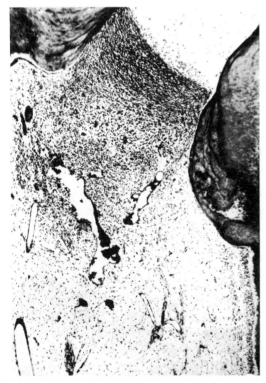

Fig. 4.16 Pulp capping. A wide exposure has been capped. Reactionary dentine production has continued, forming rounded masses extending across from either side and narrowing the exposure. A localised chronic inflammatory reaction has developed on the surface of the pulp, but the amount of secondary dentine formation indicates that vitality has been retained for a long period. The exposure appears to have been too wide for successful capping, and the material used is unknown ($\times$ 40).

After pulp capping, follow-up is essential to ensure that

1. the vitality of the pulp is undiminished
2. the periapical tissues remain radiographically normal
3. the root forms normally in the case of teeth with open apices.

Summary

1. Pulpitis is caused by infection or irritation of the pulp, usually by caries.
2. Pulpitis is the most common cause of dental pain and should be looked for in any dentate patient complaining of pain.
3. Severe stabbing pain in a tooth, brought on by hot or cold food or starting spontaneously, indicates acute irreversible pulpitis. Chronic pulpitis is often without symptoms.
4. The pulp appears to have considerable powers of repair, but untreated pulpitis leads ultimately to death of the pulp and spread of infection to the periapical tissue.
5. The treatment of pulpitis in an anterior tooth is usually by extirpation of the pulp and root canal treatment or, sometimes, extraction of the tooth. The treatment of pulpitis in a posterior tooth is usually by extraction of the tooth or, less often, root canal treatment.
6. Capping or partial amputation of the pulp can be used for 'clean' exposures of a healthy pulp, especially in teeth with open apices.

EFFECTS OF RESTORATIVE PROCEDURES ON THE PULP

The final state of the pulp after restoration is the summation of the effects of caries, cavity preparation and the filling material. The effect of caries (if not too acute) is to cause the pulp to protect itself by forming barriers between itself and the infection, but adequate preparation of a cavity necessitates the cutting of adjacent healthy dentine, the tubules of which may be widely patent. The pulp is more easily injured through normal dentine and in extreme cases, such as the prepara-tion for a jacket crown, the tubules of the crown may be severed.

Cavity preparation

The cutting of dentine during cavity preparation damages the odontoblast processes and may generate enough heat to injure the pulp. However, if cavities are cut abnormally slowly or the bur is cooled with a water spray, no significant reaction is found in the pulp. By contrast, a temperature of 600°C applied to the floor of a cavity for 10 seconds causes extensive destruction of pulp tissues and blisters of oedema. Higher temperatures or longer application cause correspondingly severe damage or death of the pulp. Burs running at anything up to 400 000 r/min inevitably cause great heat production.

In the absence of effective cooling, excessive heat production and the severity of pulp damage during cavity preparation is related to

1. The rate of cutting
2. The amount of pressure on the instrument
3. The size of the bur or stone
4. The size and duration of the preparation
5. The depth of the cavity
6. The size of the pulp or thickness of reactionary dentine.

All of these can be prevented by water spray cooling of the bur, and damage can be further limited by reducing the amount of tooth tissue removed. However, additional causes of pulp damage during restorative procedures are:

1. Blasts of air which dehydrate the tubules
2. Dehydrating or irritant chemicals used in 'cavity toilet'
3. Irritant filling materials
4. Infection resulting from leakage round the filling.

Histologically, these procedures can lead to

1. Aspiration of odontoblasts into the tubules as a result of dehydration
2. Disorganisation of the odontoblast layer
3. Oedema of the odontoblast layer (sometimes with 'wheatsheafing' of odontoblasts)

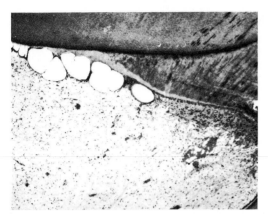

Fig. 4.17 Oedema of the pulp. Beads of fluid have formed among the odontoblasts under a cavity. To the right, pioneer organisms of caries are extending along the dentinal tubules towards the pulp (× 30).

4. Death of odontoblasts and dead tract formation
5. Pulpitis
6. Pulp death.

Effects of restorative materials on the pulp

Experimental testing of the effects of filling materials on the pulp has shown that with several materials previously regarded as being irritant, inflammation was often caused by microleakage of bacteria rather than by the material itself. To show this it was necessary to use germ-free animals because small numbers of bacteria, leaking past fillings, are usually undetectable by routine histology. Such experiments have also shown that considerable trauma to the pulp also causes no significant inflammation.

In practice therefore, in addition to precautions against damaging the pulp during cavity preparation, it is important to seal the floor of cavities with a material which will exclude infection.

Cellular responses of the pulp to dental materials

The pulp can only show a limited repertoire of responses to restorative materials. These responses can be summarised as follows

1. No response
2. Odontoblast displacement or damage
3. Inflammation, either acute or chronic
4. Necrosis as an initial reaction, or preceded by inflammation
5. Calcific change ('dentine bridging')
6. Dentine formation.

New restorative materials are constantly being introduced with alleged or real advantages, and by no means all of them have been extensively tested. However, the main findings with the more important restorative materials are as follows.

Zinc oxide and eugenol in a deep cavity or in direct contact with the pulp (contrary to earlier beliefs) causes persistent inflammation, but, as a cavity liner, it forms an effective bacteria-proof sealant. EBA cements are better tolerated by the pulp.

Calcium hydroxide has a pH of 11 but is well tolerated by an uninfected pulp. Calcium hydroxide in water can be used as a cavity liner or pulp dressing and will promote remineralisation of the floor of deep cavities or promote dentine bridge formation in exposed pulps.

The limitation of calcium hydroxide is that it does not form a bacteria-proof seal. This seal may be better with proprietary preparations but the response of the pulp may be affected by the vehicle. In one such preparation the calcium hydroxide was found to be effectively bound to the other components and biologically inactive.

Zinc polycarboxylate cement has a pH of about 5 when set. Though strongly adhesive, it appears not to form a good seal. It is not irritant as a cavity liner but may cause inflammation and necrosis when in direct contact with the pulp.

Zinc phosphate cement typically consists of zinc and magnesium oxides which, when freshly mixed with phosphoric acid and placed in the cavity, has a pH of 2 and may damage the pulp, but it is nearly neutral when set. It reportedly causes mild to severe inflammation of the pulp, but it is not clear whether this is caused by bacteria or by the material's acidity.

Despite its apparent limitations, zinc phosphate cement remains the most satisfactory luting material for inlays.

Silicophosphate and silicate cements are largely or entirely obsolete because of their tendency to cause pulpitis. Silicates must have an effective lining such as calcium hydroxide or zinc polycarboxylate but then can have a useful life of up to 20 years. Advantages are that they have a coefficient of expansion similar to that of enamel and recurrent caries at their margins is rare. They appear to be coming back into use in the USA, but acid production due to poor plaque control limits their durability.

Composite resins are dimethacrylates based on bis-GMA resin or one of its derivatives, with a filler such as quartz or borosilicate glass.

In deep cavities, composites can cause pulpitis but it is not clear whether the material allows microleakage as a result of shrinkage (their coefficient of expansion is approximately three times that of enamel) or is irritant in itself. These resins are not truly adhesive but flow into microscopic interstices of the dental tissues; bonding can therefore be improved by acid etching the enamel walls. Acid etching of dentine should be avoided as causing increased permeability of the tubules and possible irritation of the pulp. Protective linings are therefore necessary under composites.

Glass ionomer cements consist of an aluminosilicate glass mixed with polyacrylic and related acids. The set material consists of glass particles in a matrix of polyacrylate.

Glass ionomers have an enamel-like translucency and are adhesive to tooth tissues and metal fillings. However, in spite of these apparent advantages, bacteria have been reported between these materials and the cavity floor. Experimentally also, they cause inflammation when in contact with the pulp. Glass ionomers therefore require a lining such as calcium hydroxide, in deep cavities. Another disadvantage is that they are brittle.

Cermets are metal-filled glass ionomers which should resist wear better and are radiopaque. Their effects on the pulp are unlikely to be different from those of unfilled glass ionomers.

Fluorides may be present in various cements and be released into the tooth. Fluorides have also been applied to cavity floors with the aim of enhancing remineralisation of carious dentine and preventing recurrence of caries at the margins.

4% sodium fluoride appears to be well tolerated even when the dentine floor is very thin. By contrast 8% stannous fluoride (pH 2.6) applied for 5 minutes can cause pulpitis and necrosis. Fluorides have been incorporated with calcium hydroxide in pulp-capping materials and are well tolerated. However, it is likely that most of the fluoride is bound to the calcium hydroxide.

Amalgam has such high thermal conductivity that a lining is mandatory in all but the shallowest cavities. In deeper cavities, if thermal irritation is not too severe, unlined amalgams provoke reactionary dentine formation.

Histologically, amalgam accidentally embedded in the tissues (amalgam tattoos—Ch. 16) frequently causes no reaction. Experimentally also, mercury when in contact with the pulp provokes minimal reaction and may stimulate calcific repair.

Modern amalgams shrink little on setting and have a lower coefficient of expansion than composites, but do not bond to tooth substance. However, they form satisfactory filling material apparently because sulphide and other corrosion products with saliva form an effective seal at their margins.

Possible systemic effects of mercury in amalgams are discussed in Chapter 25.

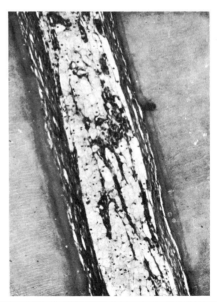

Fig. 4.18 Fatty change. Cells filled with granular, fatty material have replaced most of the normal pulp. The rest of the pulp, just beneath the dentine, has been replaced by fibrous tissue (× 40).

Regressive changes in the pulp

Several types of degenerative change have been described in the pulp. They are mostly accidental findings in extracted teeth, and their clinical importance is negligible.

They include the following.

1. *Wheat-sheafing and blistering of the odontoblast layer*. This change is an early response to irritation and follows traumatic cavity preparation and irritant filling materials. The appearance is due to fluid exudate between the cells; these are pushed aside and become bunched together. The oedema is due to increased permeability of the capillaries, a common response to irritation. Exudate in the pulp may be quickly followed by the appearance of inflammatory cells.
2. *Fatty change*
3. *Fibrous replacement*
4. *'Reticular degeneration'*. These appearances are an artefact produced by poor fixation.

Calcification within the pulp

Pulp stones. These may form rounded nodules, or large masses that almost fill the pulp chamber. They are of lamellated structure and may contain a few irregular tubules or be hyaline in appearance. Pulp stones may be found in any teeth, deciduous or permanent, unerupted or functioning. The larger specimens may be seen in radiographs of adult teeth. They are of no clinical significance unless they interfere with root canal treatment.

Diffuse calcification. Deposits of granular calcific material scattered along the fibres of the pulp are a common finding. They are most frequent in the root canals but may extend up into the coronal pulp or may form large masses. These calcifications stain purple with haematoxylin in decalcified sections. They are possibly an age change, a result of gradual ischaemia of the pulp.

Internal resorption: 'Pink Spot'. In this rare condition, osteoclastic activity in the pulp results in localised resorption of overlying dentine (Ch. 5).

Footnote

It is not of course of the slightest importance, but an excess of pulp stones is a characteristic of Ehlers–Danlos syndrome,

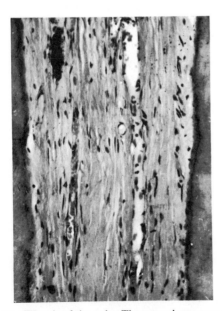

Fig. 4.19 Fibrosis of the pulp. The normal structure of the pulp have been entirely replaced by longitudinally arranged bundles of collagenous fibrous tissue (× 60).

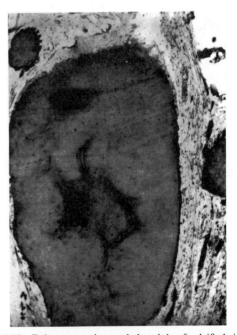

Fig. 4.20 Pulp stones. A rounded nodule of calcified tissue in which some irregular tubules may be seen. Smaller stones and amorphous calcifications surround the main mass (× 40).

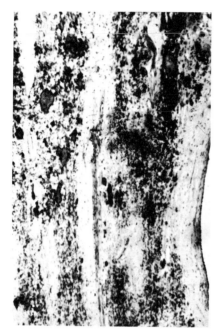

Fig. 4.21 Calcifications in the pulp. Granular deposits of amorphous calcified material lie along the line of the blood-vessels in the root canal. Larger masses are forming by fusion of smaller deposit (× 40).

where the main and most obvious abnormality is laxity of the connective tissues. This connective tissue abnormality can be—and often is—exploited to allow people with this syndrome to become contortionists.

In the unlikely event that anyone should become interested in pulp stones, these are therefore the people who might be investigated. On the other hand, one cannot easily imagine that fairground and circus workers would prove very sympathetic to research of this sort.

It is puzzling, however, that something so trifling as pulp stones may not be merely local phenomena but should have these genetic and metabolic connotations, and odd that pulp stones should have this special association with a somewhat bizarre occupation.

SUGGESTED FURTHER READING

Cawson R A 1987 Oral pathology—colour aids in dentistry. Churchill Livingstone, Edinburgh

Cawson R A, Eveson J W 1987 Oral pathology and diagnosis. William Heinemann Medical Books, London and Gower Medical Publishing, London

Cunnington S A 1990 An update on endodontics: 1. endodontic diagnosis and preparation. Dental Update 15: 95–1023

Eriksen H M, Buonocore M G 1976 Marginal leakage with different composite restorative materials: effect of restorative techniques. J Am Dent Assoc 93: 1143–1148

Harty F J 1990 Endodontics in clinical practice, 3rd edn. Wright, Bristol

Heys D R et al 1980 The response of four calcium hydroxides on monkey pulps. J Oral Pathol 9: 372–379

Negm M M, Combe E C, Grant A A 1981 Reaction of the exposed pulps to new cements containing calcium hydroxide. Oral Surg, Oral Med, Oral Pathol 51: 190–204

Paterson R C 1981 Pulp response in sound and carious teeth: a pilot study. Oral Surg, Oral Med, Oral Pathol 51: 209–212

Paterson R C, Watts A 1981 Caries, bacteria, the pulp and plastic restorations. Br Dent J 151: 54–58

Rölling I, Hasselgren G, Tronstad L 1976 Morphologic and enzyme histochemical observations on the pulp of human primary molars 3 to 5 years after formocresol treatment. Oral Surg, Oral Med, Oral Pathol 42: 518–528

Smith B G N, Wright P S, Brown D 1986 The clinical handling of dental materials. Wright (IOP Publishing Ltd), Bristol

Watts A, Paterson R C 1981 Cellular responses in the dental pulp: a review. Int Endodontic J 14: 10–21

5. Apical periodontitis, resorption, hypercementosis and acute injuries to the teeth

Periapical inflammation is usually due to spread of infection following death of the pulp. The characteristic symptom is tenderness of the tooth in its socket.

In most cases inflammation remains localised. Further spread of infection can cause inflammation of the surrounding bone (osteomyelitis) or cellulitis but only exceedingly rarely.

Local (periapical) periodontitis must be distinguished from chronic (marginal) periodontitis, in which infection and destruction of the supporting tissues spread from chronic infection of the gingival margins (Ch. 6).

The main causes of apical periodontitis are as follows.

1. *Infection* is by far the most common cause. The usual sequence of event is caries, pulpitis, death of the pulp and periodontitis.
2. *Trauma.* The pulp sometimes dies from a blow which damages the apical vessels. The necrotic pulp probably becomes infected by bacteria from the gingival margins, leading to apical periodontitis.

A high filling, or biting suddenly on a hard object, sometimes cause an acute but usually transient periodontitis.

During root canal treatment, instruments may be pushed through the apex or side of the root, damaging the periodontal membrane and carrying infected debris from the pulp chamber into the wound.

3. *Chemical irritation.* Irritant antiseptics used to sterilise a root canal can escape through the apex and damage the surrounding tissues. A root-canal filling may also extend beyond the apex with similar effect.

Progress of virulent infections

Occasionally more virulent organisms reach the periapical region. The inevitable consequence is acute inflammation and abscess formation, but pressure is soon relieved and spread of infection prevented by resorption of the thin overlying bone (usually the buccal plate). Partial drainage is established and, with rare exceptions, once the soft tissues are reached, infection remains localised.

Unusually virulent infections can cause osteomyelitis or cellulitis (Ch. 18).

Healing of periapical lesions

Though chronic lesions are often virtually symptomless and infection is of low pathogenicity, there is no spontaneous healing of periapical periodontitis because of the persistent reservoir of infection in the root canal. Healing only follows extraction or effective root canal treatment.

Cyst formation

Proliferation of the epithelial rests of Malassez in the periodontal membrane is characteristic of chronic apical periodontitis. Epithelial activity may be sufficient to lead ultimately to cyst formation and this is the most common cause of cysts in the jaws.

ACUTE APICAL PERIODONTITIS

The periapical region is the usual site, but occasionally infection reaches the periodontal ligament through the side of a tooth if there is a lateral root canal or if penetrated by an instrument during root canal therapy.

Clinical features

The patient may give a history of pain due to previous pulpitis. When periodontitis develops, escape of exudate into the periodontal membrane causes the tooth to be extruded by a minute amount and the bite to fall more heavily on it. The tooth is at first uncomfortable, then increasingly tender. Hot or cold substances do not cause pain in the tooth. As inflammation becomes more severe and pus starts to form, pain becomes intense and throbbing in character.

On examination, there is often a large carious cavity or filling in the affected tooth, or it may be

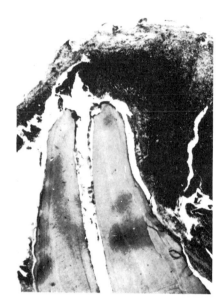

Fig. 5.1 Acute local periodontitis. The section shows the massive collection of inflammatory cells, mainly polymorphonuclear leucocytes, at the apex of a dead and infected tooth (× 15).

discoloured due to death of the pulp some time previously. The characteristic sign is tenderness of the tooth to percussion, or even to touch. At this stage the gum over the root is red and tender, but there is no swelling while inflammation is confined within the bone.

The overlying bone and periosteum may be penetrated by exudate a day or so after the onset of pain; pressure is then relieved. Pain is quickly reduced but exudate distends the soft tissues to form a swelling. When an upper canine is affected, the swelling quickly spreads to the eyelid and may close the eye on that side. In spite of the alarming appearance, the swelling is due only to oedema. It subsides when the tooth is extracted or the periapical infection is drained.

The regional lymph nodes may be enlarged and tender; there may occasionally be a degree or two of fever and a little malaise, but general symptoms are usually slight or absent.

Radiographs give little information because bony changes have had too short a time to develop. Immediately round the apex the lamina dura may appear slightly hazy and the periodontal

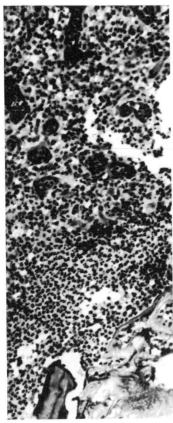

Fig. 5.2 Acute local periodontitis. A section at higher magnification showing the tip of the apex and necrotic debris, surrounded by polymorphonuclear leucocytes and dilated vessels filled with inflammatory cells (× 80).

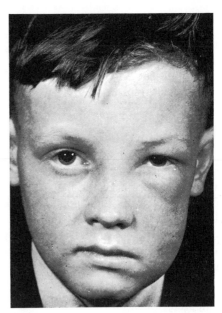

Fig. 5.3 Oedema due to acute periodontitis. An acute periapical infection of a canine has perforated the buccal plate of bone causing oedema of the face; this quickly subsided when the tooth was extracted.

space may be slightly increased. In cases where acute periodontitis is due to exacerbation of a chronic infection, the original lesion can be seen as an area of radiolucency at the apex.

Treatment

Extraction of the diseased tooth removes the source of infection and drains the exudate. This is the simplest and most effective treatment, and antibiotics should not be given for simple acute periodontitis if immediate dental treatment is available. Alternative treatment is to retain the tooth by root canal treatment, which also serves to drain the infection.

Root canal treatment for acute periodontitis

In the presence of acute periodontitis, local infiltration of a local anaesthetic is contraindicated and ineffective. Anterior teeth can usually be opened without anaesthesia by careful handling: namely, by supporting the tooth and using a diamond bur in an air-turbine handpiece. Once the canal has been opened the necrotic pulp remnants can be removed with care not to push infected material through the apex. The root canal is irrigated with 1% sodium hypochlorite, dried and a sterile paper point sealed into the canal to absorb inflammatory exudate. The opposing tooth should be ground to relieve biting on the tender tooth, and an analgesic given. In most cases symptoms subside within 24 hours; once this has happened, root canal treatment can be carried out in the normal way.

In the most severe cases where a periapical abscess has formed, longer drainage may be necessary. The root canal is opened as before and left open to allow exudate to drain. The patient must be careful not to let the root canal become blocked by food debris.

CHRONIC APICAL PERIODONTITIS

Chronic periodontitis is usually a mild infection causing little or no symptoms; it may follow an acute infection that has been inadequately drained and incompletely resolved.

Pathology

Chronic periodontitis is a typical chronic inflammatory reaction characterised by the presence of lymphocytes, macrophages and plasma cells. Infection is confined by inflammatory cells, and granulation tissue surrounds the area. The granulation tissue grows into a rounded mass, (a 'granuloma'), and osteoclasts resorb the bone to accommodate it.

Epithelial proliferation

A characteristic feature of apical granulomas is the epithelial proliferation of the rests of Malassez, forming irregular strands or loops. Sometimes a microscopic cyst cavity, with a lining of hyperplastic epithelium, forms and represents the earliest stage of a periodontal (radicular) cyst. In other cases the epithelium is scanty or destroyed by the inflammation.

Abscess formation

Polymorphonuclear leucocytes migrate into the area until it is densely packed; the dead cells liquefy and pus may reach the surface by resorption of the bone (usually on the buccal surface of the gum) immediately over the apex of the tooth. A nodule of granulation tissue forms in response to the irritation by pus and marks the opening of the sinus.

Clinical features

Frequently there are no symptoms and the lesion is found by chance on a radiograph. In other cases there is mild and intermittent pain. The tooth is slightly tender to percussion and the gum tender to pressure over the apex. If pus is forming, there may be a reddish, localised swelling on the buccal gum or a sinus where pus has reached the

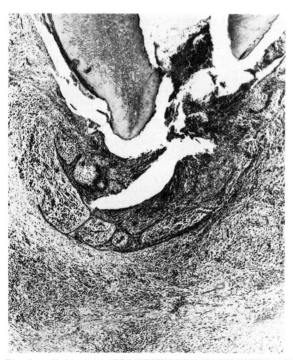

Fig. 5.4 Epithelial proliferation in a periapical granuloma. A network of hyperplastic epithelium surrounded by chronic inflammatory cells and proliferating connective tissues is seen at the apex of a dead and infected tooth (× 44).

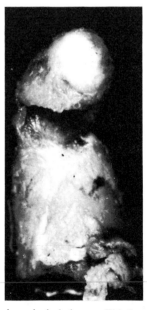

Fig. 5.5 Chronic periapical abscess. This has been removed intact; the fibrous sac being firmly attached to the tooth.

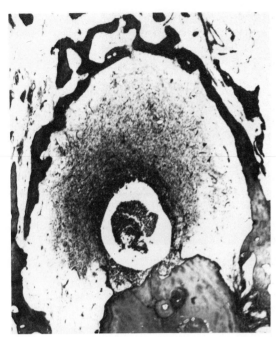

Fig. 5.6 Chronic periapical abscess. At the apex of the affected tooth is a minute abscess cavity surrounded by a thick fibrous wall (granuloma). Periapical bone has been resorbed and the trabeculae re-oriented around the mass.

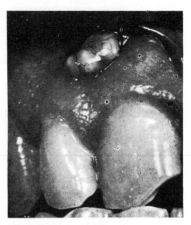

Fig. 5.8 Chronic local periodontitis. The pulp of the central incisor has died as a result of a blow some time previously, as indicated by the chipped incisal edge. There is a chronic periapical infection and formation of an abscess pointing on the buccal surface over the apex producing a pus-filled nodule.

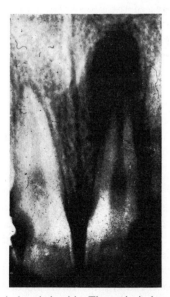

Fig. 5.7 Apical periodontitis. The periapical area of radiolucency corresponds with the changes shown in the previous picture.

surface. The pulp of the tooth is of course dead and does not respond to vitality tests.

In a radiograph, chronic local periodontitis is seen as an area of radiolucency due to bone resorption round the granuloma. The area is usually about 5 mm in diameter and has fairly well-defined margins. A sharply defined outline may suggest that a cyst is forming, but this cannot be distinguished without a biopsy.

Treatment

The treatment of chronic periodontitis is by extraction or root canal treatment which, if competent, also leads to healing even if cystic change has started. Persistence of chronic periodontitis after root canal treatment is usually due to technical faults, and apicectomy may be required.

Apicectomy

Persistent periapical periodontitis in spite of treatment is usually the result of failure to fill or seal the root canal effectively. Indications for apicectomy may include the following:

1. An apical delta, lateral branches, or perforations of the wall

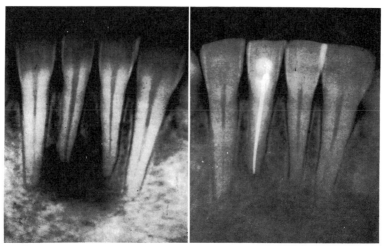

Fig. 5.9 Treatment of local periodontitis by root canal therapy. There is a considerable area of radiolucency with ill-defined margins round the apex of the affected tooth, which has also undergone resorption. Further up the root there has been some hypercementosis, giving the root a slightly irregular shape.

The root canal has been widened and straightened to remove infected material, and accurately filled. As a result, after some months, the periapical lesion has healed and the normal trabecular pattern of the bone has been restored.

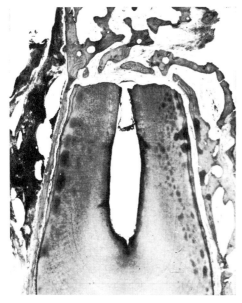

Fig. 5.10 Apicectomy. The infected tip of the apex has been excised; the periapical tissues have entirely healed; inflammatory changes have disappeared; new bone trabeculae have replaced the tissue lost and a scar has formed over the end of the root canal filling (× 10).

2. Severe curvature or dilaceration
3. Obstructions such as calcification or fragment of an instrument
4. Overfilling of the root canal, with a symptomatic reaction
5. Inadequate root filling associated with an irremovable post crown
6. Fractured apical third of a root, if there are indications for its removal.
7. Open apices that have not responded to treatment
8. Persistent symptoms despite apparently satisfactory root filling.

In essence, apicectomy, which is usually carried out under local anaesthesia, comprises raising a mucoperiosteal flap over the affected area and removing sufficient bone to get good access to the apex. The latter is then resected and the root filling modified as necessary.

In spite of the number of possible indications, apicectomy is remarkably rarely needed unless the operator is unusually incompetent at root canal treatment.

Skin sinuses

An occasional complication of periapical periodontitis is the tracking of a sinus onto the skin surface. This most frequently happens on or near the chin as a result of a long-forgotten blow and death of a lower incisor. In these circumstances the crown of the damaged tooth may be chipped and is usually discoloured. A radiograph shows the periapical area of bone destruction.

Many patients fail to associate the sinus with dental infection and consult a doctor. The result can be prolonged but ineffective dermatological treatment. Effective root canal treatment causes the sinus to heal remarkably quickly.

RESORPTION OF TEETH

The deciduous teeth are progressively loosened and ultimately shed as a result of progressive resorption of the roots as a physiological process arising from the pressure of the underlying successors.

Resorption of permanent teeth is always pathological. Whenever resorption takes place, there is virtually always some attempt at repair by apposition of cementum or bone. In the case of

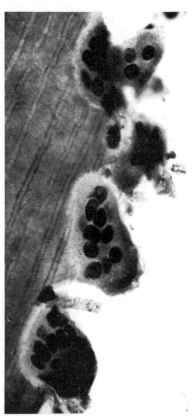

Fig. 5.12 Resorption of dentine. The process is active and osteoclasts can be seen with the cytoplasm sometimes appearing to be merging into the tissue ($\times$ 500).

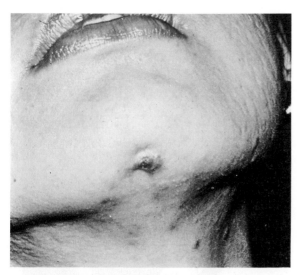

Fig. 5.11 A persistent skin sinus from a lower incisor killed by a blow some time previously. This young woman was seen and treated unsuccessfully for two years by her doctor, surgeons and dermatologists before anyone looked at her teeth.

buried teeth, for example, the processes tend to alternate, though to an unequal extent. During resorption of the deciduous teeth a period of resorption is followed by one of repair, so that clinically the looseness of these teeth varies before they are shed.

Resorption is rarely of serious significance except very occasionally as an indication of some destructive process such as a tumour. Hypercementosis is also rarely of importance but may occasionally be a cause of difficult extractions.

Mechanism of resorption

The most important factor seems to be the effect of pressure. However, in some cases no cause is apparent. Resorption is mainly carried out by osteoclasts which, during the active phases of the process, can be seen lying in lacunae in the hard

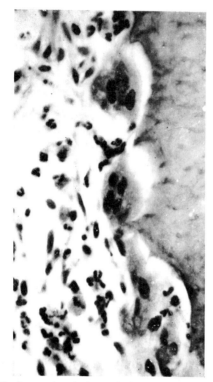

Fig. 5.13 Resorption during periapical periodontitis. Active osteoclastic resorption of dentine is going on in the presence of inflammatory exudate. This is a common change but usually minor in extent (× 500).

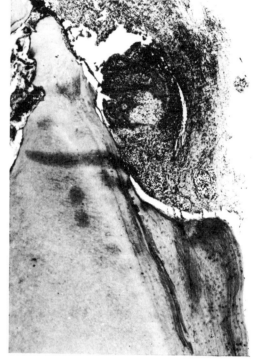

Fig. 5.14 Periodontitis. The shape of the apex (top left) is irregular due to resorption in the main area of inflammation; further away (lower right) layers of cementum have been deposited.

tissue with which their cytoplasm appears to merge. When resorption is very slow, osteoclasts may not be seen and, being intermittent in their action, disappear during inactive periods. It is also apparent that bone at least can be resorbed by the action of humoral factors, particularly prostaglandins.

Resorption of deciduous teeth

Resorption of deciduous teeth occasionally leads to a few minor complications such as the following.

1. *Ankylosis*. In the resting stages of resorption excessive repair tissue may be deposited until the root becomes fused to the adjacent bone. This may prevent the tooth from being shed and the permanent successor from erupting. If not removed the ankylosed tooth becomes partially submerged by the continued growth

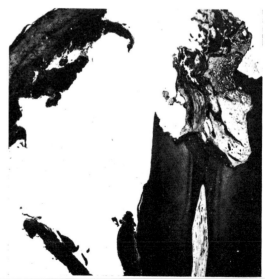

Fig. 5.15 Resorption in a dentigerous cyst. The patient was elderly and there were inflammatory episodes in the cyst. This may account for the unusual degree of resorption destroying the whole of the crown of the tooth (× 10).

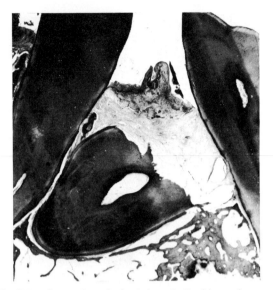

Fig. 5.16 Resorption of a buried tooth. In this specimen from an elderly patient, a buried canine has undergone complete resorption of the crown during the course of many years. Fragments of enamel remaining can be seen as spaces in the connective tissue against the root of the lateral. Inflammatory changes are absent (× 5).

of the surrounding alveolar ridge. The tooth should be removed, surgically if necessary, to allow the successor to erupt.

2. *Separation of an apex.* Resorption may be irregular so that part of the tooth is cut off. The fragment remains buried or eventually appears on the surface.
3. *Failure of resorption.* This is usually the result of absence or misplacement of a permanent successor. The deciduous tooth in these cases may remain in the arch for many years.

Resorption of permanent teeth

Permanent teeth can be resorbed by the same mechanism as that affecting deciduous teeth but only as a result of some pathological stimulus. Resorption is usually limited in extent, but may on rare occasions destroy a large part of a tooth. Causes of resorption of permanent teeth include the following.

1. *Periapical periodontitis.* This is by far the most common cause but is usually minor.

2. *Neoplasms* and, occasionally, cysts involving the roots of the teeth.
3. *Impacted teeth* pressing on the root of an adjacent tooth. Cementum is most readily resorbed while enamel is the most resistant. When an impacted tooth presses on the roots of another, these are resorbed while the crown of the impacted tooth usually remains intact.
4. *Unerupted teeth.* During the course of years these may become resorbed or undergo hypercementosis, or both.
5. *Replanted teeth.* These are sometimes rapidly and grossly resorbed.

Idiopathic resorption

Generalised radicular resorption

On very rare occasions resorption may start, apparently spontaneously, on the surface of the root near the apex, and affect many teeth. Over the course of years, more than half the root may be destroyed. The lost tissue is partially repaired by bone-like tissue.

The cause of this change is unknown and treatment is ineffective.

Peripheral resorption

This is also uncommon. A localised area of the root is attacked from its external surface and resorption goes on until the pulp is reached.

Internal resorption (pink spot)

In this curious and uncommon condition the dentine is resorbed from within the pulp. Resorption tends to be localised, producing the characteristic sign of a well-defined rounded area of radiolucency in the crown. This may affect an incisor tooth, and a rounded pink area appears where the vascular pulp has become visible through the attenuated hard tissue.

The cause is unknown but it may possibly be a late result of damage to the blood supply of the pulp by a blow.

Idiopathic internal resorption can affect any part of other teeth but causes no clinical signs until the

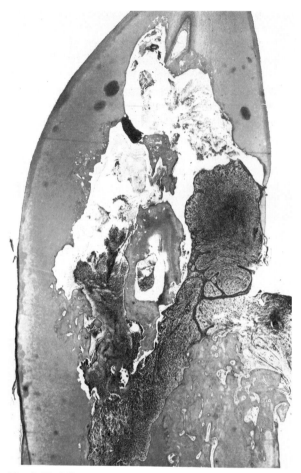

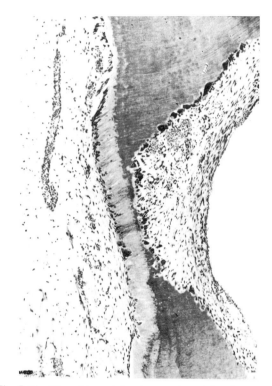

Fig. 5.18 Idiopathic peripheral resorption. A localised area of destruction of dentine produced by osteoclastic activity. The cavity is filled with proliferating connective tissue with giant cells lying in the dentine. The pulp shows no reaction apart from thickening of the predentine layer ($\times$ 40).

Fig. 5.17 Idiopathic internal resorption. A central incisor showing gross resorption that has widely enlarged the pulp chamber and perforated the labial aspect of the crown. Infection has entered, and the pulp has been replaced by granulation tissue. Extensive bony repair tissue has been laid down above the exposure ($\times$ 5).

pulp is opened and allows access to infection. Alternatively resorption may be detected by chance in a routine radiograph.

Histologically vascular granulation tissue replaces the normal pulp, with osteoclasts bordering the affected dentine or enamel. Inflammatory changes may be superimposed if the pulp chamber has been opened by destruction of its walls. Irregular repair with bone or cementum may take place.

Treatment. If a 'pink spot' in an incisor tooth is noticed at an early stage the pulp should be removed and the tooth root-filled before the pulp chamber becomes exposed.

Hypercementosis

The apposition of excessive amounts of cementum is not uncommon. Its cause and significance are unknown. Localised hypercementosis may develop under the following circumstances.

1. *Periapical periodontitis.* Close to the centre of the inflammatory focus, at the apex of the tooth, there is usually a little resorption. Further away (coronally) cementum is laid down, forming a shoulder on the root. (See Fig. 5.14).
2. *Functionless teeth: Unerupted teeth.* These teeth may also undergo resorption.
3. *Paget's disease of the jaws.* The cementum may undergo similar changes to those in the

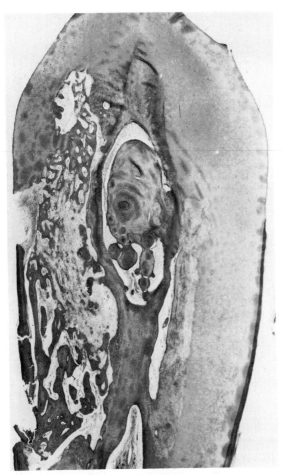

Fig. 5.19 Idiopathic resorption. There has been extensive external resorption of this incisor and replacement of the lost dentine by irregular deposition of bone.

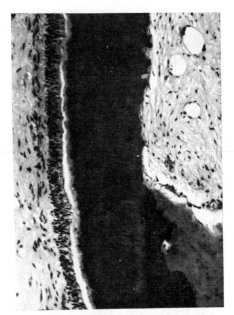

Fig. 5.20 Idiopathic resorption. The same specimen as Fig. 5.19, showing resorption to be no longer active and bony repair tissue laid down on the dentine (below right). The pulp (left) shows no reaction ($\times$ 100).

surrounding bone. Alternating, irregular apposition and resorption, with apposition predominating, produce an irregular mass of cementum on the root which on section has a 'mosaic' pattern.

4. *Cementomas.* These lesions are discussed in Chapter 11.

Increased thickness of cementum is not itself a sign of disease, and no treatment is necessary. If hypercementosis is gross, as it may be in Paget's disease, extractions become difficult.

False gemination

An uncommon complication of hypercementosis is the fusion of the roots of adjacent teeth by means of the excessive tissue. This is known as false gemination and is rarely noticed until an attempt is made to extract one of the teeth; the two teeth are then found to move in unison, and surgical intervention becomes necessary.

INJURIES TO TEETH AND SUPPORTING TISSUES

With the widespread decline in dental caries and the increase in violence, particularly both in the streets and within the home, injuries to the teeth have become an increasingly frequent clinical problem. In children they may be one of the signs of child abuse. The mouth may also be injured during anaesthesia, and damage to the teeth is the most common cause of litigation against anaesthetists in the USA.

The upper incisors, being most prominent, are the most frequently damaged and may suffer fractures of the crown or root, dislocation with death of the pulp, or avulsion. Injuries to the teeth are

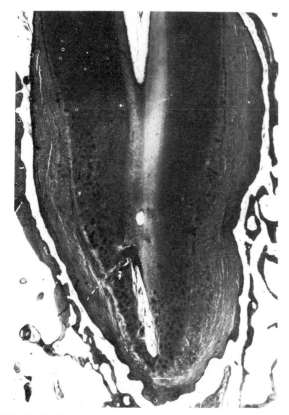

Fig. 5.21 Regular hypercementosis. Regular layers of cementum have been laid down on the apical half of the roots. This is a common change in elderly patients (× 9).

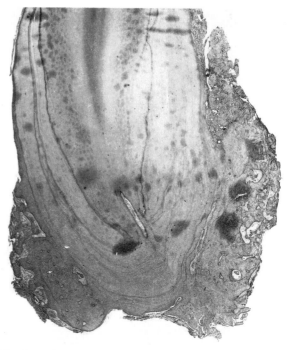

Fig. 5.22 Hypercementosis in Paget's disease. On the many even layers of cementum an irregular, craggy mass of bone-like tissue has formed (× 10).

frequently associated with injuries to the soft tissues and sometimes to the jaws.

Injuries to the crown

Fractures of crown may involve enamel alone or expose the dentinal tubules or pulp. Pulpitis can result from exposure of dentinal tubules, which allows access of infection or other irritants, and is inevitable if the pulp chamber is opened.

Displacement of a tooth, even if momentary, can tear the apical vessels, particularly when the apex is fully formed, and cause pulp death. This may be painless and unnoticed until later when the crown becomes discoloured by extravasated blood. In addition the necrotic pulp becomes infected, presumably from the gingival margins, and apical periodontitis develops. This also may not be noticed until later (Fig. 5.11). Vitality tests are

therefore required, and the management of the non-vital pulp has been described above.

In very many cases the force causing a fracture of the crown is dissipated in this way and the apical vessels are undamaged. By contrast, if the energy of the blow is sufficient to dislocate or avulse teeth, the apical vessels are torn but the crown usually remains undamaged.

Fractures of roots

If the fracture line is deep to the gingival margin, it may remain uninfected, and healing is possible provided that the coronal fragment can be immobilised. However, fractures of the coronal third of the root usually fail to heal because of exposure to infection or inadequate periodontal attachment and mobility of the crown.

Healing of fractured roots

Fractured roots can heal by a process essentially similar to fractures of bone. Bleeding along the

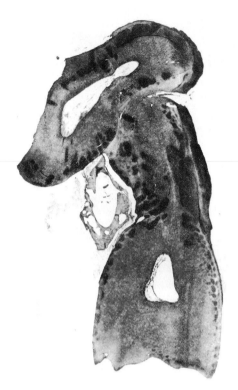

Fig. 5.23 False gemination. An upper second molar has become fused to a buried third molar by the apposition of many layers of cementum (× 5).

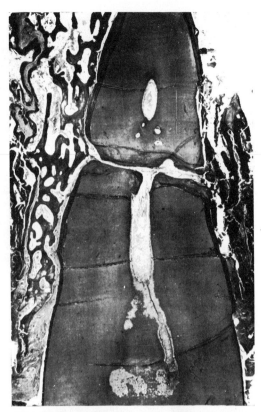

Fig. 5.24 Fracture of the root. This happened some unknown time previously. The fragments are joined by connective tissue; the tooth has remained vital and in good function, and the patient was unaware of the damage (× 8).

fracture line is followed by organisation of the clot. The fracture surfaces undergo osteoclastic resorption and deposition of cementum. However, solid union is uncommon and the fragments are frequently only joined by fibrous tissue. The pulp in the coronal third can remain vital as a result of a new blood supply via the fracture line.

Such healing is only possible if the crown can be protected from occlusal stress, and this is particularly important when the fracture is in the middle of the root.

Injuries to the periodontal ligament

Dislocation of a tooth causes tearing of periodontal ligament fibres and bleeding. This results in swelling of the periodontal ligament, partial extrusion of the tooth, and acute periodontitis.

If not seriously infected, the periodontal ligament usually heals, particularly if it can be protected from continued movement of the tooth

and tearing of the newly forming connective tissue and blood vessels. The tooth should therefore be splinted, but grinding the incisal edge clear of the bite can give temporary relief.

Less violent trauma can also tear periodontal ligament fibres and periodontitis without necessarily dislocating the tooth.

Injuries to the bone

A blow to the mouth may be sufficient to fracture the alveolar bone. When this happens, several teeth move in unison when tested for mobility, or the fracture will be evident on a radiograph. In such circumstances the teeth themselves typically remain intact but the apical vessels may be torn. Vitality testing at intervals should therefore be carried out.

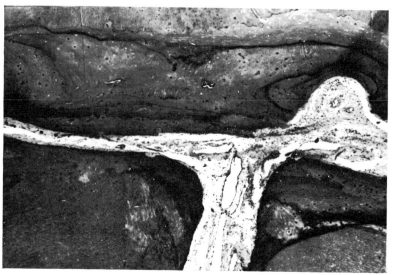

Fig. 5.25   Fracture of the root. The section shows the same specimen as the previous illustration. Along the fracture line the dentine has been resorbed; successive layers of cementum have been deposited but without uniting the fragments. The tissue between the fragments has become vascularised, and the coronal pulp (below) has obtained a new blood supply from this source (× 25).

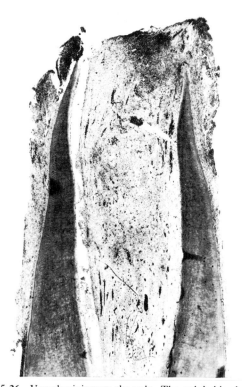

Fig. 5.26   Vascular injury to the pulp. The pulp's blood supply has been damaged by a severe blow; the pulp is undergoing necrosis, with loss of the normal architecture and of the normal staining properties of the cells (× 12).

Injuries to the soft tissues

There is often bruising and swelling of the lip. The mucosa may be lacerated by the teeth and may need to be sutured, but the possibility that a fragment of tooth or filling may have been implanted in the wound should not be overlooked.

More extensive lacerations require wound toilet, prophylactic antibiotics and careful suturing to prevent unsightly scarring.

Injuries to developing teeth: dilaceration

If a tooth with an incompletely formed root is dislocated, the blood supply occasionally remains undamaged. Root formation then continues but is occasionally at an angle to the coronal fragment, and the tooth becomes, in effect, bent (dilacerated).

Histologically the moment of injury is marked by cessation of dentine formation and a line of demarcation where dentine has started to form again. Poorly formed, irregular dentine may also form in the coronal part of the pulp chamber.

Dilaceration is a rare but a possible cause of a difficult extraction.

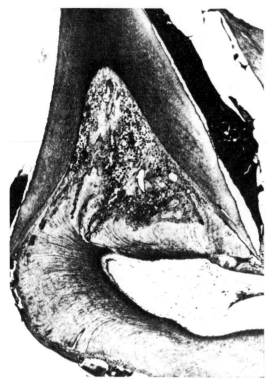

Fig. 5.27 Dilaceration. There is interruption of dentine formation at an early stage, with a sharp line of demarcation where normal development temporarily ceased. The coronal part of the pulp chamber is filled with irregular dentine; later tubular dentine formation has started again but with the remainder of the root at right angles to the axis of the crown ($\times$ 22).

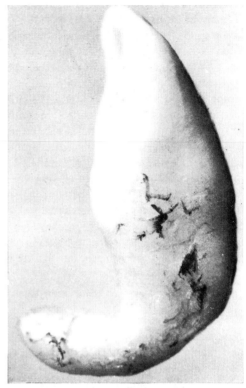

Fig. 5.28 Dilaceration. Normal tooth formation was interrupted by a blow after about half the root had formed. The remainder is at an angle to the original axis and smaller than normal.

Management considerations

Preservation of damaged teeth is desirable but it may be more important to exclude the possibility of other more severe injuries first. Also the child may have been badly frightened by the violence, accidental or deliberate. If tearful, uncooperative, or in a state of mild shock they should be comforted and allowed to recover before starting definitive treatment.

The history—head and other injuries

Details of the accident should be obtained from the patient or any witness. A blow from a small object, such as a ball, usually causes only localised injury. However, a fall on the face or a vehicle accident can result in more serious injuries. Even

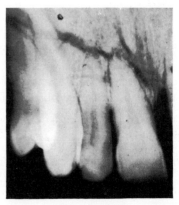

Fig. 5.29 Fracture of the alveolar process. The teeth themselves appear undamaged clinically, but the line of the alveolar fracture runs close to the apices and has damaged the apical vessels.

a fall from a bicycle can cause a skull fracture, which may be apparent only on a radiograph. Skull radiographs are particularly indicated if there has been loss of consciousness, however brief. Fractures of the facial bones and mandible should also be excluded by clinical examination and radiography. Child abuse (Ch. 23) and the current fad for trick riding on BMX machines, are important causes of multiple injuries including the teeth.

The history should also establish the time that has elapsed since the accident, and it helps, for example, as a guide to the chance of survival of a replanted tooth. If there has been pain, its origin from the pulp or periodontal tissues must be determined. Loss of sensation usually indicates death of the pulp. However, sensation may be temporarily impaired by a blow to a tooth, so that vitality tests may provide evidence of recovery.

Oral examination

The general state of care of the mouth will indicate whether saving an isolated tooth is justified or likely to be successful.

Careful clinical examination is necessary to decide the treatment category, as discussed later. Injuries to be looked for include fractures or displacement of any teeth, or disturbances of occlusion due to fractures of the alveolar bone.

Fractures involving the superficial dentine may be difficult to see or may be indicated by stabs of pain on exposure to hot or cold stimuli. Later, typical symptoms of pulpitis may develop, or absence of symptoms can result from death of the pulp. Rarely, a tooth is split longitudinally.

Mobility of a tooth may be due to dislocation and damage to the periodontal ligament. The usual consequence is periodontitis and death of the pulp. Alternatively there may be a fracture of the root or of the alveolar bone as described earlier.

Radiographs

Assessment must be made on a dry film; root fractures may be overlooked on a wet film. Points to be looked for are:

1. The stage of root development and whether the apices of affected teeth are open or closed

2. Whether and in what position the root has fractured
3. Widening of the periodontal ligament space
4. Damage to adjacent or opposing teeth
5. Other coincidental disease and, in late cases, periapical periodontitis.

Principles of treatment

The supporting tissues and alveolar bone usually heal readily, especially if immobilised by splinting the teeth. Damage to the pulp creates a more difficult problem, especially in the younger child where the roots are incomplete. In these cases every attempt should be made to maintain the vitality of the pulp at least until the roots are fully formed. If this fails, the remains of the pulp must be extirpated, but filling the widely patent root canal is difficult. The immediate emergency measures, as a consequence, are to splint the teeth and to protect the pulp or exposed dentine with a sedative dressing.

The apical tissues appear to be fairly robust; they heal readily in these circumstances. Calcium hydroxide dressings encourage calcific scar formation, closing the aperture even if root formation is not completed.

All cases must be followed up to ensure that the tissues have healed or to deal with any complications. Vitality tests must be repeated after a few weeks at first, then every few months. Radiographs should be taken at the same time to detect signs of periodontitis or the formation of a dentine bridge after pulpotomy. Healing of a root fracture is rarely seen on radiographs but, after splinting, the tooth may become firm and functional.

Minor damage to the crown can usually be repaired using composite resin and acid etch technique to build up the lost tissue.

Treatment categories

As a guide to treatment, injuries to the teeth and periodontal tissues may be classified as follows:

- *Class I*: Traumatised tooth without fracture of crown or root
  A. Tooth firm

B. Tooth loosened
- *Class II*: Coronal fracture
  A. Of enamel only
  B. Of enamel and dentine
  The tooth may be firm or loose
- *Class III*: Coronal fracture with exposure (or near exposure) of pulp
  A. Teeth with open apices
  B. Teeth with closed apices
- *Class IV*: Root fracture (with or without coronal fracture)
  A. Fracture of coronal third of root
  B. Fracture of apical third
- *Class V*: Complete displacement of tooth (avulsion).

Class I: Injury without fracture of the tooth

If the tooth is firm and not displaced, patients often ignore the injury and are not seen until later when a complication such as periodontitis has developed. Absence of damage to the crown is usually due to the supporting tissues having absorbed the force of the blow; periodontal fibres may have been torn or apical vessels damaged. If the apex is closed the pulp often dies but may survive if the apex is open. Vitality tests should be carried out and repeated at intervals. If the pulp has died, root canal treatment must be carried out.

Loosened or displaced teeth. These cases are usually seen early. A displaced tooth can usually be manipulated back into position by digital pressure without anaesthesia.

If the apex is open, healing of the pulp is possible though not invariable, but, if the apex is closed, death of the pulp is certain.

The teeth should be immobilised by splinting to allow the supporting tissues to heal and this may also allow the pulp to recover. If the pulp has died, root canal treatment must be carried out, and if the apex is closed this is by conventional methods. If the apex is still widely patent, root canal filling has special problems which are considered later in relation to exposure of the pulp (Class III).

Splints may be made of vacuum-formed plastic and should be kept in place for 2 to 3 months.

If, after about 3 weeks, the tooth still fails to respond to vitality tests, root canal treatment should be carried out and is facilitated at this stage by partial healing of the periodontal tissues.

Class II: Fracture of the crown

Fracture of enamel only. The same considerations apply in these cases as to those in Class I but there is a greater chance that the pulp has survived. The rough enamel edge should be ground smooth and the tooth splinted if necessary. Vitality should be checked at intervals.

Fracture of enamel and dentine. Exposed, patent tubules must be protected immediately by a sedative dressing to prevent pulp infection. A paste of calcium hydroxide is used and must in turn be protected by a layer of cement; this can be held in place by a contoured stainless steel band or pre-formed crown. Three months should

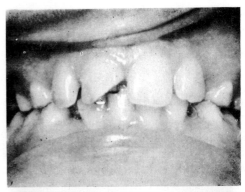
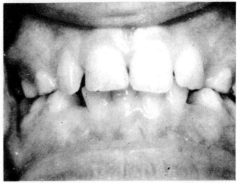

Fig. 5.30 Class II: fracture of enamel and dentine. The oblique fracture of the crown of the right central was sustained without damage to the pulp or apical vessels. Later repair of the incisal edge using an acrylic faced inlay restored the patient's appearance.

be allowed for the pulp to recover and an adequate layer of secondary dentine to form.

If there has been loosening of the teeth or partial dislocation, the tooth also has to be splinted.

Class III: Exposure of the pulp

The chances of survival of the pulp are small when a long period has elapsed since the accident, when the exposure is gross, when the apex is closed, and when there are complicating factors such as displacement, though the latter is unusual in these cases (see Fig. 5.31).

Exposure of pulp, with open apex. If there is no gross infection or displacement the treatment of choice is vital pulpotomy. With a pulp dressing

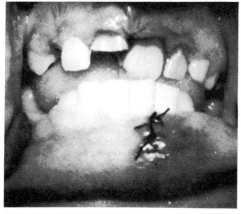

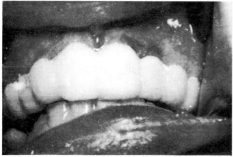

Fig. 5.31 Class III and alveolar fractures. (Upper) The pulp of the central has been widely exposed. The right central and lateral are displaced due to the alveolar fracture, and their apical vessels may have been severed. An associated laceration of the lip has been explored and sutured. (Lower) Splinting. This acrylic splint immobilises the damaged bone and periodontal tissues and will hold in place dressings applied to exposed dentine. Access must be made through the palatal aspect for root canal therapy of exposed pulps.

such as calcium hydroxide, the radicular pulp should heal and complete root formation.

Afterwards, regular vitality tests and radiographs should be taken to confirm (a) continued root formation and apical closure, (b) formation of a calcified layer on the pulp surface, (c) absence of symptoms or radiological signs of pulpal or periapical inflammation, (d) absence of root resorption.

Treatment of teeth with necrotic pulps. If pulpotomy fails or if the pulp is already necrotic, it may be possible to preserve the tooth by root filling. Necrotic tissue is removed and antibiotic paste inserted. Guttapercha is moulded to fit the root canal as closely as possible and sealed in with zinc oxide and eugenol paste.

A dressing of calcium hydroxide placed at the apical aperture may encourage calcific tissue to form. This can reduce the size of the apical aperture enough to make root canal treatment easier.

In some cases extraction may be unavoidable and may be indicated in a badly neglected mouth.

Exposure, with closed apex. Preservation of a vital pulp is rarely possible, and conventional root canal treatment is effective.

Class IV: Fracture of the root

When the fracture line is in the coronal half of the root, conservation is usually impractical; the fracture may involve the gingival crevice, and there is usually insufficient periodontal attachment to support the crown. The situation is irreparable if there is also coronal exposure of the pulp. Occasionally, in the absence of these complications, an attempt at conservation is justified.

The main measures are to reduce displacement by manipulation of the crown to appose the fragments, and to immobilise them by splinting, usually for 2 to 3 months. The pulp's vitality should be regularly tested. Should the pulp die, root canal treatment and apicectomy can be carried out if the fracture is in the apical third.

If the fracture does not involve the gingival margin it may be feasible to join the fragments with a vitallium endodontic splint (with the usual precautions for root canal treatment) or, if this fails, to use a Diodontic pin which extends through the apex into the bone to immobilise the fragments.

Class V: Complete displacement

The two main lines of treatment are:

a. Space maintenance with replacement of the missing tooth later
b. Replantation of the avulsed tooth.

Space maintenance. This must be carried out before the adjacent teeth start to drift into the space (within a few days). A partial denture is not an effective space maintainer in a developing dentition unless firmly clasped to the posterior teeth to give adequate rigidity.

Replantation. A tooth should be replanted as soon as possible to have any great chance of success. It is likely to fail if remaining cells on the root have died. This will happen if the tooth is allowed to dry, or if it has been grossly contaminated or subjected to misguided good intentions such as soaking in a disinfectant.

The root surface cells may survive for up to an hour if the tooth is wrapped in Clingfilm. Longer survival is provided by storing it in fresh, pasteurised milk which is sufficiently bacteria-free and is of appropriate pH and osmolarity.

The tooth should be gently replaced in the socket, after being gently rinsed in normal saline and with care to touch only the crown. It can be temporarily stabilised with aluminium foil or, if available, a cyanoacrylate tissue adhesive such as Histoacryl to bond the crown to the gum only. The tooth should be splinted as soon as possible and should be kept immobilised for 2 to 3 weeks.

After replantation there is usually some resorption of the root surface, but the periodontal tissues should repair within 2 weeks. Infection worsens the prognosis; a systemic antibiotic such as amoxycillin should be given, and the mouth should be rinsed 2 or 3 times a day with 0.2% chlorhexidine to control plaque round the implant. A booster dose of tetanus toxoid may be advisable if the tooth has fallen onto the ground out of doors.

After successful replantation, the pulp may recover if the apex is still widely open; otherwise root canal treatment is necessary.

After-care

Whenever there has been an injury to the teeth they should be kept under observation to detect and treat any deterioration in its earliest stages. If the pulp is alive, vitality tests should be made every three months and radiographs taken of the apical region. If the pulp dies, root canal treatment will be necessary; by this time, apices, open at the time of the accident, may have closed. In those cases in which the pulp has to be extirpated, regular radiographs should be taken to ensure that the apical region remains healthy.

When an incisor is lost it is important to fit a space-retainer, rigidly fixed to adjacent teeth. Otherwise the adjacent teeth drift together and may tilt, and it will be impossible to fit a presentable restoration later on.

No permanent restoration such as a jacket crown or a bridge should be made until after adolescence, when the chance of further injury is reduced. By this time the smaller pulp allows the preparation to be made with less fear of damage.

In cases of coronal fractures it is often possible to restore the crown using acid etch technique to bond a strong composite resin to the dental tissues.

Acute injuries to the teeth—summary

1. Immediate treatment is essential, provided that the child's general condition allows it.
2. When the periodontal tissues are injured the tooth should be supported and protected from occlusal stresses.
3. Fractures of the teeth should be looked for clinically and on radiographs. The pulps should be tested for vitality.
4. In teeth with open apices the pulp must, if at all possible, be preserved by pulp-capping or pulpotomy.
5. If the pulp is exposed or the apical vessels damaged in teeth with closed apices, they must usually be root-filled.
6. If anterior teeth have to be extracted, a space-retainer must be fitted.
7. After-care by regular examinations to make sure that healing is going on and pulp vitality is maintained, is essential.

Fractures of teeth in older persons

Part or the whole crown may fracture off as a

result of overlarge restorations. Crowning or extracting may be required according to circumstances.

Rarely, as a result of extreme abrasion weakening a tooth, it may fracture at the neck. The pulp is likely to have been obliterated by reactionary dentine formation, and post-crowning is unlikely to be feasible.

Chronic injuries to the teeth

Attrition and abrasion slowly destroy the enamel and dentine. The effects are therefore rarely seen until late in life (Ch. 24).

Erosion

Erosion is the progressive dissolution of tooth substance usually by acid solutions but sometimes of unknown cause.

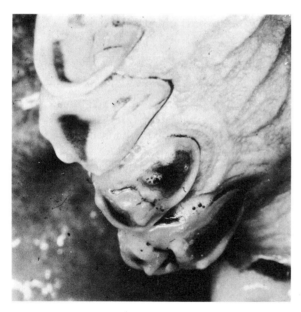

Fig. 5.32 Erosion. This is acid erosion due to recurrent gastric regurgitation, leaving destruction of enamel and dentine on the palatal aspect of the teeth.

Erosion of the labial surfaces of the teeth is occasionally an occupational disease where there is exposure to acid fumes. The habitual sucking of citrus fruits may have a similar effect, and many soft drinks have an acid reaction.

A few patients suffer from chronic regurgitation of acid gastric contents. Under these circumstances, the lingual surfaces, particularly of the upper teeth, are most severely affected.

Another uncommon type of erosion of unknown cause that is occasionally seen in young people is characterised by shallow polished depressions usually of the labial or buccal enamel of the incisor teeth. The cause of this change is not known but though the polished appearance suggests that toothbrushing may be partly responsible, it must be presupposed that the enamel is abnormally softened. This in turn may be due to the taking of excessive quantities of pure lemon juice or of acid soft drinks, particularly if these are sucked past the teeth instead of being quickly swallowed in the usual way.

Anorexia nervosa and bulimia

Anorexia nervosa is a psychogenic disease of unknown cause but characterised by an obsession with body weight, self-imposed starvation and, eventually, emaciation and secondary metabolic changes. Women in their late teens or twenties are affected. Bulimia is a preoccupation with food and body weight. It is characterised by episodes of gross overeating punctuated by self-induced vomiting or, sometimes, purgative abuse to control weight. The erosion of the teeth is similar to those seen in other types of recurrent vomiting and may be the way in which the disorder is recognised. However, patients rarely admit to their abnormal behaviour.

SUGGESTED FURTHER READING

Cawson R A 1987 Oral pathology — colour aids in dentistry. Churchill Livingstone, Edinburgh
Cawson R A, Eveson J W 1987 Oral pathology and

diagnosis. William Heinemann Medical Books, London and Gower Medical Publishing, London
Clokie C, Metcalf I, Holland A 1989 Dental trauma in anaesthesia. Can J Anaesth 36: 675–680
Cunnington S A 1990 An update on endodontics: 1.

endodontic diagnosis and preparation. Dental Update 17: 95–103

Gill Y, Scully C 1988 The microbiology and management of acute dentoalveolar abscess: views of British oral and maxillofacial surgeons. Br J Oral Maxillofac Surg 23: 452–457

Iwu C, MacFarlane, MacKenzie D, Stenhouse D 1990 The microbiology of periapical granulomas. Oral Surg, Oral Med, Oral Pathol 69: 502–505

Lewis M A O, MacFarlane T W, McGowan D A 1986 Quantitative microbiology of acute dento-alveolar abscesses. J Med Microbiol 21: 101–104

Mackie I C, Warren V N 1988 Dental trauma: 1. General aspects of management and trauma to the primary dentition. Dental Update 15: 155–159

Mackie I C, Warren V N 1988 Dental trauma: 2. Coronal fractures of immature permanent incisor teeth. Dental Update 15: 242–247

Mackie I C, Warren V N 1988 Dental trauma: 3. Splinting, displacement injuries and root fracture of immature permanent teeth. Dental Update 15: 332–336

Mackie I C, Warren V N 1988 Dental trauma: 4. Avulsion of immature incisor teeth. Dental Update 15: 406–409

Smith B G N, Wright P S, Brown D 1986 The clinical handling of dental materials. Wright (IOP Publishing Ltd), Bristol

Wellbury R R, Murray J J 1990 Prevention of trauma to teeth. Dental Update 15: 117–121

6. Periodontal disease

Periodontal disease has been defined as any pathological process affecting the periodontal tissues, but almost invariably refers to inflammatory disease: namely, gingivitis and periodontitis. Both conditions are caused by accumulation of bacterial plaque at the dentogingival junction. *Gingivitis* often starts in childhood, is confined to the marginal gingiva and there is no loss of connective tissue attachment to the tooth surface or bone. *Periodontitis* is characterised by destruction of the periodontal ligament and alveolar bone, and leads ultimately to loosening and loss of the teeth. Periodontitis is invariably preceded by gingivitis.

This is not to say that gingivitis always progresses to periodontitis, but in many cases progress may be insidious and relentless. However, there is no clinical predictor of progression which has sufficient tooth site and subject specificity to be useful. Eventually damage to the supporting tissues becomes so severe that the teeth loosen and can no longer function adequately. Chronic periodontitis is the main cause of loss of teeth as age advances.

The normal periodontal tissues

The gingivae are divided into anatomical and histological regions. The anatomical parts of the gingivae are: (i) the free gingiva; (ii) the attached gingiva and (iii) the reflected mucosa.

The free (marginal) gingiva

This comprises the marginal gingivae and the papillary gingivae between the teeth. The free gingiva is separated from the crown of the tooth by a shallow sulcus ('crevice') about 0.5 mm deep in the healthy state. The floor of the sulcus and the boundary of the free gingiva in an apical direction is formed by the junctional epithelium described below. On the external aspect the free gingiva extends about 1 mm to the gingival groove.

The attached (stippled) gingiva

This extends between the free gingiva and the alveolar mucosa, that is from the gingival groove to the mucogingival junction. The attached gingiva is firmly bound down to the underlying bone to form a tough mucoperiosteum. The stippled appearance of the surface of the attached gingiva is due to the intersections of the underlying epithelial ridges at the junction with the connective tissue, rather than the attachment of collagen bundles as was once thought.

The alveolar mucosa

This is continuous with the attached gingiva but is sharply demarcated and can be recognised by its smooth surface, darker colour and its increasing separation from the bone.

Though the gingival epithelium forms a continuous layer, it is divided into three main parts. These are: (i) oral epithelium; (ii) sulcular epithelium and (iii) junctional epithelium.

1. *The oral epithelium* extends from the mucogingival junction to the crest of the gingival margin. It is moderately thick, its deep surface is indented by the dermal ridges and it is supported by connective tissue fibres radiating from the crest of the alveolar bone and circular fibres forming the so-called marginal ligament.
2. *The sulcular epithelium* lines the gingival

sulcus and is morphologically part of the oral epithelium which it joins at the crest of the free gingiva. At the floor of the sulcus the sulcular epithelium joins the junctional epithelium.

3. *The junctional epithelium* joins the internal surface of the gingiva to the tooth and forms a cuff or collar round the neck of the tooth. The union of the epithelium with the tooth is formed by the epithelial attachment.

The epithelial attachment. The attachment apparatus consists of a basal lamina and hemidesmosomes. This epithelium, which resembles flattened stratified squamous epithelium, has a relatively high turnover rate and the epithelial attachment is probably actively maintained and reformed. This enables the attachment to migrate in an apical direction.

The epithelial attachment is firmly adherent to the tooth surface, so that mechanical damage (which would tend to pull the epithelium from the tooth) causes, instead, tears extending between the epithelial cells (Fig. 6.2). Since the junctional epithelium can be split in this way, attempts to measure the gingival sulcus by passing an instrument down towards its floor usually record a greater depth than is seen in histological preparations.

The function of the epithelial attachment is to form an effective seal at the interface between tooth and gingival epithelium.

With the development of periodontal disease the junctional epithelium gradually migrates in an apical direction.

The gingival sulcus and junctional epithelium

The enamel of a newly erupted tooth is covered by an adherent cuticle and the reduced enamel epithelium which meets and fuses with the epithelium of the gum as the tooth erupts. The epithelium is attached round the clinical neck of the tooth, forming a collar, but before eruption is complete the epithelial attachment is wholly on the enamel. Under normal conditions the epithelial attachment of the fully erupted tooth extends no further than the amelocemental junction. In later life, if the occlusal surfaces wear down, overeruption

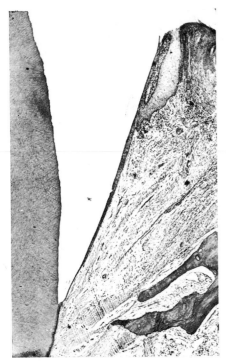

Fig. 6.1 Gingival sulcus and epithelial attachment. This sagittal section of a specimen from a woman of 27 shows the normal appearances. Enamel removed by decalcification of the specimen has left the triangular space. The epithelial attachment forms a straight line from the top of the papilla to the amelocemental junction; its enamel surface, the actual line of attachment, is sharply defined. The gingival sulcus, minute in extent, is formed where the papilla curves away from the line of the enamel surface. Here there is a minor infiltration with inflammatory cells and epithelial proliferation (× 26).

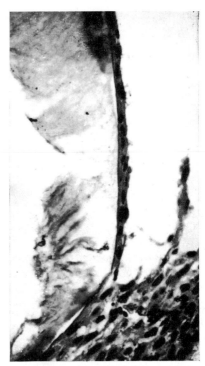

Fig. 6.2 The epithelial attachment. This specimen (from a woman aged 22) shows, on the left, the enamel matrix after decalcification and, attached to its surface, a layer of epithelial cells. The epithelium has been torn but the tear is in the junctional epithelium which has left some of its cells still adherent to the enamel. The space on the right side has been made by this tear, and the full thickness of the junctional epithelium can be seen at the bottom of the picture (× 400).

of the tooth is accompanied by maintenance of the position of the junctional epithelial attachment to the tooth surface. There is, therefore, an increase in the width of the attached gingiva since the level of the mucogingival junction remains static. The junctional epithelium may migrate apically in these circumstances when there is concurrent inflammation due to plaque or trauma.

The junctional epithelium forms the floor of the gingival sulcus. Immediately deep to it are the most superficial of the periodontal fibres attached to the tooth. Thus in the healthy state an unbroken layer of epithelium attached to the tooth protects the underlying connective tissue of the gingivae. The superficial fibres of the periodontal membrane, in turn, resist the detachment of epithelium.

With the development of periodontal disease the junctional epithelium gradually migrates in an apical direction. With pocket formation the original epithelial attachment is lost but progressively reforms as the epithelium migrates. The junctional epithelium becomes attached in this way to cementum, and histologically this attachment can be seen as a clear cuticle.

The gingival col

The interdental gingiva is wedge-shaped but dips down beneath the contact points to form a col with a peak bucally and lingually forming the visible gingival papillae. The col beneath the contact point is the part of the gum least accessible to cleansing; stagnation of plaque and, therefore, inflammatory changes are most severe in this area. Contrary to earlier views, there is little or no evidence that the epithelium of the col provides any less effective a protective barrier than the junctional epithelium.

The gingival and periodontal connective tissues

The principal fibres of the periodontal ligament form fibrous bundles between which is loose connective tissue containing blood vessels and nerves. These components of the periodontal ligament provide a complex viscoelastic supportive mechanism resisting both compressive and tensile forces. The normal thickness of the periodontal ligament is between about 0.1 and 0.3 mm. The thickness is reduced in nonfunctional teeth.

The principal fibres are arranged in a series of fairly well-defined groups. The *oblique fibres* form a suspensory ligament from the socket to the root in a coronal to apical direction. At its neck, the tooth is attached to the rim of the socket by a dense group of *horizontal fibres*. The *transeptal fibres* of the horizontal group are not attached to the alveolar bone but pass superficially to it and join adjacent teeth together. These fibres therefore protect the interdental gingiva by resisting forces that would otherwise separate the teeth and open the contact points. The *gingival fibres* form a cuff round the neck of the tooth supporting the soft tissues; these fibres therefore tend to resist the separation of the gingivae from the tooth and help to prevent the formation of pockets.

The principal fibres are embedded in the cementum at their inner ends. New fibres replacing those which have aged, or forming in response to new functional stresses, are attached by apposition of further layers of cementum which increases in thickness progressively with age.

At their outer ends the periodontal fibres are embedded in the lamina dura, a layer of compact bone continuous, at the mouths of the sockets, with the cortical bone of the jaw. The radiological appearance of a lamina dura has limited diagnostic value in periodontics as its presence is largely dependent upon the alignment of the X-ray beam.

Gingival collagen

In the clinically normal gingiva the quantity of newly synthesised non-cross-linked collagen is apparently several times greater than that of the skin or of adjacent tissues such as the palate. The rate of collagen production, maturation and breakdown have also been measured in animals using radioactive proline. The newly synthesised immature collagen fraction appears not to be progressively degraded, as in most other tissues, but persists and is comparable in amount to that in actively proliferating granulation tissue. The insoluble collagen component of gingival connective tissue is also, apparently, unusually unstable, and it is suggested that the gingival connective tissue behaves more like that of healing wounds than that of fully formed tissues.

The implications of these findings are that gingival and periodontal ligament connective tissue have an unusually high rate of turnover, with fibroblasts continually producing a pool of newly synthesised molecules which can be used for maintenance and repair. The insoluble collagen fraction, in turn, is relatively unstable and changes rapidly. These findings are compatible with, and may explain, the obvious power of the gingiva to regenerate and repair under a variety of conditions, including tooth eruption, movement of the teeth, and inflammatory disease. This instability of the connective tissue would also help to explain how collagen can be rapidly lost in the process of chronic gingivitis and periodontal disease once its metabolism has been disturbed by disease.

Gingival fluid (exudate)

In health, a minute amount of fluid can be collected from the gingival margins. It differs in composition from saliva, particularly in its immune globulin content. Saliva contains IgA while gingival fluid has a variable but significant content of IgG, IgM and leucocytes. Unlike saliva, gingival fluid is not a secretion (there are no glands in this region) but is inflammatory exudate. It therefore increases greatly with the development of clinical inflammation.

Nomenclature and classification of periodontal disease

The term periodontal disease—whatever the academic definitions may be—should be used to refer only to diseases (predominantly inflammatory in nature) of the supporting tissue alone. A wide variety of diseases of the oral mucous membrane can affect the gingivae occasionally, and conditions as diverse as tuberculosis or lichen planus can produce lesions in this area. Such conditions do not play any significant part in the development of periodontal disease in its accepted sense. A clear distinction must therefore be made between simple periodontal disease and systemic or mucosal disease which may fortuitously affect this area. It is essential, therefore, that such diseases be recognised and not treated as unusually severe or intractable gingivitis or periodontal disease merely because they also produce inflammation or periodontal destruction.

Chronic gingivitis is, in all but a few cases, the preliminary stage to the development of periodontal disease, but, clinically, no sharp dividing line can be drawn between chronic gingivitis and the onset of periodontitis. Nevertheless, the distinction is of practical importance in that chronic gingivitis can in general be cured but the effects of chronic periodontitis are largely irreversible. Alveolar bone may occasionally re-form in some localised defects when there has been resolution of inflammation, but this is unpredictable and never happens supracrestally. Most attempts to encourage re-formation of periodontal ligament attachment to affected root surfaces have failed. Some recently described methods may be more successful in this respect, as discussed below in relation to surgical aspects of treatment.

Destruction of the tissues supporting the teeth is the characteristic feature of chronic periodontitis.

Classification

There is no definitive classification of periodontal disease, and the number of classifications that have been put forward in the past reflects only the variety of personal interpretations of the limited knowledge available.

The following are therefore the main *clinical* types of periodontal disease grouped together on the basis of what seems to be the predominant pathological process.

1. Inflammatory periodontal disease

a. Gingivitis
  (i) Acute gingivitis
    — Acute ulcerative gingivitis
    — Acute non-specific gingivitis
  (ii) Chronic gingivitis
b. Periodontitis
  (i) Acute periodontitis
  (ii) Chronic periodontitis
  (iii) Juvenile periodontitis
  (iv) Other (proposed) subdivisions
2. Miscellaneous periodontal disorders
a. Gingival hyperplasia and swelling
b. Periodontal atrophy

To reduce the matter to its simplest terms, the most common type of periodontal disease is inflammatory, that is the sequence of chronic gingivitis and chronic periodontitis. Other factors may modify this inflammatory process, but rarely to a conspicuous degree.

ACUTE ULCERATIVE GINGIVITIS

(Acute necrotising ulcerative gingivitis. Vincent's gingivitis)

Acute ulcerative gingivitis is a distinct and specific disease characterised by rapidly progressive ulceration typically starting at the tips of the interdental papillae, spreading along the gingival margins and going on to acute destruction of the periodontal tissues.

Microbiological aspects

Aetiology

The bacteria responsible are a complex of spirochaetes and fusiforms traditionally termed *Borrelia vincentii* and *Fusobacterium nucleatum*. These organisms may be present in small numbers in the healthy gingival flora, though spirochaetes may be so few as to be undetectable. With the onset of ulcerative gingivitis, both bacteria proliferate to such an extent as to dominate the bacterial picture seen in smears from the lesions. There is little question about the pathogenicity of *F. nucleatum* especially, which is one of the most frequent causes of serious anaerobic infections in man. Moreover, the overwhelming proliferation of the spirochaete and fusobacterium at the site of tissue destruction, in-

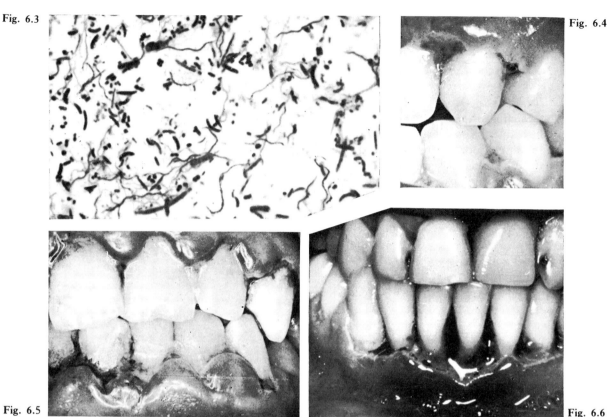

Fig. 6.3 *Borrelia vincentii* and *Fusobacterium nucleatum*. A smear from a patient with acute ulcerative gingivitis. The loose irregular shape of the spirochaetes, and the plumper, curved fusiform bacilli can be seen among other bacilli and cocci (× 700).

Fig. 6.4 Early acute ulcerative gingivitis. The interdental papillae are swollen due partly to pre-existing chronic gingivitis and partly to the acute inflammatory oedema. Blood and slough exude from the gingival margins, and an early ulcer at the tip of the papilla between the upper canine and lateral can be seen.

Fig. 6.5 Acute ulcerative gingivitis. The characteristic features of the ulcers are shown in this enlarged photograph. The ulcers start at the tips of the interdental papillae, are crater-shaped, have a pale margin and are covered by a slough. Removal of the slough leaves a raw, bleeding surface.

Fig. 6.6 Advanced ulcerative gingivitis. The gingival and periodontal tissues, especially of the lower central incisors, have been destroyed leaving triangular spaces between the teeth. The condition can be said to have reached the stage of acute periodontitis.

vasion of the tissues by spirochaetes (shown by electron microscopy) and the sharp fall in their numbers with effective treatment strongly suggest that they are the responsible agents. Despite these facts, these is still uncertainty as to whether this spirochaetal complex is the cause of ulcerative gingivitis. However, the question is less that of whether they are the cause but, rather, that their precise nature is unclear. For example, *Bacteroides intermedius* has been isolated in large numbers and

it has also been suggested that the fusiform bacterium is *Leptotrichia buccalis*, hitherto thought to be a harmless oral commensal.

Like other anaerobic infections, ulcerative gingivitis is a mixed infection with the main pathogens to some degree dependent on other bacteria. The role of the latter may be to lower the local oxygen tension or to provide specific nutrients. It is probable that factors such as these explain the failure of attempts (when the microbial physiology of anaerobic infections was less well understood) to reproduce this infection by inoculating the fusospirochaetal complex experimentally.

Despite doubts about the nature of the fusospirochaetal complex, there can be no question that ulcerative gingivitis is an anaerobic infection. This is shown by the almost immediate response to metronidazole, a drug which is effective only against obligate anaerobes.

Since local factors are likely to be of overwhelming importance in the establishment of ulcerative gingivitis, this infection does not appear to be transmissible. However, at various times the disease has been almost epidemic, but its transmissibility can hardly be said to have been thoroughly tested.

Host factors

Ulcerative gingivitis is a disease of otherwise healthy young adults usually with dirty, neglected mouths. In developed countries children are not affected. This may in part be because the child's oral flora is less favourable to the growth of anaerobes. The latter appear in greater numbers as plaque accumulates as a result of poor oral hygiene.

Though the majority of patients are otherwise healthy, ulcerative gingivitis may develop in children having immunosuppressive treatment and in patients with HIV infection.

Predisposing factors

Ulcerative gingivitis has been prevalent at various times, particularly during the First and Second World Wars.

Ulcerative gingivitis was exceedingly common among the troops in the 1914–1918 war when it was called 'trench mouth' and among civilians subjected to bombing in the 1939–1945 war when the disease was known as 'shelter mouth'. Though it was suggested that malnutrition was a factor there was nothing to support such an idea. However, the conditions of life of both these groups can (reasonably enough) be regarded as stressful, and there is some other evidence that chronic anxiety may be associated with or be a predispos-

ing factor in this infection. Smoking and upper respiratory infections have also been implicated.

A possible pathogenic mechanism that has been proposed therefore is that enhanced sympathetic activity associated with anxiety and the peripheral vasoconstrictor action of nicotine might cause some ischaemia, particularly at the tips of the interdental papillae which are supplied by the fine terminations of a capillary network.

Overall, however, little is known about the predisposing causes of acute ulcerative gingivitis, which appears to be a fusospirochaetal infection usually without obvious or gross depression of host defences.

Summary

1. Ulcerative gingivitis is an anaerobic infection, as shown by the rapid response to metronidazole.
2. The bulk of evidence indicates that the fusospirochaetal complex putatively of *Fusobacterium nucleatum* and *Borrelia vincentii* are the responsible pathogens.
3. Though ulcerative gingivitis has been almost epidemic during the two world wars it does not appear to be readily transmissible.
4. Apparently healthy young males with dirty mouths are predominantly affected, but the essential predisposing factors remain unidentified.

Clinical features

As mentioned earlier, ulcerative gingivitis in the Western world affects young adults, usually those with neglected mouths. Smoking, anxiety and upper respiratory infections are frequently associated.

General signs of infection are slight or absent. Most patients have no fever, do not feel particularly unwell and the lymph nodes are not usually enlarged.

Though at one time common, ulcerative gingivitis is infrequently seen in Britain now.

Soreness and gingival bleeding are the main complaints. Bleeding from the gums after minimal trauma, conspicuously more severe than from chronic gingivitis, and excessive salivation are typical. The breath usually smells particulary unpleasant as might be expected of an anaerobic infection causing tissue necrosis.

Most patients have neglected mouths with accumulations of plaque and calculus. The accumulation of plaque may partly be a result of the pain which prevents effective toothbrushing after the onset of the infection.

The local lesion

Crater-shaped or punched-out ulcers form primarily at the tips of the interdental papillae. The edges are sharply defined by erythema and oedema of the margins, while the surface of the ulcer is covered by a greyish or yellowish tenacious slough. Removal of the slough causes free bleeding.

Spread of ulceration

Ulceration can spread in several directions but the lesions remain restricted to the gingivae and supporting tissues almost exclusively. Though it is rare, contact ulcers may develop in severe cases where the soft tissues are in apposition to the gingival ulcers. Generalised stomatitis is not seen and, in all but a few cases, the gingivae are exclusively affected.

The main directions of spread are:

1. laterally along the gingival margins
2. deeply to destroy interdental soft and hard tissues, and
3. across the attached gingiva (rarely).

The usual picture is that of combinations of lateral and deep spread. Lateral spread produces linear ulceration of the gingival margins. Deep spread can cause rapid destruction of both soft tissues and bone, producing triangular spaces between the teeth if treatment is delayed. The end-result may therefore be considerable distortion of the normal gingival contours, which may predispose to increased stagnation and recurrences, or chronic periodontal disease.

Course of the infection

Though gingival damage may be severe, there are no worse consequences. Many patients are subject to continued neglect of oral hygiene together with increased stagnation following the initial damage to, and distortion of, the gum margins. If also heavy cigarette smoking is as important as has been suggested, this is likely to have gone on unchanged.

Children are not affected in developed countries but infection may be seen in those having immunosuppressive treatment. Children may also be severely affected in some parts of Africa such as Nigeria. There the infection may progress to massive necrosis of the facial tissues (Cancrum oris) with exposure of bone of the jaw. Cancrum oris (Chapter 8 was seen in Europe in the past but not now.

Differential diagnosis and investigation

In the great majority of cases the clinical picture is well defined, following the pattern described. A swab taken from the depths of the lesion or the deep aspect of the slough shows a heavy predominance of spirochaetes and fusiform bacilli. This picture is characteristic of ulcerative gingivitis, but care should be taken to sample the lesion rather than associated mature plaque which may contain significant numbers of these organisms.

If the patient is pale or shows obvious malaise, haematological examination should be carried out, particularly to exclude anaemia, leucopenia, acute leukaemia or AIDS.

In the differential diagnosis two conditions in particular must be considered. These are *primary herpetic stomatitis* and, more rarely, *acute leukaemia*.

The clinical picture, particularly the distribution of the lesions, the absence of significant systemic disturbance and the fusospirochaetal complex seen in a direct smear are usually, however, adequate to make the diagnosis.

By contrast, herpetic stomatitis, agranulocytosis and acute leukaemia—all of which can cause gingival ulceration—are typically associated with systemic symptoms and produce different clinical oral features (Ch. 15 and 20).

Patients with AIDS are susceptible to the development of acute ulcerative gingivitis as well as rapidly progressing periodontitis, as described later, and this indicates the importance of the immune response in protecting the periodontal tissues.

Treatment

Three main aspects of treatment are as follows:

1. Physical (oral hygiene) measures
2. Metronidazole
3. Use of oxidising antiseptics.

Oral hygiene measures (surgical débridement) are the most important aspect of treatment and the use of drugs should not be considered as as alternative.

Starting at the patient's first visit, plaque and calculus must be removed by careful and thorough scaling and irrigation. If this cleaning is done sufficiently thoroughly it should be adequate treatment in itself for any but advanced and exceptionally severe cases, and drugs should be unnecessary. The limitation of this treatment is that it is difficult to carry out fully because of the tenderness of the tissues and is very time-consuming.

Home care should continue this programme by toothbrushing and frequent use of mouthwashes of a hot dilute antiseptic.

Metronidazole is the drug of choice in that (a) it is very rapidly effective; (b) unlike penicillin is not sensitising; (c) is not prone to promote super-infection, and (d) side-effects are few and rarely significant (see Ch. 8). The usual dose is 200 mg by mouth three times a day for three days. The tablets should be taken after food.

Oxidising antiseptics were widely used before the introduction of specific antimicrobials. The most commonly used was hydrogen peroxide applied directly to the gingiva in association with general cleaning up the mouth. In association with cleaning up the mouth such measures are frequently effective but should not be persisted with if 2 or 3 applications are not successful.

The effect of antiseptics does not, incidentally, appear to be entirely non-specific. Thus povidone iodine and chlorhexidine, both of which are otherwise useful antiseptics, appear to be ineffective in ulcerative gingivitis.

Follow-up treatment—rehabilitation of the mouth

Once the acute phase has subsided the state of oral hygiene should be brought to as high a standard as possible. Oral hygiene instruction must also be given. Where there has been damage causing distortion of the gingivae and inaccessible stagnation areas, surgery may be needed to make the dentogingival margin accessible to oral hygiene.

The patient is managed in the same way as any other with incipient or established periodontal disease. The basic problem is only that many patients who get ulcerative gingivitis have neglected mouths and are too intransigent to bother with anything other than to seek relief from the acute symptoms.

Vincent's angina

Vincent's angina is a necrotising pharyngitis caused by the same fusospirochaetal complex as ulcerative gingivitis with which it may be associated. The appearance is clinically somewhat similar to diphtheria but there is typically little systemic upset.

Vincent's angina was common at the times when ulcerative gingivitis was widespread but seems to have disappeared from Britain. Its chief relevance here is that the medical profession when speaking or writing of ulcerative gingivitis frequently and incorrectly call it 'Vincent's angina'.

Acute non-specific gingivitis

Acute gingivitis is commonly associated with herpetic stomatitis or may occasionally accompany an acute streptococcal sore throat or other febrile infections. Gingivitis in these conditions does not seem to be a specific infection and is probably no more than an exacerbation of pre-existing chronic gingivitis. The gingivae tend to be bright red and oedematous. The swelling causes the surface to lose its stippling and to appear glossy. There may be slight soreness of the gingivae, or symptoms may be absent.

The treatment is that of the underlying infection and measures to improve oral hygiene.

Rare special types of gingivitis that may accompany systemic diseases such as scurvy or acute leukaemia are described with the individual diseases.

CHRONIC GINGIVITIS AND PERIODONTITIS

Chronic gingivitis, an almost universal disease, is a persistent low-grade infection resulting from the accumulation of bacterial plaque round the necks of the teeth. Adequate toothbrushing will remove the deposits from the teeth and eliminate chronic gingivitis. Failure to prevent the accumulation of these deposits is usually followed by spread of infection and inflammation, together with increasing damage to the periodontal membrane and alveolar bone. The condition of chronic periodontitis with progressive destruction of the supporting tissues thus becomes established.

Nevertheless, the factors affecting the transition from chronic gingivitis to destructive periodontal disease are far from clear.

Pathogenesis of chronic gingivitis and periodontitis

The tissues involved in the initiation and progress of periodontal disease are:

1. The junctional epithelium and epithelial attachment
2. The fibrous connective tissue of the gingival margin and the periodontal membrane
3. The alveolar bone.

The junctional epithelium and epithelial attachment

The junctional epithelium forms an attachment apparatus (Fig. 6.2). It is not merely in apposition to the enamel in the healthy state but effectively prevents the seepage of saliva and microorganisms along the interface.

In addition to the adhesion between epithelium and tooth, which prevents the ingress of foreign material between them, the epithelium also presents a barrier to the penetration of bacteria into the underlying connective tissue.

In the healthy state therefore the epithelium forms an unbroken protective layer covering the connective tissues and extending in continuity from the adjacent mucosa via free and attached gingivae to the enamel surface. The epithelial attachment extends in the healthy state, from the gingival margin (or floor of the gingival sulcus) to the apical limit of the junctional epithelium at or near the amelocemental junction. Bacterial plaque is in contact with the epithelium at the gingival margin. At the point where the gingival epithelium is reflected onto the tooth surface it usually forms an angle with the enamel (the gingival crevice or sulcus). This produces in effect a minute ledge where, in neglected mouths, plaque can collect more thickly. It appears that the earliest changes of periodontal disease develop beneath the gingival sulcus, and it seems likely that the initiation of the inflammatory response is the result of bacterial antigens passing through the epithelium to provoke the release of mediators. Antigens from plaque can be detected by immunofluorescence both in the periodontal tissues and in gingival macrophages when periodontal disease has become established.

Periodontal ligament and alveolar bone

Damage to these connective tissue structures is an essential feature of periodontal disease. Though the transition from chronic gingivitis to destructive periodontal disease is imperceptible, it is usually a point of no return. Loss of periodontal fibres leads to pocketing and conditions more favourable to plaque accumulation. Ultimately the destruction of these supporting tissues leads to mobility and loss of the teeth.

The mechanisms of periodontal destruction are not understood, but there appear to be three main factors. It is not known which is the most important, and probably all contribute in greater or lesser degree. These are:

1. Bacterial damage
2. Immunological mechanisms
3. Other factors.

Microbiological aspects

Very many detailed studies have been carried out on the microbiology of bacterial plaque in relation to periodontal disease. The aim has been to discover whether specific pathogens could be identified and whether their elimination would lead to the control of periodontal disease. An alternative view is that plaque is non-specific in its effects and that individual pathogens are of relatively little importance.

More recently the importance and some of the properties of *biofilms* (Ch. 2) have become recognised. It seems possible therefore that periodontal plaque may behave as an organised entity, and the properties of individual bacterial components in isolation may have little relevance to the overall effects of plaque in which they are present. Certainly, identification of individual pathogens in periodontal pockets has had little influence as yet on the management of periodontal disease.

The bacterial population of periodontal plaque is vast and mixed. There are basic difficulties in any attempt to characterise the bacterial population and to identify all individual members, some of which may be fastidious in their growth requirements and difficult or as yet impossible to culture in the laboratory. An even greater difficulty is to determine which of these microorganisms are pathogenic in this environment and responsible for periodontal tissue destruction. In an attempt to solve this problem an effort has been made to quantify some types of bacteria in relation to the stage of the disease and the clinical periodontal state. The technical difficulties are nevertheless formidable, and it has to be admitted that the results so far have been inconclusive.

It is important to emphasise that the mere presence of important pathogens such as fusobacteria and bacteroides species does not of itself indicate that they necessarily cause tissue damage *in this environment*. An analogy may be drawn between the periodontal and the bowel flora. The bowel flora also includes many Gram-negative bacteria and anaerobes but these do no harm unless they are, for example, released into the peritoneal cavity. Lethal peritonitis can then result. In the bowel the pathogens are (so to speak) kept under control by innumerable other organisms as well as by the defences of the bowel wall. If, however, this balance is disturbed the bowel wall itself may be damaged, sometimes with fatal results. The classic example is the effect of clindamycin, which may occasionally destroy so many bowel bacteria

that pathogenic clostridia (especially *C. difficile*) can proliferate and cause destructive colitis.

Bacteria isolated from plaque are shown in Table 6.1, but this picture is far from complete, especially as some plaque bacteria have as yet eluded identification.

Variations in plaque bacteria with stage of disease

Healthy (uninflamed) gingivae. The plaque is supragingival and thin (1 to 20 cells thick). Grampositive bacteria appear to predominate and

Table 6.1   Some bacteria isolated from periodontal plaque

Actinobacillus actinomycetemcomitans

Actinomyces bifidus, A. israelii, A. naeslundii, A. odontolyticus, A. viscosus

Arachnia propionica

Bacillus cereus

Bacterionema matruchotii

Bacteroides melaninogenicus, B. gingivalis, B. intermedius, etc.

Bifidobacterium species

Campylobacter sputorum

Capnocytophaga species including *C. ochracea*

Clostridium species

Corynebacterium species

Eikenella corrodens

Escherichia coli

Fusobacterium nucleatum, F. polymorphum

Lactobacillus species

Leptotrichia buccalis

Neisseria species

Peptococcus species

Peptostreptococcus species

Propionibacterium acnes

Rothia dentocariosa

Selenomonas sputigena

Streptococcus mitis, S. mutans, S. intermedius, S. salivarius, S. sanguis and group D streptococci (enterococci)

Staphylococcus epidermidis

Treponema denticola, T. macrodentium, T. socranskii, etc.

Veillonella alcalescens, V. parvula

Vibrios (especially anaerobic vibrios)

Wolinella recta

include actinomyces species, Rothia, viridans streptococci and *S. epidermidis*.

In elderly patients who are periodontally healthy, Gram-positive bacteria, particularly streptococci, form the largest single group (50% of the predominant cultivable flora), while Gram-negative bacteria only account for 30%. The latter, however, include bacteroides and fusobacterium species.

Early (and experimental) gingivitis. If plaque is allowed to accumulate as a result of stopping toothbrushing for several days the plaque increases in thickness and is typically 100 to 300 cells thick. In these earliest stages the number of bacteria increases but the plaque remains Gram-positive in character and actinomyces species become predominant.

Chronic gingivitis. With the passage of time, persistence of plaque leads to chronic inflammation, and as this happens Gram-negative organisms become increasingly prominent and veillonella, fusobacterium and campylobacter species are conspicuous.

Destructive periodontitis. With the development of pocketing and formation of subgingival plaque there is a great increase in the number of bacteria of all kinds. Subgingival plaque seems to have a dense zone attached to the tooth surface where the bacteria are mainly Gram-positive. The zone of plaque related to the gingival surface, by contrast, is less densely packed but includes large numbers of Gram-negative bacteria (including anaerobes and spirochaetes). Organisms particularly associated with destructive disease include *Bacteroides gingivalis**, *A. actinomycetemcomitans*, *B. intermedius*, *Wolinella recta*, spirochaetes with axial filaments, or in other cases *Eikenella corrodens*, and other corroding bacteria. The latter are so named because on culture their colonies cause pitting ('corrosion') of the surface of the agar. Also present are *Fusobacterium nucleatum* and as yet unidentified anaerobic vibrios and spirochaetes.

Where there is severe and relatively acute bone loss in young adults, for example, associated with severe inflammation, *Actinobacillus actinomycetemcomitans* and *Bacteroides gingivalis*, *Clostridium*

malenominatum* and *Clostridium sporogenes* appear to be particularly important.

Where inflammation is minimal in spite of extensive bone loss there may be greater numbers of *Bacteroides melaninogenicus* and *Eikenella corrodens*.

It is perhaps worth emphasising again that many of the bacteria implicated in destructive periodontitis, such as *Fusobacterium nucleatum* and bacteroides species, are potent pathogens and the most frequently isolated from severe or lethal anaerobic systemic infections. More recently *Capnocytophaga ochraceus*, *Selenomonas sputigena* and *Eikenella corrodens* have been implicated in life-threatening infections, particularly in patients with granulocytopenia.

In human periodontal disease attempts to incriminate particular bacteria as specific pathogens have not yet yielded clear answers. Moreover, if anaerobes are the main pathogens, the infection will virtually inevitably be mixed in character because of the dependence of many anaerobes on other bacteria for production of an anaerobic environment and, often, essential growth factors.

It may therefore be that the empirical method of reducing the total bacterial population by removing dental plaque may be the most satisfactory method of control of the disease.

The ability of individual species of bacteria to damage the periodontal tissues can, however, be tested in gnotobiotes.

Periodontal disease in gnotobiotes

Inoculation of particular bacteria into the mouths of germ-free animals has yielded somewhat unexpected results. Thus, various Gram-positive bacteria typically produce large amounts of plaque but Gram-negative bacteria do not. Certain bacteria of either group could induce or accelerate periodontal tissue damage but there was typically little in the way of an inflammatory response or lymphocytic infiltrate in the tissues. In Gram-positive infections also, few osteoclasts were seen. Among the latter, *A. viscosus* has been shown to produce a bone-resorbing factor. Gram-negative bacteria, however, seem more likely to stimulate osteoclastic activity, and numerous osteoclasts were seen at the sites of tissue destruction.

The possibility that individual species of bac-

---

* termed *Bacteroides asaccharolyticus* in earlier classifications

teria may be responsible (in part at least) for periodontal tissue destruction is also suggested by the report that in monkeys the severity of periodontal damage correlated well with the numbers of *Bacteroides gingivalis* which could be isolated. Further (it was reported) anti-microbial treatment that suppressed *B. gingivalis* lead to healing and bone regeneration. Increased numbers of *B. gingivalis* have also been reported to be associated with increased periodontal disease activity in humans.

Bacterial mediators of tissue damage

Periodontal destruction may result from the actions of bacterial products (such as collagenase for example) or indirectly from immunologically mediated processes or from both in varying degree.

Bacterial products (virulence factors) that may contribute to tissue damage include the following:

1. Enzymes
2. Lipopolysaccharides (endotoxins) and lipoteichoic acid
3. Bone-resorbing factors
4. Interference with host defences.

Enzymes. In view of the destruction of periodontal fibres, bacterial collagenases have been subjected to extensive study. Bacteroides species, for example, produce collagenase, trypsin, fibrinolysin, hyaluronidase, chondroitin sulphatase, heparinase, ribonuclease and deoxyribonuclease. Cytotoxic metabolic products such as indole, ammonia and hydrogen sulphide may also be important. Bacteroides species, especially *B. gingivalis*, are regularly associated with human destructive periodontitis.

Toxins. Bacterial toxins have been traditionally divided into exotoxins and endotoxins. Exotoxins are proteins released by bacteria and capable of causing severe and usually specific damage to certain types of cells. The neurotoxin produced by *Clostridium tetani* in tetanus is a classic example. Very few bacteria associated with periodontal disease produce exotoxins of pathogenic significance, but certain strains of *Actinobacillus actinomycetemcomitans* produce a powerful leukotoxin, and

Bacteroides gingivalis and *B. intermedius* produce an epitheliotoxin.

Endotoxin is a lipopolysaccharide (LPS) component of Gram-negative bacteria cell walls. It is released primarily after cell lysis, and its lipid region is responsible for direct toxicity. It can cause release of lysosomal enzymes from phagocytes and activates complement via the alternative pathway. Endotoxins can therefore mediate an inflammatory response. Endotoxins from some bacteria have been shown to enhance osteoclastic resorption to variable degrees. For instance endotoxin from *B. gingivalis* is ten times as potent as that from *A. actinomycetemcomitans* in this activity.

The Gram-positive cell wall component, lipoteichoic acid (LTA) is also a potent mediator of inflammation and enhances bone resorption.

Bone resorbing factors. Actinomyces viscosus was among the first bacteria to be shown to produce factors which cause decalcification of bone in vitro. Lipopolysaccharide can also produce bone resorption under experimental conditions, as can crude soluble extracts of human supragingival plaque and some other bacterial products. Bacterial factors can also cause bone resorption by stimulating release of, or acting synergistically with, the lymphokine, osteoclast activating factor and prostaglandin E_2.

Interference with host defence mechanisms

Other virulence factors act by interfering with host defences. Substances (leukotoxins) cytotoxic for human leucocytes are produced by *A. actinomycetemcomitans* in particular. This organism is involved in juvenile periodontitis and is a cause of osteomyelitis and infective endocarditis in humans.

Other bacterial factors potentially capable of damaging host defences are immunoglobulin proteases. It has long been known that *N. gonorrhoea* can produce IgA proteases which seem likely to help it overcome mucosal defences and to contribute to the inability of infected persons to develop protective immunity. Several of the oral viridans streptococci have also been shown to produce IgA proteases.

Lipopolysaccharides, dextran and levan may also have immunosuppressive properties, but under different circumstances may be immunopotentiating.

Immunological aspects

General considerations

There is little doubt that plaque antigens trigger immune responses—it would be abnormal if they did not. However, these responses are for the most part protective (as in most infections), and their contribution to tissue damage, though widely assumed, is more controversial.

Periodontitis is a typical chronic inflammation in which there may be acute exacerbations interspersed with periods of tissue repair. The inflammatory and immune responses are both local and systemic. They involve the mucosal immune system, phagocytic cells (neutrophils and macrophages), the complement system, lymphocytes, antibody production and immunoregulatory mechanisms. There are complex interactions between these arms of the immune system, and, therefore, involvement of even one component in tissue destruction can quite readily involve the others. The literature is replete with claims for greater importance of one component rather than another.

Though it is widely believed that immunological reactions contribute to tissue damage in periodontitis it has not proved possible to distinguish the effects of the microbes from those of the immune response.

Mucosal immunity

Bacteria are important in periodontal disease particularly because of their ability to colonise non-shedding tooth surfaces. Later in the disease, when pockets have formed, bacteria may also colonise the epithelium of the pocket lining. Antibodies which are important in prevention of bacterial adherence to oral surfaces are IgA class and are derived from two sources. Secretory (salivary) IgA is produced within the salivary glands and is secreted in saliva. Minute amounts of serum IgA are present in the gingival inflammatory exudate and can be detected in whole saliva. Mucosal immunity may be important in preventing bacterial invasion of the tissues in addition to the defence afforded by phagocytes. However, it has been shown that putative periodontal pathogens, notably *Bacteroides gin-*

givalis and Capnocytophaga species produce enzymes able to cleave and inactivate IgA and IgG and may therefore seriously damage immune defences.

Phagocytes, complement and antibodies

Phagocytosis of bacteria by neutrophils and macrophages is a basic protective response. These cells are capable of phagocytosis and killing of microorganisms by both oxygen-dependent and oxygen-independent mechanisms; the latter may be of value within the anaerobic environment of the periodontal pocket. Patients with neutrophil defects such as agranulocytosis, Chediak–Higashi disease and lazy-leucocyte syndrome have more severe periodontal disease than normal persons, and this makes it clear that the function of neutrophils is largely protective. Further evidence comes from patients with localised juvenile periodontitis who have depressed neutrophil chemotaxis and phagocytosis. However, phagocytes may also cause tissue damage by extracellular release of their enzymes during phagocytosis and after cell death. This causes tissue destruction in acute abscesses and may promote the progression of periodontitis if it should lead to short acute bursts of inflammation, as suggested by some workers. It is possible that such an event could be consistent with tissue invasion by bacteria which is normally prevented by the phagocytes.

Bacteria have been demonstrated in the tissues in periodontitis and occasionally within phagocytes. The fact that bacteria enter the tissues is hardly surprising as bacteraemias are known to be a frequent consequence of minimal trauma, such as toothbrushing. However, definitive proof of bacterial invasion would require the demonstration of bacterial proliferation within the tissues. This has not been shown in periodontitis.

As mentioned earlier, complement can be activated by endotoxin via the alternative pathway or by immune complexes via the classical pathway. Activation of complement by immune complexes is an essential feature of type 3 (immune complex) hypersensitivity reactions, but the evidence for this mechanism of tissue damage in periodontitis is unconvincing. Increased levels of complement components are found within gingival fluid in diseased sites, and the presence of C3 and Factor B cleavage products is evidence of local activation via the alternative pathway. The complement system produces most of its effects by active peptides produced within a cascade system. Neutrophil and macrophage chemotaxis is enhanced by C5a. Phagocytosis is facilitated by adherence brought about by C3b which acts synergistically with IgG. Inflammation is potentiated by C3a and C5a which cause histamine release from mast cells and basophils, thus increasing vascular permeability. Complement components may also be involved in cell killing, lysosomal enzyme release, bone resorption and lymphokine production, all of which have potentially damaging effects.

Antibodies, like most components of the immune system are protective. They can enhance

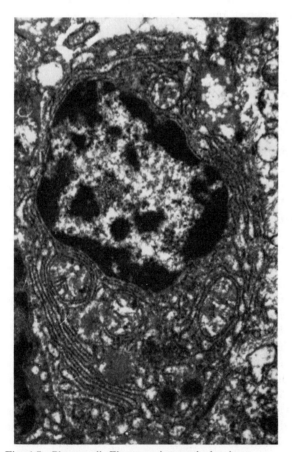

Fig. 6.7 Plasma cell. Electron micrograph showing a plasma cell from the gingiva. The much folded endoplasmic reticulum is indicative of protein synthesis (antibody formation).

phagocytosis by opsonisation of specific bacterial antigens. Significantly higher levels of IgG to putative periodontal pathogens such as *Bacteroides gingivalis* are found in the serum of some adult periodontitis patients, although there is considerable variation among individuals. There is a good correlation between serum antibody levels and bacterial species within the pockets. High levels of antibodies to *A. actinomycetemcomitans* and its leukotoxin have been found in localised juvenile periodontitis and likewise to *B. intermedius*, and to spirochaetes in acute ulcerative gingivitis. Antibody levels within gingival fluid may be higher than serum levels because of a local production by the many plasma cells within the diseased tissue (Fig. 6.7). Much of the locally produced antibody may be non-specific polyclonal/mitogen-induced, but currently used highly sensitive techniques have demonstrated specific antibodies.

In addition to antibody production against periodontal bacteria, antibodies against bacteria entering other parts of the body are detectable in serum leaking into periodontal pockets. There is also evidence of polyclonal B cell activation in periodontal disease but, again, the role of such phenomena in periodontal tissue destruction remains speculative.

Immunoregulatory substances

Early studies concentrated on cell-mediated immunity and showed lymphocyte transformation and lymphokine production in response to various plaque bacteria. However, it was not appreciated that non-specific stimulation by mitogens or polyclonal activation could be induced, particularly by Actinomyces antigens. It has been suggested that killing of fibroblasts by cytotoxic T cells or natural killer cells may operate in periodontitis but that the major effects result from lymphokine production. Lymphokine production following stimulation was largely thought to be a T lymphocyte response but it is now known that B lymphocytes may produce far greater amounts. Lymphokines include alpha-lymphotoxin, which can cause fibroblast cell death, macrophage activating factor, which increases collagenase secretion by macrophages, and osteoclast activating factor, which is homologous with Interleukin

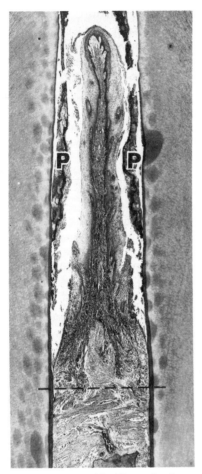

Fig. 6.8 Advanced periodontitis. The pocket has extended well below the amelocemental junction, and heavy deposits of subgingival plaque (P) can be seen on either side of the gingival tissue. It will be obvious that the inflammatory infiltrate is concentrated in the vicinity of the plaque (above dotted line) and the connective tissue above the alveolar bone is virtually free of immunologically active cells.

2. Interleukin 2 is detectable in gingival fluid and is an important mediator of inflammation by its involvement in antigen presentation to T cells. The fibrosis seen in periodontitis may be enhanced by the lymphokine, fibroblast–activating factor.

There has been much controversy as to whether cell-mediated immunity or humoral immunity is more important in progression of periodontitis. The stable lesion of gingivitis in children is dominated by T lymphocytes, while in established periodontitis B lymphocyte and plasma cells predominate. The widely used terms 'B cell lesion' or 'T cell lesion' have little meaning in im-munological terms except in relation to lymphomas, but in relation to periodontitis they are meant to imply predominantly humoral or cell-mediated reactions, respectively. The importance of these differences in cell populations may possibly be clarified when our understanding of immunoregulatory processes increases. For example, it has been proposed that local tissue alterations in immunoregulation could lead to tissue destruction or, on the other hand, protection.

As mentioned earlier, control of B cells is mediated by T cells which can be subdivided into helper (T4 or CD4) and suppressor (T8 or CD8) subsets. Immunoregulation also involves interactions with antigen-presenting cells which express Class II major histocompatibility antigens. In early gingivitis and childhood gingivitis the T4:T8 ratio is approximately 2:1. In periodontitis this ratio has been reported to be about 1:1, but other studies have shown a decreased proportion of T8 cells. Whether any changes in the balance of immunoregulatory activities are the cause or the result of the disease, however, remains a matter for speculation.

The clinical significance of immunological phenomena in periodontal disease

Abnormally severe periodontitis develops in patients with neutrophil abnormalities and in AIDS where there is severe depression of cell-mediated immunity.

Reduced neutrophil chemotaxis and phago-cytosis in some diabetics may be responsible for more severe periodontitis and a tendency to develop abscesses. In Down's syndrome there are typically multiple immunodeficiencies which also include depressed neutrophil phagocytosis. As a result there is increased susceptibility to infection and, in particular, periodontal destruction which starts in childhood. Rapid periodontal destruction can also result from acute leukaemia and, as mentioned earlier, can be a feature of AIDS.

Immunosuppressed patients, typically those on drugs for organ transplants, have reportedly no change in susceptibility to periodontal disease when compared to matched control subjects. Many studies on these patients took no account of the anti-inflammatory properties of these drugs

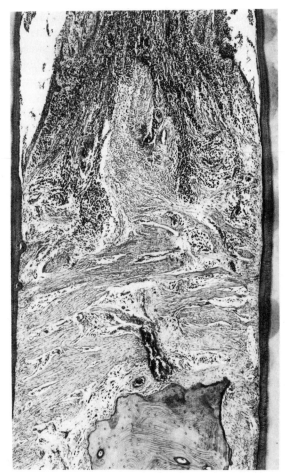

Fig. 6.9 A higher power view of the previous specimen shows the cell-free zone above the alveolar bone.

which inevitably suppressed the clinical signs of gingivitis. However, more prolonged studies have suggested that the rate of periodontal destruction is not necessarily accelerated.

The overall progress of periodontitis in the long term is almost immeasurably slow in most cases. Thus, even in the presence of chronic, uncomplicated periodontal disease, destruction of 10 mm of attachment often takes 50 years. This is an average of 1 mm in 5 years and is therefore undetectable in radiographs taken at yearly intervals. Attempts to measure clinical progress of disease by probing measurements are greatly hampered by inherent measurement errors, due to alterations in the position and angulation of the probe, force applied

and tissue resistance. Thus it has been suggested that the probing depth has to increase by at least 3 mm before it can be certain that the disease has progressed. That is not to say that there has been 3 mm true loss of attachment but that the change is greater than the expected measurement error. Problems such as this have created renewed interest in hypotheses suggesting that periodontitis progresses in short bursts rather than as a slow insidious process. There is such variability among individuals and among sites within the same individual that the disease could progress in either or both ways.

Under these circumstances it is practically impossible to correlate laboratory findings of immunological phenomena with the progress of periodontal destruction. Moreover this insidiously slow process (in most persons) in the presence of innumerable bacterial pathogens in plaque, strongly suggests that immune responses in periodontal disease are predominantly protective*.

Immunological aspects of periodontal disease—summary

1. Immune responses to plaque antigens are the formation of antibodies and development of cell-mediated immunity. Complement may also be activated.
2. There is a good correlation between serum antibody levels and specific pocket bacteria.
3. Immune responses are in the main protective, but immunologically mediated tissue damage might be mediated by any of the 4 types of hypersensitivity reaction.
4. Immunologically mediated tissue damage cannot be recognised by any direct means. It is to be expected that there are immune responses to plaque antigens—it would be abnormal if there were not—but such responses are not in themselves indicative of immunologically mediated tissue damage.

---

* Those who are not committed to immunological theorising about the causes of oral disease may, incidentally, wonder why the current fixation seems to be that immune responses to dental caries are 'good' (protective) but in periodontal disease are 'bad' (destructive). Such diametrically opposite biological responses to diseases that have the same basic cause (bacterial plaque) seems remarkably capricious.

5. In gnotobiotes, various plaque pathogens cause severe periodontal destruction, but there is little histological evidence of the participation of immunologically active cells in this process.

6. In human periodontal disease also, the histological findings are not particularly suggestive of immunologically mediated injury.

7. The reported reduction in the severity of gingivitis in patients having immunosuppressive treatment (as evidence of immunological mechanisms in periodontal disease) is no more than a manifestation of the anti-inflammatory actions of corticosteroids and other immunosuppressive drugs. This finding provides no information about the rate of tissue destruction in immunosuppressed patients.

8. Immunodeficiency is typically associated with accelerated microbial tissue damage and is strikingly shown by the early onset of destructive periodontitis in Down's syndrome and, especially, in AIDS.

9. The very slow progress of chronic periodontitis in most persons, in spite of the presence of innumerable pathogenic bacteria in plaque, strongly suggests that immune responses are predominantly protective in periodontal disease.

10. The many reported immunological findings in periodontal disease have no practical implications for its management, which remains dependent on conventional methods of controlling plaque.

Other factors

There is no doubt that gingivitis develops if plaque is allowed to accumulate for a day or two. It is also readily demonstrable that gingivitis subsides when plaque is removed.

Nevertheless, the severity of periodontal disease shows wide variation not directly related to the severity of the deposits on the teeth. This was confirmed by an extensive study on American adults where the combined effects of age, plaque and cal-

culus accounted statistically for only about 32% of the variation in scores for loss of attachment.

In more extensive (though less detailed) surveys in Britain (Ch. 26) it is apparent that, though women generally have lower scores for deposits on the teeth and gingivitis, nevertheless they lose their teeth significantly earlier and more women are edentulous than men. It also appears that the prevalence of gingivitis does not correspond closely with the proportion of people with deposits on the teeth.

Pregnancy is an important example of a physiological change which nevertheless leads to an abnormally severe response to gingival plaque.

Stagnation areas which allow plaque to accumulate also do not necessarily aggravate periodontal disease. In conditions characterised by fibrous gingival hyperplasia, inflammation, in spite of gross false pocketing, is often inconspicuous.

In the case of prepubertal periodontitis, where destruction of the supporting tissues may start almost as soon as the teeth erupt, there is typically a phagocyte defect. It can affect both dentitions and usually leaves the patient totally edentulous in early adolescence.

In one rare syndrome (Papillon Lefevre) rapid periodontal destruction is associated with hyperkeratosis of the palms and soles of the extremities. In Ehlers-Danlos syndrome (type VIII) also, early and rapid periodontal destruction is associated with a defect of synthesis of the collagen molecule.

Clearly in these, admittedly uncommon, types of periodontal disease mere accumulation of plaque is inadequate to explain the rapidity of tissue destruction.

While these findings can do no more than raise doubts as to whether plaque is all important in the causation of periodontal disease, they should at least suggest that other factors (such as abnormal lability of bone, cementum or collagen, but as yet unidentified) may play a part.

Systemic and other disorders which may affect periodontal disease

Systemic disease rarely plays any important role in chronic periodontitis but *occasionally* it may be contributory.

Nutritional deficiencies. Vitamin deficiency,

particulary severe and prolonged vitamin C deficiency (scurvy), can produce a characteristic haemorrhagic gingivitis in the advanced stages of the disease but this is hardly ever seen now. Protein and calcium deficiency may also contribute to loss of periodontal supporting tissues, but these also are rarely encountered in Britain and other Western countries.

Endocrine factors. In pregnancy, gingivitis is often exacerbated and there may be proliferative inflammatory changes producing a so-called pregnancy tumour (epulis). Though gingivitis is worsened during this period it does not appear to produce any persistent periodontal damage post-partum. The main consideration is to make sure that good oral hygiene is maintained during pregnancy.

Uncontrolled diabetes mellitus is associated with increased susceptibility to infection and this includes aggravation of gingivitis. Periodontal disease is more severe and periodontal abscesses are common, but the changes are non-specific.

Blood diseases. Acute leukaemia, particularly the myelomonocytic variety, can produce characteristic swelling and ulceration of the gingivae as described later. Though it is uncommon, acute leukaemia should be suspected in a patient with gingival swelling or acute deterioration of gingival disease, particularly when accompanied by pallor of the oral mucosa and petechiae. Swelling and ulceration of the gingivae in a child of recent onset is an especial cause for anxiety on this score; blood examination can quickly confirm or exclude this diagnosis.

Mucocutaneous disorders. Acute primary herpetic stomatitis may be associated with severe gingivitis as described in Chapter 15 but this usually produces a clear-cut clinical picture and makes no lasting contribution to chronic periodontal disease.

Lichen planus, when it affects the gingivae, is usually predominantly of the atrophic type and can produce inflammatory changes extending from the gingival margin across the attached gingiva to the sulcus and sometimes beyond. In addition the soreness of the gingivae, caused by this disease, makes toothbrushing painful. Plaque and gingivitis in turn appear to worsen the lichen planus, and a vicious circle may be set up. Lichen planus is considerably more common than most of the con-

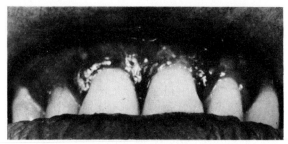

Fig. 6.10 Gingival lichen planus. The atrophic form of this disease has produced the picture of typical 'desquamative gingivitis'.

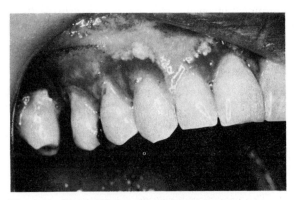

Fig. 6.11 Gingival lichen planus. Another variant characterised by patchy atrophic changes at the gingival margins together with minute white plaques at the borders.

ditions previously mentioned, but, though it can produce severe inflammation of the attached and sometimes the marginal gingivae, its main significance here is that the tenderness of the gingivae may make control of plaque more difficult. Lichen planus does not otherwise appear to aggravate periodontal destruction, and it therefore provides a convincing demonstration that gingival inflammation may not necessarily be caused by plaque accumulation or contribute to periodontal deterioration.

Mucous membrane pemphigoid can produce particularly severe gingival changes as described in Chapter 15. The erosions thus produced also greatly interfere with normal toothbrushing. Mucous membrane pemphigoid is not, however, common; it predominantly affects elderly people and is less likely therefore to cause difficulties in managing periodontal disease.

Lichen planus and mucous membrane pemphigoid are the main causes of so-called *'desquamative gingivitis'*.

Drug treatment. Phenytoin is the most widely used drug which produces significant gingival changes. In susceptible patients (between 30% and 50%) there is more or less severe gingival hyperplasia. A few other drugs such as cyclosporin have a similar effect, as discussed later; but, despite the deep false pocketing that they may induce, inflammation is frequently not apparent clinically or is disproportionally slight.

Immunodeficiencies. As mentioned earlier, immunodeficiency states frequently lead to gross acceleration of periodontitis and tissue destruction. Examples are acute leukaemia, uncontrolled diabetes mellitus, Down's syndrome and, in particular, HIV infection as discussed later. Rapidly progressive or early periodontitis may also be associated with a more minor defect of immune function.

AETIOLOGY OF CHRONIC GINGIVITIS AND PERIODONTITIS SUMMARY

1. Accumulation of bacterial plaque at the gingival margins quickly leads to an inflammatory response and the establishment of gingivitis.
2. Removal of plaque at the gingival margins is followed by subsidence of the inflammation.
3. Plaque consists of microorganisms in a matrix of bacterial polysaccharides. There is some evidence that anaerobes and Gram-negative bacteria are important in causing periodontal damage but the microbiology of plaque is exceedingly complex.
4. Destruction of the supporting tissues (chronic periodontitis) is the usual sequel to chronic gingivitis if sufficiently longstanding. Nevertheless the events leading to the transition from gingivitis to periodontitis are not understood.
5. Although plaque causes gingivitis, epidemiological evidence indicates that variations in the level of oral hygiene account for only part of the variation in the severity of periodontal disease when large groups of people are followed-up over a long period.
6. The mechanisms underlying destruction of the supporting tissues in chronic periodontitis are not firmly established. It is widely believed that tissue damage is caused by plaque bacteria and their products, especially enzymes and endotoxin.
7. It is postulated that tissue destruction by plaque bacteria may be mediated by a variety of immunological mechanisms, but, though a variety of immunological reactions can be detected in vitro in association with periodontal disease, their clinical importance has not been established.
8. Immune responses are, in most cases, predominantly protective and it seems likely that this function may be more important than any (postulated) contribution to tissue damage.
9. Depressed immune responses as in AIDS and Down's syndrome may be characterised by greatly enhanced destruction of periodontal tissues.
10. Definable systemic disorders can—but in fact rarely do—accelerate the progress of periodontal disease.
11. In the present state of knowledge, therefore, management of periodontal disease is by control of plaque.

CHRONIC GINGIVITIS

Histological changes

The stagnant debris round the necks of the teeth can be seen to consist of a dense mass of microorganisms. These provoke chronic inflammatory changes in the gingival margin. The epithelium is hyperplastic and the epithelial ridges ('rete pegs') are elongated. The blood-vessels are dilated and some extend up through the epithelium almost to the surface. Accompanying the blood-vessels are inflammatory cells, mainly plasma cells and lymphocytes, which densely infiltrate the gingival connective tissue.

A heavy predominance of plasma cells is com-

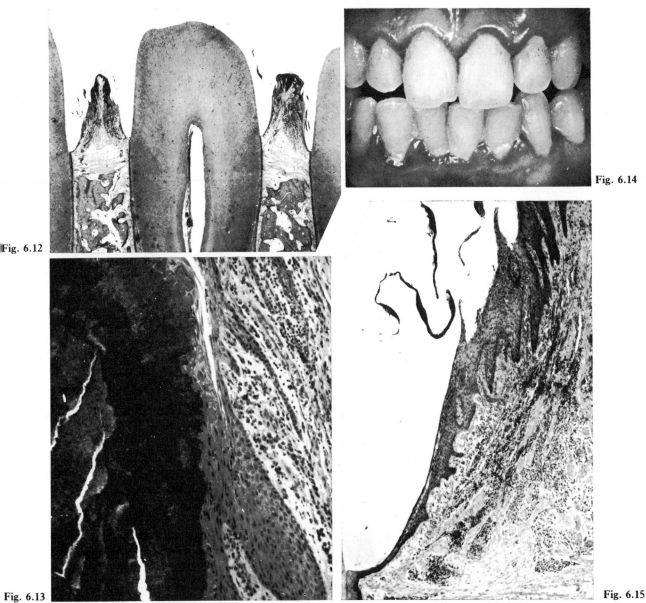

Fig. 6.12

Fig. 6.14

Fig. 6.13

Fig. 6.15

Fig. 6.12 Chronic gingivitis. The gingival tissues, from a woman of 35, show typical changes of chronic marginal gingivitis. Inflammatory changes are entirely localised to the interdental papillae; the upper periodontal fibres and alveolar crest are intact and undamaged and changes do not extend below the amelocemental junction (× 10).

Fig. 6.13 Calculus and the gingival tissues. Calculus can be seen to be built up of successively formed layers, and its basis to be a felted mass of filamentous microorganisms. The gingival epithelium is in close apposition, and chronic inflammatory changes, indicated by the presence of lymphocytes and plasma cells, are present in the underlying tissues (× 65).

Fig. 6.14 Chronic gingivitis. The gingival margins are red and swollen. The lower incisor region, where the teeth are irregular, is more severely affected, and plaque lies along the gingival margin. Traces of blood from the gingival margin are present between some of the upper teeth.

Fig. 6.15 Chronic gingivitis. Part of an interdental papilla from Fig. 6.12 is shown at higher magnification. The junctional epithelium extends to the amelocemental junction; inflammatory changes are most intense in the upper part of the papilla, but groups of inflammatory cells are extending more deeply between the bundles of connective tissue. The sharply defined outline of the epithelial attachment is formed by the enamel cuticle. The curly strips of darkly stained material at the top of the enamel space are bacterial plaque displaced during preparation of the specimen (× 45).

mon in chronic gingivitis and periodontitis, and is associated with local antibody production.

Inflammatory cells spread mainly along the loose connective tissue between the principal fibres which eventually become surrounded by the infiltrate. The gingival margins are oedematous and slightly swollen so that the gingival crevice is deepened. As a consequence stagnation and its effects become progressively more severe. At this stage the periodontal ligament and alveolar bone are undamaged.

Calculus

Calculus is a hard deposit formed on the teeth by calcification of bacterial plaque. Calculus seen on superficial examination (supragingival calculus) is present in greatest amount on the lingual surfaces of the lower anterior teeth and, to a lesser extent, on the buccal surface of the upper molars. These areas are opposite the orifices of the main salivary glands whose secretions are the main source of calcium and other salts which form the hard substance of calculus. Supragingival calculus is usually whitish or creamy in colour but may be more darkly stained. In the lower anterior region calculus starts to form interstitially and along the lingual gingival margins. From here the deposit spreads over the lingual surfaces of the teeth and overhangs the gum. In children little calculus forms.

Histologically, calculus consists of a filamentous bacterial plaque; chemically, calculus consists mainly of calcium phosphates, of which the greater part are in the form of apatite. The mechanisms by which plaque becomes calcified are unknown but several possibilities exist.

When saliva is secreted into the mouth it loses carbon dioxide and becomes more alkaline. This rise in pH may cause calcium salts to be precipitated.

A somewhat similar theory also suggests that the precipitation of calcium salts is due to a local rise in pH but that the alkaline environment is created immediately around the teeth by bacteria breaking down proteins and liberating ammonium ions.

The gingival cells secrete phosphatase. This enzyme may break down organic phosphates from the saliva so that phosphate ions are liberated and calcium phosphates are deposited.

Some filamentous bacteria such as Actinomyces sp. can concentrate calcium intra- and extracellularly and promote crystal growth by a seeding process. The importance of calculus is in the bacteria it harbours, but it should be appreciated that, though calculus is a common accompaniment of gingivitis, it is not a primary cause; it is itself a consequence of stagnation around the teeth and deposition of plaque.

Clinical features

Gingivitis often starts in childhood, and early signs are usually seen at adolescence. There may be complaint of bleeding from the gums, but the patient is often unaware of the disease. The earliest visible change is a darkening of the gingival margin from its normal pale pink to red or even a purplish hue, due to congestion. Plaque is visible along the gingival margins. The gingivae are slightly swollen, soft, smooth and glazed, and the normal surface pattern is lost. Slight pressure on the gums, which are not tender, causes bleeding.

Chronic oedematous ('hyperplastic') gingivitis

In younger patients, especially those who are mouth-breathers or whose mouths are particularly dirty, the gingival margins are swollen and the interdental papillae become bulbous. In this way deep stagnation areas (false pockets) are formed between the gingival margins and teeth. The condition is known as chronic hyperplastic gingivitis, but the swelling is mainly caused by inflammatory oedema. Chronic oedematous ('hyperplastic') gingivitis differs mainly in the degree of the inflammatory changes rather than in its essential nature from chronic simple gingivitis. A distinction must, however, be made between gingival swelling mainly due to inflammatory oedema and true gingival hyperplasia. In the latter there is fibrous overgrowth but inflammatory changes are of a minor degree or secondary to the false pocketing. The distinction is important in that the differences in underlying pathology inevitably affect the management.

Progress of gingivitis

Without adequate treatment or care by the patient, chronic gingivitis usually progresses to chronic periodontitis, namely destruction of the supporting tissues and true pocket formation. There is no finite dividing line between the two conditions, but periodontitis is regarded clinically as being present when the pocket extends on to cementum. Development of the process is usually slow, and in some patients chronic gingivitis may never progress to periodontitis or it may take many years.

Gingival bleeding

Bleeding from the gums is a common complaint and in most cases is due to chronic gingivitis. Occasionally, gingival bleeding may be the result of some systemic disease; the causes of this symptom therefore include the following.

1. *Local disorders*
   a. *Chronic gingivitis and chronic periodontitis*
   b. *Acute ulcerative gingivitis*

These are by far the most common causes of gingival bleeding.

2. *Systemic diseases*
   a. *Acute leukaemia.* In this disease there may be acute gingivitis as a result of the lowered resistance to infection, or haemorrhagic tendencies so that bleeding from the gums is sometimes an early symptom.
   b. *Haemorrhagic disorders.* There is sometimes persistent oozing of blood from the gingival margins in haemophilia, while severe and rapid bleeding from the gums of sudden onset is a well-recognised feature of idiopathic purpura. It may occasionally be the first symptom.
   c. *Scurvy.* Grossly swollen, bleeding gums are characteristic of advanced scurvy, but the disease is rarely seen now and most of the patients are elderly and edentulous.

When bleeding is due solely to gingival disease, the patient's history, the fact that he is otherwise well, and examination of the mouth will make the diagnosis clear. If, however, the history or clinical findings, such as purpura or anaemia, suggest more serious disease, haematological examination must be carried out and will usually provide the diagnosis.

ACUTE PERIODONTITIS

Acute periodontitis is relatively uncommon and is of short duration.

Traumatic periodontitis. Biting suddenly on a hard object or a high restoration causes minor damage to periodontal fibres and localised inflammation with tenderness of the tooth. Removal of the cause is quickly followed by resolution.

Periodontal abscess. This is a localised acute or subacute complication of periodontal disease, characterised by rapid deepening of a pocket and abscess formation in its depth. Periodontal abscess is described later.

Ulcerative gingivitis. If unchecked, infection rapidly and progressively destroys gingiva, alveolar margins and periodontal fibres. This tends to be most severe interdentally, and the deep cratered ulcers, after healing, leave triangular gaps between the teeth where the supporting tissues have been destroyed. One or more segments may be involved

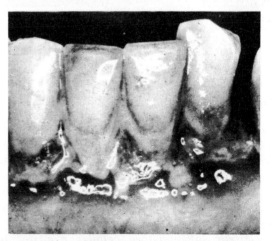

Fig. 6.16 Acute periodontitis in acute ulcerative gingivitis. Rapid destruction of interdental papilla, periodontal ligament and alveolar bone during the course of severe acute ulcerative gingivitis. Necrotic tissue remains between the teeth where the gingival margin stood only a short time previously (see also Fig. 6.6).

but the condition is rarely so severe as to cause generalised periodontal destruction.

CHRONIC PERIODONTITIS

Chronic simple periodontitis is the most common and important type of periodontal disease and is the main cause of loss of teeth in later adult life.

Aetiology and pathology

Conditions predisposing to stagnation of debris and the maintenance of infection at the gingival margins have been discussed in connection with chronic gingivitis. Chronic periodontitis is usually regarded as a continuation of the process of chronic gingivitis. Persistence of infection at the gingival margins leads to progressive inflammation and usually to destruction of the supporting tissues. The disease may progress more rapidly in patients with poor resistance to infection, but this is rarely due to identifiable disease, and in most cases local factors are more important in the development of chronic periodontitis.

There are five main features of the pathology of chronic periodontitis; these are:

1. Inflammation
2. Destruction of periodontal membrane fibres
3. Resorption of alveolar bone
4. Migration of the epithelial attachment along the root towards the apex
5. Formation of pockets around the teeth.

Histological changes

In established chronic periodontitis the following features can be seen on histological examination.

Plaque. On the surface of the tooth and extending into the pocket is bacterial plaque, a dense mat of microorganisms. Some of the plaque is calcified forming calculus and shows a laminated appearance with altered staining.

Chronic inflammatory cellular exudate. Inflammatory cells, mainly plasma cells and lymphocytes, infiltrate the connective tissue and spread between the principal fibres. Dense masses of these cells accumulate, especially under the epithelium in the connective tissue superficial to the alveolar bone. Plasma cells are always present, often predominate and are sometimes virtually the only cells seen.

Pocketing. Formation of pockets is a characteristic and essential feature of chronic periodontitis and is due to the fact that the gingival soft tissues are not destroyed at the same rate as periodontal ligament and bone. By contrast, where the gingival tissue is thin, it may be lost at the same rate as the supporting tissues, and gingival recession therefore results. Pockets round the teeth provide a protected environment in which bacteria can grow freely; there is no effective drainage of septic material, and the wall of the pocket presents a large area where bacteria or their products can irritate the tissues.

Pockets may also favour the growth of anaerobes which probably play an important role in the destructive changes characteristic of periodontal disease.

Pockets surround the tooth; one wall is formed by cementum covering the root, the other by soft tissue replacing the destroyed bone and periodontal fibres. The outer wall consists of connective tissue infiltrated by chronic inflammatory cells and lined by epithelium continuous with the gingival epithelium at the mouth of the pocket. The epithelial attachment forms the deep boundary. The epithelium is hyperplastic but often attenuated, with blood vessels extending through it almost to the surface. 'Ulceration' of the lining (areas of complete destruction of epithelium) is often described but is rarely seen histologically, and in some cases the epithelial lining is surprisingly thick.

Epithelial migration. The epithelium migrates down from the enamel onto and along the cementum, forming the floor of the pocket. The attachment to cementum is strong, and mechanical tears of the epithelium run between the cells, leaving a layer still attached to the cementum. A clear refractile cuticle can sometimes be seen joining the epithelium to the root surface. The length of the epithelial attachment is variable but may be several millimetres long.

Destruction of periodontal fibres. Periodontal fibres are destroyed progressively from the gingival margin towards the apex, down to the level of the

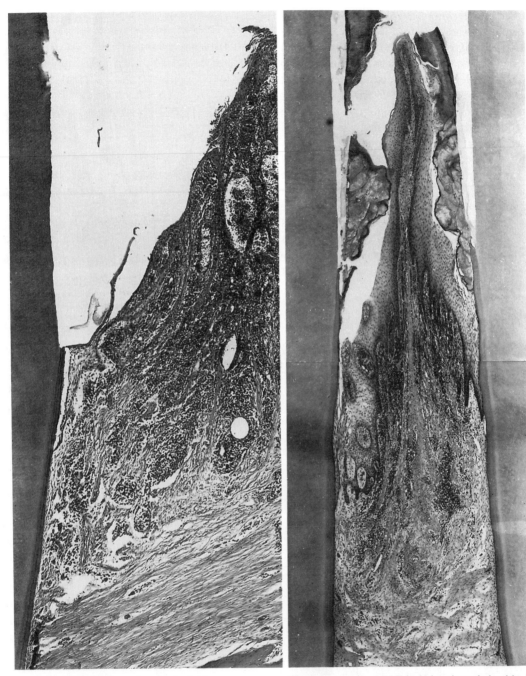

Fig. 6.17   Left: transition from chronic gingivitis to periodontitis. Pocket formation has not yet started but the epithelial attachment has extended onto the cementum and inflammation has spread deeper still.

Fig. 6.18   Right: established chronic periodontitis. In this woman of 33, there are heavy deposits of plaque, shallow pockets have developed and the epithelial attachment has extended considerably more deeply along the cementum. The pockets have a thick, intact epithelial lining and inflammatory cells do not extend significantly beyond the deeper limits of the epithelial attachment. Nevertheless there has been considerable bone loss.

floor of the pocket; more deeply, the fibres retain their normal appearance.

Loss of alveolar bone. The alveolar bone is destroyed and the process starts at the alveolar crest. The usual level of the remaining bone is just deep to the floor of the pocket where the most superficial fibres of the periodontal membrane are attached. The inflammatory focus is separated from the underlying bone by a zone of fibrous tissue. This so-called fibrous walling-off is typical of chronic inflammation and is invariably present. It has been suggested that the inflammatory lesion may extend beyond this to affect the alveolar bone and remaining periodontal ligament during periods of active disease, but histological evidence of this is lacking. Osteoclasts are rarely seen, probably because their action is intermittent and the rate of bone destruction extremely slow.

Subgingival calculus

Subgingival calculus forms within periodontal

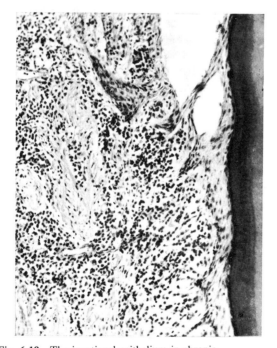

Fig. 6.19 The junctional epithelium in chronic periodontitis. The epithelium has migrated along and gained a firm attachment to the cementum. A tear in the upper part of the junctional epithelium has run between the epithelial cells, leaving a layer adhering to the cementum. Deep to the epithelial attachment are chronic inflammatory cells, mainly plasma cells (× 120).

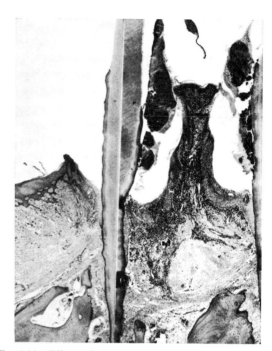

Fig. 6.20 Effects of plaque and stagnation. The mesial and distal aspects of the same tooth are shown. On the right the adjacent tooth is present, stagnation is severe interstitially beneath the contact point, heavy accumulations of plaque are present associated with pocketing and a dense inflammatory cellular exudate extending from the tip of the papilla almost to the bone. On the left, the distal tooth has been removed; the area is accessible to cleansing, plaque is absent, inflammatory changes have virtually disappeared and there is no appreciable pocketing (× 20).

pockets. The deposits are thin, are more widely distributed, harder, darker and more firmly attached than supragingival calculus. The chemical composition of subgingival and of supragingival calculus is similar but the colouring may be due to breakdown products from blood cells oozing into the pockets.

Subgingival calculus is an important feature of chronic periodontitis. It forms a source of plaque, helping to perpetuate inflammatory changes, and it acts as a barrier to healing.

Further progress of chronic periodontitis

The process of chronic periodontitis once established is self-perpetuating. The pockets cannot drain effectively and favour proliferation of bacteria; the epithelial lining, plaque and subgingival calculus effectively prevent healing. Further destruction of the periodontal membrane and alveolar bone causes the pockets to deepen. The natural termination of the process is loosening and exfoliation of the teeth.

Clinical features

The patient may complain of bleeding from the gums or of an unpleasant taste. In the late stages the complaint may be of recession of the gums or loosening of the teeth. The infection is often a cause of foul-smelling breath.

There is chronic gingivitis, and the congested gingival margins become purplish-red, flabby and swollen. The interdental papillae 'split' and can be detached from the teeth. Later the papillae are destroyed and the gingival margin tends to become straight with a swollen, rounded edge. Pressure on the gingival margins causes bleeding, and sometimes pus can be expressed from round the necks of the teeth. Bacterial plaque and calculus are widespread.

Loss of attachment generally leads to pocketing so that a probe can be passed down between teeth and gum. The depth to which the probe passes is a measure of the severity of the disease and is referred to as 'the probing depth' since the true pocket depth cannot be measured accurately by clinical means.

Loss of attachment is measured from the amelocemental junction. In the pockets the rough surface of the subgingival calculus can be felt. In

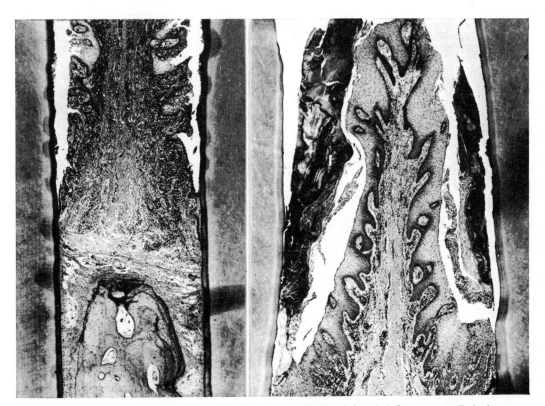

Fig. 6.21 (left) Advanced chronic periodontitis. The dense infiltrate of chronic inflammatory cells is shown in relation to the pockets, the irregularly hyperplastic but somewhat attenuated epithelial lining, and the crest of the alveolar bone. The latter is not infiltrated by lymphocytes, and osteoclasts are also absent; the outline is smooth due to apposition of small amounts of repair tissue (× 25).

Fig. 6.22 (right) Slowly advancing chronic periodontitis. This specimen from a man of 52 may be contrasted with the previous one. In spite of the very large deposits of plaque the pockets are shallow, involving only about 3 mm of cementum. The papilla is covered by a continuous thick layer of epithelium and there is only a mild infiltration of chronic inflammatory cells (× 33).

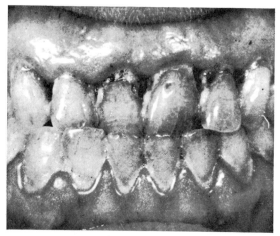

Fig. 6.23 Chronic gingivitis and chronic periodontitis. There is well-established chronic periodontitis in the upper jaw. The gingival margins are red, swollen, rounded and have a rolled appearance: the interdental papillae have been destroyed, and the gingival margin is almost a straight line. There is deep pocketing around the teeth.

In the lower jaw there is chronic gingivitis; the attached gingiva retains its stippled appearance and pale colour, and inflammatory changes are restricted to the gingival margins.

the late stages, the teeth become increasingly loose and dull to percussion.

Radiological changes

The earliest change is loss of definition and blunting of the tips of the alveolar crests. Bone resorption usually progresses in a regular manner and its level remains the same along a row of teeth. A straight line can be drawn along the edge of the alveolar bone at almost any stage of the disorder, and the bone loss is said to be horizontal. This is the characteristic radiological feature of simple periodontitis.

Complex patterns of bone loss are seen in periodontitis, probably due to the effects of variable degrees of loss of attachment superimposed upon the underlying anatomical features. Thus in areas where the bone is thin, its destruction results in horizontal bone loss, whereas in situations where the alveolar bone is thicker, partial destruction gives rise to vertical or angular bone defects.

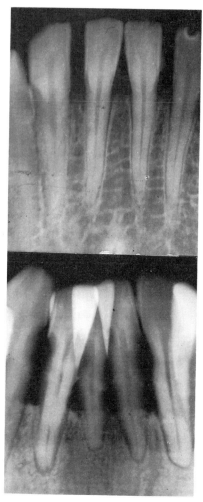

Fig. 6.24 Radiographs showing very early loss of alveolar crest bone (upper) in contrast to typical severe horizontal bone loss of advanced periodontal disease (lower).

GENERAL PRINCIPLES OF MANAGEMENT OF CHRONIC GINGIVITIS AND PERIODONTITIS

The management of periodontal disease can be regarded as comprising three main components. These are:

1. Control of bacterial plaque

2. Establishment of healthy gingiva which is accessible to oral hygiene measures
3. Maintenance of periodontal attachment.

It may be depressing for the reader who has steeped himself in the mysteries of the immunopathogenesis of periodontal disease to find that its management still depends on time-honoured, mechanical methods of plaque control.

Effective daily plaque removal by the patient is essential for successful treatment. This is achieved by mechanical removal of plaque by toothbrushing and interdental cleaning aids such as floss, wooden sticks, or small brushes. This simple measure will bring about complete resolution of simple gingivitis. However, various factors may hinder patient plaque control, and other factors may modify the disease process, including the following.

1. Calculus. Supragingival calculus which usually forms opposite the orifices of the major salivary glands in the lower incisor and upper first molar areas cannot be removed by the patient and provides a rough plaque-retentive surface which prevents the patient from cleaning the dentogingival junction. Calculus should be removed by scaling.

2. Restorations. Poor quality restorative dentistry can promote plaque retention. These defects include overhanging restoration margins, poorly fitting crowns, carious cavities, badly contoured restorations and poorly designed partial dentures. These faults are harmful because of plaque retention rather than any mechanical injury. Restoration overhangs should be removed, defective restorations replaced, or more satisfactory dentures provided. Occasionally, however, direct mechanical damage is produced by partial dentures, particularly lower free-end saddle designs with inadequate tooth and ridge support. These may cause some stripping of the gingiva. This is rarely seen in the upper jaw, where gingival recession under partial dentures is usually due to plaque-induced inflammation in areas of thin gingival tissue. This is particularly likely in patients who wear dentures at night.

3. Irregularities of the teeth. Crowded, irregularly placed teeth are an additional handicap to effective plaque removal. Imbricated incisors are a common

example. Orthodontic treatment may produce more perfect alignment of the teeth, but there is little evidence that this results in any improvement in periodontal health. Interdental spaces between closely approximated roots (most commonly affecting rotated lower canine/lateral incisor and upper first and second molars) may suffer from more severe destruction when affected by periodontitis. They are extremely difficult to treat.

4. Food packing. Food packing in areas where the contact points are poor contributes to plaque retention if the patient allows the impacted material to remain in place.

5. Mouthbreathing. Mouthbreathing or inability to keep the lips closed leads to partial drying of the front of the mouth. The drying of gingiva may alter the vascular response within the tissue, and lack of salivary protection may make gingivitis more severe.

6. Trauma. Overvigorous use of a toothbrush with a sawing motion over the years may be associated with gingival recession. Thin gingiva is more susceptible to this type of damage, which is commonly found on teeth which are prominent in the arch. It is noticeable, however, that the gingival margins usually remain firm and healthy. Occasionally, a patient also complains of sore gums due to traumatic abrasions produced by brushing the attached gingiva. The lesions are usually close to the gingival margin, and some individuals cause sufficient damage to cause bleeding.

Patients, of course, commonly complain that that the gums bleed when the teeth are brushed. This bleeding is, however, invariably a consequence of established gingivitis where the inflamed and engorged gingiva bleed at the slightest contact. It must therefore be explained to the patient that it is not the toothbrushing itself which causes the bleeding but, rather, that oral hygiene has been inadequate to control the gingivitis.

7. Occlusal trauma. Abnormal occlusal forces acting on teeth with normal supporting tissues (primary occlusal trauma) does not cause gingivitis or established gingivitis to progress to periodontitis. Whether excessive occlusal forces acting upon established periodontitis cause more rapid destruction is open to question. Experimental evidence has been provided both for and against this hypothesis. The results are difficult to interpret, since the experimental periodontitis produced in animal models and the methods of applying excessive forces are not directly comparable with the human clinical situation.

Under certain special conditions occlusal relationships can cause *localised* damage to the supporting tissues. This is seen, for instance, when the lower anterior teeth bite directly onto the palatal gingival margins of the upper incisors in class II incisor relationships.

8. Pockets. The most important hindrance to effective plaque control by the patients is the periodontal pocket. The periodontal pocket can be treated by either promoting readaptation of the detached pocket wall to the root surface or surgical removal of the pocket.

Treatment of the periodontal pocket

Successful treatment depends upon effective supragingival plaque removal by the patient and thorough subgingival plaque removal by the dentist or hygienist. Subgingival plaque consists of a firmly adherent, thick mass of bacteria which in many areas calcifies to form hard, black or brown subgingival calculus. Its removal is termed *subgingival scaling*. Effective scaling probably requires the removal of at least some of the root surface cementum to ensure plaque elimination from surface irregularities; the term *root planing* is then usually applied, though, in practical terms there may be no difference from subgingival scaling. The aim of treatment is to produce a 'biologically acceptable' root surface: namely, one to which the detached gingival tissue will adhere. It has been suggested that bacterial endotoxin is an important root surface contaminant which prevents fibroblast and epithelial adherence. Recent work, however, has shown that most endotoxin is located in surface plaque and only minute amounts are found in the underlying cementum. Elimination of subgingival plaque results in resolution of inflammation in the pocket wall. The junctional epithelial attachment to the root surface may increase in length in a coronal direction, and there is usually shrinkage of the gingival margin thus exposing more root surface. The clinical result is increased recession, decreased probing depth and less bleeding on probing. Reduction in the probing attachment levels is also seen—this means that the probe passes less deeply, subgingivally, when measured from a fixed landmark such as the amelocemental junction. Failure to achieve these clinical improvements is due to either a lapse in plaque control by the patient or failure by the dentist to remove subgingival plaque.

Various factors can compromise adequate subgingival plaque removal; these include the following.

1. *Depth of pocket.* The chances of successful débridement decrease with increasing pocket depth. It has been suggested that pockets over 5 mm are unlikely to be adequately scaled.
2. *Root anatomy.* Root grooves, concavities and, particularly, furcations on posterior teeth are very difficult to instrument.
3. *Tooth position.* Treatment is more successful on anterior teeth because, in addition to having a more favourable root morphology, they are easier to reach by both patient and dentist.
4. *Appropriate instruments.* Complex root forms may require specialised instruments. However, studies have shown little difference between conventional hand instruments and ultrasonic scalers.
5. *Operator skill.* As in any dental procedure some operators are more proficient than others.

It should be appreciated that there is great variation in individual response to a given degree of plaque removal. Following subgingival scaling/root planing, and where it is clear that the patient is achieving a good standard of supragingival plaque control (as shown by a healthy-appearing gingival margin), any of the following must be taken as evidence of progressive disease or, at the least, persistence of subgingival inflammation caused by retained plaque:

1. Bleeding or exudation of pus on probing the depth of pocket
2. Increasing probing depths
3. Radiographic deterioration of bone levels.

Under such circumstances, periodontal surgery

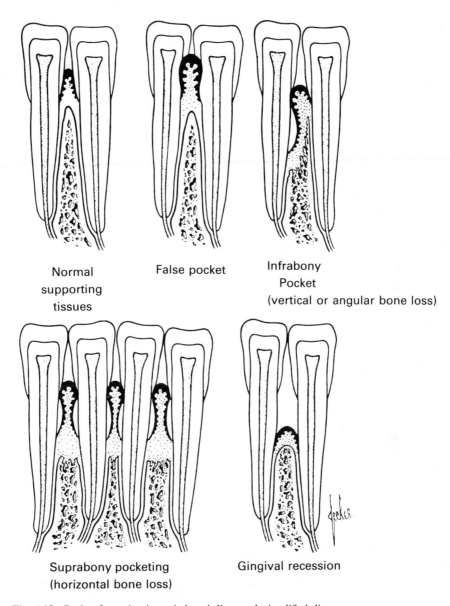

Normal supporting tissues

False pocket

Infrabony Pocket (vertical or angular bone loss)

Suprabony pocketing (horizontal bone loss)

Gingival recession

Fig. 6.25 Pocket formation in periodontal disease. A simplified diagram to show the relationship between periodontal soft tissues and alveolar bone in the different types of periodontal disease.

is often recommended. Surgery can be used to excise the pockets to enable the patient to keep the root surfaces clean. Surgery can also allow access to root surfaces which have proved impossible to render biologically-acceptable by conventional closed instrumentation.

Gingivectomy

The earliest form of excisional or resective surgery was gingivectomy. This is still a useful procedure, particularly in patients with false pockets which fail to resolve with simple treatment. This is often

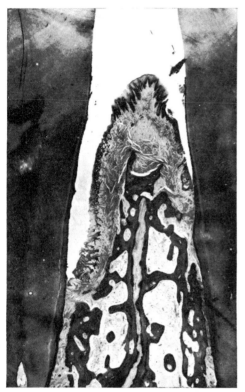

Fig. 6.26 An infrabony pocket. The pocket, with a thick epithelial lining, has extended deeply between the root and alveolar bone on the left, and to a slight extent on the right. The aim of a reattachment operation in this sort of case would be to remove the lining, infected tissue and calculus in the pocket so that the periodontal membrane might reform between the alveolar bone and the cementum. The specimen is from a man of 55 ($\times$ 7).

the case with fibrous gingival overgrowth associated with phenytoin treatment.

The value of gingivectomy is limited when (i) pockets extend beyond the mucogingival junction such that excision would remove all the keratinised gingiva and (ii) the base of the pocket is apical to the bone crest (infrabony pockets— Fig. 6.25). Under such circumstances gingivectomy is not recommended, although it can be argued that keratinised gingiva is not necessary for gingival health and any remaining infrabony pockets can be treated by curettage and root planing.

Gingivectomy for deep pocketing also exposes the necks of the teeth and a 'horse tooth' appearance unacceptable to most patients.

Flap operations

Currently, the most widely used surgical approaches depend upon the elevation of flaps and are designed to remove the inner lining of the pocket whilst preserving the outer keratinised gingiva. Remaining inflamed tissue is curetted away and the root surfaces cleaned. The flaps are then sutured back around the necks of the teeth. There are, in essence, two alternative positions to place the flap. It can be replaced at or near the preoperative level or it can be repositioned apically so that it just covers the alveolar crest. The former approach requires that the flap must reattach to the denuded root surface, whereas the latter aims to eliminate the pocket.

Pocket elimination surgery in its purest form often requires removal of bone to eradicate infrabony pockets. There is obviously a limit to which bone can be removed, and under more difficult circumstances the operator has to rely upon 'reattachment' in the deeper parts of infrabony defects. Apical displacement of the flap may also produce an aesthetically undesirable result, and exposure of complex root forms does not always facilitate plaque control by the patient.

Reattachment type surgery

This has as its ultimate goal the formation of new cementum attaching periodontal ligament fibres to the previously diseased root surface. This ideal result is called 'new attachment' and would obviously be the most satisfactory method of treatment. Unfortunately its attainment has been largely unsuccessful, mainly as a consequence of rapid re-epithelialisation of the root surface and the production of a long junctional epithelium. Until recently, methods designed to retard or redirect epithelial migration at the healing dento-gingival junction have not been successful. Current research suggests that a new connective tissue attachment will only form if repopulation of the root surface by cells from the remaining healthy periodontal ligament is facilitated. This is achieved by the insertion of a barrier membrane between the flap and root surface to prevent epithelial and gingival connective tissue ingrowth and is called 'guided tissue regeneration'. Histological evidence has been produced of new attachment formed after this procedure but in relatively small amounts.

Limitations of periodontal surgery

Periodontal surgery has limitations, particularly in the treatment of multirooted teeth with furcation involvements. Where the pattern of disease has affected one root more than another, more complex treatment involving removal of the affected root (root resection) or half the tooth (hemisection) may be successful.

Despite all these considerations, clinical trials comparing gingivectomy and various flap procedures have shown minimal differences in results under conditions where a high standard of plaque control is maintained. If plaque control is poor they are equally ineffective and may lead to greater loss of periodontal support. Most patients with periodontal disease can be successfully treated with a non-surgical approach, and very similar results have been obtained when studies have compared surgical and non-surgical treatment. Surgery tends to have advantages when treating deep pockets, while the non-surgical approach is better for treating shallower pockets.

Antibiotics in the control of plaque bacteria

Antibiotics reaching the periodontal plaque cause considerable disturbance of the bacterial flora and have the potential for destroying important pathogens. It might seem that this effect would be transient, but it must be borne in mind that the complex mixed bacterial flora of plaque associated with periodontal disease is built up over a period of years.

Another limitation is the development of resistance by plaque bacteria but, though this undoubtedly happens, anaerobes have, in general, maintained patterns of antibiotic sensitivity that do not change as readily as in the case of aerobes.

In the USA especially, antibiotics have been used experimentally, particularly for the management of periodontal disease poorly responsive to conventional treatment.

Overall tetracyclines seem so far to be the most promising agents. They have the widest spectrum of antibacterial activity of all antibiotics, and the side-effects, particularly of topical applications, are minimal. Even when given systemically tetracyclines may reach concentrations in the gingival sulcus several fold greater than serum levels. They also bind to calcified tissues such as cementum.

In several studies tetracyclines have been reported to produce significant changes in the composition of plaque and to improve the clinical state, particularly when used in conjunction with conventional treatment such as root planing. Most recently, tetracycline-containing plastic fibres have been placed in the gingival sulcus for direct delivery of a high local concentration of the drug. In one report at least, putative plaque pathogens such as bacteroides species and other anaerobes were not found to have repopulated the plaque within the period of follow up.

The use of antibiotics as an adjunct to the management of periodontal disease is still controversial, but there is the reasonable hope that in spite of the inevitable development of resistance by many bacteria the disturbance of the composition of plaque may produce long-term reduction in its pathogenicity by interfering with the complex bacterial interactions, allowing proliferation of less harmful species. With the small doses used in topical applications, significant adverse effects are unlikely to be troublesome.

Treatment of advanced periodontal disease

Once pocketing has gone beyond the point where surgical treatment can have any useful effect the teeth should be extracted. Deep pockets are a source of sepsis which may have remote effects such as infective endocarditis and if infection is allowed to persist, excessive resorption of the alveolar bone may result. This may cause difficulties in making satisfactory dentures.

Before extracting these teeth an attempt should be made to reduce the amount of infection in the pockets, as large numbers of bacteria may otherwise be released into the bloodstream. Care should be taken during the extractions as the teeth are often unexpectedly firmly attached in spite of severe bone-loss and, in older patients especially, the roots of the teeth are frequently sclerosed and brittle.

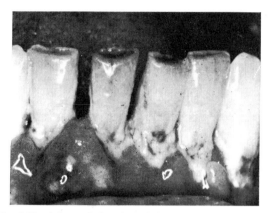

Fig. 6.27 Advanced chronic periodontitis. There is severe destruction of alveolar bone and the teeth are drifting apart; thick accumulation of plaque covers the necks of the teeth, the gingival margins are swollen and inflamed and a periodontal abscess is pointing below the gum margin.

Periodontal traumatism

Damage to the periodontal tissues can be caused by abnormal stresses imposed on the teeth. A blow on the tooth or biting on a high filling may cause damage to the periodontal membrane, acute inflammation and pain (acute periodontitis).

Occasionally, intermittent excessive occlusal forces damage the ligament; this is referred to as 'the lesion of occlusal trauma'. Compression of the ligament fibres and thrombosis of the blood vessels lead to an area of avascular necrosis: the loss of definition of the fibre bundles is described as hyalinisation. The adjacent alveolar bone is resorbed both from its surface and from within the marrow spaces, ('undermining resorption'). This results in widening of the ligament space and increased mobility of the tooth. In this way the ligament gradually adapts to the forces and a normal histological appearance is restored except for the increased width. This may also be apparent radiographically. When applied to a tooth with a normal healthy periodontium this is called 'primary occlusal trauma'. The same response is seen in teeth with reduced but healthy support, except that there appears to be a limit at which the adaptive capability of the remaining ligament is exceeded. Under these circumstances the tooth suffers from ever-increasing mobility to the point

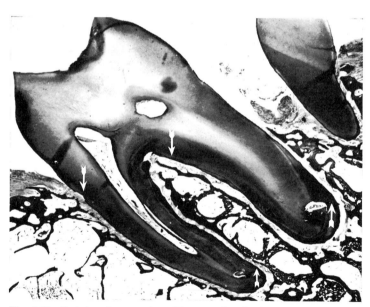

Fig. 6.28 Periodontal traumatism. The second molar has erupted at an angle, and abnormal, oblique stresses are imposed on the supporting tissues. The force of occlusion imposes a tilting movement compressing the periodontal membrane most severely in the direction of the arrows where there is active resorption of the bone and widening of the periodontal membrane ($\times$ 4).

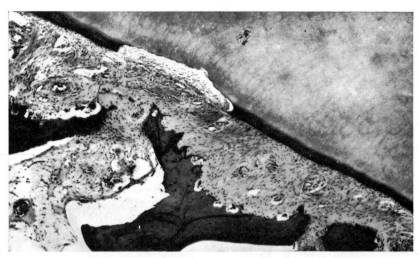

Fig. 6.29 Periodontal traumatism. Part of the previous specimen from near the gingival margin shows the effect of excessive pressure on the supporting tissues. There is resorption of the normally smooth lamina dura by osteoclasts and of dentine and cementum. The periodontal membrane has thus become widened. The specimen is from a woman of 37 ($\times$ 48).

where its loss becomes inevitable. This may be prevented by splinting, and is one of the few indications for this form of treatment. However, this situation should not be confused with the much more common one where increasing tooth mobility is due to failure to treat a progressing plaque-induced periodontitis effectively. The tooth may also be subjected to excessive occlusal forces which could act in a codestructive fashion with periodontitis. Splinting in this case is largely palliative, as it is unlikely to slow progression of disease, and extraction becomes inevitable sooner or later.

The subject of 'occlusion' has been inflated until some seem even to believe that it is a branch of dentistry in its own right. As a result, complicated procedures have been devised to bring about complete occlusal harmony. Unfortunately, there is little scientific evidence that these procedures are of any benefit, particularly if the supporting tissues are initially healthy. Nevertheless removal of obvious sources of occlusal imbalance or disharmony can presumably do no harm and may do some good when periodontal disease is also present. The more logical alternative view is that if the periodontal disease is adequately treated by

plaque removal then the occlusal forces cannot act codestructively.

Periodontal (lateral) abscess

Periodontal abscess is a complication of periodontal disease and results from acute infection of a pocket.

The causes of this acute exacerbation of inflammation are uncertain but it may be the result of some change in the pocket flora or damage by a foreign body such as a fish bone driven through the floor of a pocket. Food packing down between the teeth with poor contact points may also contribute. Drainage through the mouth of the pocket is poor, and is made worse by inflammatory oedema and swelling of the soft tissues.

The pocket deepens rapidly by destruction of periodontal fibres, sometimes to the apex of the tooth, and extends beyond the epithelial lining of the pocket.

The alveolar bone in the floor of the original pocket is destroyed, and the pocket extends between the tooth and alveolar bone. In some anatomical circumstances an infrabony pocket is thus formed. The vertical surface of the bone

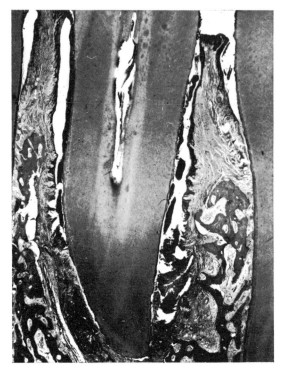

Fig. 6.30 Acute periodontal abscess. There is well-advanced chronic periodontitis, but acute inflammatory changes have developed in this pocket with destruction of periodontal ligament and alveolar bone extending to the apex with formation of an abscess and a deep infrabony pocket. From a man of 55 (× 8).

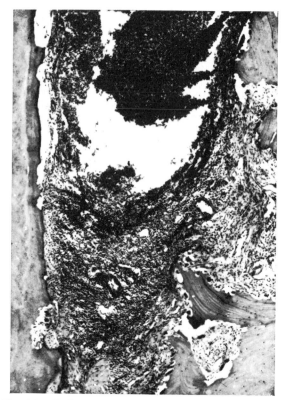

Fig. 6.31 Periodontal abscess. The floor of the abscess shows acute inflammatory changes with dense infiltration of the tissues by polymorphonuclear leucocytes and suppuration. The lamina dura has been destroyed and the alveolar bone is being actively resorbed by osteoclasts; the abscess is extending both laterally and deeply; the cementum has been resorbed in many places (× 48).

forming the wall of the pocket is actively resorbed, and many osteoclasts can be seen. There is a dense infiltration of polymorphonuclear leucocytes and suppuration.

Clinical features

The onset is rapid; there is soreness of the gum which soon develops into throbbing pain. The tooth affected is usually vital and is tender to percussion. The overlying gum is red, swollen and tender to touch. Pus may be seen exuding from the pocket, but a more deeply formed periodontal abscess may point on the buccal mucous membrane forming a sinus. The vitality of the tooth and its less severe tenderness usually distinguish a lateral abscess from acute apical periodontitis. More generalised chronic periodontitis is usually associated. The great depth of the pocket from which pus may be seen to come, helps to make the diagnosis clear.

Changes are not visible radiologically until the condition has been present for about a week; an area of radiolucency may then be seen beside the tooth.

Treatment

A periodontal abscess may be drained and infected tissue removed by subgingival curettage, and the root surfaces thoroughly débrided. Occasionally a surgical approach is needed if access is difficult. Alternatively the affected tooth may be extracted, and this is the most suitable method of treatment if, as it often is, periodontal disease affecting adjacent teeth is severe.

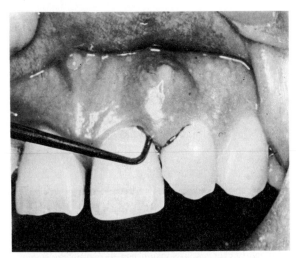

Fig. 6.32 Periodontal abscess. The abscess is pointing on the gum well above the gingival margin. The probe is inserted deeply in the pocket communicating with the abscess.

Prognosis in periodontal disease

It is impossible to make reliable predictions about the results of treatment but some indication of the likelihood of success can be gained from the following considerations.

1. *Severity of disease*
   — degree of attachment loss
   — pocket depth
   — bone loss.
2. *Age.* In patients with the same amount of destruction of supporting tissues, the older the patient the better the prognosis will be because, presumably, the disease is of slower progress.
3. *Oral hygiene status.* The degree of destruction can be related to the degree of insult that the tissues are receiving. Individual susceptibility varies enormously and ranges from patients with gross plaque accumulations and minimal disease to those with advanced destruction but little plaque. The former obviously have a much more favourable prognosis than the latter.
4. *Tooth factors*
   — tooth type
   — root length

— root anatomy/degree of furcation involvement
— restorative/endodontic status
— prosthetic status.
5. *Patient motivation.* Is the patient sufficiently motivated to carry out an effective standard of plaque control and willing to subject themselves to treatment?
6. *Unidentifiable individual factors.* Despite intensive investigation, there remains, for no clear reasons, a 'high risk' group for periodontitis who suffer more extensive bone loss than others of similar age.

Juvenile periodontitis and periodontosis

Juvenile periodontitis is an uncommon condition with a prevalence of about 1:1000, affecting males and females equally, and not predominantly females as was earlier believed. Its onset is supposedly around puberty or earlier, and it is characterised by rapid periodontal destruction often in the absence of overt gingival inflammation. The term periodontosis was often applied to this condition when its aetiology was more obscure. However, the terms juvenile periodontitis and periodontosis are used more or less synonymously.

Juvenile periodontitis most often affects the permanent first molars and incisors in its localised form and rarely is more generalised. The generalised form appears to be a less clearly definable disease entity, and differentiation from other rare forms of early onset periodontitis is far from clear. Several systemic diseases can cause early onset periodontal destruction but the term 'juvenile periodontitis' is reserved for cases in which clinically significant organic disease is absent.

Aetiology and pathology

There is a familial predisposition but it is also believed that the immediate cause is a specific bacterial infection and an associated neutrophil defect. The bacterium commonly found in the diseased sites is *Actinobacillus actinomycetemcomitans*, strains of which produce a potent leukotoxin. Antibodies to the organism and the leukotoxin are found in

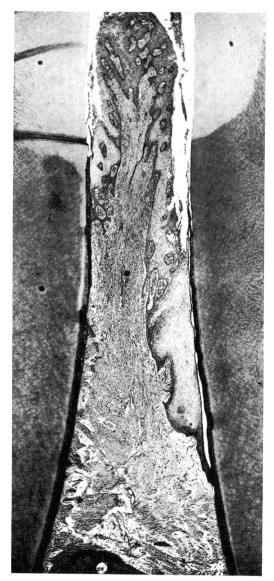

Fig. 6.33 Periodontosis. The periodontal tissues in a man of 32, showing severe loss of alveolar bone and gross overgrowth of the epithelial attachment but striking absence of inflammatory changes and minimal pocketing (× 26).

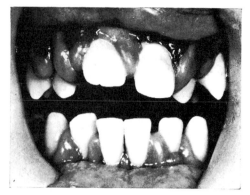

Fig. 6.34 Juvenile periodontitis. The patient, a girl of 11 in good general health, shows drifting and displacement of the teeth, many of which were loose. There is chronic hyperplastic gingivitis which, together with the slight inflammatory changes, was insufficient to explain the state of the supporting tissues.

the serum and gingival fluid. Neutrophils from many patients suffer from a defect in chemotaxis and reduced surface receptor binding capacity. The defect may be genetically determined, while acquisition of the organism is presumably from other family members.

From the small amount of material that has become available for histological examination it appears that there is degeneration of the principal fibres of the periodontal membrane, which become replaced by a loose oedematous network of connective tissue, and resorption of the alveolar bone.

Clinical features

The incisor and first molar teeth are usually the most severely affected and the main feature is drifting and loosening, most noticeable in the front of the mouth. The teeth may also tilt or become extruded. There is a tendency for the condition to slow down or burn-out in some individuals in their twenties. This is referred to as post-juvenile periodontitis.

Radiological features

The main features of periodontosis are deep, angular bone-loss and the displacement of the anterior teeth that has been described. The remarkable symmetry seen in this condition is often such as to make each side of the mouth appear almost as a mirror image of the other.

Treatment

Severely affected teeth may require extraction. Currently, early surgical treatment and tetracycline administration are advised. Surgical

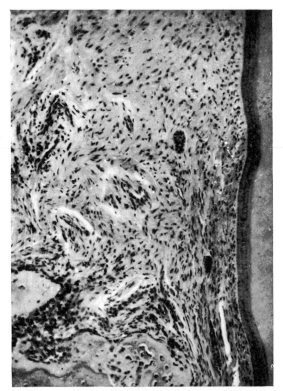

Fig. 6.35 Juvenile periodontitis. A specimen from the same patient as in Figure 6.34 shows, on section, that the alveolar bone and principal fibres of the periodontal membrane have disappeared. In their place is loose, cellular connective tissue without any functional orientation of the fibres. The epithelial rests of Malassez can be seen to have drifted laterally away from the surface of the root. At the bottom of the picture (about two-thirds of the way down the root) there is some bone, but even here the normal structure of the periodontal ligament has disappeared and the fibres between bone and root run vertically (× 100).

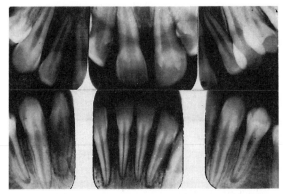

Fig. 6.36 Juvenile periodontitis. Radiographs of the same child show the gross and irregular ('vertical') bone destruction which is most severe in the incisor and upper first molar regions.

excision of the pocket lining may help to eradicate bacteria colonising the epithelial lining and possibly bacteria within the diseased tissue, which have also been described. Tetracycline is effective against *A. actinomycetemcomitans* and is given for 2 to 3 weeks. This treatment can be dramatically successful in the early stages of the disease. Treatment not involving these modalities has also been successful.

Other causes of early-onset periodontal destruction

Very rarely, severe periodontal destruction may affect the deciduous and permanent dentition in a condition called 'prepubertal periodontitis'. These children have profound neutrophil or monocyte dysfunction or both and suffer from other infections such as otitis media. Another form of generalised severe periodontitis which affects young individuals in their twenties and early thirties may also be associated with a phagocyte defect and is referred to as 'rapidly progressive periodontitis'.

Recognised causes of premature destruction also include the following:

1. Immunodeficiency disorders
   a. Down's syndrome
   b. Leucopenia (various causes)
   c. Severe, uncontrolled diabetes mellitus
   d. HIV infection
2. Genetic syndromes
   a. Hypophosphatasia
   b. Hyperkeratosis palmaris et plantaris
   c. Ehlers Danlos syndrome (type VIII)
3. Eosinophilic granuloma (Langerhans' cell histiocytosis)

All (except Down's syndrome) are uncommon or rare, but are important to distinguish from 'idiopathic' juvenile periodontitis in that there is an underlying disorder which may threaten the patient's health or life.

Immunodeficiencies

Some types of immunodeficiency are associated

with premature destructive periodontitis. Down's syndrome (Ch. 23), in which there are multiple immunodeficiencies, is the most common example.

Agranulocytosis and acute leukaemia (Ch. 20) may also be associated with necrotising gingivitis. Agranulocytosis is mainly a disease of adults, while the common childhood type of acute leukaemia (acute lymphocytic leukaemia) typically does not show periodontal destruction.

The importance of cyclic neutropenia (Ch. 20) has been greatly exaggerated. It is so rare as to be no more than a pathological curiosity and even of the few cases that are seen, not all suffer from early-onset periodontitis.

It should be emphasised that early-onset periodontitis in patients with immunodeficiency disorders (unlike 'idiopathic' juvenile periodontitis) is, in general, associated with increased susceptibility to other (non-oral) infections.

Hypophosphatasia

Hypophosphatasia is a rare genetic disorder which can have severe effects on the skeleton as a result of failure of development of mature bone. There may also be failure of formation of cementum and loosening or exfoliation of the teeth without signs of gingivitis or periodontitis. Premature loss of the deciduous teeth, especially the incisors, is characteristic and is occasionally the only overt manifestation of the disease.

Hyperkeratosis palmaris et plantaris and Ehlers Danlos syndrome have been discussed earlier.

Eosinophilic granuloma

The clinical features of eosinophilic granuloma may be characteristic in that the periodontal destruction typically also involves the gingival soft tissues and exposes the roots of the teeth. In addition there is widespread destruction of the bone of the jaw with formation of a tumour-like mass, with recognisable histological features (Ch. 11).

HIV-associated periodontal disease

The main effects, seen in varying combinations, of the immunodeficiency appear to be:

1. Atypical gingivitis (HIV-associated gingivitis)
2. Ulcerative gingivitis and rapidly progressive periodontitis (HIV-associated periodontitis).

HIV-associated gingivitis is characterised by intense erythema of the free and attached gingivae and alveolar mucosa. This erythema may be punctate or coalescent. It can also be band-like, extending 2 to 3 mm apically from the free gingival margin to the attached gingiva. Bleeding is both spontaneous and profuse on probing. There is typically little response to conventional oral hygiene measures.

HIV-associated periodontitis is characterised by gingivitis of the type described above, together with soft-tissue necrosis and rapid destruction of the periodontal attachment and bone, which is typically intensely painful. There is little deep pocketing because soft tissue and bone are lost virtually simultaneously. More than 90% of the attachment can be lost within 3 to 6 months, and the soft-tissue necrosis can lead to exposure of bone and sequestration.

The pain of HIV-associated periodontitis is usually aching in character and felt within the jaw rather than in the gingivae. It may be felt before tissue destruction becomes obvious.

The gingivitis and periodontitis are usually generalised but are sometimes localised to one or more discrete areas.

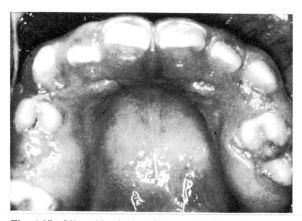

Fig. 6.37 Idiopathic gingival fibromatosis. There is gross enlargement of the whole of the gingivae producing a general broadening of the 'ridge'. The teeth are partly buried but the gums are firm and pale.

Microbiological sampling of both HIV-associated gingivitis and periodontitis has isolated *Bacteroides gingivalis* and *B. intermedius*, *F. nucleatum* and *Actinobacillus actinomycetemcomitans*. Thus the bacterial picture resembles that of classical periodontitis but not gingivitis in HIV-negative persons.

Management. Débridement and removal of any sequestra under local anaesthesia, chlohexidine mouth rinses, systemic metronidazole and analgesics are reported to be effective. Additional broad-spectrum antibiotics have been recommended by some but increase the risk of thrush to which these patients are particularly susceptible. If thrush is present or develops, antifungal drugs are required.

MISCELLANEOUS PERIODONTAL DISORDERS

Fibrous gingival hyperplasia

Hereditary gingival fibromatosis

There are several heritable disorders in which gingival fibromatosis is a feature. All are rare but the most common type is the syndrome of gingival fibromatosis, hypertrichosis and mental retardation—an autosomal dominant disorder.

The onset of gingival enlargement may be early in infancy preceding eruption of the teeth or may not develop until later in childhood. The gums may be so grossly enlarged as completely to bury the teeth and are pale, firm and smooth or stippled in texture.

The gingival tissue consists histologically of thick bundles of collagenous connective tissue with little or no inflammatory exudate.

The facial features may also be coarse and thickened, simulating acromegaly, and there may be excessive hairiness (hypertrichosis). Epilepsy or mental retardation are rare features.

The excess gingival tissue can only be removed by surgical excision but is likely to re-form. Gingivectomy should be delayed as long as possible, preferably until after puberty when the rate of growth of the tissues is slower. Attention must be paid to oral hygiene to prevent infection being superimposed, but, in spite of deep false pocketing, inflammation may be insignificant.

Drug-induced hyperplasia

Some patients taking phenytoin (Epanutin*) for epilepsy develop gingival hyperplasia. The overgrowth principally involves the interdental papillae which become bulbous and overlap the teeth. Typically the gums are firm and pale, and the stippled texture is exaggerated producing an orange-peel appearance. Clinically and histologically similar changes are seen with the immunosuppressive drug cyclosporin and the antihypertensive agent nifedipine, but less frequently. There are also isolated reports of the same changes associated with analogues of nifedipine and the anti-anginal agent diltiazem.

Though inflammation is frequently not apparent and the microscopic appearances are similar to those of idiopathic fibromatosis, infection appears to play a part, and in some patients overgrowth of the gingivae can be kept under control by rigorous oral hygiene. Frequently, however, gingivectomy becomes necessary or is demanded by patients who are embarrassed by what they regard as a stigma of their disease.

Gingival swelling

True hyperplasia (fibrous overgrowth) is uncommon. Swelling of the gingivae is far more often inflammatory in origin, and precipitated by infection at the gingival margins, though the response may be modified by systemic factors.

The causes of swelling of the gingivae therefore tend to fall into two main groups, and the distinction is important as the differences in pathology determine the management.

The main causes of gingival swelling are:

1. *Fibrous hyperplasia*
   a. Idiopathic or hereditary
   b. Drug-induced.
2. *Inflammatory*
   a. Chronic 'hyperplastic' gingivitis
   b. Pregnancy gingivitis
   c. Leukaemic gingivitis

---

* Phenytoin is sometimes referred to as Dilantin by a generation that has not caught up with current drug names. Dilantin is an American proprietary name for phenytoin and does not exist in Britain.

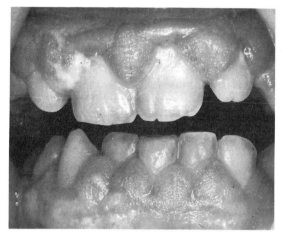

Fig. 6.38 Gingival hyperplasia due to phenytoin. The characteristic features are fibrous swelling of the interdental papillae, which become bulbous but remain firm and pale. The stippling of the attached gingiva becomes exaggerated.

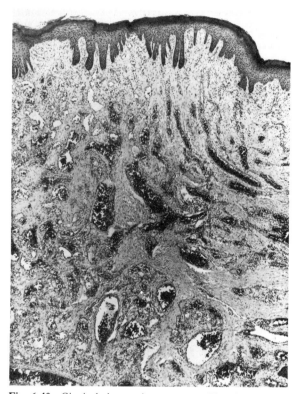

Fig. 6.40 Gingival changes in pregnancy. The gingiva is swollen and oedematous, and there are many dilated vessels. Near the surface against the tooth (left), the vessels are congested and there are many chronic inflammatory cells (× 48).

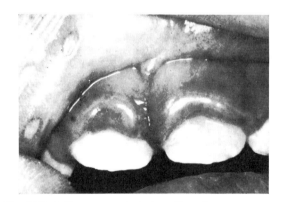

Fig. 6.39 Inflammatory gingival swelling. Acute non-specific gingivitis characteristic of primary herpetic infection. Typical herpetic ulcers are present inside the upper lip on the left.

d. Sarcoidosis (see Ch. 20 Fig. 20.17)
e. Scurvy.

Chronic 'hyperplastic' gingivitis

This is the most common cause of gingival swelling; it mainly affects young people. Delayed passive eruption where the gingival margin

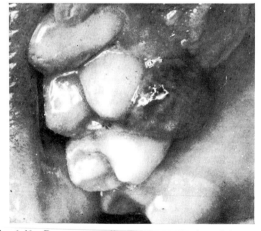

Fig. 6.41 Pregnancy epulis. The hyperplastic nodule is soft and red, and is a vascular oedematous overgrowth of connective tissue probably initially provoked by local irritation and infection.

remains nearer the incisal edge for a long time after eruption may be an additional factor. The gingival margins are swollen, smooth, oedematous and congested. The management is essentially that of rigorous oral hygiene to control gingival infection since the swelling is mostly due to oedema.

Gingivitis in pregnancy

During pregnancy the gingival margins may sometimes become swollen and pre-existing gingivitis is aggravated. Hormonal changes exaggerate the vascular response. There are no entirely specific features, but in typical cases there is redness and swelling sharply restricted to the interdental papillae and gingival margins, which may have a fringed appearance. Exaggeration of these changes may produce a localised nodule (pregnancy 'tumour'). The gingival changes are initiated by local infection, but gingivitis may be more difficult to control at this time. After parturition the gingivitis is likely to improve and a pregnancy epulis may resolve, partially or completely, if oral hygiene is good. Histologically the gingivae show chronic inflammatory changes and highly vascular, oedematous connective tissue. Somewhat similar changes may also be seen at puberty.

Acute leukaemia

Acute myelo-monocytic leukaemia is most likely to be associated with gingival swelling. The abnormal white cells are unable to carry out their normal defensive function and can no longer control infection at the gingival margins. The abnormal leucocytes infiltrate the area until the gingivae become packed and swollen with leukaemic cells. These cells are so defective that infection progresses, leading to ulceration and breakdown of the tissues.

Clinically the gingivae are swollen, shiny and pale or purplish in colour; ulceration may develop. Other signs of leukaemia (pallor, purpura or lassitude) may also be seen.

Intensive topical use of antibiotics may lead to regression of the swelling, but the patient's general prognosis is poor.

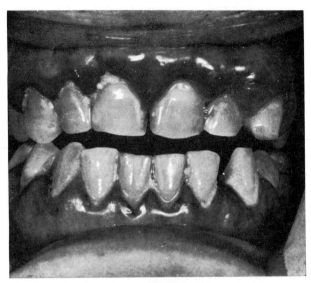

Fig. 6.42 Acute myelo-monocyte leukaemia. The gingival margins are swollen, soft and have a purplish colour.

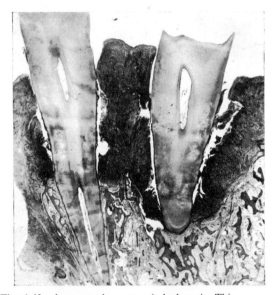

Fig. 6.43 Acute myelo-monocytic leukaemia. This specimen from the patient shown in Fig. 6.42 shows the gingival swelling to be due to the dense packing of the gingivae with leukaemic cells. These cells are infiltrating deeply into the tissues, suggesting that the supporting tissues are breaking down as a result of the poor resistance to infection (× 3).

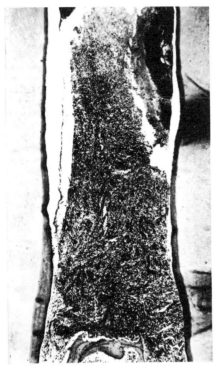

Fig. 6.44 Acute myclo-monocytic leukaemia. At higher power it can be seen that the gingival epithelium interdentally has been destroyed and the papilla is so densely infiltrated with leukaemic cells that the normal structure is obliterated. The scalloped crest of the alveolar bone indicates that bone is being actively resorbed (× 32).

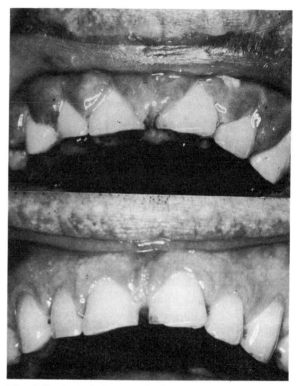

Fig. 6.45 Acute leukaemia. Gross swelling, causing the gingival margins to reach the incisal edges of the teeth, is seen in the upper picture.
  The lower picture shows the effects of an antibiotic mouthrinse (tetracycline with amphotericin) and oral hygiene. The swelling has entirely subsided and the gingivae have regained their normal firm texture and pale colour.

Sarcoidosis and other granulomatous diseases

Sarcoidosis is a granulomatous disease predominantly affecting the lungs but with a predilection also for salivary glands. It is an uncommon cause of soft painless gingival swelling involving several or many teeth. Diagnosis depends on biopsy showing the typical granulomas, and on other signs of the disease. However, in the absence of the latter, other causes of granuloma formation (Ch. 20) must be considered.

Scurvy

Grossly swollen and congested gums are a classical sign of scurvy, but only of advanced disease and are rarely seen, even among the very few patients with scurvy who are not edentulous.

The gingival swelling is due to a combination of chronic inflammation and an exaggeration of the inflammatory congestion due to scorbutic purpura. The diagnosis should only be made on clear evidence of dietary deficiency and of purpura. In these cases treatment with vitamin C and adequate oral hygiene relieves the gingival condition.

Keratinisation and gingival health

There seems to be a persistent fantasy that gingival health depends on keratinisation and that this in turn is produced by toothbrushing. This idea seems to be based on a somewhat facile analogy with cornification of the hands caused by manual labour, where the increased keratinisation can be regarded as protective.

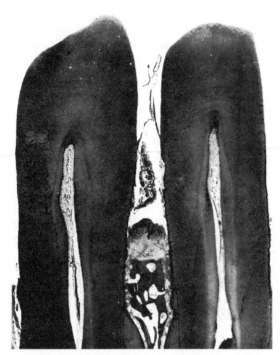

Fig. 6.46 Gingival recession. This specimen from a man of 72 shows general recession of gingivae and alveolar bone. There is no pocketing, and the periodontal tissues, though reduced in amount, are healthy. The strips of plaque which mark the site of the enamel surface indicate the extent of the recession.

It is true that the healthy masticatory mucosa, including the gingival margins and attached gingiva (unlike the buccal mucosa), shows a tendency to keratinisation, but this is minimal and of minor degree in comparison with the skin. Toothbrushing can increase slightly the thickness of the stratum corneum, but this is unimportant unless it can be shown that increased keratinisation enhances the barrier function of epithelium. Unfortunately keratin is *more* permeable to water and a less efficient barrier to a variety of substances than the thinner, normal stratum corneum.

The value of toothbrushing is by removing plaque. If this is done thoroughly there may be slightly increased keratinisation, but this is quite incidental and of no measurable benefit.

Gingival recession

Recession of the gingival margins and gradual ex-posure of the roots is common and certainly increases with age. However, gingival recession is not an invariable feature of ageing, and some individuals are more predisposed to it than others. The major predisposing factor is thinness of the gingival tissue. This is readily damaged by trauma from forceful toothbrushing and plaque-induced inflammation. A recent hypothesis suggests that epithelial proliferation of the junctional epithelium in inflammation results in an epithelial 'bridge' extending to the external gingival epithelium across the narrow band of inflamed connective tissue. This is followed by remodelling of the gingival margin. It seems reasonable to assume that plaque-induced loss of attachment in areas of thick tissue can lead to pocket formation, whereas thin tissue is destroyed entirely. The resulting receded gingival margins often appear relatively uninflamed.

Gingival abrasion

Abrasion, usually by vigorous toothbrushing, causes recession of the gingivae and damage to the teeth. The change is seen in its early stages in some young adults and severe examples are seen in later life. Forceful toothbrushing with a stiff brush used with a sawing motion across the teeth is the most usual cause, and in a right-handed person the most severe damage is in the left canine

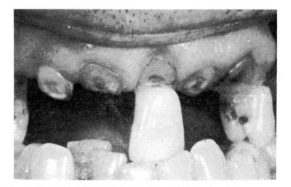

Fig. 6.47 Gingival abrasion. Severe damage has been done to the teeth by vigorous toothbrushing over the course of many years. The teeth have been so deeply cut into that several have snapped off, but the gingival margins have stood up well to this heavy wear; they have receded to a small extent but remain firm, pale and healthy.

region. Grooves are worn into the necks of the teeth, and reactionary dentine is formed under the damaged area. Eventually the neck of the tooth may be cut so deeply that the crown breaks off, but the pulp remains covered by reactionary dentine. The gingival margins recede but it is conspicuous that they remain firm, pale and healthy where they are hit by the toothbrush. Nearby, in the interstitial spaces where the toothbrush may not reach, there is sometimes chronic gingivitis.

Treatment of gingival recession

Recession of the gingivae sometimes causes patients to fear that they will soon lose their teeth. In older patients, where enough alveolar bone remains, the teeth can be kept in useful function for many more years and the patient can be reassured. The main consideration is to keep the gingival margins clean, especially in the enlarged interstitial spaces. In the case of abrasive gingival recession the treatment is the same, but the patient must also be shown how to keep the teeth clean without causing further damage.

Various surgical procedures have been devised to correct localised areas of gingival recession or to produce thicker zones of gingiva which, it is hoped, are more resistant to recession.

An early result of abrasive damage to the teeth is exposure of the dentine, which may be hypersensitive.

Many treatments for hypersensitive dentine have been introduced, and the number of such preparations is indicative of their limitations. Traditional remedies are topical applications of strong astringents such as zinc chloride or silver nitrate. More recent proprietary preparations such as Tresiolan and Durophat, however, appear to be more effective.

SUGGESTED FURTHER READING

Abel S N, Andriolo M 1989 Clinical management of HIV-related periodontitis: report of a case. JADA Supplement: 35S–36S

Aeppli D, Pihlstrom B L 1989 Detection of longitudinal change in periodontitis. J Periodont Res 24: 329–334

Artzi Z, Gorsky M, Raviv M 1989 Periodontal manifestations of adult onset histiocytosis X. J Periodontol 60: 57–66

Astemborski J A, Boughman J A, Myrick P O et al 1989 Clinical and laboratory characterization of early onset periodontitis. J Periodontol 60: 557–563

Beal M, Broawnstein C N 1988 Antimicrobial agents in the prevention and treatment of periodontal diseases. Dental Clinics of North America 32: 217–236

Carlos J P, Wolfe M D, Zambon J J, Kingman A 1988 Periodontal disease in adolescents: some clinical and microbiological correlates of attachment loss. J Dent Res 67: 1510–1514

Cawson R A 1987 Oral pathology—colour aids in dentistry. Churchill Livingstone, Edinburgh

Cawson R A, Eveson J W 1987 Oral pathology and diagnosis. William Heinemann Medical Books, London and Gower Medical Publishing, London

Dzink J L, Socransky S S, Haffajee A D 1988 The predominant cultivable flora of active and inactive lesions of destructive periodontal diseases. J Clin Periodontol 15: 316–323

Elsberg J 1987 Regeneration and repair of periodontal tissues. J Periodont Res 22: 233–242

Embery G, Last K 1989 Biochemical markers of periodontal tissue destruction. Dental Update 16: 167–177

Genco R J, Christersson L A, Zambon J J 1986 Juvenile periodontitis. Int Dent J 36: 168–176

Griffiths G S, Wilton J M A, Maiden M F J et al 1988 Detection of high-risk groups and individuals for periodontal diseases. J Clin Periodontol 15: 403–410

Hagel-Bradway S, Dziak R 1989 Regulation of bone cell metabolism. J Oral Pathol Med 18: 344–351

Heasman P A, Smith D G 1988 The role of anatomy in the initiation and spread of periodontal disease: 1. Dental Update 15: 192–197

Heasman P A, Smith D G 1988 The role of anatomy in the initiation and spread of periodontal disease: 2. Dental Update 15: 250–255

Hillman J D, Socransky S S, Shivers M 1989 The relationship between streptococcal species and periodontopathic bacteria in human dental plaque. Arch Oral Biol 30: 791–795

Hirsch R S, Clarke N G 1989 Infection and periodontal disease. Rev Infect Dis 11: 707–715

Holbrook W P, Cawson R A 1990 The problem of the taxonomy of the fusiform bacillus of acute necrotizing ulcerative gingivitis (Vincent's gingivitis). Antonie van Leeuwenhoek 57: 55–58

Hugoson A, Thorstensson H, Falk H, Kuylenstierna J 1989 Periodontal conditions in insulin-dependent diabetics. J Clin Periodontol 16: 215–223

Lindhe J, Okamoto H, Yoneyman T et al 1989 Longitudinal changes in periodontal disease in untreated subjects. J Clin Periodontol 16: 662–670

Listgarten M A 1987 Nature of periodontal diseases: Pathogenic mechanisms. J Periodont Res 22: 172–178

Manson J D, Eley 1989 The prevention of periodontal disease. Dental Update 16: 189–196

Moore L V H, Moore W E C, Cato E P et al 1987 Bacteriology of human gingivitis. J Dent Res 66: 989–995

Moore W E C 1987 Microbiology of periodontal disease. J Periodont Res 22: 335–341

Murray P A, Grassi M, Winkler J R 1989 The microbiology of HIV-associated periodontal lesions. J Clin Periodontol 16: 636–642

O'Leary T J, Barrington E P, Gottsegen R 1988 Periodontal therapy. A summary status report 1987–1988. J Periodontol 59: 306–310

Page R C 1986 Current understanding of the aetiology and progression of periodontal disease. Int Dent J 36: 153–161

Papapanou P N, Wennstrom J L 1989 Radiographic and clinical assessments of destructive periodontal disease J Clin Periodontol 16: 609–612

Reynolds M A, Minah G E, Peterson D E et al 1989 Periodontal disease and oral microbial successions during myelosuppressive cancer chemotherapy. J Clin Periodontol 16: 185–189

Ries W L, Seeds M C, Key L L 1989 Interleukin-2 stimulates osteoclastic activity: Increased acid production and radioactive calcium release. J Periodont Res 24: 242–246

Ripamonte U, Petit J-C, Penfold G, Lemmer J 1986 Periodontal manifestations of acute autoimmune thrombocytopenic purpura. J Periodontol 57: 429–432

Sanholm L, Swanljung O, Rytomaa et al 1989 Periodontal status of Finnish adolescents with insulin dependent diabetes mellitus. J Clin Periodontol 16: 617–620

Skrinjaric I, Miljenko B 1989 Hereditary gingival fibromatosis: Report on three families and dermatoglyphic analysis. J Periodont Res 24: 303–309

Slots J 1986 Bacterial specificity in adult periodontitis. J Clin Periodontol 13: 912–917

Smith D G, Seymour R A 1989 Periodontal disease and treatment in the elderly: 1. Dental Update 16: 18–25

Smith D G, Seymour R A 1989 Periodontal disease and treatment in the elderly: 2. Dental Update 16: 58–64

Suzuki J B 1988 Diagnosis and classification of the periodontal diseases. Dental Clinics of North America 32: 195–215

Tew J, Engel D, Mangan D 1989 Polyclonal B-cell activation in periodontitis. J Periodont Res 24: 225–241

Theilade E 1986 The non-specific theory in microbial etiology of inflammatory periodontal diseases. J Clin Periodontol 13: 905–911

Watanabe K 1990 Prepubertal periodontitis: a review of diagnostic criteria, pathogenesis and differential diagnosis. J Periodont Res 25: 31–48

Weiss S J 1989 Tissue destruction by neutrophils. New Engl J Med 320: 365–376

Williams R C 1990 Periodontal disease. New Engl J Med 322: 373–382

Winkler J R, Murray P A, Grassi M, Hammerle C 1989 Diagnosis and management of HIV-associated periodontal lesions. JADA Supplement: 25S–34S

7. Prevention of dental disease

Dental caries can be completely prevented, but it is less certain that periodontal disease can be equally effectively controlled.

Prevention of dental disease involves constant effort by the patient. This in turn means that the patient must be highly motivated and constantly encouraged to maintain good habits. Unfortunately, so much restorative dentistry usually needs to be done and so many dentists become absorbed by the technical aspects of the subject that effective preventive dentistry often falls by the wayside. The application of sound principles of preventive dentistry is, however, possible in everyday practice, though it requires a vigorous approach, some dedication to the idea and, inevitably, some effort.

While the ideal remains that preventive measures be applicable on a community-wide scale, there are few effective public health measures available. Every effort is therefore justified in helping those who want to preserve a healthy dentition. In addition it is desirable to make sure that as many as possible are fully in-formed about the nature of dental disease and its prevention. Among those that respond the results can be rewarding.

Awareness and motivation

If dental disease is to be prevented patients must both understand the causes of dental disease and genuinely want to achieve dental health by the application of this knowledge.

A major difficulty is that dental disease, particularly periodontal disease, is so insidious that even total neglect may produce no obvious ill effects for many years. For the same reason even the most assiduous care by the patient produces little in the way of visible results—and any benefits only become apparent much later.

It would be more encouraging for the patient perhaps if, with the present faith in pills and injections, the dentist could be seen to be making a more obvious contribution. In many patients, motivation is also weak and ideas about prevention of dental disease are often confused, as shown by

155

the extensive surveys that have been carried out (Ch. 26). The dentist therefore plays a crucial role in educating and motivating the patient, limiting the spread of caries, monitoring plaque control and providing regular, meticulous periodontal care. Nevertheless, despite such efforts, it appears that even of those who claim to have regular dental care too many people are undismayed at the prospect of losing all their teeth, whilst others have no more than emergency treatment.

Another difficulty is that dentures often look acceptable and can function so well that loss of teeth has no adverse effect on health. Even poorly made dentures, however horrible they may look, rarely affect nutrition. Similarly, diseased teeth can also function adequately and fail to cause troublesome symptoms. Many people with neglected mouths have been lucky enough not to experience pain, as the teeth have decayed and died without symptoms.

It must be accepted therefore that a significant number of patients are not, and probably some cannot, be motivated. They see no point in saving their teeth and no disadvantage in having dentures. Some probably think of regular habits of dental care as a mark of a decadent, middle-class and disciplinarian society. A few may be handicapped in various ways such as low intelligence or poor manual dexterity.

Initiation of preventive measures

Ideally, preventive dentistry should be started as early as reasonably possible, preferably when the child is between $2\frac{1}{2}$ and 3 years of age. At this age the child has no preconceptions about the horrors of dentistry and no natural fear of it. Bad habits such as compulsive sweet-eating should not have become established and it is easier to inculcate good habits both of diet and of oral hygiene.

At this early age little dental treatment is usually needed and small cavities can be prepared and restored virtually painlessly. This helps the child to get used to dental treatment. Similarly, gingival health is usually good and, though early gingivitis may be detectable, it is readily reversed.

A young child may, however, find it difficult to understand what it is all about and also does not have the necessary skill to brush the teeth effec-tively. Parents must therefore be made to understand what is at stake and what must be done to prevent dental disease. Parent and child together must learn the techniques of plaque control using any available teaching aids. In addition to making sure that parents can teach the child to brush the teeth effectively they must also clearly understand the harmful effects of sweets. Ideas that sweets can be used as bribes, rewards or presents should be eradicated.

If the parents are unprepared to adopt a constructive, cooperative attitude the chance of establishing good preventive habits in a child are slight. Parents must therefore be made to understand that it requires active effort on their part to maintain the child's oral health and to give him a reasonable chance of retaining a healthy dentition later in life. To a large extent the way in which the parents respond may affect their offspring's dental health for the next fifty or more years.

Another advantage of treating a child as early as this is that the need for future orthodontic treatment, which itself may affect periodontal health and caries, can be assessed.

PRACTICAL ASPECTS OF PREVENTIVE DENTISTRY

As discussed in Chapter 26, a high proportion of the population have ambivalent ideas about preserving a healthy dentition. Even among those who seek regular dental treament, many express no distress at the idea of losing all their teeth. Many are also ignorant of, or have confused ideas about, how dental disease can be prevented.

As already discussed, preventive dentistry can be successful only if

1. The patient genuinely wants to preserve a healthy dentition.
2. The dentist genuinely believes in the effectiveness of preventive dentistry, is completely confident that he can achieve its aims and knows how to do so.
3. The dentist can convey his confidence to the patient.
4. All the rest of the staff, particularly hygienists, are equally confident of the need for and effectiveness of preventive dentistry

and do not regard scaling alone as an end in itself.

5. The dentist appreciates the necessity for continuous active intervention, particularly the encouragement of well-motivated patients. Regular meticulous inspection of the mouth is also essential, particularly to make sure that plaque is being controlled. Successful preventive dentistry does not result from handing out pamphlets, toothbrushes, fluoride tablets and all the rest, then letting patients get on with it themselves on their own. The 'preventive dentistry kit' is no more than an aid to the dentist's efforts, to be used like any other teaching aid.

6. The dental team appreciates that the prevention of both periodontal disease and dental caries are equally important and act accordingly.

7. Preventive measures are easy for patients to carry out and the dental team are fully capable of carrying out all the measures that are their responsibility.

8. Patients understand the basis for all the preventive measures, and the factors determining dental disease must be explained in simple fashion. The use of pictures of plaque, for instance, and of the stages of dental decay and periodontal disease can be helpful for this purpose. Patients must also be disabused of the many misapprehensions about the causes and prevention of dental disease.

9. Patients appreciate that practical preventive dentistry is a continuous process and that this hard work has to continue for the rest of life.

10. Patients understand above all, their own involvement in dental health care and that, in many ways, it is *they* who carry out the most essential part of the programme. However skilled and well intentioned the dentist may be, he cannot prevent dental disease without the continuous active co-operation of the patient. It is even possible for the highly motivated and skilled patient, once adequately instructed, to maintain an adequate standard of oral health without intervention from the dentist, though this is unusual.

Some statistical data on the numbers of people who try to maintain dental health, and the amount of help given by dentists is given in Chapter 26.

PREVENTION OF DENTAL CARIES

Prevention of dental caries depends on understanding its causes, as outlined in Chapter 3. These suggest therefore that the disease can be prevented or at least mitigated by the following types of measure:

1. Antibacterial measures
2. Dietary measures (control of sugar intake)
3. Modifying plaque metabolism
4. Increasing resistance of the tooth to attack.

These methods vary widely in their effectiveness and the ease with which they can be used. They are by no means all practical propositions.

Antibacterial measures

The use of antibacterial agents seems superficially to be the most obvious and logical approach, but these agents have serious limitations. The main examples are:

1. Antibacterial drugs
   —Antibiotics and antiseptics (chlorhexidine)
2. Immunisation.

Antibiotics

Penicillin depresses caries activity in animals. In humans also, long-term administration of penicillin for the prevention of rheumatic fever reduces caries incidence by 50%. However, antibiotics are not a feasible method of preventing caries, because of possible toxic effects and promotion of resistant bacteria.

Chlorhexidine

Chlorhexidine is a cationic antiseptic which acts by damaging the cell membrane of a wide variety of bacteria. Its effective antibacterial action in the mouth was first demonstrated in 1959.

Chlorhexidine binds on to the enamel surface, oral mucosa and plaque components. It is slowly released to have an antibacterial effect lasting several hours. This can inhibit bacterial colonisation of the teeth and plaque formation.

When used as a daily mouth rinse (0.1% or 0.2%) chlorhexidine reduces the amount of plaque formed and helps to prevent gingivitis. As long as chlorhexidine is used in this way it appears that the salivary flora is decreased by 20–50%, and most notably the numbers of *Strep. mutans* that can be isolated also decline. These effects have been maintained in studies lasting 2 or more years. On the other hand, the oral flora and plaque formation revert to normal very quickly after use of chlorhexidine is stopped.

However, chlorhexidine does not enter stagnation areas and has not been shown to reduce caries activity. Its main value is in the control of gingivitis as discussed later.

The main disadvantages of chlorhexidine are its unpleasant flavour and its tendency to cause brownish staining of the teeth and anterior restorations. This can be removed with polishing paste.

The toxicity of chlorhexidine seems otherwise to be low, though soreness of the mouth is an occasional complaint.

Immunisation

Since dental caries is an infective disease but difficult to prevent, immunisation is an attractive possibility. Difficulties include those of identifying with certainty a single bacterial cause for the disease and the fact that the teeth are relatively inaccessible to humoral and, particularly, cell-mediated defences.

Vaccines may theoretically be produced to act in a variety of ways; for example by inhibiting the causative bacteria, by blocking the activity of glucosyl transferase or by interfering with their attachment mechanisms.

Salivary immunoglobulins

In quantitative terms, secretory IgA is the main immunoglobulin of saliva, but minute amounts of IgG and IgM reach the mouth in the gingival exudate. The amounts of this exudate and of the immunoglobulins it contains depend on the severity of the gingival inflammation.

Some workers have reported a positive correlation between salivary IgA levels and caries activity. Nevertheless the raised IgA levels found in the saliva of those with active dental caries do not seem to have impeded the progress of the disease. Other workers have failed to find any such relation between salivary immune globulin levels and dental caries activity.

The function of salivary IgA has been suggested as being directly antibacterial, and in favour of this is the finding that bacteria adsorb IgA onto their surfaces. However, IgA, unlike other antibodies, cannot fix complement, and complement-dependent bacteriolysis does not appear to be possible.

Another action of salivary IgA may be to inhibit the adherence of the oral flora to epithelial or dental surfaces by coating these surfaces within the mouth. By coating mucosal surfaces, salivary IgA might also function as a blocking antibody and interfere with the absorption of bacteria and other antigens through the mucosa. This might not, however, be wholly advantageous; blocking the absorption of antigens might be protective—on the other hand it might be the reason for the apparent lack of natural immunity to these antigens.

IgG and IgM antibodies are likely to have greater antibacterial activity, but the minute amounts of these antibodies that leak into the mouth with the gingival exudate are likely only to reach the interstitial surfaces of the teeth. They are probably too greatly diluted to have any effect on the occlusal surfaces which are the most common sites of attack. However, it seems unreasonable to encourage the patient to develop gingivitis in order to provide a better supply of IgG and IgM to protect the teeth.

There have been several reports of immunisation of monkeys by injection of preparations of *S. mutans* with an adjuvant. In such cases interstitial caries was reduced more than occlusal caries. This suggests that antibodies reached the teeth mainly from the gingival crevice.

However, one problem that has transpired from these experiments is that a proportion of animals under test produce antibodies slowly. Cavities therefore develop and progress before effective concentrations of the antibody appear. This finding may explain the negative results of other workers.

Purified protein antigens from *S. mutans* (antigens I and I/II with an adjuvant) given by injection have been reported to reduce caries by over 50% in rhesus monkeys fed a 15% sucrose human-type diet. Immunisation was associated with the appearance of IgG antibodies to the antigens in the serum and with a reduction in the numbers of *S. mutans* in dental plaque. More recently, monoclonal antibodies against *S. mutans*, applied topically, have been reported to be effective.

Despite some encouraging results in animal experiments and after more than 20 years of research and the expenditure of millions of pounds, no anti-caries vaccine has reached the stage of clinical trials in humans.

In addition to the technical difficulties associated with the production of safe vaccines, other questions—which may ultimately prove to be theoretical—remain unanswered; these include the following.

1. Elimination of *S. mutans* might in the long term result in other serotypes or different bacteria becoming cariogenic,
2. As in some animals, the human response to a vaccine may be weak.
3. With the decline in the incidence of dental caries, it may be asked whether a vaccine is needed at all.
4. For so minor a disease as caries, any vaccine must be 100% safe. Vaccines are needed for systemic diseases such as measles or smallpox which cause significant morbidity or mortality and for which there is no effective treatment. For such diseases, the risk of side-effects from vaccines has to be accepted. Unlike them, caries hardly affects health, is largely preventable by other means and, if not prevented, is not difficult to treat. Any risks from a vaccine against such a disease are totally unacceptable.
   Possible risks from an anticaries vaccine include antigens in common with other streptococci and the development of

antibodies cross-reacting with cardiac tissue. Some evidence has been produced that this may be the case and, as with other vaccines, additional adverse effects are unpredictable. To show that a vaccine was completely safe would therefore require trials in perhaps 100 000 persons.
5. Even if (unlike every other vaccine) an anticaries vaccine completely without adverse effects can be produced, its acceptability is likely to be questionable. There is anxiety about the safety of vaccines in general, and, for example, confidence in whooping cough vaccine is only slowly being restored after the publicity given to the risk of encephalitis. In Texas, when diphtheria immunisation was not obligatory, it was not taken up and minor epidemics resulted.

Equally important is that those in most need of additional anticaries measures—namely, the most poorly educated—are the least likely to take up an anticaries vaccine, as they are of other dental preventive measures (Ch. 26).

Finally, many are doubtful about whether an effective anticaries vaccine is a practical possibility since it has never been shown unequivocally that natural immunity to the disease develops. It is difficult to establish that a caries-free mouth is the result of immunity rather than many other variables such as the diet or dental structure.

Dental caries also does not seem to be promoted by immunodeficiency. Children with Down's syndrome (Ch. 23) who suffer multiple immunodeficiencies and gross plaque accumulation have low caries activity. Despite the suggested protective effect of salivary IgA mentioned earlier, the many persons who are congenitally IgA deficient (Ch. 20) have not been shown to suffer rampant dental caries. Finally, dental caries remains virtually the only infective disease that does not run out of control as a direct result of the lethally severe immunodeficiency of AIDS.

DIETARY MEASURES

Limitation of sugar intake

Sugar, particularly sucrose, is the most important cariogenic substrate. Caries is most active when

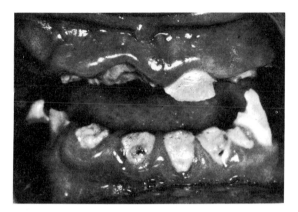

Fig. 7.1   Rampant dental caries. A 10-year-old girl, a compulsive sweet-eater, all of whose teeth have been destroyed by caries.

sugar is taken at frequent intervals or in such a form as to adhere to the teeth and remain available to the plaque for a long period.

Severe or complete sugar restriction is the simplest, safest and most effective way of preventing dental caries. It represents, however, an act of self-denial unacceptable to the vast majority and is a practical measure only for the dedicated few. Ideally, sweet eating—sweets include candy bars and all such confectionery with a high sugar content—should be stopped altogether. Almost as effective is to stop sweets and sweet snacks between meals; if such things must be eaten they can be taken at the end of meals as a dessert.

If sweets or sugary foods are eaten sufficiently infrequently, sugar reaches plaque on so few occasions that plaque pH remains safely at a high level for the greater part of the day. After meals the plaque pH falls temporarily, but thereafter cariogenic bacteria have to depend on reserve carbohydrate, and caries activity is low.

Sweet foods can be particularly cariogenic if taken just before going to sleep. During sleep salivary secretion and buffering power fall to negligibly low levels. Sugar clearance from the mouth is therefore greatly impaired. Foods such as sweet biscuits eaten as bedtime snacks may therefore have a more severe effect than during the day.

Alternatives to sucrose

Glucose, which is slightly less sweet than sucrose,

is made synthetically by hydrolysis of starch and is used commercially in a wide variety of food and drinks. Experimentally, glucose is appreciably (up to 30%) less cariogenic than sucrose when added to drinking water. However, there have been no clinical trials substantiating the benefits of glucose.

Fructose is also made on a vast scale by hydrolysis of starch. It is sweeter than sucrose and is used particularly in soft drinks. Fructose also seems to be less cariogenic than sucrose—a 2-year clinical trial showed a 25% reduction in caries in comparison with sucrose—but has disadvantages. Used in large amounts fructose can cause gastrointestinal upsets; it is also suspected of being more prone to promote the development of atherosclerosis than sucrose.

Xylitol is a sugar alcohol produced synthetically from birchwood. It is as sweet as sucrose, but in an extensive clinical trial extending over 2 years caries was reduced by 90% compared with a high-sucrose diet. The disadvantage of xylitol is that it is very expensive; in animal experiments gastrointestinal upsets have also been reported, but in the clinical trial fewer than 1% complained of diarrhoea.

Saccharin is a widely used synthetic sweetening agent, particularly for beverages. It is not metabolised by plaque bacteria and is not cariogenic. Saccharin cannot be used for making sweets as a large part of the structure of sweets and candies depends on the sugar.

Increasing numbers of artificial sweeteners such as aspartame and acesulfacme-K continue to be introduced in the profitable business of low-calorie food production. Most of them are not metabolised in plaque and are non-cariogenic. Interestingly manufacturers have found it worthwhile to introduce soft drinks containing artificial sweeteners rather than sugar, but these are sold as low-calorie beverages. It seems therefore profitable to take advantage of people's anxiety to lose weight, but it is obviously not felt that there is comparable interest in preventing dental decay.

Summary

Severe limitation of sugar intake is by far the most satisfactory and effective means of preventing dental caries. Unfortunately, few people find this measure acceptable, and there are no non-cariogenic substitutes which do not have considerable disadvantages in practical use.

Modification of plaque metabolism

Chlorhexidine

As mentioned earlier, chlorhexidine depresses or inhibits plaque production but has not been shown to have a significant effect on caries activity.

Phosphates

The addition of phosphate compounds has been shown under experimental conditions, in both animals and man, to reduce the cariogenicity of sugar.

Experimentally calcium phosphate and, particularly, calcium glycerophosphate have shown most promise and when added to cariogenic diets have reduced caries in animals by 60% or more. Results in clinical trials have been variable, but in general they have produced less satisfactory results than in experiments on animals. Thorough clinical trials have not, however, been carried out on these agents.

AGENTS AFFECTING THE RESISTANCE OF THE TOOTH

Background to the use of fluorides

Fluorides have had a major effect in reducing the prevalence of dental caries, as a result of the widespread use of fluoridised dentifrices.

The unlikely beginning of the history of fluorides in dental tissue was its discovery in the teeth of a disinterred mammoth at the beginning of the 19th century. Fluoride was detected in human enamel as early as 1805 and in water in 1822. Without any clinical basis for the idea, the belief spread that fluorides were protective, and by 1897 it was hypothesised that they increased caries-resistance by an anti-enzymic or an antibacterial effect. Fluoride-containing preparations to protect the teeth were available by the end of the 19th century. Thereafter the matter seems to have been completely forgotten until the 1930s.

Mottled enamel

Mottling is a specific defect of the enamel with the characteristic feature that it is endemic in certain areas while nearby communities are often unaffected. Severely mottled teeth have opaque, stained, brittle and pitted enamel as described in Chapter 2. The importance of mottling is that it is associated with reduced susceptibility to caries in spite of obvious structural defects of the enamel.

Mottling is associated with high concentrations of fluorides (over 2 ppm) in the drinking water.

Mottling affects only those persons who have lived in a high-fluoride area during the period of dental development. Individuals more than about 7 years old coming from a low-fluoride area to one where mottling is endemic do not develop the characteristic dental changes, and are also more susceptible to caries than the indigenous population. The deciduous teeth are not affected by mottling unless the concentration of fluorides is very high.

Mottled teeth are relatively common in the USA, and the many affected communities have provided material for detailed study of the disorder.

Field studies on mottled enamel and dental caries

Mottling of the teeth was first described in Mexico and soon afterwards in Naples, though the cause was not then understood. Similar defects were noticed by McKay in Colorado at the beginning of this century. In spite of the grossly defective enamel structure, it was noticed that these teeth were no more susceptible to decay than normal teeth, though it was not appreciated that they were more resistant. It was not until 1931 that Churchill, in trying to solve the cause of mottling of teeth in Bauxite, Arkansas found that in this area the water supply had an unusually high level of fluoride.

In 1933 Ainsworth carried out a study in Maldon and adjacent areas of Essex which established that caries experience was lower in areas where teeth were mottled. He found that the prevalence of carious teeth in children aged 5 to 15 was 7.9% in Maldon compared with an average of 13.1% for all districts examined, since many of the other towns had water with a lower fluoride content. The fluoride content of the water at Maldon was then over 4 ppm but there has since been progressive dilution of high-fluoride water supplies.

The relationship between caries prevalence and the fluoride content of the drinking water was finally established on a quantitative basis by the extensive epidemiological surveys carried out by Trendley Dean and his associates (1942). In this survey they examined 7257 children, 12 to 14 years old, in 21 towns where the fluoride levels ranged from undetectable to 2.6 ppm. Where the fluoride level was from 1 to $1\frac{1}{2}$ ppm, the prevalence of caries of the permanent teeth was about a third of that in areas where there were negligible amounts of fluoride, and there were no conspicuous defects due to mottling.

In Britain, Weaver showed that in North Shields, where the fluoride content of the water was less than 0.25 ppm, the prevalence of caries in 5–12-year-old children was almost twice as high as in South Shields, where the fluoride content of the water was 1.4 ppm. The teeth which showed the greatest improvement were the upper incisors, and Weaver suggested that the caries-inhibiting factor was not sufficiently powerful to confer a high degree of protection to the more susceptible molar teeth.

In West Mersea (F = 5.8 ppm), Burnham-on-Crouch (F = 3.5 ppm), Harwich (F = 2.0 ppm) and Slough (F = 0.9 ppm) Forrest found that the prevalence of caries in 12–14-year-old children was about a third of that in children of the same age living in Saffron Walden (F = 0.1 ppm) or in Stoneleigh and Malden in Surrey (F = 0.1–0.2 ppm). Some of the children in Mersea and Burnham showed severe mottling of the enamel, but Forrest found the prevalence of enamel defects to be slightly higher in the low-fluoride towns than in Harwich and Slough, where she considered that the enamel appeared better formed.

With regard to the duration of protection given by fluorides, it has been shown that caries experience increases with age but that protection persists into adult life.

Fluoridation of water supplies

Final confirmation of the value and safety of fluorides in caries prevention has been provided by the addition of fluoride to the drinking water of communities to provide the optimum level (1 ppm).

In 1944 three towns—Grand Rapids and Newburgh in the United States, and Brantford in Canada—were chosen for experimental fluori-

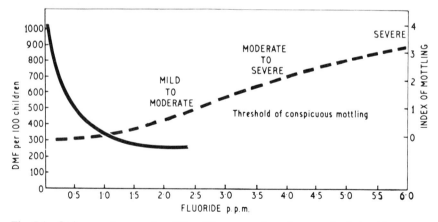

Fig. 7.2 Caries prevalence and mottling. The curves show the general relationship between the prevalence of caries (continuous line) and the severity of mottling (broken line) in persons continuously exposed to various levels of fluoride in the water during dental development. The optimum level of fluoride can be seen to be about 1 part per million. Higher concentrations of fluoride cause increasing incidence and severity of mottling without a comparable improvement in resistance to caries. The index of mottling is obtained by giving an arbitrary value for each degree of mottling and relating the numbers of patients in each grade with the total number examined.

dation of the water supply. All these towns had less than 0.1 ppm of fluoride in their water. Nearby cities having water with a similar fluoride content were used as controls. These were Muskegon, as a control for Grand Rapids, Kingston for Newburgh, and Sarnia for Brantford.

Several thousand children were examined in each of these towns to establish the prevalence of caries before the start of the experiment. In 1945 the fluoride content of the water of Grand Rapids, Newburgh and Brantford was raised to 1 ppm, and in the following years information has accumulated upon the effects of this concentration of fluorides on the prevalence of caries, on mottling and on the general health both of those who have lived in these towns before the start of the experiment, and also of newcomers.

After 10 years the children of Newburgh between 6 and 9 years old (born since the beginning of the experiment) showed 58% less caries than their counterparts in Kingston. Children of 16, whose first 6 years preceded fluoridation, showed 41% less caries in Newburgh than in Kingston. Similar findings have been made in the other towns. No ill-effects of any sort due to fluoridation have been detected. There has been a low incidence of 'slight' or 'very slight' enamel opacities due to fluorosis in Newburgh but a greater number of enamel defects (non-fluoride opacities) in Kingston.

The findings in Grand Rapids and Brantford have been similar to those in Newburgh. Other cities in America and elsewhere have followed the example of these pioneers. In Britain, trials of fluoridation of the water supply were carried out in Watford, Anglesey and Kilmarnock. After 5 years, comparison with control areas showed the expected reduction in the incidence of caries in young children in the fluoridated areas. Nevertheless progress in fluoridation has been slow.

Kilmarnock has abandoned fluoridation, but it has been extended in Anglesey and is continuing in Watford. Birmingham and Newcastle are the only large cities to have introduced fluoridation.

By 1987, 10% of the total population of Britain had fluoridated water, but no further progress has been made. According to a World Health Organization (1969) survey, fluoridation programmes were in progress in 30 countries, affecting over

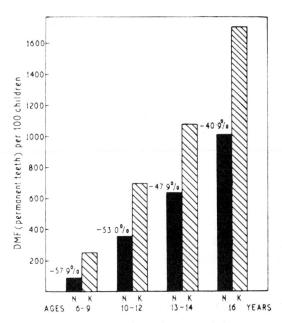

Fig. 7.3 Effects of artificial fluoridation. Some of the findings after 10 years of the Newburgh–Kingston caries-fluorine study. The incidence of caries (decayed, missing or filled permanent teeth) per hundred children of different age-groups is shown in each of the two towns together with the percentage reduction in caries in Newburgh in comparison with Kingston, the control town.

120 000 000 people. The conclusions of the WHO were that the safety and effectiveness of fluoridation of water were fully established and that member states should try to use this measure whenever possible.

Alternatives to water fluoridation

Where fluoridated water is not available fluoride can be ingested when incorporated in milk or table salt, or as fluoride tablets. Other alternatives are to apply fluorides topically to the teeth. By these means, those who wish can have some of the benefits of fluoridation, while those who object to the idea can be spared. These alternatives are, however, less satisfactory for a variety of reasons.

Addition of fluoride to salt and milk

The use of table salt as a vehicle for fluoride has been mainly tried in Switzerland. The variations in individual intake of salt are not well known, and hence the level of fluoridisation of salt has to be relatively low. Nevertheless the risk of fluoride intoxication from excessive salt intake is small. The level of fluoride included in salt provides a mean daily dose of about half to a third that which would have been received from fluoridated water by the average person.

After a 5-year trial it was found that the prevalence of dental caries in children between 7 and 12 years was reduced, but the benefit was only approximately half that expected from fluoridated water.

Fluoridisation of milk has also been tried on only a small scale. Fluoride is absorbed slightly more slowly from milk than from water, presumably because of interaction between the calcium and fluoride, but the final percentage absorbed is almost the same.

The results of fluoridised milk have been variable, but about 30% reduction in caries has been reported. As milk has been condemned by some as contributing to atherosclerosis, it might be considered inappropriate to recommend extra milk merely for caries prevention.

Yet another alternative to fluoridation of water supplies has been some pilot experiments in the USA, whereby fluoridated water has been available only at schools. In these circumstances water is fluoridated at about 5 ppm to make up for the absence of fluoride in the water at home. Clearly, however, this is a relatively expensive method to implement.

Fluoride tablets

Fluoride can be taken as tablets, but it requires intelligent cooperation by the parents to ensure that the tablets are taken regularly and to take precautions against accidental overdose.

When fluoride tablets are chewed or sucked there is the dual advantage of systemic effects because of absorption from the gut together with a topical effect after the teeth have erupted.

A variety of proprietary fluoride tablets, oral drops and mouthrinses is available. However, they cannot be prescribed by dentists in the National Health Service. The tablets each contain from 0.55 mg to 2.2 mg fluoride for use according to the child's age but they do not appear to be necessary before the age 6 months.

When taken by pregnant mothers fluoride tablets do not provide so useful a degree of protection of the child's teeth against caries.

Studies on transmission of fluoride across the placenta have produced somewhat conflicting results. It is apparent, however, that the placenta accumulates fluoride from the maternal blood, and most studies, including the more recent ones, show that the placenta acts as a partial barrier to fluoride. In addition excess fluoride is taken up by the mother's skeleton. The fluoride content of fetal blood is therefore low and probably never greater than a third of that of maternal blood.

Dosage of fluoride tablets

The recommended dosage of fluoride tablets has varied over the years, especially since there is wide individual variation in response, and, even in low fluoride areas, 0.5 mgF/day from birth up to the age of 2 years and 1.0 mgF/day thereafter can cause mild or, occasionally, disfiguring mottling. A suggested regimen is therefore as shown in Table 7.1.

Table 7.1 Recommended dosage (mg/d) of fluoride tablets

Concentration of fluoride in the drinking water (ppm):	0.2	0.3–0.7	>0.7
Age			
6 mths–2 yrs	0.25	0	0
2–4 yrs	0.50	0.25	0
4–16 yrs	1.00	0.50	0

The fluoride content of the local water supply should be available from the Health Authority for the area and must be taken into account before prescribing fluoride tablets as indicated.

Timing of optimal fluoride effects

Benefit is obtained from the intake of fluoride during the period of the formation and calcification of the enamel matrix. Systemic fluoride intake over 2 years of age can also provide significant benefit, particularly to interproximal tooth surfaces. With pit and fissure caries, systemic fluoride must be used soon after birth to have a beneficial effect. But whenever and however fluoride is taken, the benefits are greatest for the smooth interproximal surfaces and much less for pit and fissure caries. The evidence indicates that there is still a significant uptake of fluoride by the enamel within a period of about 12 months before eruption. This means that a child of 4 or 5 years of age can begin a fluoride tablet regime and gain benefit, even in the case of the first permanent molars.

Objections to the use of fluoride tablets

The objections to, and limitations on, the value of fluoride tablets are as follows.

1. *Overdose.* If a child should take a handful of fluoride tablets in mistake for sweets, toxic effects could result. However, an enormous number of tablets have to be taken to have any serious effects. The estimated lethal dose for adults is 2.5 g (1000 × 2.5 mg tablets) but the lethal dose for a child is not known. The treatment of acute overdose is discussed below.
2. *Mottling.* As mentioned earlier, fluoride tablets, in addition to fluoride from other sources, can raise the total intake to a level capable of causing mottling even in areas where there is little natural fluoride in the drinking water. Since the quantities of fluoride in all extraneous sources cannot be quantified, the recommended levels of dosage have been lowered, as explained earlier.
3. *Compliance.* The protective effect of fluoride tablets depends on their being taken regularly over a long period. This demands motivation on the part of the parents and cooperation by the children. The use of fluoride tablets, though generally safe and effective, is therefore feasible only for a minority.

Treatment of overdose

If the overdose is relatively small, the child should be made to drink a large volume of milk. This greatly slows absorption by interacting with the fluoride ions. If the level of overdose is not known, or if many tablets have been taken, the child should preferably be taken to hospital and can be given calcium chloride or lactate dissolved in water, followed by an emetic. Alternatively the stomach may have to be washed out.

Gross accidental overdose of fluoride can be lethal and has occasionally caused deaths.

Topical use of fluoride tablets

A high local concentration of fluoride is obtained by allowing tablets to dissolve slowly in the mouth. A 1 mg tablet held in the mouth at bedtime can provide a local fluoride concentration of up to 1000 ppm. This high concentration in contact with the teeth for a prolonged period has been reported to reduce caries activity by 80–90%. In a group of children with cleft palate where this measure was supplemented by regular application of APF gel and use of fissure sealants, a reduction in caries of 95–99% was reported.

Fluoride tablets can be made sufficiently pleasantly flavoured for children to enjoy sucking them. Cooperation can reasonably therefore be expected to be good.

Topical application of fluorides

Topical fluorides are indicated mainly for highly caries-prone children, the handicapped, or adults with xerostomia (Ch. 17). The usual technique is to apply the fluoride solution after cleaning and drying the teeth, and isolating them with cotton wool rolls. Alternatively, fluoride gels such as APF can be applied to the teeth in preformed trays to allow more prolonged contact of fluoride with the teeth.

Sodium fluoride

Sodium fluoride is usually used as a 2% solution. Its advantages are that (i) it is stable but may have to be stored in plastic bottles because it may attack glass, (ii) its flavour is acceptable and (iii) it is not irritating to the gingivae and does not stain the teeth.

Stannous fluoride

Stannous fluoride in 2% to 8% solutions appeared in some clinical trials to be more effective than 2%

sodium fluoride. Experimentally also, stannous fluoride retards the solution of enamel by acid. Though the clinical benefits of stannous fluoride have not been fully confirmed, some still regard it as the most effective topical preparation and it is available as a 4% gel.

Disadvantages of stannous fluoride are that (i) it is unstable in aqueous solution and a fresh solution should be made up on each occasion; (ii) it has an unpleasant and astringent taste; (iii) it sometimes causes gingival irritation and blanching; (iv) it frequently stains the teeth—this might mask caries.

Acidulated phosphate fluoride (APF)

Initial clinical trials with APF (a solution of sodium fluoride in weak phosphoric acid) indicated better caries protection than other fluorides. Experimentally, APF confers better uptake of fluoride by enamel than stannous or neutral sodium fluoride. However, the clinical benefits of APF have not been confirmed.

Otherwise the advantages of APF are essentially the same as those of sodium fluoride, and its disadvantage is its considerably greater cost.

Fluoride varnish

Sodium fluoride (50 mg/ml) suspended in a special base (Duraphat) adheres to the teeth long enough to allow better penetration of fluoride ions.

Fluoride-containing dentifrices

Toothpastes containing fluoride salts are widely available, heavily advertised and the way in which fluorides are most widely used. Use of fluoride salts in dentifrices has advantages, in that toothpaste is usually used every day and the material may be brought into close contact with the teeth, assisted by the abrasive in the dentifrice.

Initially there were technical problems in formulation of these dentifrices, in that the fluoride reacted with the usual abrasive (calcium carbonate) and was soon inactivated. In fact even the currently available dentifrices tend to become inactivated after a time and should be used as fresh as possible.

There are several formulations, and fluoride is used as stannous fluoride, sodium fluoride or sodium monofluorophosphate. Compatible abrasives include calcium pyrophosphate, insoluble sodium metaphosphate or plastic particles. The level of fluoride in these dentifrices is usually in the region of 0.1%, to reduce the danger of excessive quantities being swallowed by children.

In clinical trials fluoride-containing dentifrices have given variable results but can on average be expected to reduce caries by about 30%. The regular use of these preparations over many years, however, is likely to have a cumulative effect. Though (inevitably) some dispute the fact, it seems certain that the striking decrease in caries prevalence among children in recent years is the result mainly of the virtually universal use of fluoridised dentifrices.

The effect of fluoride toothpastes on caries prevalence has probably been most convincingly demonstrated in Japan, where their market share changed from only 10% to 15% between 1979 and 1983 and there was no change in DMFT levels in 12-year-old children between 1975 and 1980. By contrast, the market share of fluoride dentifrices had already reached 95% by 1977 in Britain, and caries showed a 36% decline between 1973 and 1983. This change has been noted despite the fact that the per capita sugar consumption in Britain was nearly twice that of Japan.

In France also DMFT levels at 12 years had not changed between 1975 and 1982. Here too the market share of fluoride toothpastes had risen from 10% in 1970 to only 58% in 1982.

Mode of action of fluorides against dental caries

The main value of fluorides was originally thought to be the result of their incorporation in enamel structure as fluorapatite, particularly during dental development. However, fluorides affect the teeth in a variety of ways, such as enhancing remineralisation, and their topical action is also important. However, the mode of action of fluorides in protecting teeth against dental caries is not fully understood. The three main theories are:

1. By promoting remineralisation of enamel after the carious attack
2. By making enamel more resistant to solution by acid
3. By interfering with bacterial metabolism in the plaque.

Effect of fluorides on remineralisation.
Fluorides are preferentially concentrated in bacterial plaque, and their presence either in plaque or within the enamel may favour precipitation of calcium and phosphate ions in the form of apatite rather than as more soluble calcium phosphates. When hydroxyapatite is attacked the calcium salts removed may be secondarily precipitated as calcium fluorapatite on the surface of the enamel crystallites. This may then reduce the rate of movement of hydrogen ions into the crystals and their rate of solution.

Effect of fluoride on the solubility of enamel.
There is some evidence that under the influence of fluoride larger apatite crystals are formed with fewer imperfections. The crystal lattice is therefore more stable and less susceptible to dissolution. Enamel also has a lower carbonate content in the presence of fluoride and this also reduces solubility.

Nevertheless it is by no means certain that the initial rate of dissolution of hydroxyapatite is any higher than that of fluorapatite.

Effect of fluoride on plaque metabolism.
Fluorides are concentrated in the plaque at much higher levels than would be expected from the fluoride content of the drinking water or saliva. The fluoride content of plaque may be anything from 6 to 100 parts per million. These levels of fluoride, in ionic form, will inhibit bacterial enzyme systems.

Fluoride in plaque, however, is predominantly in bound form and, unless it is bound to enzymes, is likely to be biologically inactive. There is nevertheless some evidence that up to 10% may be in ionic form. If this is so, fluoride could affect bacterial metabolism and depress acid production if the fluoride content of the plaque were sufficiently high. This, however, also remains unconfirmed.

It has also been suggested that fluorides may reduce the amount of plaque formed, or deposited on the teeth. Clinical trials have in general failed to demonstrate a plaque-reducing effect of this sort.

The evidence therefore indicates that fluoride probably achieves its optimal effect when incorporated into enamel during the course of its formation and by enhancing remineralisation.

Whatever the precise mechanism of protection by fluoride may be, its effectiveness is usually appreciably less when applied topically, especially after enamel has matured. Plaque may act as a barrier to absorption of fluoride by enamel in spite of, or perhaps because of, the fact that plaque can concentrate fluoride. However, the extent by which plaque interferes with the protective effect of topical fluorides remains unclear.

Fluorides in the prevention of dental caries—summary

1. Fluorides are the most widely used and effective measure for the control of dental caries. This effect was first shown in Britain in 1933.
2. Fluoridation of water supplies has been carried out in at least 30 countries, but only about 10% of the population of Britain have fluoridated water.
3. Fluoride at a level of 1 ppm in the water reduces the prevalence of caries by up to 60% in those exposed to it during dental development.
4. No adverse effects from fluoridation of water have been detected after its introduction in America in 1945.
5. Fluorides added to milk or table salt are alternatives to, but less effective than, fluoridation of the water.
6. Fluoride tablets taken during dental development effectively reduce susceptibility to caries, but the dosage must be carefully controlled because of the risk of mottling.
7. Allowing fluoride tablets to dissolve slowly in the mouth has an additional effect from the high (1000 ppm) concentration locally, in addition to the absorbed fluoride.
8. Sodium, stannous or acidulated phosphate fluorides can be used for direct topical

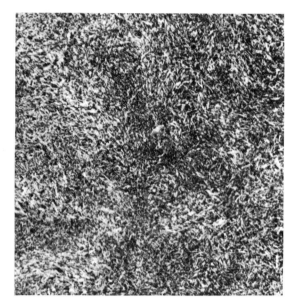

Fig. 7.4 Fluoride-containing enamel exposed to acid. An electron photomicrograph of a section of enamel from a patient from a high-fluoride area. The enamel has been exposed to a dilute acid but, unlike the specimen shown in Fig. 3.18, shows a uniform appearance without loss of the prism cores; both components of the matrix have remained intact and the apatite crystallites remain unaffected. This suggests that one effect of fluorine may be upon the organic matrix, and in this way it increases the resistance of the enamel to solution by acid ($\times$ 7500). (From a photograph kindly lent by Dr K. Little).

application to the teeth in high-risk patients. The effectiveness depends to a large degree on the frequency of application.

9. Sodium fluoride (0.2 to 0.6%) or APF mouthrinses used weekly by children may reduce caries by up to 50% but the effect declines rapidly after rinsing stops.

10. In Britain, by far the most common use of fluorides is in dentifrices which reduce caries by about 30%.

11. The mechanism of protection by fluoride is controversial but it may be by incorporation into the enamel structure, making it more resistant to acid attack and by enhancing remineralisation.

12. Fluoride is concentrated in plaque, but the effect of this on caries is uncertain.

Fissure sealants

Fissure sealants are used in a quite different way from other preventive measures. Their purpose is to obliterate the stagnation areas of occlusal pits and fissures.

The occlusal surfaces of molar teeth are the sites most vulnerable to caries and with few exceptions are attacked soon after eruption. These surfaces are also less well protected than the interstitial surfaces by fluorides, particularly when taken in the drinking water.

Fissure sealants have (obviously) to seal pits and fissures making it impossible for plaque to become established and to cut off plaque already formed from dietary substrate.

Effective sealing of many materials is achieved by preliminary etching of the enamel surface with phosphoric acid. This forms a submicroscopic mechanical key into which the liquid sealant penetrates. The sealant is then polymerised by local exposure to blue light or by addition of a catalyst.

New materials, the glass-ionomers, are true adhesives (form a chemical bond to the surfaces), and preliminary acid etching is not essential.

Examples of sealants are dimethacrylate resins which are unfilled or lightly filled, based on bis GMA (glyceridyl methacrylic acid).

Complete or almost complete retention of fissure sealants for up to 2 years in over 80% of cases has been reported. There has nevertheless been some controversy regarding their long-term effectiveness, but newer materials may overcome the problems of adhesion and durability.

An important limitation of fissure sealants is that there must be no faults in application (such as imperfect preparatory cleansing and drying of the enamel surface) whereby the seal is defective. This allows leakage of bacteria and saliva under the plastic and caries to progress unseen and unsuspected. Fissure sealants can therefore produce a false sense of security and do more harm than good.

Fissure sealants do not of course protect the interstitial surfaces, and parents must understand that normal preventive measures must continue to be used. These materials are therefore probably most appropriate for use in cooperative patients with a genuine desire for prevention.

PREVENTION OF DENTAL CARIES—SUMMARY

1. Complete prevention of dental caries is feasible but depends on motivation: namely, that patients genuinely want to save their teeth and are prepared to maintain the necessary effort.
2. The simplest, safest and most effective measure is to cut off the supply of sugar to the bacteria of the plaque. Sweets and candy bars in particular should be forbidden. Eating sweet stuffs between meals must be stopped, and sticky sweets, particularly caramels, must be avoided.
3. No foods have a useful natural protective effect and parents or patients must be disabused of ideas that milk, calcium supplements, or vitamins will counteract the effects of sweet eating.
4. Toothbrushing alone has little effect on caries except as a means of applying fluoride salts.
5. Directly antibacterial measures (antibiotics) are effective but are not of practical usefulness. Chlorhexidine has a theoretical potential for reducing caries activity but this has not been realised in practice.
6. Work continues on the development of vaccines against caries, but none has yet reached the stage of clinical trial. The effectiveness and safety of such vaccines in humans therefore remain speculative.
7. Fissure sealants are a supplementary measure that can be used to protect the highly vulnerable occlusal pits and fissures of molars. They should be used only in conjunction with other accepted preventive measures.
8. The main standby in caries prevention is the use of fluorides. Waterborne fluoride at 1 ppm should give about 60% reduction, while topical fluorides either in dentifrices or applied by the dentist can give 20% to 40% reduction or even more, according to how carefully and frequently they are used.

PREVENTION OF PERIODONTAL DISEASE

The attitudes of mind of both patient and dentist necessary for the prevention of both dental caries and periodontal disease are the same. Periodontal disease, however, presents a different kind of challenge, in that its progress is so insidious that failure to institute effective plaque control measures as early as possible may lead to irreversible destruction of supporting tissues. This may not become obvious until far advanced, when treatment may be too late to save the teeth. By contrast, even if no serious attempt is made at prevention, the damage from dental decay can usually be controlled by skilful restorative dentistry. Even after the pulp is involved, the tooth can usually be preserved.

Inspections twice a year are frequent enough to prevent excessive damage by decay in most patients. In contrast, the month-by-month progress of periodontal disease is often undetectable. In England and Wales the proportion of totally edentulous persons more than *trebles* between the ages of 40 and 70, when periodontal disease usually starts to have severe effects. For example, a person of 60 with 8 mm of bone loss round the lower incisors would (assuming steady progress over 50 years) have lost on average a mere 0.16 mm of bone per year. The difficulty of detecting bone loss at this rate with the crude methods available is only too obvious. Alveolar bone loss therefore only makes itself apparent when well established or when destruction accelerates. This in turn may indicate that treatment is less likely to be successful.

An exceptional level of vigilance is therefore essential to keep track of the rate of advance of periodontal disease, but to monitor the effectiveness of the patient's oral hygiene habits is easier. In most cases the progress of periodontal disease cannot be measured directly but has to be assessed indirectly by looking for traces of plaque or gingivitis.

Control of periodontal disease is therefore very much more difficult than controlling the effects of dental caries and demands more effort by the patient. At the risk of repetition, therefore, effective management of periodontal disease depends on the following.

1. Awareness of the problem by the dentist and constant vigilance to detect the most minor changes.
2. Adequate assessment of the patient. The main consideration is the patient's motivation, but the possibility of physical disability has also to be taken into account.
3. Making the patient understand the causes and effects of periodontal disease, motivating the patient to establish the necessary preventive habits and making it clear that these habits must be life-long.
4. Deciding on the optimal treatment plan for each patient, explaining the reasons for these decisions and training the patient accordingly.
5. Giving the patient an initial trial period of treatment to determine the response.
6. Reassessment of plaque control, showing patients where they have failed, reconsideration of the level of cooperation by patients, and vigorous encouragement when progress is made.

As discussed earlier, the proof of the pudding is shown by how the patient responds. If the patient is intelligent enough and has no other disability (and assuming also that the dentist is competent) the results after two or three visits will show whether or not the attempt is going to be successful. If, therefore, there has been adequate—and it really must be adequate—instruction and encouragement on each occasion, but after the third or fourth visit no visible progress has been made, the dentist will probably have to accept that he is fighting a losing battle.

Practical aspects

The management of periodontal disease is mainly preventive—by plaque control to prevent its onset if possible, but at least to try to prevent further progress. Most of this treatment is in the hands of the patient. Ancillary treatment measures, particularly periodontal surgery to eliminate pockets to facilitate scaling and to make the patient's own oral hygiene measures more effective. Diseased root surfaces should also be planed and any complications dealt with.

It is particularly important for the patient to acquire the habits necessary for plaque control early in life before tissue damage becomes irreversible.

Oral hygiene measures

The measures at the patient's command are: (1) toothbrushing; (2) use of dental floss; (3) use of wood sticks; (4) ancillary measures. The most important of these, particularly in the undamaged mouth, is toothbrushing.

Toothbrushing

Many toothbrushing techniques have been devised, but it must be accepted that many of these techniques are based on somewhat futile theorising as to the purposes or effects of toothbrushing or on nebulous concepts such as 'massaging the gums'. Often, these toothbrushing techniques demand manual dexterity far beyond the average patient's capabilities. Even when expertly performed these techniques have not been shown to remove plaque more effectively than simpler methods. The sole criterion of the quality of toothbrushing is whether plaque is completely removed.

There is *no* right or wrong way to brush the teeth, and it is irrelevant whether the patient brushes his teeth twenty times a day or in any particular direction if plaque still remains. This too must be explained to the patient. A small circular scrubbing action with the toothbrush bristles directed towards the gingivae is frequently recommended.

The most convincing means of assessing the effectiveness of plaque control is to get the patient to brush his teeth in the surgery, then to apply a disclosing agent. This shows the amount of residual plaque to the patient in dramatic fashion.

Any deficiencies in the patient's technique can be corrected. The patient can then use disclosing agent at home after toothbrushing until he has (a) acquired the necessary skill, (b) is spending enough time in toothbrushing to remove all accessible plaque and (c) is doing this sufficiently

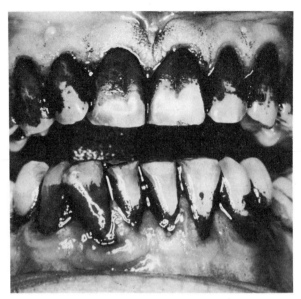

Fig. 7.5 This shows 24 hours accumulation of plaque stained by disclosing solution. The dramatic appearance that the latter produces impresses on the patient both the severity and distribution of plaque deposition.

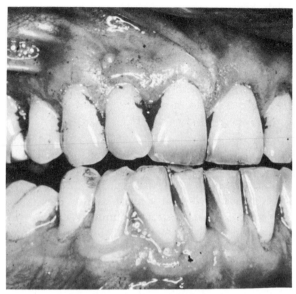

Fig. 7.6 This shows residual plaque interstitially in the same patient after fairly effective toothbrushing.

frequently and consistently to keep plaque under control. Thereafter the patient can use the disclosing agent at intervals (say once a month) to make sure that standards are being maintained. Use of disclosing agent is essential in the assessment of plaque control.

The patient must be disabused of the idea that toothbrushing 'makes the gums bleed'. Bleeding with toothbrushing is the result of gingivitis, and until this subsides bleeding is inevitable—indeed if there is gingivitis, absence of bleeding with toothbrushing means only that toothbrushing is ineffective.

Choice of toothbrush

The brush should have:

1. Synthetic (nylon) multitufted filaments. These do not absorb water, are cleaner and can be made to an exactly consistent quality of firmness and flexibility.
2. 'Medium' or 'medium soft' texture. The filaments should be fine and flexible enough to reach the depths of embrasures. Very soft

brushes such as badger hair are virtually useless and have little effect on plaque.
3. A short head (about 1 inch) to enable it to reach the inner aspects of a narrow or small arch.

Again, the final criterion is the ability of the patient to remove plaque with the chosen brush.

Automatic (electric) brushes

These have small brush heads with fine multi-tufted filaments allowing good access to the embrasures in all parts of the mouth. The rapid arcuate (rolling) oscillation also cleans effectively, and less manual dexterity or effort is needed than with an ordinary brush.

An electric toothbrush is therefore of special value to those with physical disabilities such as arthritis of the hands or who seem unable to acquire manual skills.

Patients must nevertheless be taught carefully how to use an automatic brush and must be able to show, with disclosing agent, that they can effectively remove plaque. It is a fallacy to assume that the purchase of an automatic brush immediately solves all toothbrushing problems as clinical trials have shown them to be no more effective than conventional toothbrushes.

Automatic brushes must be rechargeable or mains operated, otherwise the power falls off too rapidly. Even at full power they are relatively weak compared with manual brushing and can do no harm to the teeth or gums.

Dentifrices

In theory toothpastes are not necessary except for the removal of extrinsic staining. Plaque can be effectively removed with a brush alone. This is so unpleasant, however, that volunteers cannot be made to do without toothpaste, for experimental purposes, for any long period.

The refreshing taste and sensation left by the flavouring matter of the toothpaste makes the whole dreary business of toothbrushing more pleasant and makes one feel that something has been achieved, even (unfortunately) if it has not.

Dentifrices therefore have a very important role in encouraging toothbrushing. In addition the abrasive and detergent contribute to the removal of plaque. Pharmacologically active agents, particularly fluorides, can also be included in toothpastes, but so far no agent of proven value in the control of periodontal disease has been produced.

Other measures

Dental floss

Dental floss is the only means by which patients can remove plaque at and around interdental contact points. The danger of flossing in the young patient is that it can damage normal interdental gingivae. Flossing is therefore more appropriate after some gingival recession has developed.

Wood points

Wood points are needed when there has been gingival recession sufficient to expose the embrasures. These areas are inaccessible to toothbrushing. The sides of the wood points are used to rub plaque from these surfaces. The tip of the wood point must be directed slightly coronally when the stick is pushed between the teeth otherwise it can damage the interdental gingivae.

Bottle brushes

Miniature bottle brushes are useful for those with spaces between the teeth and where there are difficult concavities on the approximal surfaces.

Chlorhexidine

Chlorhexidine is available in Britain as a mouth rinse (0.1–0.2%) and as a gel (1%). It has been incorporated into dentifrices for experimental purposes. These are not yet generally available but the gel can be applied on a toothbrush.

Many studies have shown that regular use of chlorhexidine reduces plaque scores and gingivitis. A few studies have, however, failed to confirm these effects. Plaque formation quickly reverts to normal after the use of chlorhexidine is stopped. It must therefore be used regularly and continuously.

The many reports of studies on chlorhexidine that continue to appear suggest perhaps that its optimal mode of use and long-term value as a practical rather than as an experimental measure are not yet fully established for the following reasons.

1. Chlorhexidine has some value in the control of gingivitis but apparently only if patients' toothbrushing is not very effective. The effect of chlorhexidine on plaque or gingivitis cannot, for instance, be demonstrated in those who are skilled in plaque control. Nevertheless, since the majority of the population are neither very careful nor skilful in this activity chlorhexidine could be helpful.
2. Chlorhexidine is effective only against supra-gingival plaque and hence it is of little or no value in retarding the progress of pockets once they have formed.
3. The effect of chlorhexidine on plaque in stagnation areas inaccessible even to the conscientious toothbrusher is questionable. However, irrigation devices have been developed to deliver chlorhexidine subgingivally.

4. Chlorhexidine will not remove existing plaque, and every trace of the latter must be removed if chlorhexidine is to be effective.

To be effective, chlorhexidine should preferably be used twice a day in association with toothbrushing using a conventional dentifrice. The latter contributes to plaque control by mechanical means and also minimises staining of the teeth by the chlorhexidine.

Chlorhexidine itself has an unpleasant flavour but most patients seem quite quickly to accept it.

At the moment it seems that regular use of chlorhexidine as a mouth rinse or in gel form is useful mainly as supplementary aid for those whose plaque control is poor. In these chlorhexidine may help to control gingivitis to some degree.

Diet

Sugar consumption should be kept to a minimum, particularly to control caries and, in addition, to discourage plaque formation. Sticky carbohydrates should be avoided as far as possible.

PREVENTION OF PERIODONTAL DISEASE—SUMMARY

The success of long-term preventive measures depends mainly upon the following factors.

1. Careful assessment of the patient is essential to determine whether motivation is adequate and also to take into account physical factors which can occasionally affect the progress of periodontal disease.
2. Patients must be made to understand the purpose of plaque control, be trained (with the help of a disclosing agent) how to achieve it and be made to appreciate that only they can keep effective control of plaque on a day-to-day basis.
3. The patient must be sufficiently highly motivated; that is, there must be a strong and genuine desire to retain a healthy dentition regardless of the effort involved.
4. The dentist must exercise meticulously careful supervision of plaque control and watch for the slightest signs of failure (as indicated by disclosing solution) and the onset of gingivitis. Regular checks should be made on the thoroughness of brushing. Retraining should be given at intervals. Constant encouragement of the patient is also necessary.
5. Factors contributing to stagnation and accumulation of plaque should be eliminated as far as possible.
6. Plaque control is mainly by regular, skilful and careful toothbrushing. There should also be regular scaling and polishing by a skilled hygienist.
7. Ancillary measures are the use of woodpoints and flossing of interdental surfaces.
8. Chlorhexidine, preferably used twice daily, may help if toothbrushing is not of a high standard.

SUGGESTED FURTHER READING

Ainsworth N J 1928 Mottled teeth. Royal Dental Hospital Magazine, February
Ainsworth N J 1933 Mottled teeth. Br Dent J 60: 233–250
Anderson R J 1989 The changes in dental caries experience of 12-year old schoolchildren in two Somerset schools. A review after 25 years. Br Dent J 167: 312–315
Arnold F A Jr et al 1962 Fifteenth year of the Grand Rapids fluoridation study. J Am Dent Assoc 65: 780–785
Ashley F P, Sainsbury R H 1981 The effect of a school-based plaque control programme on caries and gingivitis. Br Dent J 150: 41–45
Ast D B et al 1956 Newburgh-Kingston caries-fluorine study XIV. Combined clinical roentgenographic dental findings after ten years of fluoride experience. J Am Dent Assoc 52: 314–325
Carlos J P 1982 The prevention of dental caries: ten years later. J Am Dent Assoc 104: 193–197
Carmichael C L et al 1980 The effect of fluoridation upon the relationship between caries experience and social class in 5-year-old children in Newcastle and Northumberland. Br Dent J 149: 163–167
Cawson R A, Stocker I P 1984 A note on the early history of fluorides. Br Dent J 157: 403–404
Choi S H, Stinson M W 1989 Purification of a Streptococcus mutans protein that binds to heart tissue and to glucosaminoglycans. Infect Immun 57: 3834–3840
Churchill H V 1931 Occurrence of fluorides in some waters of the United States. Ind and Eng Chem 23: 996–998

Creanor S L, Strang R Fluoridated dentifrices and early enamel lesion remineralisation. Dental Update 16: 9–17.

Dean H T 1938 Endemic fluorosis and its relation to dental caries. Public Health Reports 53: 1443–1452

Dean H T, Arnold F A Jr, Elvove E 1942 Domestic water and dental caries, V, additional studies of the relation of fluoride domestic waters to dental caries experience in 4,425 white children aged 12–14 years, of 13 cities in 4 states. Public Health Reports 57: 1155–1179

Diesendorf M 1986 The mystery of declining tooth decay. Nature 322: 125–129

Ferretti J J, Shea C, Humphrey M W 1980 Cross-reactivity of Streptococcus mutans antigens and human heart tissue. Infection and Immunity 30: 69–73

Forrest J R 1956 Caries incidence and enamel defects in areas with different levels of fluoride in the drinking water. Br Dent J 100: 195–200

Grenby T H, Paterson F M, Cawson R A 1973 Dental caries and plaque formation from diets containing sucrose or glucose in gnotobiotic rats infected with Streptococcus strain IB–1600. Br J Nutr 29: 221–228

Grenby T H 1977 Caries inhibiting chemicals. Nutr and Food Sci 46: 8–11

Grenby T H 1989 Latest state of research on lactitol and dental caries. Int Dent J 39: 25–32

Gustaffson B E et al 1954 The Vipeholm dental caries study. Acta Odontol Scand 11: 232

Health Education Authority. The scientific basis of health education, 3rd edn. Health Education Authority, London

Hepworth A 1973 Some implications of attitude research and motivation theory for the dentist–patient relationship. In: Davis H C, Forrest J O (eds) Review of dental practice 1972. Dental Publications, Epsom

Hobdel M H, O'Hickey S 1989 Public Water fluoridation in Ireland: twenty five years on. Br Dent J 195: 36–38

Hoffman R et al 1980 Acute fluoride poisoning in a New Mexico elementary school. Pediatrics 65: 897–900

Holloway P J, Mellor A C 1989 Capitation: an alternative payment system for the treatment of children in the General Dental Service. Dental Update 16: 234–240

Kay E 1988 The psychology of behaviour change and dental health. Dental Update 15: 386–388

Krasse B, Emilson C-G, Gahnberg L 1987 An anticaries vaccine: report on the status of research. Caries Res 21: 255–276

Manson J D, Eley B M 1989 The prevention of periodontal disease. Dental Update 16: 189–196

Murray J J 1976 Fluorides in caries prevention. Wright, Bristol

McCall D, Stephen K W, McNee S G 1981 Fluoride tablets and salivary fluoride levels. Caries Res 15: 98–102

McCann D 1989 Fluoride and dental health; a story of achievements and challenges. JADA 118: 529–540

McKay F S 1928 The relation of mottled teeth to caries. J Am Dent Assoc 15: 1429–1437

Palmer J D 1980 Dental health in children—an improving picture? Br Dent J 149: 48–50

Randal J 1990 USA: Another flap over fluoride. Lancet 335: 282–283

Rugg-Gunn A J 1990 Prevention of dental caries. Dental Update 17: 24–28

Rugg-Gunn A J 1990 Current issues in the use of fluorides in dentistry. Dental Update 17: 154–160

Rugg-Gunn A J 1990 Diet and dental caries. Dental Update 17: 198–201

Silverstone L M 1973 Plaque control. Dental Update 1: 147–159

Silverstone L M 1974 Topical fluorides: development and clinical trials. Dental Update 1: 401–405

Silverstone L M 1976 Topical fluorides: Mouth rinses, dentifrices, pastes and varnishes. Dental Update 3: 107–110

Silverstone L M 1977 Fissure sealants: 2. Dental Update 4: 73–83

Sims W 1970 The concept of immunity in dental caries. I. General considerations. Oral Surg, Oral Med, Oral Pathol 30: 670–677

Stephen K W, Macfadyen E E 1977 Three years of clinical caries prevention for cleft palate children. Br Dent J 143: 111

Stephen K W, McCall D R, Tullis J I 1987 Caries prevalence in northern Scotland before and 5 years after water defluoridation. Br Dent J 193: 324–326

Stephen K W 1989 Criteria for efficacy of plaque control agents for caries. J Dent Res 68 (Spec Iss): 1672–1676

Weaver R 1944 Fluorosis and dental caries on Tyneside. Br Dent J 76: 29–40

Welbury R R Prevention of trauma to teeth. Dental Update 1990; 17: 117–122

World Health Organization 1958 Report of Expert Committee on water fluoridation. WHO Technical Report Series 146

World Health Organization 1969 Fluoridation and dental health. WHO Chronicle 23: 505–512

8. Major oral, perioral and related systemic infections

Despite the frequent presence of dangerous pathogens, particularly in periodontal pockets, dental infections are mostly minor and localised, as described in the previous chapters. Nevertheless, more serious oral or perioral infections can be caused by these bacteria, and under certain circumstances they can cause systemic infections, such as infective endocarditis. Another factor which can promote serious oral infections or systemic spread of oral bacteria is immunodeficiency and, in particular, AIDS.

MAJOR ORAL AND PERIORAL INFECTIONS

Acute osteomyelitis of the mandible

Acute osteomyelitis of the jaw is typically a disease of adult males and in most cases the infection has a dental source. However, the infection can originate from any of the following.

1. Acute periapical infection
2. A periodontal pocket when the jaw is fractured
3. Acute gingivitis or pericoronitis (very rarely)
4. The skin or other external sources (open fractures or gunshot wounds).

Predisposing causes

Now that 'spontaneous' severe infections in or around the jaws have become rare in the normal population, predisposing conditions have become relatively more important. The main examples include.

175

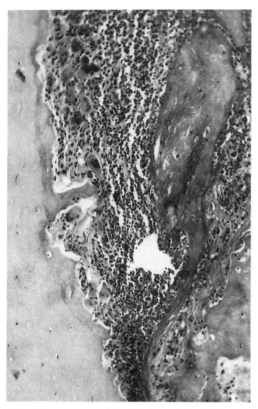

Fig. 8.1 Acute osteomyelitis. The bone is bathed in pus; bone to the right is dead and on its surface is pale-staining amorphous material which consists largely of bacteria. To the left the bone is undergoing active resorption and many osteoclasts can be seen (× 60).

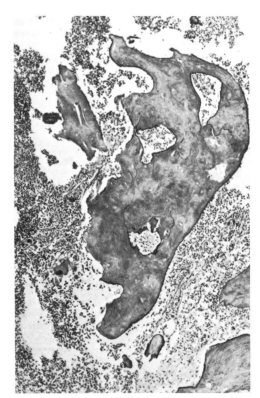

Fig. 8.2 Acute osteomyelitis. This is a sequestrum; the bone is dead (the lacunae are empty of osteocytes), irregular in shape due to resorption and lying free in the inflammatory exudate (× 60).

1. Local damage to, or disease of, the jaws
   a. open fractures, including gunshot wounds
   b. radiation damage
   c. Paget's disease
2. Impaired immune defences: examples are acute leukaemia, AIDS, immunosuppressive treatment, uncontrolled diabetes mellitus and malnutrition and/or chronic alcoholism. In such cases, and particularly in alcoholics, serious infection of the bone is typically precipitated by injury, sometimes of a minor nature.

Microbiology

Acute osteomyelitis of the jaws is caused by oral bacteria, particularly anaerobes such as Bac-

teroides species, and is typically a mixed infection. However, strict care in sampling techniques is necessary to isolate anaerobes, and for this reason they may not be found and were not considered in the past. Gram-negative infections have also been reported.

Unlike osteomyelitis of long bones, *Staphylococcus aureus* is rarely the cause of osteomyelitis of the jaw unless it comes from an external source, such as the skin, as a result of an open fracture or gunshot wound.

Pathology

On the rare occasions that osteomyelitis follows an extraction it must be presumed that the infection was unusually virulent or resistance is impaired. Delay in carrying out the extraction may give an opportunity for infection to spread along the marrow cavity. Extraction no longer then provides adequate drainage, and osteomyelitis becomes established.

Fractures of the tooth-bearing regions of the jaw are invariably open to the oral cavity through torn mucoperiosteum. When the fracture involves the periodontal ligament, however, infection can spread from a pocket. When the injury is a gun-shot wound there may be the combined effects of gross trauma, foreign bodies implanted in the wound and infection from the skin.

The process comprises, in brief, an initial stage of spread of infection and of acute inflammation in bone and death of an area of bone. The necrotic tissue becomes separated by osteoclastic action along its junction with healthy bone and forms a sequestrum. New bone forms outside the infected area, and, after the sequestrum has been shed, repair follows.

In the early stages a typical acute inflammatory response leads to dilatation of blood vessels and outpouring of fluid and cellular exudate which carries infection further. The rigid bony canals cause the exudate to compress blood vessels; thrombosis and obstruction can then lead to further bone necrosis. This dead bone is readily recognisable microscopically by lacunae empty of osteocytes and the presence of pus cells. Bacteria can proliferate in this dead avascular tissue and are then relatively inaccessible to many antibiotics such as the penicillins.

Pus formed by liquefaction of necrotic soft tissue and inflammatory cells are forced along the medulla but pus is eventually able to escape by osteoclastic resorption of bone to form sinuses. Distension of the periosteum by pus leads to sub-periosteal bone formation but perforation of the periosteum by pus and formation of sinuses on the skin or oral mucosa is rarely seen now.

At the boundary between the infected and healthy tissue, osteoclasts resorb the margins of the dead bone, which thus eventually becomes separated as a sequestrum.

Healing of bone infections

Once the infection has become localised, new bone forms around it, particularly subperiosteally as mentioned earlier. In the past this could lead to involucrum formation and enclosure of sequestra; however, no more than a rim of new bone below the lower border of the mandible is usually seen now.

Where bone has died and been removed, healing is by granulation with formation of coarse fibrous bone in the proliferating connective tissue. Gradually the fibrous bone is replaced by compact bone and remodelled to restore normal morphology to some extent.

Clinical features

Males are predominantly affected and the mandible is almost exclusively involved. This is probably due to the more limited blood supply and the denser nature of the mandible with its thick cortical plates and coarse trabeculae. Pain and swelling are early complaints. The pain is severe, throbbing and deep-seated. The external swelling is at first due to inflammatory oedema, but later distension of the periosteum with pus, and, finally, subperiosteal bone formation cause the swelling to become progressively firmer. The overlying gum is red, swollen and tender.

Teeth in the area are tender, or in severe cases may become loose and pus may exude from round their necks or from an open socket.

Muscle oedema causes difficulty in opening the mouth and swallowing. The regional lymph nodes are enlarged and tender and there may be anaesthesia or paraesthesia of the lower lip.

During the acute phase there may be fever, malaise and leucocytosis but frequently the patient remains surprisingly well. A severely ill, or very pale patient suggests underlying disease which should be investigated.

Radiographic changes

Bony changes do not appear until after at least 10 days. The sharp trabecular pattern of the bone is lost where bone has been resorbed, and areas of radiolucency indicate bone destruction. These areas have ill-defined margins and have a fluffy or moth-eaten appearance. Areas of dead bone appear relatively dense and become more sharply defined as they eventually separate as sequestra. Later, there is subperiosteal new bone formation: this is most often seen in young patients and appears as a thin, curved strip of new bone below the lower border of the jaw.

Management

The main principles are as follows.

Bacteriological diagnosis. A specimen of pus or, failing that, a swab from the depths of the lesion should be cultured and the sensitivity of the organisms tested.

Antibiotics. Initially penicillin, 600 mg to 1200 mg daily, should be given by injection provided that the patient is not hypersensitive. The bacteriological findings may, however, dictate a change of treatment.

Drainage. Pressure within the bone must be relieved by tooth extraction, bur holes or decortication, and exudate should be drained into the mouth or externally as necessary.

Removal of sequestra. The acute infection must first be controlled: dead bone should not be forcibly separated, and vigorous curetting is inadvisable. Teeth should be extracted only if their attachments have been destroyed and they are loose.

Complications

1. Involvement of the inferior dental nerve may cause anaesthesia of the lower lip. This is relieved when the infection resolves.
2. Pathological fracture may be caused by severe bone destruction.
3. Cellulitis, due to spread of exceptionally virulent organisms, is rare.
4. Septicaemia is almost unknown in the present day unless the patient is immunodeficient.

Acute osteomyelitis in infancy

Exceptionally rarely now, acute osteomyelitis involves the maxilla in neonates or infants and is a consequence either of birth injuries (due to forceps, for example) or uncontrolled middle ear infection.

Chronic osteomyelitis

If inadequately treated, osteomyelitis may oc-

casionally become chronic; rarely, chronic osteomyelitis may develop without any apparent acute episode and may be a response to low-grade infection or result from high local resistance. The infection is localised, but persistent because bacteria growing in dead bone are inaccessible to host defences.

Pain is mild but may be punctuated by acute exacerbations and intermittent discharge of pus. Sequestra may often be felt by probing along a sinus; they give a characteristic rough, grating sensation. Small sequestra may continue to be shed for months.

Radiographically, the area of bone destruction is usually limited and there may be sclerosis of surrounding bone, together with subperiosteal new bone formation. Treatment is usually by combinations of antibiotics, and decortication and/or exposure to hyperbaric oxygen may be helpful.

Chronic osteomyelitis with proliferative periostitis (Garré's osteomyelitis)

This rare reaction, usually to periapical infection in young persons, is characterised by mild pain

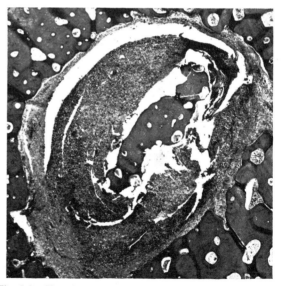

Fig. 8.3 Chronic osteomyelitis. A sequestrum has become trapped in a cavity within the bone. The eroded appearance of the sequestrum can be clearly seen and it is surrounded by granulation tissue containing chronic inflammatory cells. New bone is being deposited on the walls of the cavity. Surgical intervention is needed to remove an infected sequestrum such as this ($\times$ 15).

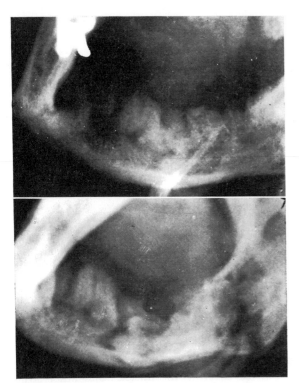

Fig. 8.4 Osteomyelitis of the mandible following dental extractions. In the upper picture the outlines of the extraction sockets can be seen and there are early signs of bone destruction extending along the jaw. In the lower picture, taken about two months later, there is extensive bone destruction and sequestration with loss of the normal trabecular structure of the jaw.

and later a non-tender bony swelling, usually of the mandible. Radiographically there is a lucent area surrounded by a sclerotic laminated cortex, best seen in an occlusal film. Treatment of the causative infection leads to gradual resolution.

Diffuse sclerosing osteomyelitis

This is of uncertain aetiology. It resembles gigantiform cementoma (florid osseous dysplasia) radiographically and is thought by many to be a variant of the latter. However, it may be associated with severe periodontal disease and give rise to episodes of pain.

Radiographs show areas of diffuse or nodular sclerosis, resembling the cotton-wool radiopacities of Paget's disease, often bilaterally, and sometimes involving both the mandible and the maxilla.

Microscopy shows dense, irregular bone with a pagetoid ('mosaic') pattern of reversal lines and patchy infiltration by chronic inflammatory cells.

Diseased teeth should be extracted and antibiotics given. If the dense masses form sequestra they should be removed. However, healing is slow.

Chronic focal osteomyelitis

This is a rare reaction to periapical infection and may cause mild pain. It is usually seen as a sclerotic area at the apex of a dead tooth in a young patient.

Microscopically, the bone is typically empty of osteocytes and may show a pagetoid pattern of reversal lines. Extraction of the infected tooth should lead to resolution.

Sclerotic bone islands

Areas of bone sclerosis may sometimes be seen radiographically in a healthy jaw and appear to be a normal variant. In the absence of signs of inflammation or symptoms they should not be interfered with.

Radiation-associated osteomyelitis

Radiation for cancer of the mouth can cause death of an area of bone of the jaw (osteoradionecrosis). This bone is dense and avascular but can remain buried and asymptomatic until it becomes infected. Infection can gain entry via pulpal or periodontal disease or, particularly, extractions or any minor injuries which allow the entry of dental bacteria. There appears to be a close relationship between the health of the dentition before irradiation and subsequent infection, which, once it has gained entry, spreads widely.

The mandible is usually affected. It has dense cortical plates and trabeculae, and its blood supply via the periosteum may become even more limited in the elderly.

Clinical features

Irradiation-induced osteomyelitis is persistent and intractable as a result of the ischaemia resulting from radiation-induced arteritis. There is extensive necrosis of bone, periosteum and mucosa. The overlying tissues may slough away exposing the bone within the mouth or externally or both. Sequestra are often large, densely radiopaque and fail to separate normally. The periosteum may also fail to form new bone.

Treatment is difficult and prevention is essential (Ch. 22). Extractions before radiotherapy are unlikely to cause serious complications, but 10 to 14 days is usually allowed to permit healing before irradiation. However, such delay is probably not essential if treatment is urgent (see also Ch. 16).

Management

Treatment should be conservative. Any intraoral wounds should be frequently irrigated, and the patient must maintain meticulous oral hygiene with frequent mouthrinses to dislodge food debris.

Sequestra should be allowed to separate spontaneously, since active curettage promotes extension of the infection. Only loose bony sequestra should be removed, but sharp edges or spicules of bone should be smoothed off to prevent irritation of the soft tissues. Approximately 50% of cases ultimately heal spontaneously by natural sequestration and granulation if infection can be controlled. However, separation of dead bone may take many months or even years because of the affected bone's poor blood supply.

The slow healing makes the value of antibiotic therapy uncertain, and the avascularity of the tissues limits the access of many antibiotics apart from clindamycin and a few others. However, some advocate long-term administration of tetracycline or sodium fusidate, and metronidazole may be included. In the majority of cases, pain is not severe or can be controlled with simple analgesics.

Indications for surgical intervention are uncontrollable severe pain or infection. Failure of healing may also result from residual or recurrent tumour which becomes apparent when dead bone is removed. If resection is undertaken, the margins should be within healthy bleeding bone or further necrosis follows.

Chronic specific osteomyelitis

Syphilitic, actinomycotic and tuberculous osteo-myelitis of the jaws are recognised entities, but unlikely to be seen now.

Cervicofacial cellulitis

Cellulitis is a spreading infection of connective tissue, characterised by gross inflammatory exudate and oedema, together with fever and toxaemia which may be severe and, if not promptly and vigorously treated, can be quickly fatal.

Aetiology and pathology

Cervicofacial cellulitis has become rare in many parts of Britain but appears to be considerably more common among West Indians. Such patients are fit, well nourished young male adults, frequently with apical periodontal abscesses but no apparent systemic predisposing factors other than sickle cell trait in some cases.

The organisms mainly responsible are beta-haemolytic streptococci and various anaerobes.

Fasciae covering the muscles and other structures are normally in close apposition. If these fascial planes are separated artificially a space is created. Such spaces contain little except loose connective tissue and are almost avascular. If, therefore, virulent organisms get between the fascial planes, inflammatory exudate is poured out from nearby vessels but, failing to localise the organisms, opens up the fascial space, carrying infection with it. Infection may thus spread through one or more fascial spaces until their natural boundaries are reached.

The main cause of cellulitis of the neck is infection arising from the region of the lower molars. Several fascial spaces are accessible from this area, and the following factors are contributory.

1. The apices of the second and, more especially, the third molars are often close to the lingual surface of the mandible.
2. The mylohyoid attachment inclines upwards as it runs forward; the apices of the third molar are usually, and the second molar are often, below this line.
3. The posterior border of the mylohyoid is close to the sockets of the third molars. At this point the floor of the mouth consists

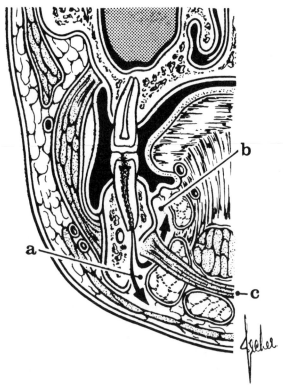

Fig. 8.5 Paths of infection from lower molars. By penetrating the lingual plate of the jaw below the attachment of mylohyoid (c), infection immediately enters the submaxillary space (a). Below the mylohyoid is the main body of the submaxillary salivary gland with its deep process curving round the posterior border of the muscle; infection from the third molar can follow the same route to enter the sublingual space (b).

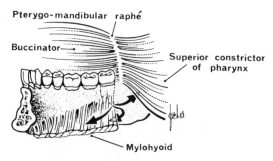

Fig. 8.6 Paths of infection from the third molar. The diagram shows the lingual aspect of the jaw and indicates how infection penetrating the lingual plate of bone can enter the sublingual space above, or the submaxillary space below the mylohyoid muscle which forms the major part of the floor of the mouth. Moreover, since this point is at the junction of oral cavity and pharynx, infection can also spread backwards to reach the lateral surface of superior constrictor, i.e. the lateral pharyngeal space.

only of mucous membrane covering part of the submandibular salivary gland.

For these reasons, a virulent periapical infection of a lower third molar may penetrate the lingual plate of the jaw and is then at the entrance to several fascial spaces. In front of this point are the submandibular and sublingual spaces, while behind it are the parapharyngeal and pterygoid spaces. Infection in this area may also spread from an acute pericoronitis, particularly when the deeper tissues are opened to infection by extraction of the tooth during the acute phase.

Cellulitis can be a complication of acute osteomyelitis of the jaws due to spread of an exceptionally virulent infection, but this is hardly ever seen now.

In general, cellulitis around the jaw is only likely to develop when the tissues are infected by virulent and invasive organisms at a point where there is access to the fascial spaces. Since the predisposing causes do not often coincide, cellulitis is uncommon. Cellulitis in the region of the upper jaw is even more uncommon, but fascial space infections may develop in various sites as the result of infected local anaesthetic needles.

General clinical features

The characteristic features of cellulitis are diffuse, brawny swelling, pain, fever and malaise. The swelling is tense, tender, with a characteristic boardlike firmness. The overlying skin is taut and shiny. Pain and oedema cause difficulty in opening the mouth and, often, difficulty in swallowing.

Constitutional upset becomes severe with increasing fever, toxaemia and leucocytosis. The regional lymph nodes are swollen and tender.

Sublingual cellulitis

The sublingual space lies between the mucous membrane of the floor of the mouth above, and the mylohyoid below and laterally; medially the space is bounded by the geniohyoid and genioglossus muscles. In front of the tongue, the left and right sublingual spaces are continuous. A deep extension of the space lies between the genial muscles.

Posteriorly, on either side, the sublingual space is open, communicating round the posterior border of the mylohyoid with the submandibular space below, and with the parapharyngeal space behind. The sublingual space contains the sublingual gland and related arteries and nerves.

Clinical features. The source of infection is usually a mandibular molar, but occasionally infection from a tooth nearer the front of the mouth may penetrate the lingual plate of bone. Sublingual cellulitis is characterised by gross swelling of the floor of the mouth. The mucous membrane is red or purplish and is pushed upwards level with the occlusal surfaces of the teeth, which indent it. Swallowing is difficult because of oedema of the muscles of the tongue, which becomes swollen and elevated.

Infection may remain localised in the sublingual space or may spread backwards towards the parapharyngeal, pterygoid, or submandibular space.

Submandibular cellulitis

The submandibular space contains the submandibular salivary gland and is formed by the splitting of the deep cervical fascia above the hyoid bone. The submandibular space is bounded laterally and below by the superficial layer of the deep cervical fascia which extends from the hyoid bone to the mylohyoid and forms the superior and medial boundary of the space.

The intercommunications of the three main fascial spaces in this area are shown by the deep process of the submandibular gland. This extends round the posterior border of the mylohyoid, jutting into the entry to the parapharyngeal space and curving forward onto the superior surface of the mylohyoid and comes to lie within the sublingual space.

Clinical features. Submandibular cellulitis is typically caused by infection from the second or third molars. The swelling is centred upon the upper part of the neck, mainly along the lower border of the mandible. Infection may spread into the sublingual or parapharyngeal spaces as already indicated.

Ludwig's angina

Ludwig's angina is a severe form of cellulitis which usually arises from the lower second or third molars; it involves the sublingual and mandibu-

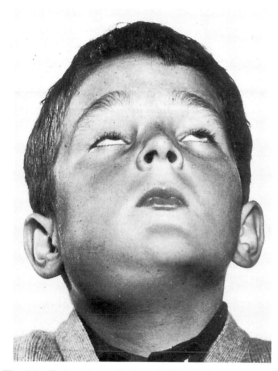

Fig. 8.7 Early submandibular cellulitis. A firm inflammatory swelling occupies the whole of the right submandibular region.

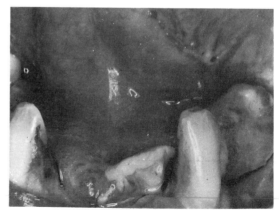

Fig. 8.8 Sublingual cellulitis in Ludwig's angina. The floor of the mouth is pushed up to the level of the teeth and is dark and oedematous.

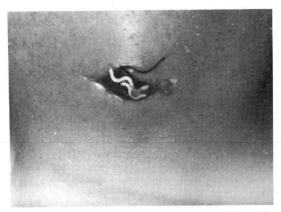

Fig. 8.9 Ludwig's angina. The same patient as in Fig. 8.8 showing the swelling of the neck due to simultaneous submaxillary and sublingual cellulitis. The incision in the front of the neck was to relieve the pressure of exudate to allow the patient to breathe. The neck is grossly swollen, shiny (due to the tension on the skin) and dusky in hue; the edges of the wound have pulled apart indicating the distension of these normally lax tissues.

lar spaces bilaterally almost simultaneously and readily spreads into the pharyngeal and pterygoid spaces.

The parapharyngeal space extends backwards from the lingual aspect of the third molar region, between the superior constrictor of the pharynx medially, and the internal pterygoid laterally. Above the mylohyoid line the space is limited anteriorly by the pterygomandibular raphe. Below, the parapharyngeal space is bounded by the muscles arising from the styloid process. Within this space lies the carotid sheath.

The pterygoid space lies lateral to the pharyngeal space. Its lateral border is the mandibular ramus, and the medial pterygoid muscle is medial to it. Above, it communicates with the infratemporal fossa.

Clinical features. Ludwig's angina is characterised by rapid development of sublingual and submandibular cellulitis with painful, brawny swelling of the upper part of the neck and the floor of the mouth on both sides. When the parapharyngeal space becomes involved the swelling tracks down the neck, and oedema readily spreads into the loose connective tissue round the glottis.

There is difficulty in swallowing, opening the mouth may be limited and the tongue may be pushed up against the soft palate. Oedema of the glottis causes increasing respiratory obstruction. The patient soon becomes seriously ill, with fever, headache and malaise.

Signs of respiratory obstruction are noisy breathing and restlessness, going on to violent efforts at respiration and darkening cyanosis. A patient with cellulitis of the neck may die quickly from this cause, or later from the effects of spread of infection to the mediastinum via the carotid sheath.

Any patient with a brawny swelling of the mouth or neck, fever and malaise, requires urgent admission to hospital. The mainstay of treatment of cellulitis is vigorous use of antibiotics. Provided that the patient is not hypersensitive, intravenous penicillin (not less than 600 mg) should be given every 6 hours. Metronidazole may also be given. Early drainage is necessary to relieve the pressure of exudate, particularly if the swelling is so large and tense as to force the tongue into the airway. The swelling should be opened widely and multiple corrugated drains inserted. Little fluid is produced at first but exudate continues to dribble away.

Emergency tracheostomy may be necessary to maintain the airway but general anaesthesia is hazardous if the airway is becoming obstructed.

The tooth from which the infection started should be extracted as soon as the patient's condition allows.

Soft-tissue abscesses

An abscess may form as a result of direct spread from a periapical infection or be the result of localisation of a fascial space infection. The palate is more frequently affected than other sites. The microbial causes are those of the preceding infection.

Palatal abscess

Infection may spread from a lateral incisor because of its backward-sloping root, or from the palatal root of a molar. The swelling is rounded, discrete and tender. It is usually close to the offending tooth but may occasionally spread to the posterior border of the hard palate from a lateral incisor.

Buccal abscess

The abscess may be either medial or lateral to the buccinator and can result from periapical infection on a molar tooth, breaking through the buccal plate of the jaw deep to the buccal sulcus. There is pain, swelling, redness and tenderness of the cheek. The swelling, though not easily defined because of the thickness of the cheek, is more localised than that of cellulitis, and systemic effects are minimal. Later the swelling becomes fluctuant as pus localises.

Submasseteric abscess

Rarely, infection from a lower third molar tracks backwards, lateral to the mandibular ramus, and pus localises deep to the masseter attachment. Such an abscess deep to the thick masseter muscle produces little visible swelling but causes profound muscle spasm and limitation of opening.

Management. Antibiotic therapy may be unnecessary if the abscess is small and well localised, as in the case of many vestibular or palatal abscesses. Otherwise 600 mg of penicillin, if the patient is not allergic, should be given to hasten localisation.

The infected tooth should be extracted or the root canal opened, and, most important, the abscess should be drained via an intraoral incision.

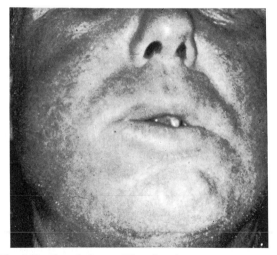

Fig. 8.10 Buccal abscess. There is a firm rounded swelling of the cheek pulling the angle of the mouth to one side and containing a collection of pus.

Principles of drainage of an abscess

The main principles are as follows.

1. Make sure that a localised collection of pus has formed and is accessible. Signs of localisation are a well-defined area of inflammation becoming fluctuant in the centre.
2. The opening must be in the most dependent part to give good gravitational drainage and be wide enough to drain the whole cavity. Any locules of pus should be opened.
3. The incision must avoid important vessels and nerves, especially branches of the facial nerve.
4. Whenever possible the opening should be intraoral but, when external, the direction of the incision should be such as to leave as little visible scarring as possible.
5. The incision must be kept open with a drain for an adequate period; usually 2 or 3 days.

A neglected abscess will eventually point and discharge spontaneously, sometimes with an unsightly facial sinus and subsequent scarring.

Cavernous sinus thrombosis

Cavernous sinus thrombosis is a serious but rare complication that can result from spread of infection, usually from an upper anterior tooth but sometimes from infections of the upper lip or anterior nares. Infected thrombi in the anterior facial vein or, less commonly, the pterygoid plexus of veins communicate with the cavernous sinus via either the ophthalmic veins or via the foramen ovale, respectively.

Clinically, there is gross oedema of the eyelids together with pulsatile exophthalmos due to venous obstruction. Venous stasis also leads to cyanosis. The superior orbital fissure syndrome rapidly develops, the facial vein is dilated and the conjunctiva is oedematous. There are papilloedema and multiple retinal haemorrhages. The patient is ill with rigors and a high swinging pyrexia. Initially one side is affected, but, without treatment, infection rapidly spreads to the opposite side.

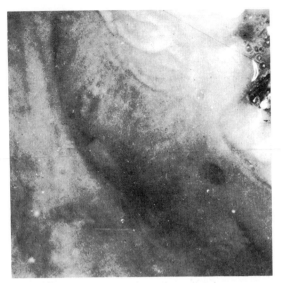

Fig. 8.11 Palatal abscess. Infection has spread under the periosteum from the palatal root of a molar causing a swelling extending to the median raphe (left).

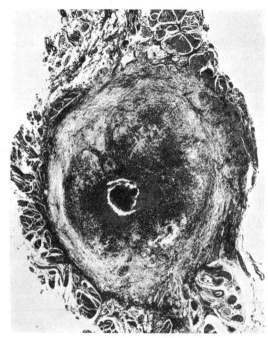

Fig. 8.12 Actinomycosis. This single, complete loculus was from an early case of actinomycosis that followed dental extractions. The colony of actinomyces with its paler-staining periphery is in the centre, around it is a dense collection of inflammatory cells, surrounded in turn by proliferating fibrous tissue. It will be apparent that an antibiotic cannot readily penetrate such a fibrous mass and must be given in large doses to be effective ($\times$ 10).

Management

A combination of anticoagulants, antibiotics, drainage of pus and the elimination of the source of infection is essential. There is a 50% mortality, and, of those who survive, half lose the sight of one or both eyes.

Actinomycosis

Actinomycosis is an uncommon, chronic, suppurative infection caused by a filamentous bacterium and characterised by formation of multiple sinuses and widespread fibrosis. The soft tissue in the region of the angle of the jaw and adjacent neck is the most common site.

Aetiology and pathology

The causative organism is usually *Actinomyces israelii*, but other bacteria may occasionally be responsible. In culture, pathogenic actinomyces grow slowly on enriched media under anaerobic conditions to form a mass of branching filaments. Actinomyces are present in the normal mouth, and, in some cases, injuries, especially dental extractions or fractures of the jaw, provide a path-way into the tissues for the organism, and precede infection. Nevertheless, it is unclear why actinomycosis so rarely follows extractions or hardly ever becomes established in bone. Most patients are apparently otherwise healthy, and, though actinomycosis is a recognised complication of AIDS, it is not common even in this group.

A. israelii spreads by direct extension through the tissues and excites a chronic inflammatory reaction with suppuration. In the tissues, colonies of actinomyces form rounded masses of filaments, at the periphery of which radially-arranged thickenings, or clubs, develop. Polymorphonuclear leucocytes mass around the colonies; pus forms centrally, chronic inflammatory cells surround the focus and an abscess wall of connective tissue is formed.

The abscess eventually points on the skin, discharging pus in which 'sulphur granules' (colonies of actinomyces) may be visible. The abscess continues to discharge, and the surrounding tissues become fibrotic; this is nevertheless insufficient to localise the infection, which spreads causing further abscess formation. Eventually, in the absence of effective treatment, the area may become honeycombed with abscesses and many sinuses, and widespread fibrosis, but this is unlikely to be seen now. The infection is only rarely seen within the bone of the jaw.

Clinical features

Men are predominantly affected, typically adults between the ages of 30 and 60. The complaint is usually of a chronic soft-tissue swelling near the angle of the jaw and neck. There may be a history of dental extractions, especially of lower molars, several weeks previously. The swelling is dusky-red or purplish in colour, firm and slightly tender. The skin becomes fixed to the underlying tissues and eventually breaks down as the characteristic sinuses and discharge appear. There is often difficulty in opening the mouth, but pain is mild or absent.

Healing is associated with scarring and puckering of the skin, and, in the absence of treatment, a large fibrotic mass may form, covered by scarred and pigmented skin on which several sinuses open.

The lymph nodes are not affected but occasionally may become involved by local spread of the actinomyces, or by secondary infection.

Fully developed cases, as just described, are very rarely seen, and currently the more usual clinical features are a persistent subcutaneous collection of pus or a sinus, unresponsive to conventional (short) courses of antibiotics.

Diagnosis and management

For bacteriological confirmation of the diagnosis a fresh specimen of pus is necessary to obtain the organism for culture. Sulphur granules are rarely obvious but may be seen when a specimen of pus is first washed with saline. A positive diagnosis can rarely be made in the absence of sulphur granules.

It is important to warn the laboratory that actinomycosis is suspected, in order that the appropriate media are used and the culture maintained long enough for the organisms to grow.

Frequently, small amounts of penicillin have been given earlier. These are insufficient to control the infection but make bacteriological diagnosis difficult.

The mainstay of treatment is penicillin, erythromycin or tetracycline: 2 g of oral penicillin a day should be given, and continued from 4 to 6 weeks or occasionally longer; pockets of surviving organisms may persist in the depths of the lesion to cause relapse after a short course of treatment. Abscesses should be drained surgically as they form.

Complications

The most dangerous complication is spread of the infection, particularly to the lungs, but is rare.

Cancrum oris (noma)

Cancrum oris is a gangrenous infection spreading outwards from the mouth to cause extensive facial destruction and, often, death.

The disease is virtually only seen in countries, such as parts of Africa, where malnutrition, poor oral hygiene and debilitating diseases such as measles are contributory. Children under the age of 10 are mainly affected.

The microbial cause appears to be the Gram-negative anaerobic fuso-spirochaetal complex of ulcerative gingivitis which is the initial manifestation of the disease. This is associated with extensive oedema, and infection spreads outwards to cause rapid destruction of the facial soft tissues and bone. The gangrenous process starts as a painful, small, reddish-purple spot or indurated papule which ulcerates. Diffuse oedema of the face, foetor oris and profuse salivation are associated. As the overlying tissues become ischaemic the skin turns blue-black, and the area of gangrene becomes increasingly well demarcated. It ultimately sloughs away with subsequent sequestration of bone and exfoliation of teeth. In survivors, the infection gradually resolves, but is grossly mutilating.

The combination of destructive periodontitis and necrotising stomatitis in a patient with AIDS has been reported to be similar to cancrum oris.

General management

Underlying diseases must be treated. A combination of penicillin and metronidazole usually then controls the local infection.

The wound should be frequently irrigated and the sloughs and sequestra allowed to separate spontaneously. Ultimately, reconstructive surgery is often required.

CHOICE OF ANTIBIOTICS

The penicillins

The penicillins remain the most useful and widely used antibiotics in dentistry. Though the natural penicillins, benzyl and phenoxymethyl, have been supplemented by a wide range of semi-synthetic penicillins, the latter are only of use in specific circumstances which rarely apply in dentistry.

The commonly used penicillins are remarkably non-toxic, but all share the common problem of allergy. Minor reactions such as rashes are common, while severe reactions, particularly anaphylaxis, though rare, can be lethal. In the USA penicillin is still one of those that heads the list of drugs causing fatal reactions.

Allergy to one penicillin is shared by all the penicillin analogues, and in general the drug should not be given to a patient who gives a history of a reaction, even a minor one, to any of this group.

If, during a course of penicillin, a rash, urticaria, or other reaction develops, the drug should be stopped and the patient told that they should not have penicillin in the future.

Benzyl penicillin

This is given by injection; absorption is rapid, and within a matter of minutes there is a high bactericidal concentration of the drug in the blood. This is highly effective in spite of rapid excretion. Severe infections should be treated initially by injection of not less than 300 mg of benzyl penicillin 6 hourly.

Phenoxymethyl penicillin

This is resistant to gastric acid and is absorbed from the gut, obviating the need for injections. It is best absorbed from an empty stomach. Oral penicillin is especially useful for infants and children, but severe infections should be treated by giving benzyl penicillin by injection because of the certainty and rapidity of absorption.

Oral penicillins only rarely causes severe reactions in allergic patients, and there is a longer delay before the onset of the reaction while the drug is being absorbed. The same precaution, (a careful history) must be taken before prescribing an oral penicillin.

Depot penicillins

Procaine penicillin is relatively insoluble and slowly absorbed, after intramuscular injection the blood concentration is usually sufficient to remain bacteriostatic to sensitive organisms for 24 hours. Fortified procaine penicillin injection contains benzyl penicillin in addition, to give an initial high blood concentration that may be bactericidal while the procaine sustains a more prolonged bacteriostatic effect. Penicillin Triple Injection (a mixture or benzyl, benethamine and procaine penicillins) gives an initial high blood concentration which remains at least bacteriostatic for a longer period (for 2 or 3 days).

Depot penicillins are of limited value but may be useful, initially at least, for children who are acutely ill in whom oral absorption is likely to be poor. Penicillin Triple Injection could also be used for a patient postoperatively, particularly if it is thought that the patient may not take penicillin by mouth sufficiently regularly.

The broad-spectrum penicillins

Penicillins such as ampicillin and amoxycillin are effective against many Gram-negative bacilli, such as those in the gut, as well as the organisms sensitive to benzyl penicillin. These penicillins are resistant to gastric acid and can be taken by mouth.

Amoxycillin is regarded as the drug of choice in the prophylaxis of infective endocarditis for most patients and for other dental infections because of its excellent absorption and slow excretion.

Penicillinase-resistant penicillins

These penicillins, such as cloxacillin, are highly effective against penicillinase-producing staphylococci but are relatively ineffective against most other organisms. Suppurative parotitis can be caused by a penicillinase-producing staphylococcus, in which case flucloxacillin is useful.

Side-effects

It should be emphasised again that all penicillins show cross sensitivity, and, if a patient is allergic to one, then they should all be avoided.

Amoxycillin and other antibiotics can interfere with the action of oral contraceptives by a variety of possible mechanisms, but evidence that this interaction can lead to unwanted pregnancies is very scanty.

Ampicillin and amoxycillin can cause irritating rashes unrelated to penicillin allergy, particularly in patients with glandular fever or other lympho-proliferative diseases.

Hypersensitivity to penicillin

Allergy is the most important side effect of penicillin. As mentioned earlier, it is essential whenever penicillin is to be given to ask whether it has ever been given before and whether there were any ill effects of any sort. If signs of sensitivity (such as a rash or urticaria) develop, the drug should be stopped immediately and the patient told that penicillin should not be given again in future. The common type of hypersensitivity reaction to penicillin is a rash; anaphylactic reactions are much less common but dangerous, as discussed in Chapter 21.

The cephalosporins

The cephalosporins have a nucleus somewhat similar to that of penicillin. Two examples are *cephradin*, which can be given by injection, and *cephalexin*, which is only given by mouth.

The cephalosporins have a broad spectrum of activity somewhat similar to ampicillin, but are also effective against many penicillinase-producing staphylococci.

Clinical applications

The range of activity of the cephalosporins is not particularly relevant to dental infections. They should be reserved for specific infections where the bacteriological findings suggest that they are the most effective drug.

About 10% of patients allergic to penicillin may also be allergic to the cephalosporins. It is therefore safer to give a drug such as erythromycin which is completely different in structure. Another disadvantage is that viridans streptococci tend to develop cross resistance to both penicillin and the cephalosporins. Cephalosporins are not, therefore, suitable alternatives for a patient who has recently had penicillin and is at risk from infective endocarditis. The cephalosporins are also prone to cause superinfection, particularly by *Candida albicans*.

Erythromycin

Erythromycin has a range of activity very similar to that of penicillin. It is useful, therefore, for patients allergic to penicillin.

Erythromycin has few serious side-effects. Its disadvantages are its erratic absorption and that a dose of 2 g (for prophylaxis of infective endocarditis) often causes nausea. Erythromycin by injection is painful partly because of its large volume (10 ml). It can be given intravenously, but should then be given by slow infusion over a period of 15 minutes.

Clindamycin

Clindamycin is effective against many organisms causing oral infections. An advantage of clindamycin is the effectiveness of absorption when given by mouth, even when the stomach is full. It is also particularly effective in penetrating poorly vascular tissues, notably bone and connective tissue.

Allergy is exceedingly rare, and hypersensitivity to penicillin is not shared. There is also no cross resistance by bacteria to these two antibiotics.

Clindamycin is frequently the drug of choice for infections due to Gram-negative anaerobes of the bacteroides group. These are common in the mouth, probably play a role in infections involving the gingivae and periodontal tissues and can cause severe infections of the head and neck.

The chief side-effect of clindamycin is diarrhoea, which is relatively common. On rare occasions it may also cause colitis characterised by abdominal pain and passage of mucus or blood in the stools. In elderly or debilitated patients on multiple drug treatment, colitis can be severe and, rarely, fatal. Colitis due to this drug is the result of proliferation of resistant, toxigenic strains of clostridia (*C. difficile*) but usually responds to oral vancomycin. Colitis occasionally follows the use of many other antibiotics including penicillin or ampicillin.

Despite many useful features, clindamycin is a drug for specialist use in, for example, oral surgery, because of the risk of pseudomembranous colitis. However, clindamycin *as a single dose only*, is currently recommended for patients allergic to penicillin, as an alternative to erythromycin because of its better absorption and low incidence of nausea or vomiting. As a single dose, clindamycin appears to present no significant risks.

The tetracyclines

The tetracyclines have the widest spectrum of activity of all antibiotics, and the only groups of organisms which are completely resistant are the viruses and fungi. The tetracyclines have the disadvantage that they are bacteriostatic, but in addition very many organisms have now become resistant.

There are now very many tetracyclines but they share a similar spectrum of antibacterial activity and are all absorbed when given by mouth.

Clinical applications

Tetracyclines now have little use in dentistry. Their main applications are for severe chronic periodontitis as an adjunct to surgical measures such as root planing, and as a mouth rinse for oral ulceration.

An important side effect of the tetracyclines is the promotion of candidosis (thrush) particularly when used topically. When given systemically during the period of dental development tetracyclines can cause irreversible staining of the teeth.

Vancomycin

Vancomycin is a potent but highly toxic antibiotic whose only application in dentistry is for prophylaxis of endocarditis in certain, high-risk patients allergic to penicillin. For this purpose it has to be given as an intravenous infusion over a period of an hour.

Vancomycin's other uses are for serious Gram-positive bacterial infections, including some multiresistant staphylococci. It is also effective given by mouth for clindamycin-induced pseudomembranous colitis.

Toxic effects include allergic and febrile reactions, renal damage on more prolonged use, and histamine release (red man syndrome) on rapid injection.

Teicoplanin

Teicoplanin is similar to vancomycin but can be given as a single intravenous or intramuscular injection. It seems likely therefore to become a better alternative to vancomycin for the prophylaxis of infective endocarditis.

The sulphonamides and cotrimoxazole

Sulphonamides, to which many microbes have become resistant, have largely been replaced by less toxic and more effective antibiotics. Sulphonamides have the major advantage that (unlike penicillin, for example) they cross the blood–brain barrier, and sulphadimidine or co-trimoxazole can be given as prophylaxis against meningitis after severe maxillofacial injuries with tearing of the dura. However, even here, many of the bacteria causing meningitis are now resistant.

Nevertheless, for some infections, co-trimoxazole has been shown to be more effective than antibiotics such as broad-spectrum penicillins or the cephalosporins, and it is not inactivated by pus. Co-trimoxazole can therefore be used in many cases where an alternative to penicillin is required or where sensitivity tests show it to be the antimicrobial of choice. The risk of toxic effects such as rashes or, rarely, agranulocytosis is somewhat greater, but an important use of co-trimoxazole now is for the treatment of *Pneumocystis carinii* pneumonia, one of the most lethal complications of AIDS.

Metronidazole

Metronidazole is effective only against obligate anaerobes which are common, for example, in periodontal pockets. One of its uses in dentistry is for the treatment of acute ulcerative gingivitis (200 mg, 3 times a day for 3 days) for which it is outstandingly effective in conjunction with local débridement. Metronidazole's advantages are that its limited spectrum is more specifically related to this infection and it does not promote proliferation of penicillin-resistant bacteria or cause severe allergic reactions.

Metronidazole is effective for other dental infections such as pericoronitis. However, it should be noted that metronidazole is not effective against *all* anaerobes and that other antibiotics such as the penicillins may be more effective against some of them. A useful combination for troublesome dental infections, because of their mixed bacterial nature, is therefore a penicillin such as amoxycillin with metronidazole. Further, clindamycin is the drug of choice for some Bacteroides species which can cause severe dental and other infections.

The side-effects of metronidazole include gastrointestinal upset, an unpleasant taste in the mouth, a furred tongue and, occasionally, transient rashes. Metronidazole also interferes with the metabolism of alcohol, and if this is taken during a course of treatment there may be severe nausea, flushing and palpitations. Nevertheless, an important advantage of metronidazole is that (assuming it is effective) side-effects are few and minor.

Fungal and viral infections

The use of antifungal drugs for candidal infection, and of acyclovir for herpetic infections, is described in Chapter 15.

THE DEEP MYCOSES

The deep mycoses are rare in Britain, but are most likely to be seen in immunodeficient patients, particularly those with AIDS, or in those who have come from endemic areas such as South America.

Examples of deep mycoses are mucormycosis, aspergillosis, histoplasmosis and cryptococcosis. Of these only aspergillosis is a common complication of immunodeficiency in Britain.

Clinically, several of the deep mycoses can cause oral lesions at some stage, and often then give rise to a nodular and ulcerated mass, which can be tumour-like in appearance. The diagnosis is frequently therefore suggested by biopsy but culture is necessary for confirmation.

Microscopically the deep mycoses frequently cause granulomatous reactions which simulate tuberculosis, but the characteristic tissue form of the fungus, if it can be found and stained with PAS or silver stains, will suggest the diagnosis. Culture of the fungus should be confirmatory if fresh material is available.

Rhinocerebral mucormycosis (phycomycosis, zygomycosis)

Mucormycosis is an invasive infection caused by a variety of common moulds which grow on decaying organic material. These fungi only attack those with immunodeficiency diseases such as uncontrolled diabetes mellitus, acute leukaemia, or AIDS.

The spores are probably inhaled, and infection typically starts in the maxillary antrum. Invasion of the surrounding tissues can cause necrotising ulceration of the palate with a blackish slough and exposure of bone. Local pain and tenderness over the sinus is associated with thickening of the lining and sometimes radiographic signs of destruction of the walls of several paranasal sinuses. There may also be nasal congestion or bloody discharge.

Spread to the orbit causes blurred vision, proptosis and limitation of eye movements. Spread to the brain causes clouding of consciousness, cranial nerve palsies, blindness, coma and death, often within 2 weeks.

Microscopically the hyphae in the tissues show a characteristically irregular width, a crushed ribbon appearance and right-angled branching. They typically involve blood vessels with thromboses and haemorrhages, inflammation and tissue necrosis.

Aspergillosis

Aspergillus fumigatus

This is an important cause of opportunistic infections in immunodeficiency states but can also form harmless aspergillomas (fungus balls) in the maxillary antrum.

Rhinocerebral aspergillosis is rare and particularly affects poorly-controlled diabetics. It gives rise to a picture similar to that of mucormycosis and can produce necrotic, brown or blackish palatal ulceration. Painful, bleeding oral lesions have also been reported as a rare feature of disseminated aspergillosis.

Diagnosis is by recognition of the branching hyphae in the tissues by microscopy, but the characteristic mop-like spore-bearing structures are rarely seen. Culture is therefore also essential.

Aspergilloma

An aspergillomatous fungus ball is a rare cause of opacity of the antrum in a healthy person. The mass appears brown and dry and is recognisable only by microscopy showing the tangled mass of hyphae. Culture is confirmatory if fresh material is available. There is no invasion of the surrounding tissues.

Following removal of the fungal mass, no treatment is necessary, provided that the patient remains healthy.

Histoplasmosis

Histoplasma capsulatum

This can cause localised or generalised disease, but is usually subclinical. It is not naturally present in Britain, but can be secondary to immunodeficiency states, particularly AIDS. The main clinical types of infection are pulmonary, which may heal without symptoms, or disseminated and fatal. Oral lesions develop in up to 50% of cases of disseminated disease. They are usually painful, tumour-like and ulcerate.

Histoplasmosis of the adrenals can cause Addison's disease with oral pigmentation.

Microscopically the lesions simulate those of tuberculosis with granulomas and sometimes

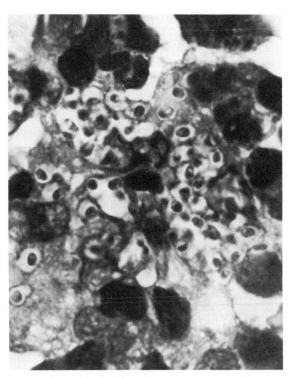

Fig. 8.13 Histoplasmosis. Part of an oral biopsy under high power, showing the typical yeast forms with their clear haloes. (From McCracken and Cawson. Clinical and Oral Microbiology. Hemisphere Press.)

caseation, in the absence of which the organism can rarely be demonstrated in epithelioid cells.

Cryptococcosis

Cryptococcosis is a common complication of AIDS and typically causes meningitis, pulmonary or disseminated infection.

Oral lesions are uncommon and mainly a complication of widespread disease. They appear as a granular swelling or necrotic ulcers.

Microscopically there are granulomas, and the organism may be seen as a spherical or ovoid spore with a halo formed by the large gelatinous capsule.

Treatment of the deep mycoses

The most effective agent overall has been intravenous amphotericin. This has a broad spectrum of activity against most of these fungi but is so toxic that it is only given when the nature of the infection has been confirmed and is life-threatening. Ketoconazole and its analogues are considerably less toxic and appear to be very promising, but remain to be more fully evaluated. Antifungal chemotherapy is usually combined with surgical excision for localised disease.

SYSTEMIC INFECTIONS

Infective endocarditis

Infective endocarditis remains one of the few ways by which a patient can die as a result of dental treatment. The disease is caused by colonisation of a heart valve by bacteria, and death can result from progressive cardiac damage or uncontrollable septicaemia.

Aetiology and pathogenesis

Infective endocarditis typically results from (1) the presence of a cardiac defect on which bacteria could settle and (2) bacteraemia. Attachment of bacteria to a cardiac defect depends on its disturbance of the normal laminar flow of blood through the heart, causing eddy currents with foci of relative stasis. Examples of such defects are shown in Table 8.1. However, the defect is not necessarily so severe as to affect the patient's health.

Dental extractions regularly release bacteria from the gingival margins into the bloodstream

and were the first recognised source of bacteria that could precipitate endocarditis. Extractions are effective at producing bacteraemia, both because of the great numbers of bacteria surrounding the teeth and because extraction has a pumping action on the vessels of the periodontal region as they are alternately stretched and compressed by the rocking of the tooth in the socket. The frequency of bacteraemias after extractions is related to the severity of gingival sepsis. Moreover any dental manipulation involving the gingival margins, including scaling or even toothbrushing, can also release bacteria into the bloodstream.

Viridans streptococci remain the most common single group of causative organisms, but currently they account for fewer than 50% of cases overall. Viridans streptococci are the most frequently isolated bacteria from the mouth, and from among this group *S. mutans* accounts in some series for a high proportion of cases of infective endocarditis. Their attachment mechanisms, including glucan production, may assist these bacteria to adhere to the endocardium.

Portals of entry for bacteria. Many, for historical reasons, still believe that dental manipulations are the main cause of infective endocarditis. However, this is no longer true and there are many ways by which bacteria can be introduced into the bloodstream, particularly as a result of invasive medical or surgical procedures. Infective endocarditis has as a result been called by one authority 'a disease of medical progress'. As a consequence, in some large series there has been preceding dental interference in only 6–10% of cases.

Factors affecting susceptibility

Little is known about what determines susceptibility to endocarditis after a bacteraemia.

For example, infective endocarditis is no longer a disease of young people and is uncommon in children. A contributory factor may be that rheumatic fever has virtually disappeared from Britain and the USA, though there remain older patients with chronic rheumatic heart disease.

Illustrative of the low risk of infective endocarditis in children is that, in Down's syndrome, congenital heart defects are common and associated with immunodeficiencies. In addition

Table 8.1 Risk factors for infective endocarditis

Congenital heart disease[1]
Rheumatic heart disease
Other types of valve lesion and heart disease[2]
Prosthetic heart valves[3]
A previous attack of infective endocarditis
Increasing age

Notes:
[1] Different types of congenital lesions vary widely in their susceptibility to infective endocarditis, but the level of risk is not predictable in any given patient.
[2] Calcific aortic degeneration is an important predisposing factor, while many other types of valve lesion such as the common floppy mitral valve are relatively rarely affected. Infective endocarditis hardly ever complicates damage by myocardial infarction.
[3] Prosthetic heart valves appear, overall, to be less frequently infected by oral bacteria than natural valves.

there is typically severe periodontal disease with accumulations of plaque. Despite this multiplicity of risk factors, there is no evidence that infective endocarditis is common in these children. Nevertheless, antibiotic cover must be given for them as for others with valve disease.

Risk factors for the elderly include calcific aortic degeneration and the poor dental state of many of them, including those undergoing heart valve surgery. However, there does not appear to be any increased risk of infective endocarditis after myocardial infarction (despite the damage to the endocardium) or to those wearing pacemakers.

The level of risk from dental procedures. Some idea of the level of risk is important, to decide when prophylactic antibiotics should be given. However, it is remarkably low in statistical terms. In the pre-penicillin era there was no effective preventive measure or treatment, rheumatic heart disease was common, many more extractions were carried out and oral sepsis was more prevalent and severe. Despite all these factors favouring the development of infective endocarditis it was, even then, a rare disease and there is no evidence that it was more common than today. In one experiment in that era, approximately 1000 extractions were carried out on patients with rheumatic heart disease without a single case of infective endocarditis as a result. In a survey of reports dating from 1909 to 1975 of no fewer than 4821 cases of infective endocarditis (the majority before the introduction of penicillin), dental procedures were implicated in only 13% and, of these, 95.5% were extractions.

Dental extractions may therefore be the most dangerous *identifiable* dental procedure in patients at risk from endocarditis, but, even with these, the danger is small and that of other procedures (even though they may cause bacteraemia) is even smaller. It has been estimated that the risk of a patient with a cardiac defect developing endocarditis after a dental operation is 1 in 5000 or even less.

This is not to suggest that antibiotic cover should not be given, but only that it should not be given unnecessarily. If antibiotics are given for negligible-risk procedures, then resistance soon develops and protection when genuinely required may not be readily possible. Thus, antibiotic cover for root canal treatment is not recommended, since infective endocarditis as a consequence of such treatment is virtually unknown.

Mortality rates

The overall mortality from infective endocarditis is about 30%, and this figure has not improved since the introduction of penicillin. The reasons are that different risk factors now operate. For example, elderly patients are now predominantly affected. Thus, the last available figures (1986) showed that out of 205 deaths from this disease, only 13 were below the age of 40, and the peak mortality was between 60 and 80. In addition, many infections are by organisms such as *Candida albicans* or *Staphylococcus aureus* that are difficult to treat. However, the mortality from infections by viridans streptococci has fallen from being uniformly fatal in the pre-penicillin era to as low as 5% in some series.

Prevention of infective endocarditis

The prevention of infective endocarditis after dental procedures depends on the following.

1. Identification of those at risk
2. Use of prophylactic antibiotics
3. Reduction in the level of oral sepsis and the amount of operative treatment
4. Clearance of teeth in selected cases
5. Ensuring early treatment if endocarditis develops (secondary prevention).

Identification of patients at risk. All patients must be asked whether they have any heart defects or a prosthetic valve, a history of rheumatic fever, previous infective endocarditis, or a heart murmur. Though rheumatic fever has become uncommon in Britain it is common in many countries from which immigrants come.

Such questions will rarely elicit information about other types of vulnerable cardiac disease, and patients can also be unaware of having a heart defect.

In the case of patients with a history of rheumatic fever or a murmur, it is desirable, if possible, to have a cardiological examination to confirm whether there is any organic valve disease.

Use of prophylactic cover. Since the risk of infective endocarditis after dental treatment is small and extractions are clearly the main hazard, the administration of antibiotics before *any* procedure that could conceivably cause bacteraemia, may do more harm than good.

Antibiotics should therefore be given to those with cardiac lesions before extractions and any operative procedures involving the gingival margins, including scaling.

Choice and timing of antibiotic cover. An antibiotic should be given only long enough before the operation to ensure maximal absorption and a bactericidal concentration of the antibiotic to meet the bacteria as they enter the bloodstream.

Antiquated ideas about 'sterilising the mouth' by giving antibiotics for several days beforehand still persist among the uninformed. Such attempts are not merely ineffective but, worse, cause resistant strains of bacteria to proliferate. Penicillin-resistant infections caused in this way have occasionally been fatal.

Oral amoxycillin (3 g) half an hour before operation is recommended for most adults who are not allergic to penicillin, but details of currently recommended prophylactic regimens are given in Appendix I.

There are theoretical advantages from giving an antibiotic by injection, but most dentists in general practice are reluctant to give antibiotics by this route. Further, patients with heart disease have been known to conceal the fact to avoid having an injection.

The advantages of amoxycillin are that it is exceptionally well absorbed when taken orally, and a 3 g dose gives bactericidal levels that are maintained for several hours.

Secondary prevention. It is of the utmost importance to warn all patients at risk (even though apparently adequate antibiotic cover may have been given) to report back if *any illness, however slight* develops after dental treatment. The majority of cases of infective endocarditis develop within a month.

The successful treatment of infective endocarditis is heavily dependent on early diagnosis but this is frequently not achieved, because initial symptoms are so slight.

Summary

1. Infective endocarditis can occasionally follow dental procedures, particularly extractions, which produce bacteraemias.
2. The frequency and severity of dental bacteraemias is related to the amount of gingival sepsis, and any disturbance of the gingivae or movement of the teeth by chewing can often produce bacteraemias.
3. Bacteraemias are rarely significant but can lead to infective endocarditis, particularly in those with valve lesions or prosthetic heart valves.
4. The overall mortality from infective endocarditis is about 30% but in the case of infections by viridans streptococci is usually 10–15%.
5. Only a very small proportion (5–15%) of cases of infective endocarditis have a documented history of recent dental treatment, but it is mandatory for the dentist to try to prevent the disease.
6. Prevention of infective endocarditis depends on (a) identifying patients at risk by taking a careful history and (b) giving an adequate dose of a bactericidal antibiotic shortly before treatment.
7. The current drug of choice for most adults is amoxycillin (3 g orally an hour before operation) if not allergic to penicillin.
8. All but a few cases of endocarditis related to dental treatment have followed extractions, but any operations affecting the gingival margin (scaling, periodontal surgery and mucoperiosteal flaps) should have antibiotic cover.
9. Most other dental procedures can cause bacteraemias but these are not of proven clinical significance, and the use of antibiotic cover on all such occasions is out of all proportion to the risk.
10. Some, such as those with prosthetic valves and allergic to penicillin, present special problems. Such patients should be referred to hospital.
11. Additional preventive measures are (a) maintenance of optimal oral hygiene and

(b) warning all patients at risk to report back if any indisposition develops after dental treatment.

12. No prophylactic regimen is of *proven* effectiveness, and the dentist should follow the published recommendations—there are no absolute rules.

Lung and brain abscesses

These are sometimes due to oral anaerobic bacteria which are probably aspirated during sleep. Brain abscesses are frequently a complication of lung abscesses, but oral bacteria can also cause brain abscesses in the absence of lung infection; how they reach this site is unknown.

Septicaemias and metastatic infections

In severe immunodeficiency states such as in organ transplant patients or those with AIDS, bacteria from the mouth are a significant cause of metastatic infections or septicaemias. Many of these are spontaneous and probably induced by chewing, but antibiotic cover is indicated for dental operations, particularly those involving the gingival margins. Unfortunately, there is no consensus as to the most appropriate prophylactic regimen, as the causes are varied and unpredictable. A combination of amoxycillin 3 g plus metronidazole 400 mg by mouth, 1 hour before operation should offer some protection and can be repeated 6 hours later, if thought desirable. In such patients optimal standards of oral hygiene should be maintained to keep the numbers of periodontal bacteria, in particular, to as low levels as possible.

Prosthetic joint replacements

These prostheses are susceptible to blood-borne infections but, despite the many thousands of joint replacements that have been performed, there has been, as far as is known, no case where infection has been of dental origin. However, if the orthopaedic surgeon demands cover for dental treatment and can indicate the antibiotics he requires, it may be prudent to agree for the peace of mind of all concerned.

THE ACQUIRED IMMUNE DEFICIENCY SYNDROME (AIDS)

Severe mucosal, soft-tissue of perioral infections are common manifestations of the acquired immune deficiency syndrome. This disease is epidemic in parts of the USA and Africa. It is worldwide in distribution, and several million persons have been infected. In 1989 there were approximately 2000 patients with the disease in Britain and 1000 deaths; it is also estimated that there are at least 14 000 asymptomatic carriers of the virus. In the same year, in the USA, the number of cases of AIDS has passed 100 000. More recent studies in the USA have reported that over 1.5% of patients in hospital for complaints unconnected with AIDS were infected with HIV and that in one hospital nearly 8% of the patients had been infected.

Although AIDS is considerably less common in women in many parts of the world, it has become the leading cause of death for women between 20 and 40 in major cities in the USA. The World Health Organization estimated that in 1990 there were $2\frac{1}{2}$ million infected women in Africa alone and that, worldwide, between 8 and 10 million people had been infected by the end of the 1980s.

The human immunodeficiency virus is transmissible to health care personnel, particularly surgeons, dental surgeons and nurses, via needles or other sharp instruments. However, the risk of acquiring the infection by this means is considerably smaller than that of hepatitis B.

Aetiology

AIDS is caused by a retrovirus, the Human Immunodeficiency Virus (HIV), mainly HIV 1. HIV 2 is as yet only widely prevalent in West Africa.

The chief mode of transmission is by male homosexual activity, and in Britain over 70% of patients are homosexual or bisexual males. Heterosexual transmission is uncommon in the Western world.

The second most common mode of transmission is by intravenous drug abuse. Blood or blood products can also contain the virus, and many haemophiliacs have acquired the disease. However, screening of donors and heat-treatment of clotting factor concentrates should have eliminated this risk. Once infected, pregnant women can also transmit the infection to the fetus and the child usually develops AIDS.

Table 8.2 shows the relative risks for different groups in Britain. In the USA, the very high prevalence of intravenous drug abuse, particularly in poor urban communities, has resulted in its accounting for a considerably higher proportion of AIDS patients there.

The incubation period

The incubation period of AIDS is highly variable and may be related to the infecting dose of virus. In the case of male homosexuals the incubation period is, on average, approximately 11 years but can be as long as 14 years. By contrast, trans-

Table 8.2 High risk groups for, and relative frequency of, AIDS in British males

Homosexual (or bisexual) males	83%
Intravenous drug abusers (IDU)	3%
Homosexual/bisexual male and IDU	2%
Haemophiliacs	6%
Recipients of blood or blood products	1%
Heterosexual contact:	
partner(s) with known risk factors	0.3%
known exposure abroad	3%
no evidence of exposure abroad	0.3%
Children of HIV-positive parent	0.3%
Others or unknown source of infection	1%

Notes: 1. Females account for only 4% of the total number of AIDS patients in the UK.

2. In the USA a significantly higher proportion of AIDS patients are intravenous drug abusers.

3. Among females, the highest proportion (26%) have acquired AIDS as a result of heterosexual contacts abroad. The second highest (17%) are intravenous drug abusers.

4 Other major risk factors for women are, equally, receipt of blood or blood products abroad or heterosexual activity with HIV-positive partners in Britain (13.4% each).

5. Overall, 41% of women with AIDS have acquired the disease abroad. (Above data modified from Communicable Disease Report 90/28 from the PHLS Communicable Disease Centre.)

6. A high proportion of HIV-positive patients are also HBV-positive, and exposure to blood from one of these individuals is far more likely to transmit hepatitis than AIDS.

mission of the virus by a blood transfusion, when very many viral particles may enter the blood, can result in rapid onset of symptoms.

Testing of apparently healthy infected persons also shows deterioriation of immune function long before the disease becomes clinically apparent, but the majority of those who develop prodromal disease such as generalised lymphadenopathy as part of an AIDS-related complex (ARC) will develop the full, lethal syndrome.

Immunology

The human immunodeficiency virus directly infects lymphocytes and other cells which carry the CD4 marker. In particular, the virus depresses the number of T helper (CD4) cells and reverses the ratio of helper to suppressor lymphocytes. Macrophages and monocytes can engulf the virus, and some monocytes also express the CD4 receptor to which the virus binds.

Antibody is produced in response to the virus but does not appear to be protective, and there is no evidence as yet that the virus is ever eliminated from the body. All HIV-infected (seropositive) persons must therefore be assumed to be carriers of the virus and capable of transmitting it. The presence of antibodies to HIV is used to detect acquisition of infection. Though the detection of these antibodies is often misnamed by the press, 'the AIDS test', it is of little value in predicting whether the full-blown disease will develop: its main use is as a marker of potential infectivity. The immune responses and serological consequences of HIV are not as yet clear, but it has become apparent that, in some patients, antibodies to HIV may not appear for periods of up to 3 *years* after infection. In others, antibodies may disappear from the blood late in the disease.

It is now possible to detect viral antigens, such as the p24 antigen, in the blood to provide a more direct and reliable indicator of infection. Moreover, minute amounts of the virus in the form of provirus DNA in lymphocytes can be detected by gene amplification using the polymerase chain reaction.

The main effect of depletion of T helper cells is increasingly deep depression of cell-mediated immunity. This can be demonstrated by such means as decreasing responses of lymphocytes to antigens in vitro, and impaired or absent delayed hypersensitivity, long before any clinical manifestations of the disease appear. The main effect of the immunodeficiency and the chief cause of death is acquisition of a wide variety of infections, particularly by opportunistic microbes.

There is also polyclonal B lymphocyte activation resulting in hypergammaglobulinaemia and auto-antibody production.

In addition to its effects on the immune system, the human immunodeficiency virus also attacks the central nervous system, cells of which carry receptors for the virus.

Clinical aspects

The possible courses of events after infection by HIV are shown in Figure 8.14, but it is still uncertain whether any symptomless carriers of the virus will ultimately remain clinically healthy.

As can be seen from Figure 8.14 the earliest clinical manifestation of infection is a transient illness resembling glandular fever; this is associated with antibody production. Thereafter, in progressive cases, markers of declining cell-mediated immunity eventually become detectable on testing, and, later, clinical syndromes termed AIDS-related complex (ARC) may develop. ARC refers to the appearance of one or more, but not all, of the clinical manifestations of AIDS. A typical example is Generalised Lymphadenopathy Syndrome, in which widespread enlargement of lymph nodes is associated with opportunistic infections which usually respond to treatment at this stage. It should be noted that the course of AIDS is highly variable, and none of the prodromal symptoms appears to be inevitable. The first clinical sign may therefore be *Pneumocystis carinii* pneumonia or Kaposi's sarcoma.

The full syndrome of AIDS is characterised by multiple infections by bacteria, fungi, parasites and viruses (Table 8.3). Many of these infections, particularly *Pneumocystis carinii* pneumonia are opportunistic and virtually unknown in normal persons.

Though infections are the main cause of death, there is also a greatly increased incidence of tumours, particularly Kaposi's sarcoma and lym-

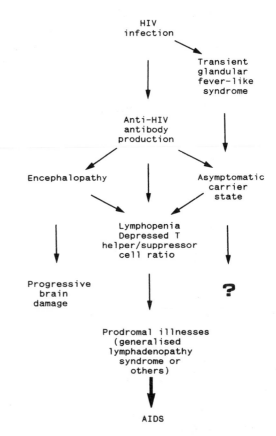

Fig. 8.14 Some of the more important possible outcomes of HIV infection. The ultimate fate of asymptomatic carriers is not as yet known.

phomas which frequently affect the oral or perioral tissues. In normal persons these tumours are not merely uncommon or rare but are particularly rare in this region.

The second major manifestation of AIDS is, in addition to opportunistic infections or tumours involving the central nervous system, neuropsychiatric disease which can range from psychiatric disturbance resembling depression, to dementia and death. These neurological disorders may be associated with, or develop in the absence of, signs of immunodeficiency.

A third but lesser manifestation of AIDS in some patients is autoimmune disease, particularly, thrombocytopenic purpura or, less frequently, a disease resembling lupus erythematosus.

Once AIDS has developed, the outcome is invariably fatal, usually within 2 to 3 years, though the course of the disease may be modified to some

Table 8.3 Opportunistic infections, neoplasms and other features of AIDS

(a) Opportunistic infections
Pneumonia or sinusitis

Pneumocystis carinii	Atypical mycobacterioses
Aspergillosis	Cytomegalovirus
Candidosis	Legionellosis
Cryptococcosis	*Pseudomonas aeruginosa*
Mucormycosis	*Staphylococcus aureus*
Strongyloidosis	*Streptococcus pneumoniae*
Toxoplasmosis	*Haemophilus influenzae*

Gastrointestinal infections
Cryptosporidiosis
Isosporiasis
Giardiasis
Microsporidiosis

Meningitis, encephalitis
JC virus
Toxoplasmosis
Papovavirus

Mucocutaneous infections
Herpes simplex
Herpes zoster
Candidosis
Staphylococcus aureus
Histoplasmosis

Disseminated infections
Atypical mycobacterioses
Avium intracellulare
Cryptococcosis
Histoplasmosis
Cytomegalovirus
Adenoviruses

(b) Neoplasms
Kaposi's sarcoma
Lymphoma (especially of the central nervous system)

(c) Other possible effects
Encephalopathy
Idiopathic thrombocytopenic purpura
Lupus erythematosus
Addison's disease
Seborrhoeic dermatitis
Embryopathy with abnormal facies

Orofacial manifestations of AIDS

More than 75% of patients with AIDS or its prodromal illnesses have orofacial manifestations, and thrush is a common early sign. Orofacial manifestations of AIDS are listed in Table 8.4 and discussed in more detail below.

Oral infections in AIDS

Candidosis. Oral thrush may be seen in over 70% of patients at some stage. It is indicative of declining immunity, and other infections may be associated or are likely to follow. In approximately 50% of such patients, AIDS is likely to develop within 5 years. Thrush may be concurrent with oral herpes to produce a confusing clinical picture.

Table 8.4 Oral disease in AIDS or its prodromes

Infections
Fungal
  Thrush and other forms of candidosis
  Mucosal lesions of deep mycoses (cryptococcosis, histoplasmosis, etc)

Viral
  Herpes simplex
  Herpes zoster or varicella
  Oral hairy leukoplakia (EBV)
  Molluscum contagiosum

Bacterial
  M. tuberculosis and nontuberculous ("atypical") mycobacterioses
  K. pneumoniae
  E. coli
  E. cloacae

Tumours
  Lymphomas
  Kaposi's sarcoma

Salivary glands
  Swelling (cystic, lymphoproliferative, or neoplastic)
  Xerostomia

Neurological
  Facial palsy
  Trigeminal neuropathy

Others
  Purpura
  Pigmentation
  Major oral aphthae
  Necrotising gingivitis
  Accelerated periodontitis
  Delayed wound healing

degree by drugs such as zidovudine and vigorous treatment of the infections.

The terminal stages of AIDS may be horrifying. In typical cases the patient is emaciated by persistent diarrhoea, suffering a multiplicity of infections, covered with skin lesions, breathless from *Pneumocystis* pneumonia, frequently with malignant tumours, and sometimes also blind and demented.

The appearance of thrush in a previously healthy, young adult male, not receiving any drugs likely to have promoted it, is strongly suggestive of HIV infection.

Most other types of candidosis, such as angular stomatitis, generalised mucosal erythema, or hyperplastic candidosis have also been reported.

Viral infections. Herpetic stomatitis is common. Severe orofacial zoster may be indicative of a poor prognosis. Cytomegalovirus has also been found in a palatal ulcer in an AIDS patient.

The possible role of the Epstein Barr virus in hairy leukoplakia is discussed below.

Papillomaviruses have been isolated from proliferative lesions, such as verruca vulgaris, condyloma acuminatum and focal epithelial hyperplasia in patients with AIDS.

Bacterial infections. A variety of infections by bacteria which rarely affect the oral tissues, such as *Klebsiella pneumoniae*, *Enterobacter cloacae*, and *Eschericia coli*, have been reported.

In the later stages, there may be oral lesions secondary to systemic infections, particularly mycobacterial ulcers.

Accelerated periodontitis and acute ulcerative gingivitis are also well-recognised features.

Deep mycoses, such as histoplasmosis or cryptococcosis can give rise to proliferative or ulcerative lesions. Histoplasmosis can also destroy the adrenal glands and occasionally cause Addison's disease with oral hyperpigmentation.

Oral lesions can also result from complex mixed bacterial and fungal infections.

'Hairy' leukoplakia. This lesion, characteristic of, but not quite unique to, HIV infection, is so-called because hair-like filaments of keratin may extend from the surface, but more commonly the hyperkeratotic surface is corrugated. The plaque is soft, usually painless and is most frequently along the lateral borders of the tongue.

Microscopically, hairy leukoplakia is characterised by hyperkeratosis with an irregular surface or, sometimes, hair-like extensions. Surface invasion by candidal hyphae is relatively common but a secondary phenomenon and other features of candidosis are lacking. More important is the presence of *koilocytes*, which are vacuolated and ballooned prickle cells with pyknotic nuclei.

The Epstein Barr virus capsid antigen can be

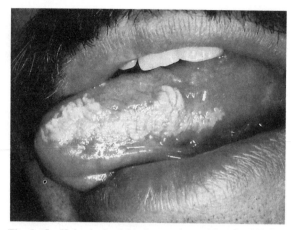

Fig. 8.15 Hairy leukoplakia in a patient with early AIDS. The surface of the lesion is corrugated and, as in many other cases, no keratin hairs are apparent. (By kind permission of Prof W. H. Binnie.)

identified in the epithelial cell nuclei, and viral particles resembling EBV can be seen by electron microscopy. Hairy leukoplakia may also respond to treatment with acyclovir, which has some activity against EBV. Langerhans' cells are reported to be few or absent, so that a defect of local immunity may be contributory.

Hairy leukoplakia appears to have no premalignant potential, but over 80% of patients with this lesion are likely to develop full-blown AIDS within 3 years.

Tumours. Nearly 50% of patients with AIDS have a malignant tumour when first seen. These tumours are varied in type but by far the most frequent are Kaposi's sarcoma and non-Hodgkin lymphomas. Unlike non-AIDS patients, these tumours are particularly common in the head and neck region.

The aetiology of AIDS-associated tumours is unknown, though it is suspected that they may be viral and secondary to the immunodeficiency.

Kaposi's sarcoma. This tumour is particularly common in male homosexuals with AIDS. Clinically a common oral site is the hard palate, where the tumour forms a purple area or, later, a nodule which bleeds readily. The histological features are described in Chapter 16.

Non-Hodgkin lymphomas can develop in intraoral sites, in the salivary glands or in the cervical

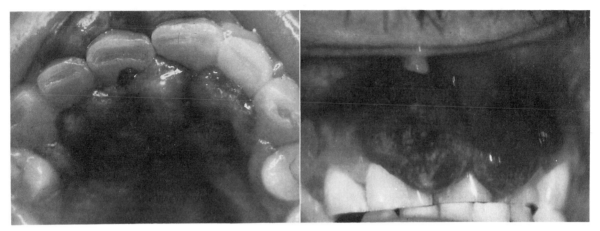

Fig. 8.16 Kaposi's sarcoma in a patient with early AIDS. As in many such cases there is a purplish area in the palate, but the tumour has extended forward to cause a purplish gingival swelling. (By kind permission of Prof. W. H. Binnie.)

lymph nodes. Typical sites within the mouth are the palate or alveolar ridge, where the tumours form soft painless swellings which do not ulcerate unless traumatised.

Microscopically these tumours frequently resemble Burkitt's lymphoma and are frequently of high-grade malignancy.

Squamous cell carcinoma of the mouth has been reported in a few patients with AIDS, but it does not seem that these tumours are particularly characteristic of the disease.

Lymphadenopathy. Enlargement of lymph nodes is particularly characteristic of AIDS and its prodromes, particularly the early glandular-fever-like syndrome and, later, Generalised Lymphadenopathy Syndrome. Cervical lymphadenopathy is probably the most common head and neck manifestation of HIV infection.

Microscopically, typical findings are decreased numbers of T-helper cells in the paracortical region associated with increased numbers of T-suppressor cells there and in the follicles. Follicles may initially be hyperplastic but later undergo involution. The lymph nodes become virtually or entirely functionless.

Enlargement of cervical lymph nodes may also be due to lymphomas.

Autoimmune disease. The most common autoimmune phenomenon in AIDS is thrombocytopenic purpura. This can appear as purple patches in the mouth and may be mistaken for Kaposi's sarcoma.

Other autoimmune diseases reported in AIDS are lupus erythematosus and salivary gland disease resembling Sjögren's syndrome, as discussed later.

Gingival disease. Severe gingival disease, secondary to the immunodeficiency, includes necrotising gingivitis and accelerated periodontitis (Ch. 6). The acceleration of periodontal infection in AIDS indicates the importance of the protective activity of the immune system, rather than as a cause of tissue damage.

Salivary gland disease. The main effects include.

1. Parotitis, possibly due to Epstein Barr or cytomegalovirus, which appears to affect children with AIDS particularly
2. A Sjögren-like syndrome in adults
3. Parotid swellings due to lymphoproliferation
4. Parotid cysts, with mural lymphoproliferation, are frequently bilateral and identifiable by CT scanning.

Orofacial neurological complications. When HIV affects the central nervous system, facial palsy and trigeminal neuropathy can result.

Miscellaneous oral lesions. *Major aphthae* are painful, can interfere with eating and can accelerate deterioration of health. Their pathogenesis is unknown but their reported response to zidovudine suggests that they may be caused by HIV.

Necrotising oral ulceration of an ill-defined nature has also been reported.

Oral hyperpigmentation may occasionally be secondary to Addison's disease due to fungal destruction of the adrenals. Alternatively the pigmentation can be a complication of treatment with zidovudine or results from an unknown mechanism.

No doubt, with the passage of time, yet other orofacial manifestations of AIDS will be reported. AIDS-related arthritis for example, was only firmly identified approximately 7 years after the disease was first characterised.

The prognosis of HIV infection

The current estimate is that at least 60% of HIV seropositive individuals will develop AIDS, but increasing evidence of silent infections with greatly delayed onset antibody production, and retrospective studies of 'pre-AIDS' stored sera, may cause such estimates to appear modest.

Haematological markers, indicative of progression to AIDS, include rising levels of viral antigens in the serum, high beta 2 microglobulin levels, and fewer than 2×10^8 CD4 (T-helper) lymphocytes per litre or a T4/T8 ratio of less than

0.5. Low levels of T-helper lymphocytes probably indicate irreversible damage to the immune system.

Clinical indicators of a poor prognosis are persistent oral thrush or other infections such as herpes zoster, hairy leukoplakia, unexplained constitutional symptoms, cutaneous anergy and lymphadenopathy. Approximately 20–70% of such patients can be expected to develop full-blown AIDS in less than 5 years.

Recognition of AIDS patients and occupational hazards

As mentioned earlier there is the possibility (however slight) of transmission of HIV during dental treatment. Oral infections and other features of AIDS or its prodromes may enable patients to be recognised by signs described above. Nevertheless, despite the frequency with which oral or perioral lesions are seen in AIDS or its prodromes, there are many other patients who are infective but without overt signs to suggest the possibility. At the time of writing there are probably between 10 000 and 20 000 antibody-positive, potentially infective persons in Britain, and the number rises each month.

As in the case of hepatitis B, *ALL patients must now, therefore, be regarded as potentially infective* and treated in the same way—namely, with full aseptic precautions. The only small crumbs of comfort are that the AIDS virus is considerably less easily transmitted than hepatitis B. Most health care workers who have developed AIDS have not acquired it as a result of their occupation. However, a few nurses have become infected as a result of needle-prick injuries and accidental self-injecting of a significant amount of infected blood. By contrast many other needle-prick injuries have apparently failed to transmit the infection.

As to the risk to dental and general surgeons, at least 2 of the latter are known to have died from the disease, acquired at operation. By contrast only one dental surgeon is known as yet to have acquired the disease as a consequence of this occupation. This dental surgeon was working in New York (by far the highest incidence area in the Western world), did not practise a high standard of infection control and had had many needle-stick

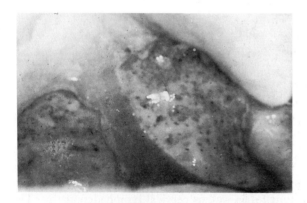

Fig. 8.17 AIDS: major aphthae such as these on the soft palate, can be a presenting feature either as worsening of minor aphthae or as new lesions which, in either case can interfere with eating and add to the patient's disabilities. (By kind permission of Prof W. H. Binnie.)

injuries. More recently it appears that a patient has become infected after a dental operation by an HIV-positive dentist in the USA.

In practical terms the risk of acquiring HIV infection from a patient appears to be related to the stage of his disease. Thus, a patient with overt manifestations such as thrush or hairy leukoplakia has higher levels of circulating virus, and the blood is more infective than that of an asymptomatic, recently infected person.

Cross-infection control is discussed in Chapter 20 and summarised in Appendix II.

Treatment

As yet only zidovudine has been shown to have any significant effect on the AIDS virus. It delays the progress of the disease but is not curative, and it has many adverse effects such as bone marrow depression. In addition, treatment with conventional antimicrobial drugs must be given for infections as they develop. However, antimicrobial treatment eventually fails.

Currently, prophylactic zidovudine is being recommended for those such as health care workers exposed to the virus. In the lower doses used for this purpose, adverse effects are less troublesome, but the degree of protection is uncertain.

ENLARGEMENT OF THE CERVICAL LYMPH NODES

Cervical lymphadenopathy, as mentioned earlier, is one of the most frequent manifestations of HIV infection. However, cervical lymphadenopathy is most commonly due to infection from the teeth, nasopharynx, or face. Dental infection should always be excluded, but the possibility of more serious infections or lymphoreticular tumours must always be borne in mind.

Causes of cervical lymphadenopathy include the following.

1. *Infections*
   a. Bacterial
      — Dental, nasopharyngeal or facial
      — Tuberculosis and non-tuberculous mycobacterioses

   — Syphilis
   — Cat scratch disease
   — Lyme disease
   b. Viral
      — Upper respiratory tract infections
      — Infectious mononucleosis
      — Herpetic stomatitis
      — HIV infection (AIDS and its prodromes)
   c. Parasitic
      — Toxoplasmosis
   d. Unknown (? viral)
      — Kawasaki's disease (mucocutaneous lymph node syndrome)
2. *Tumours*
   a. Primary
      — Lymphomas (Hodgkin's and non-Hodgkin's)
      — Leukaemia, especially lymphocytic
   b. Secondary
      — Carcinomas of mouth, salivary glands, nasopharynx or skin of the head
      — Other neoplasms, such as malignant melanoma, rarely
3. *Miscellaneous*
   — Sarcoidosis
   — Phenytoin and other drug reactions
   — Connective tissue diseases
   — Non-neoplastic lymphoproliferative diseases

Many of these diseases have been discussed earlier in this or other chapters.

Kawasaki's disease

Kawasaki's disease affects children; it is of unknown cause and is considerably more common in Japan than in Britain, where, nevertheless, more than 100 cases a year are recognised and cause at least twice as many deaths here as Reye's syndrome (Ch. 20).

Kawasaki's disease causes fever, a rash, conjunctivitis, redness and oedema of the oral mucosa with swelling of the lingual papillae (strawberry tongue) as well as cervical lymphadenopathy. The chief cause of death is myocardial infarction or myocarditis. Microscopically vasculitis is prominent.

Cat scratch disease

Cat scratch disease is a common cause of cervical lymphadenopathy in the USA and is occasionally seen in Britain. Not all cases give a history of a scratch by a cat, but the bacterium may persist on an object such as a thorn.

The causative bacterium, which has not yet been categorised, is a gram-negative bacillus, detectable at the site of injury and in the lymph nodes by means of Warthin–Starry or other special, but not conventional, stains.

The site of the injury is marked by a papule or ulcerated pustule. Lymph node enlargement may be gross, and fever or conjunctivitis may be associated. The disease is usually self-limiting after 1 or 2 weeks. Very rarely, encephalitis may develop.

The lymph nodes may suppurate and microscopically show a granulomatous reaction. The cat-scratch bacterium also appears to be the cause of a tumour-like vascular proliferation (epithelioid angiomatosis) sometimes seen in the mouth or perioral regions in AIDS.

Lyme disease

Lyme disease is caused by a spirochaete *Borrelia burgdorferi*, which is mainly transmitted by animal ticks. The disease has been reported in many parts of the world, including Britain.

The chief manifestation is a characteristic rash, erythema chronicum migrans, which spreads outwards from the site of the insect bite. Fever, enlargement of regional lymph nodes, and systemic symptoms may be associated.

The main chronic effect of Lyme disease is arthritis, especially of the knees but it can affect the temporomandibular joint: this may develop within weeks of, or more than a year after, infection.

In about 15% of patients, neurological complications develop and are typically heralded by headache and pain and stiffness of the neck. Facial palsy or other cranial nerve lesions are well-recognised features.

B. burgdorferi is sensitive to several antibacterial drugs such as penicillin or tetracycline, which should be given as early as possible. However, joint pain may recur or destructive arthritis develop.

Toxoplasmosis

Toxoplasma gondii is a parasite of man and animals, particularly cats, and worldwide in distribution. Transmission of infection is probably mainly by contaminated food. Four main clinical syndromes can result, as follows.

1. Acute toxoplasmosis in normal children or adults can cause a disease very similar to infectious mononucleosis, with cervical lymphadenopathy as the most common feature. Atypical lymphocytes are present in the blood but there is no heterophil antibody production. Usually the infection is self-limiting.
2. In immunodeficient patients such as those with AIDS, toxoplasmosis causes disseminated disease and, particularly, encephalitis.
3. In pregnant women, toxoplasmosis is an important cause of congenital abnormalities in the fetus.
4. Toxoplasmal chorioretinitis with impairment or loss of sight is usually a result of congenital infection, but can also occasionally result from severe infections in previously healthy adults.

In the lymph nodes, the microscopic changes include small clusters of epithelioid cells, follicular hyperplasia and inflammation. The merozoites of the parasite are only rarely seen. The diagnosis must be confirmed by serology.

Treatment is only required for the severe types of toxoplasmosis and is with pyrimethamine and a sulphonamide.

SUGGESTED FURTHER READING

April M M, Burns J C, Newburger J W, Healy G B 1989 Kawasaki disease and cervical lymphadenopathy. Arch Otolaryngol Head Neck Surg 115: 512–514.

Bach M C, Howell D A, Valenti A J et al 1990 Aphthous ulceration of the gastrointestinal tract in patients with the acquired immunodeficiency syndrome (AIDS). Ann Internal Med 112: 465–467

Baker P J, Evans R T, Slots J, Genco R J 1985 Antibiotic susceptibility of anaerobic bacteria from the human oral cavity. J Dent Res 64: 1233–1244

Barone R, Ficarra G, Gagliotti D et al 1990 Prevalence of oral lesions among HIV-infected intravenous drug abusers and other risk groups. Oral Surg, Oral Med, Oral Pathol 169–173

Bartlett J G, O'Keefe P 1979 The bacteriology of perimandibular space infections. J Oral Surg 37: 407–409

Beral V, Peterman T A, Berkelman R L, Jaffe H W 1990 Kaposi's sarcoma among persons with AIDS: a sexually transmitted infection? Lancet 123–127

Bergman O J 1988 Oral infections and septicemia in immunocompromised patients with hematologic malignancies. J Clin Microbiol 26: 2105–2109

Bissenden J G, Hall S 1990 Kawasaki syndrome: lessons for Britain. Brit Med J 300: 1025–1026

Bounds G A 1985 Subphrenic and mediastinal abscess formation: a complication of Ludwig's angina. Brit J Oral Maxillofac Surg 23: 313–321

Calhoun K H, Shapiro R D, Stiernberg C M, Calhoun J H 1988 Osteomyelitis of the mandible. Arch Otolaryngol Head Neck Surg 114: 1157–1162

Catto B A, Jacobs M R, Shlaes D M 1987 *Streptococcus mitis*. A cause of serious infections in adults. Ann Intern Med 147: 885–888

Cawson R A 1983 The antibiotic prophylaxis of infective endocarditis. Br Dent J 154: 183

Cawson R A 1986 Prophylaxis of infective endocarditis. Br Dent J 157: 376

Cawson R A, Eveson J W 1987 Oral pathology and diagnosis. William Heinemann Medical Books, London and Gower Medical Publishing, London

Centers for Disease Control 1990 Update: Acquired immunodeficiency syndrome—United States, 1989. J Am Med Assoc 263: 1191–1193

Chow A W, Roser S M, Brady F A 1978 Orofacial odontogenic infections. Ann Intern Med 88: 392–402

Cobb C M, Shultz R E, Brewer J H, Dunlap C L 1989 Chronic pulmonary histoplasmosis with an oral lesion. Oral Surg, Oral Med, Oral Pathol 67: 73–76

Cochran M A, Miller C H, Sheldrake M A 1989 The efficacy of the rubber dam as a barrier to the spread of microorganisms during dental treatment. J Am Dent Assoc 119: 141–145

Colman M F 1985 Invasive aspergillosis of the head and neck. Laryngoscope 95: 898–899

Cottone J A, Moliari J A 1989 Hepatitis, HIV infection and AIDS: some issues for the practitioner. Int Dent J 39: 103–107

Council on Dental Therapeutics 1988 Infection control recommendations for the dental office and the dental laboratory. J Am Dent Assoc 116: 241–248

Danchin N, Briancon S, Mathieu P et al 1989 Mitral valve prolapse as a risk factor for infective endocarditis. Lancet 1: 743–745

Davies H T, Carr R J 1990 Osteomyelitis of the mandible: a complication of routine extractions in alcoholics. Br J Oral Maxillofac Surg 28: 185–189

De Foer C, Fossion E, Vaillant J-M 1990 Sinus aspergillosis. J Cranio-Maxillo Fac Surg 18: 33–40

Dobloug J H, Gerner N W, Hurlen B et al 1988 HIV and hepatitis B in an international cohort of dental hygienists. Scand J Dent Res 96: 448–450

Dreizen S, Bodey G P, McCredie K B, Keating M J 1985 Oral aspergillosis in acute leukaemia. Oral Surg, Oral Med, Oral Pathol 59: 499–500

Emslie R D 1963 Cancrum oris. Dent Pract Dent Rec 13: 481–494

Enwonwu C O 1985 Infectious oral necrosis (cancrum oris) in Nigerian children. Community Dent Oral Epidemiol 13: 190–194

Feder H M 1990 Actinomycosis presenting as a painless jaw lump. Pediatrics 85: 858–863

Ferretti G A, Ash R C, Brown A T et al 1987 Chlorhexidine for prophylaxis against oral infections and associated complications in patients receiving bone marrow transplants. J Am Dent Assoc 114: 461–467

Friedlander A H, Yoshikawa T T 1990 Pathogenesis, management and prevention of infective endocarditis in the elderly. Oral Surg, Oral Med, Oral Pathol 69: 177–181

Glick M, Pliskin M E, Weiss R C 1990 The clinical and histologic appearance of HIV-associated gingivitis. Oral Surg, Oral Med, Oral Pathol 69: 395–398

Gould I 1990 Teicoplanin for prophylaxis of endocarditis after dental bacteraemia. J Antimicrobial Chemother 25: 501–503

Guralnick W 1984 Odontogenic infections. Br Dent J 156: 440–447

Haseltine W A 1988 Silent HIV infections. New Engl J Med 320: 1487–1488

Hein K 1990 Adolescent acquired immune defiency syndrome. AJDC 144: 46–48

Hutchison I L, Cope M, Delpe D T et al 1990 The investigation of osteoradionecrosis of the mandible by near infra-red spectroscopy. J Oral Maxillofac Surg 28: 150–154

Hutchison I L, Cullum I D, Langford J A et al 1990 The investigation of osteoradionecrosis of the mandible by 99 m TC methylene disphosphonate radionuclide bone scans. J Oral Maxillofac Surg 28: 143–149

Imperiale T F, Horwitz R I 1990 Does prophylaxis prevent postdental infective endocarditis. Am J Med 88: 131–137

Ioachim H L 1990 Biopsy diagnosis in human immunodeficiency virus infection and acquired immunodeficiency syndrome. Arch Pathol Lab Med 114: 284–294

Ioachim H L, Cronin W, Manimala R, Maya M 1990 Persistent lymphadenopathies in people at high risk for HIV infection. Am J Clin Pathol 208–218

Iwu C O 1990 Ludwig's angina; report of seven cases and review of current concepts on management. Br J Oral Maxillofac Surg 28: 189–193

Langford A, Kunze R, Timm H et al 1990 Cytomegalovirus associated oral ulcerations in HIV-infected patients. J Oral Pathol Med 19: 71–76

Leading article 1989 Oral hairy leukoplakia. Lancet 334: 1194–1195

Leading article 1989 Oral candidosis in HIV infection. Lancet 334: 1491–1492

Lehrer R I (Moderator) 1980 Mucormycosis. Ann Internal Med 93: 93–108

Lemp G F, Payne S F, Neal D, Temelso T, Rutherford
G W 1990 Survival trends for people with AIDS. J Am
Med Assoc 263: 402–406

Levy J A, Greenspan D 1988 HIV in saliva. Lancet 2: 1248

Lewis M A O, MacFarlane T W, MacGowan D A 1986
Quantitative bacteriology of acute dento-alveolar abscesses.
J Med Microbiol 21: 101–104

Lockhart P B, Crist D, Stone P H 1990 The reliability of
the medical history in the identification of patients at risk
for infective endocarditis. JADA 119: 417–422

Makkonen T A, Borthen L, Heimdahl A et al 1989
Oropharyngeal colonisation with fungi and gram-negative
rods in patients treated with radiotherapy of the head and
neck. Br J Oral Maxillofac Surg 27: 334–340

Marcus R and the CDC Cooperative Needlestick
Surveillance Group 1988 Surveillance of health care
workers exposed to blood from patients infected with the
human immunodeficiency virus. New Engl J Med
1118–1123

McNulty J S 1982 Rhinocerebral mucormycosis:
predisposing factors. Laryngoscope 92: 1140–1143

Meikle D, Yarington C T, Winterbauer R H 1985
Aspergillosis of the maxillary sinuses in otherwise healthy
patients. Laryngoscope 95: 776–779

Miller R L, Gould A R, Skolnick J L, Epstein W M 1982
Localized oral histoplasmosis. Oral Surg, Oral Med, Oral
Pathol 53: 367–374

Mitchell R, Russell J 1989 The elimination of cross
infection in dental practice—A 5-year follow-up. Br Dent
J 166: 209–211

Morduchowicz G, Shmueli D, Shapira Z et al 1986
Rhinocerebral mucormycosis in renal transplant patients:
Report of three cases and review of the literature. Rev
Infect Dis 8: 441–446

Moss A R, Bacchetti P 1989 Natural history of HIV
infection. AIDS 3: 55–61

Murphy J B, Ilacqua J, Bianchi M 1985 Diagnosis of acute
maxillofacial infections: the role of computerized
tomography. Oral Surg, Oral Med, Oral Pathol
60: 154–157

Ogundia D A, Keith D A, Mirowski J 1989 Cavernous
sinus thrombosis and blindness as a complication of an
odontogenic infection. J Oral Maxillofac Surg
47: 1317–1121

Ord R A, El-Attar 1987 Osteomyelitis in children—clinical
presentations and review of management. Br J Oral
Maxillofac Surg 25: 204–217

Pallasch T J 1989 A critical appraisal of antibiotic
prophylaxis. Int Dent J 39: 183–186

Pogrel M A 1990 Letter from California: Prophylactic
antibiotics. Br Dent J 168: 446–448

Reichart P A, Lanford A, Gelderblom H R, Pohle H D,
Becker J, Wolf H 1989 Oral hairy leukoplakia:
observations on 95 cases and review of the literature. J
Oral Pathol Med 410–415

Rogers S N 1989 A study of the dental health of patients
undergoing heart valve surgery. Postgrad Med J
65: 453–455

Rosenstein D I, Chiodo G T 1989 Recurrent herpes simplex
and the acceleration of the wasting syndrome. J Am Dent
Assoc 43S–45S

Rubin M M, Gatta C A, Cozzi G M 1989 J Oral Maxillofac
Surg 47: 1311–1313

Rubin M M, Cozzi G M 1987 Fatal necrotizing mediastinitis
as a complication of an odontogenic infection. J Oral
Maxillofac Surg 45: 529–533

Samuels R H A, Martin M V 1988 A clinical and
microbiological study of antinomycetes in oral and
cervicofacial lesions. Brit J Oral Maxillofac Surg
26: 458–463

Schild G C, Minor P D 1990 Modern vaccines. Human
immunodeficiency virus and AIDS: challenges and
progress. Lancet 335: 1081–1084

Schubert M M, Peterson D E, Meyers J D et al 1986 Head
and neck aspergillosis in patients undergoing bone marrow
transplantation. Cancer 57: 1092–1096

Scully C, Porter S M 1988 Orofacial manifestations of HIV
infection. Lancet 1: 976–977

Simmons N A, Cawson R A, Clarke C A et al 1990
Prophylaxis of infective endocarditis. Lancet 1: 88–89

Smith R D 1990 The pathobiology of HIV infection: a
review. Arch Pathol Lab Med 235–239

Smith O P, Prentice H G, Madden G M, Nazareth B 1990
Lingual cellulitis causing upper airways obstruction in
neutropenic patients. Br Med J 300: 24–25

Tempest M N 1966 Cancrum oris. Brit J Surg 53: 949–969

Tuffin J R 1989 Ludwig's angina: an unusual sequel to
endodontic therapy. Int Endodont J 22: 142–147

Van der Westhuizen A J, Grotepass F W, Wyma G,
Padayachee A 1989 A rapidly fatal palatal ulcer:
Rhinocerebral mucormycosis. Oral Surg, Oral Med, Oral
Pathol 68: 32–36

Wallace M R, Harrison W O 1988 HIV seroconversion with
progressive disease in a health care worker after
needlestick injury. Lancet 1: 1454

Weber J N, Weiss R A 1988 The virology of human
immunodeficiency viruses. Br Med Bull 44: 20–37

Wescot W B, Werksman L 1989 Kaposi's sarcoma in
patients with AIDS. J Am Dent Assoc 37S–39S

Williams C A, Winkler J R, Grassi M, Murray P A 1990
HIV-associated periodontitis complicated by necrotizing
stomatitis. Oral Surg, Oral Med, Oral Pathol 69: 351–355

9. Extraction of teeth and related problems

In most patients extraction of teeth is a simple operation rarely causing anything more than minor after-effects. Occasionally, underlying disease may make extractions difficult or dangerous.

Indications for extractions

1. *Gross caries*. Even in those teeth where the pulp is not involved, restoration may sometimes be impractical.

2. *Pulpitis*. Teeth with exposed or inflamed pulps should be extracted if endodontic treatment is impractical.

3. *Apical periodontitis*. Non-vital posterior teeth with periapical disease often have to be extracted, but anterior teeth can usually be saved.

4. *Periodontal disease*. As a rough guide, loss of about half the normal depth of alveolar bone or extension of pockets to the bifurcation of the roots of posterior teeth, or obvious mobility usually means that extractions are unavoidable.

5. *Fractured teeth*. When the fracture line passes through the coronal half of the root, or both root and crown are fractured, the tooth should usually be extracted.

6. *Fractures of the jaw*. Teeth in the line of a fracture may have to be extracted to prevent infection of the bone unless their retention is essential for stabilisation of the fracture.

7. *Misplaced and impacted teeth*. These should be extracted when they are carious, are causing pain, or are damaging adjacent teeth.

8. *Orthodontic treatment*. Extraction of selected teeth is sometimes the most effective method of treating malocclusion particularly when the arch is too small to accommodate all the teeth without overcrowding.

9. *Retained deciduous teeth*. These should be extracted if there is a permanent successor in a good position to erupt. Roots and fragments of teeth should also be removed.

10. *Prosthetic considerations*. When a partial denture has to be fitted, teeth may have to be extracted if they interfere with the fitting of the denture or detract from the patient's appearance.

11. *Supernumerary and supplemental teeth*. These may interfere with the eruption of the normal teeth or cause them to be misplaced or overcrowded.

12. *Gross neglect*. Where only a few teeth are saveable, clearance is frequently the most practical solution and may be preferred by the patient.

13. *Patients at risk from certain systemic diseases*.

Where patients are at risk from infective endo-carditis or haemophilia especially, but neglect their mouths, admission to hospital and clearance (with appropriate precautions) may be desirable (Ch. 20).

14 *Preparation for radiotherapy*. Before irradia-tion of oral tumours, teeth—especially if unhealthy and in the radiation path—may need to be ex-tracted, to reduce the chance of irradiation-associated osteomyelitis (Ch. 22).

In addition to purely practical dental consider-ations, the decision whether or not to save teeth depends greatly on the patient's attitude and pre-vious level of care. Some patients are so reluctant to lose teeth that, to preserve them, justifies prolonged and complex treatment—however there are limits to what can be done.

Causes of difficult extractions

In most cases these are unpredictable, but oc-casionally patients give a history of difficult extractions. Under these circumstances radio-graphs should be taken and instruments chosen to deal with the problem.

When unforeseen difficulties develop it is better to stop the operation, explain the situation to the patient, then take radiographs and assess the nature of the problem rather than to blunder on. Once the tooth has fractured, complications are often increased by attempts to dig out frag-ments of root via the socket.

This relatively common and often unavoidable accident is best dealt with by reflecting a mucoperiosteal flap giving direct access to the root through the buccal plate of bone.

The main difficulties include the following.

1. *Excessively strong supporting tissues*. Difficult extractions of this sort are said to be more frequent in massively built patients, but this is not a wholly reliable guide. Blacks, especially Africans, may, however, have immensely strong and tough jaws.
2. *Misshapen roots*. Roots may be widely divergent, hooked or pincer-shaped (locked). Hypercementosis causing bulbous roots rarely causes difficulties unless it is gross or massive and craggy, as in Paget's disease.

3. *Easily detached crowns*. These may be due to large restorations, deep cervical caries, or to abrasion.
4. *Brittle teeth*. With increasing age teeth become brittle and bone becomes harder ('glass in concrete'). Root-filled, and teeth involved in severe chronic periodontitis, may break very easily, but in the latter case the loss of supporting bone usually obviates the problem.
5. *Sclerosis of the bone*. The bone of the jaw may rarely be excessively dense due to long-standing chronic inflammation, or occasionally to a disorder such as Paget's disease.
6. *Buried and impacted teeth*. Lower third molars are most often affected. The management of these problems is discussed later.
7. *Ankylosis and geminated teeth*. Chronic local periodontitis may cause hypercementosis and, rarely, fusion of one tooth to another or to the jaw.
8. *Inadequate access*. If the patient cannot open the mouth fully it may be difficult to reach the posterior teeth.

Most of these conditions are apparent clinically or on radiographs. If simple forceps extraction proves impossible the operation should be post-poned until the tooth can be removed surgically. Provided that the surrounding tissues have not been seriously damaged, a broken root left in the socket does not cause pain. The patient can wait a day or two if necessary until preparations can be made for a more elaborate operation, but may need an analgesic in the interim.

Healing of extraction wounds

The healing of a socket after an extraction is by essentially the same process as the healing of a fracture and takes place in the following stages:

a. Formation of a blood clot filling the socket
b. Organisation of the clot
c. Epithelialisation of the surface of the wound
d. Formation of woven bone in the connective tissue filling the socket
e. Replacement of woven bone by trabecular bone and remodelling of the alveolus.

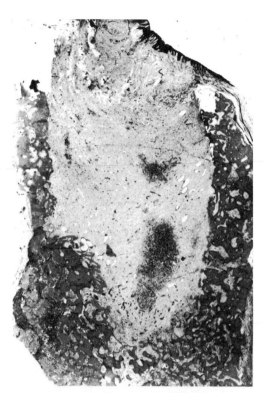

Fig. 9.1 A healing socket. This specimen, taken about a month after the extraction, shows the clot to have been replaced by connective tissue and to have been covered by epithelium. The lamina dura has been resorbed and new bone is being laid down from the periphery of the socket. The dark areas in the socket are groups of red cells which have not yet been removed (× 6).

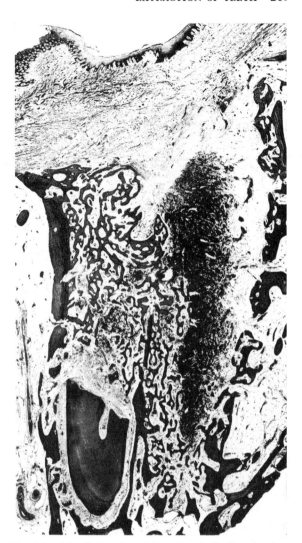

Fig. 9.2 A healing socket. A later stage in healing showing extensive new bone formation, though the outline of the socket is still clearly visible. In the mesial part there is still a good deal of unabsorbed clot as shown by the dark area of red cells; this is possibly due to later operative interference. The distal root has also fractured but remains in place and is being surrounded by new bone (× 12).

Immediately after extraction, bleeding helps to wash debris out of the socket. Torn vessels retract and, after a few minutes, the blood clots.

Tissue damage provokes a mild, subclinical inflammatory reaction; blood-vessels of the socket dilate, and leucocytes invade the clot from the periphery. Fibroblasts and capillary buds grow in from the surrounding connective tissue, until the clot is replaced by granulation tissue. Organisation is accompanied by gradual digestion of the clot by leucocytes. Epithelium begins to proliferate over the surface during the second week and eventually forms a complete, protective covering.

The increased blood supply to the socket is associated with resorption of the dense lamina dura by osteoclasts. Small fragments of bone which have been injured during extraction and have lost their blood supply are separated by osteoclasts and

eventually shed. In the connective tissue filling the socket, coarse, woven bone is laid down. In an adult this starts about a month after the extraction and may be complete in a further month. During the following months woven bone is, in turn, resorbed and replaced by trabecular bone until the normal pattern is restored. A layer of compact bone forms over the surface, and the alveolus is remodelled; it becomes narrower and its surface sinks below the adjacent parts of the ridge where teeth are still standing.

If all the teeth are lost, resorption goes on relatively rapidly at first then more slowly for some years until the alveolar bone is entirely removed. This may cause difficulty in the retention of lower dentures.

Delayed healing of extraction wounds

Delayed healing of extraction wounds may result from

1. Infection
2. Prolonged bleeding due to a clotting defect
3. Formation of an oro-antral fistula
4. Proliferation of a malignant tumour
5. Radiotherapy
6. Immunodeficiency
7. Scurvy.

Complications of dental extractions

In most cases extraction of teeth is a straightforward operation which, if competently done on healthy patients, is usually followed by remarkably little discomfort and rapid healing. Complications are uncommon and usually minor. However, a few patients are subject to serious risk when teeth are extracted, and infective endocarditis is one of the very few ways by which dental operations can have fatal consequences.

Local complications

These are often unpredictable but can sometimes be anticipated from the history. They include the following.

1. *Fracture of the tooth.* An unusually firmly attached tooth may prove almost impossible to remove intact with forceps alone as discussed earlier.

2. *Fracture of the jaw.* This is particularly liable to happen when an isolated molar or a buried tooth has to be removed from a frail edentulous mandible. In many cases, therefore, the hazard is predictable and precautions can be taken.

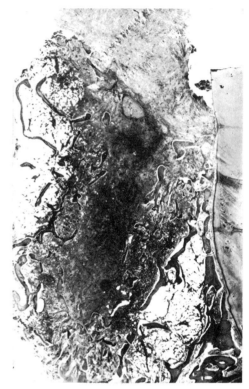

Fig. 9.3 Delayed healing of an extraction socket in acute leukaemia. The socket has become filled with a dense mass of leukaemic cells, and healing has not got beyond early organisation of the clot. The lamina dura has been resorbed, but there is no new bone formation ($\times$ 6).

3. *Damage to soft tissues.* Soft tissues may be torn when an instrument slips off the tooth. The lower lip may be crushed between the teeth, and handles of the forceps or pressure of the hand supporting the jaw can cause bruising.

4. *Opening the maxillary antrum.* This is particularly liable to happen if an attempt is made to remove a fractured root tip of an upper molar without adequate buccal access, as discussed later.

5. *Fracture of the maxillary tuberosity.* This is particularly liable to happen when attempting to remove an isolated upper 3rd or 2nd molar where the antrum has extended deeply, as discussed later.

6. *Loss of a tooth.* A tooth may occasionally be displaced into the loose tissue on the lingual

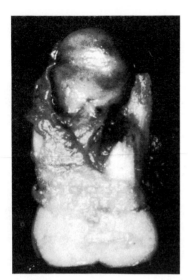

Fig. 9.4 Removal of a premolar tooth germ. The rounded, encapsulated swelling attached to the roots of a deciduous molar resembles a large periapical granuloma.

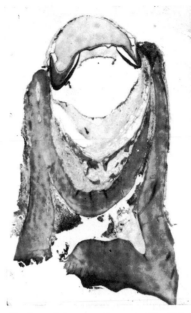

Fig. 9.5 Section of the mass shown in Fig. 9.4 shows a complete developing tooth, with a thin cap of enamel and dentine (× 6).

side of the lower molars or swallowed. A tooth can also be inhaled, particularly under general anaesthesia, and in this case more serious complications can follow, as discussed later.

7. *Removal of a permanent tooth germ.* This rarely follows extraction of a deciduous molar with apical infection, which causes the premolar tooth germ to become attached by fibrous tissue to the periodontal membrane of the overlying tooth.

8. *Excessive bleeding.* This is usually due to tissue damage, particularly if extractions are carelessly carried out, but can be the result of haemorrhagic disease.

9. *Local infection.* This is usually a painful localised osteitis (dry socket). More serious infections such as osteomyelitis are exceedingly rare.

10. *Loss of a root fragment.* The fragment may be displaced into the inferior dental canal, the medullary cavity, or antrum.

Late effects of retained roots

Contrary to popular lay belief, roots broken during extractions and left in the jaw usually cause no

pain, but any of the following can eventually happen:

1. *Eruption.* The retained root lies dormant, usually unsuspected for years, then breaks through the surface. A denture can often cause a sore, tender area as the mucosa is crushed between the denture base and the hard tip of the root. Fit and stability may be affected.

2. *Granuloma or abscess formation.* This consequence of death and infection of the pulp before the extraction may not become apparent until later. Symptoms may then start, or the retained root and the related radiolucent area may be seen in a radiograph.

3. *Cyst formation.* Occasionally, low-grade infection in the canal of a retained root stimulates granuloma formation which progresses to a periodontal cyst.

Treatment

Retained roots should be removed as soon as they make themselves apparent. By this time they have usually reached, or are close under, the surface; this makes the operation simple.

Dry socket (Alveolar osteitis)

Dry socket is by far the most frequent painful complication of extractions. Nevertheless, it is overall uncommon.

Aetiology

Dry socket is frequently unpredictable and without any obvious predisposing cause. Possible aetiological factors include:

1. *Excessive trauma.* Difficult disimpactions of third molars frequently lead to painful dry socket.
2. *Impaired blood supply.* In healthy persons dry sockets virtually only affect the lower molar region where the bone is more dense and less vascular than elsewhere.
3. *Local anaesthesia.* There is a higher incidence of dry socket in susceptible patients, even when regional blocks are used.
4. *Oral contraceptives.* The oestrogen component apparently causes increased serum fibrinolytic activity and, reportedly also, an increased incidence of dry sockets.
5. *Osteosclerotic disease.* Infected socket is a complication which must be expected after extractions in Paget's disease.
6. *Radiotherapy.* The resulting endarteritis and ischaemia of the bone makes dry socket (at the least) or osteomyelitis an almost inevitable complication of extractions.

Pathology

The initial event appears to be destruction of the clot which normally fills the socket. This was thought to be due to the action of proteolytic enzymes produced by bacteria but may be due to excessive local fibrinolytic activity. The alveolar bone and other oral tissues have a high content of activators of fibrinolysins (plasmin) which are released when the bone is traumatised.

As with other dental infections, anaerobes are likely to play a major role.

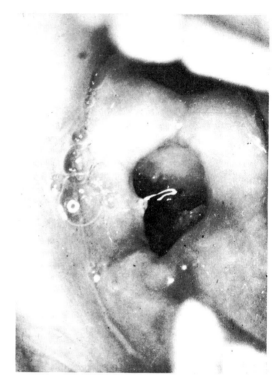

Fig. 9.6 Dry socket: A typical appearance showing the socket empty of clot but filled with saliva, and the bone of the socket wall. The patient, incidentally, was receiving systemic corticosteroids.

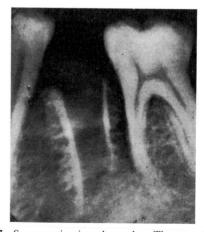

Fig. 9.7 Sequestration in a dry socket. The premolar socket has become infected, and the radiograph shows that almost the whole of the lamina dura and attached trabeculae have become necrotic, forming a sequestrum. Healing is delayed as long as this infected mass of dead bone remains in the socket. In most cases of dry socket, the sequestrum is much smaller than this.

Destruction of the clot leaves an open socket in which infected food and other debris can accumulate in direct contact with the bone. Bone damaged during the extraction, particularly the dense bone of the lamina dura, also dies. The necrotic bone lodges bacteria which proliferate freely, protected from the leucocytes unable to reach them through this avascular material. In the surrounding tissue in the vast majority of cases, inflammation localises infection to the socket walls.

Dead bone is gradually separated by the action of osteoclasts, and sequestra are usually shed in tiny fragments.

Healing is by granulation from the base and walls of the socket.

Clinical features

Pain following an extraction is usually due to a dry socket. The pain usually starts a few days after the extraction, but sometimes may be delayed for a week or more. It is deep-seated, severe and aching or throbbing in character.

The mucous membrane around the socket is red and tender. There is no clot in the socket, which contains, instead, saliva and often decomposing food debris.

When debris is washed away, whitish, dead bone may be seen or may be felt as a rough area with a probe. Sometimes the socket becomes concealed by granulations growing in from the edge, but the cavity beneath is unhealed and these granulations further hinder drainage. Pain often continues for a week or two and occasionally longer.

Prevention

Since damage to bone appears to be an important predisposing factor, it should go without saying that extraction should be carried out with minimal trauma. Immediately after the extraction the socket edges should be squeezed firmly together and held for a few minutes until the clot has formed.

In the case of disimpactions of third molars, where bone damage is inevitable and often also periosteum has to be stripped from the underlying hard tissue, a dry socket is more common. For this reason prophylactic antibiotics are often given, though their value is questionable.

There is no indication for using antibiotics topically in the socket for routine dental extractions, as in the vast majority of cases it is completely unnecessary and the value of this measure is quite unproven.

In patients who have had irradiation for cancer of the mouth every possible precaution should be taken to avoid the necessity for extractions (Ch. 8).

In patients with osteosclerotic Paget's disease the problems are less severe. Provided that the tooth can be removed surgically, causing as little damage as possible to the surrounding bone, adequate antibiotic cover usually satisfactorily localises the infection.

There remain a few patients who in every respect appear to be well but are especially prone to this complication which happens after every, or almost every, extraction under local anaesthesia. Though vasoconstrictors appear to be unimportant in the aetiology, dry socket seems to be preventable if general anaesthesia is used. It must be emphasised again that these patients are rare, and for the vast majority local anaesthesia is perfectly satisfactory.

Treatment of dry socket

Local conditions strongly favour persistence of infection, and it is more surprising that the infection is relatively so mild and well localised than that it responds poorly to treatment. It is important to explain this to patients and to warn them that they may have a week or more of discomfort. It is also important to explain that the condition is an infection not, as patients usually think, a broken root.

The aims of treatment are to keep the open socket clean and to protect exposed bone. The main measures are to irrigate the socket using mild warm antiseptic and then to fill it with an obtundant dressing containing some non-irritant antiseptic to prevent food and debris from accumulating. This should be followed by frequent use of hot mouth washes.

A great variety of dry socket dressings has been formulated. Iodoform-containing preparations are frequently used, and a convenient proprietary preparation of this kind is Alvogel. The latter is easy to manipulate, and patients report that it can convey a sensation of warmth in place of the pain. Apart from being obtundant and antiseptic, the socket dressing should preferably be soft, should adhere to the socket wall and be absorbable. Such pastes have been formulated, and the user had best decide for himself whether they have any advantages.

In many cases irrigation of the socket and replacement of the dressing has to be repeated every few days but non-absorbable dressings must be removed as soon as possible to allow the socket to heal. Most cases become free from pain after one or two dressings.

Severe infections

Infections such as osteomyelitis following extractions have become rare but are discussed in Chapter 8. The main risk factors are previous irradiation, severe immunodeficiency (as in AIDS or acute leukaemia) and some cases of diabetes mellitus.

Infective endocarditis

Extractions, particularly, can release bacteria into the bloodstream. Such bacteraemias can occasionally be followed by infective endocarditis in susceptible patients, usually with cardiac defects (congenital or acquired) or a prosthetic valve. These patients should be protected by giving an antibiotic before dental extractions and some other dental procedures (see Ch. 8).

EXCESSIVE BLEEDING AFTER DENTAL EXTRACTIONS

Prolonged bleeding after a dental operation when due to one of the more severe haemorrhagic diseases, may be difficult to manage and dangerous.

Patients are often remarkably capricious and often fail to mention peculiarities of this sort, preferring to wait until bleeding is well established before letting out their little secret. The dental surgeon is therefore sooner or later likely to regret any failure to ask patients about the results of pre-

vious extractions or to investigate a history of prolonged bleeding.

Causes of excessive bleeding after extractions are as follows:

1. *Local causes*. This is the most common cause and usually due to gross tissue damage. When there is severe bony injury and tearing of the periosteum many vessels are opened and there is little protection of the clot by the soft tissues. Secondary haemorrhage (infection of the extraction wound causing erosion of a vessel) is rare in the mouth.
2. *Systemic causes*. Haemorrhagic diseases are of two main types, namely:
   a. Purpura
   b. Clotting defects.

These are discussed in more detail in Chapter 20.

Prevention of haemorrhage after extractions

The history is the single most important aspect of the investigation of possible haemorrhagic tendencies, as discussed in Chapter 20.

It is pointless merely to ask patients whether they bleed 'abnormally' or 'excessively'. Who knows what abnormal or excessive bleeding is? It is essential therefore to try to find out some of the effects of previous extractions, surgery or injuries, how any previous episodes of bleeding were treated and especially if any other members of the family also tend to bleed excessively.

The only other requirement is that the extraction be carried out competently with minimal trauma and the socket edges neatly squeezed together.

Occasionally a dental extraction is the first manifestation of serious haemorrhagic disease such as haemophilia. In such cases, persistence of bleeding after application of routine preventive measures and suturing should prompt thorough haematological investigation.

Treatment of established bleeding

A little blood makes a lot of mess. Patients (and relatives) are often therefore disproportionately anxious but nevertheless seem frequently to choose to wait until 3 or 4 a.m. before seeking attention.

The patient and relatives should be reassured and the relatives politely got out of the way. The bleeding should be treated by clearing the mouth of clot to find the source of blood, giving a local anaesthetic and suturing the socket. A piece of oxidised cellulose (surgical) may first be placed in the socket to help clotting. Any tags of soft tissue and sharp bone fragments should be tidied up.

When the patient has thus been made comfortable and can speak more easily the history should be taken to exclude any haemorrhagic disease. If the history is suggestive (and particularly if there is a family history of bleeding), or if bleeding persists after suturing, the patient should be sent for haematological investigation.

COMPLICATIONS INVOLVING THE MAXILLARY ANTRUM

The floor of the antrum may be damaged during dental extractions in the following ways:

1. Displacement of a root or, rarely, a tooth into the antrum
2. Formation of an oro-antral fistula, with or without displacement of a root into the antrum
3. Avulsion of the maxillary tuberosity.

If the antrum is opened during an extraction, infection is common and may become chronic. This may be from a displaced infected root or by bacteria from the mouth. There is also damage to the ciliated lining and loss of the normal scavenging action which carries foreign material out of the cavity. If sinusitis becomes established and the fistula has not been closed, the walls of the passage may become epithelialised and the opening made permanent.

Displacement of a root or tooth into the maxillary antrum

The displacement of a whole tooth into the antrum is rare and can virtually only happen if the tooth is conical and considerable upward force has been used. Displacement of a root into the antrum is more common. Factors which contribute to this accident include the following:

1. A thin antral floor extending down into close relationship to the roots
2. Attempting to dig out a broken molar root through the mouth of the socket.

Clinical features

The usual sign of this accident is that the root or tooth suddenly disappears during the extraction. If the opening into the antrum is large enough the patient may notice that air comes into the mouth during swallowing, or that rinsing the mouth causes fluid to escape into the nose. Occasionally there may be bleeding from the nose on the affected side. Blowing the nose may also force air into the mouth or cause frothing of blood from the socket. Later a salty taste or unpleasant discharge may be noticed, or there may be facial pain from acute sinusitis. Rarely a swelling may appear in the mouth due to the prolapse of an antral polyp through a large opening.

Diagnosis

An opening into the antrum may be obvious from the signs and symptoms but it is important to decide whether a displaced tooth is in the antrum itself, whether or not it is mobile, and, later on, to recognise any secondary changes within the antrum.

Radiological examination. A periapical view should be centred on the infected region. This usually has to be supplemented with occlusal intraoral views, but if the root has been displaced far, and particularly if it is necessary to determine whether the root is able to move freely, then antral views with the head in two different positions are also necessary.

Principles of management

Two essentials are that the root may have to be removed from the antrum and the oro-antral opening may have to be closed.

Though entry of a root into the maxillary antrum usually causes sinusitis, this may be localised and produce no more than mucosal thickening. Severe sinusitis is less common. It may also happen that, though it appears that the root has been pushed into the antrum, it is still within the alveolar process or is lying outside the antrum between the lining and its bony floor.

There are two important principles that should be followed. The first is to *explain the nature of the accident to the patient* and how it has happened, and to give the necessary reassurance. The second is not to try to retrieve the lost root immediately by digging through the socket opening. This usually does no more than damage the antral floor and lining even further.

In many cases the tip of a root can be retained in the floor of the antrum with minimal reaction, even after several years. There is often no evidence of any reaction if the root lies between the bony wall but beneath the mucosal lining. Under these circumstances it is questionable whether it is essential to remove these roots, but many would prefer to do so rather than risk infection later. If there is a substantial piece of root or even, on rare occasions, a whole tooth within the antrum, then it should be removed, particularly if causing sinusitis.

Removal of a root or tooth from the antrum

For an elective operation, it is essential first to confirm the position of the object with radiographs and in particular that it is within the antrum itself. The second precaution is to delay the operation until any acute sinusitis has resolved.

The approach depends on the position of the root and the presence or absence of a wide oro-antral opening. The usual approach is to reflect an adequate mucoperiosteal flap in the labiobuccal sulcus and to open the bony wall of the antrum in the canine fossa. The antral lining can then be opened and the interior examined, preferably using a fibre-optic light source. Usually the best instrument for removing the tooth fragment is a sucker with a nozzle small enough to prevent the root fragment from disappearing into the suction apparatus.

If the infection is long-standing it may be necessary to remove polyps or displace granulation tissue with the sucker tip, to find the root.

After the root has been removed and any bleeding has been controlled, the antrum is irrigated with sterile normal saline and the incision sutured.

In those cases where it appears that the root is still in the socket and also in those cases where there is a persistent oro-antral opening the incision is usually made along the alveolar crest, if possible, or round the gingival margins of remaining teeth.

Wide exposure allows the socket region to be explored without entering the antrum, and the socket can if necessary be enlarged from its buccal aspect. Once the opening is large enough to allow the sucker nozzle to reach to the tooth fragment and remove it, the opening is closed by reflection of a flap over the orifice of the fistula.

Oro-antral fistula

The antrum may be accidentally opened without displacement of a tooth. Additional predisposing factors to those already discussed include the following

1. Sockets which are wide in proportion to their depth, when for instance there has been bone destruction by severe periodontal disease or extension downwards by the antral floor
2. Where periapical infection has destroyed the antral floor
3. Bony damage to the floor of the antrum during difficult extractions

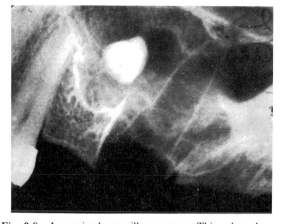

Fig. 9.8 A root in the maxillary antrum. This enlarged radiograph shows the outline of the socket, the low position of the antral floor and the fragment of root lying within the antral cavity.

4. Avulsion of the maxillary tuberosity. This is discussed later.

Once an oro-antral fistula has been created its persistence depends on the size of the opening and on the establishment of infection.

Diagnosis

The symptoms of an oro-antral fistula have been described earlier. If the fistula is so small as not to be visible, then its presence should be verified by telling the patient to blow gently while at the same time blocking the nose by pinching the nostrils together. This will cause air (detectable with a tuft of cotton wool held in tweezers), blood, pus, or mucus to be expelled from the opening into the mouth. Occasionally an opening may be blocked by a polyp.

If a swelling protrudes from a fistula into the mouth it is usually an antral polyp and is bluish or dark red (Fig. 9.9). If the opening is large enough it may be possible to push it gently back into the antrum. Alternatively a silver probe can be very gently insinuated beside the mass to enter the antral cavity to confirm the presence of a fistula. Usually a large oro-antral fistula gives adequate drainage, while a pinhole fistula will block drainage and is often associated with recurrent attacks of sinusitis.

Treatment

Ideally an oro-antral fistula should be repaired immediately.

A course of antibiotic treatment, such as oral penicillin 250 mg 4 times a day for 5 days, is usually given. The nasal ostium should also be kept patent by use of inhalations, 6-hourly, and ephedrine nasal drops 3-hourly.

In some cases, in the absence of complications, this treatment alone allows fistulae to heal spontaneously.

A simple method of managing a fresh oro-antral fistula is to suture a pack impregnated with Whitehead's varnish over the opening. This is frequently followed by closure of the fistula by proliferation of granulation tissue in about 3 weeks, and healing. If this fails, a flap can be reflected over the opening.

The established infected fistula. If the patient is not seen until late after the accident there is

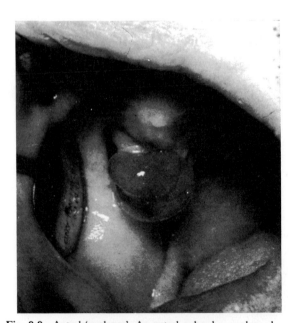

Fig. 9.9 Antral 'prolapse'. An antral polyp has prolapsed into the mouth through a large fistula caused by an extraction. The swelling is very soft, bluish in colour and can be pushed back towards the antrum.

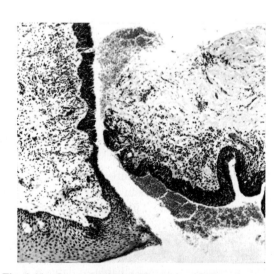

Fig. 9.10 Oro-antral fistula. The oral epithelium (lower left) has fused with the antral lining; the junction of the two different types of epithelium at the mouth of the fistula can be clearly seen. To the right an antral polyp has prolapsed (× 70).

chronic infection of the antrum, persistent discharge and proliferation of granulation tissue. The inflamed aural lining is usually much thickened, and polyps may fill part of the cavity.

The first essential is to control the chronic sinusitis by removal of any polyps with minimal damage to the remainder of the antral lining. This procedure can be carried out via opening the canine fossa (the Caldwell–Luc approach), as described earlier, or through the oral opening if the fistula is sufficiently large.

The entire epithelialised fistula can then be excised and the opening closed by reflecting a flap. This is most easily done by reflecting the soft tissue from the adjacent buccal sulcus. The tip of the flap can then be sutured to the palatal mucoperiosteum. The flap can be protected with an acrylic splint.

As an alternative, a flap can be transposed from the palate. This is somewhat more difficult and leaves a raw area, but can produce equally satisfactory results.

Postoperative treatment

It is usual to give a course of antibiotic treatment, usually penicillin, for 5 days and a 10-day course of decongestant nose drops and inhalations. Frequent hot mouth washes may also be helpful. The patient should be warned against blowing the nose.

If an oro-antral fistula is dealt with systematically in this way there is no point in carrying out an intranasal antrostomy, which is of no benefit and causes more damage to the antrial lining.

Fracture of the maxillary tuberosity

Occasionally the maxillary tuberosity may be fractured and torn away when extracting an upper second or third molar. This has two ill-effects: it may make a wide opening into the antrum, and it makes difficult the fitting of a satisfactory upper denture.

The accident is especially liable to happen if the molar is isolated and subject to the full force of the bite, and if the antrum extends down towards the roots of the teeth, weakening the ridge.

Chronic infection round the tooth may also cause sclerosis of the surrounding bone.

Management

If the bone is felt to move in unison with the tooth during the extraction, the operation should be stopped. Ideally the tooth should be preserved in place until the fracture has healed, that is, for several months if possible. The tooth may then be removed by surgical means that impose no force on the bone. It is, however, rarely possible to preserve the tooth once the bone has been injured, unless the tooth is unopposed, or can be supported and protected from the force of the bite.

If the tuberosity has already been removed—and this will be obvious when the tooth is seen, embedded in the characteristically shaped piece of bone—the wound should be sutured immediately. An acrylic plate should preferably be made to protect the wound.

UNERUPTED, MISPLACED AND IMPACTED TEETH

Mandibular third molars and upper canines are the teeth most often misplaced and have difficulty in erupting.

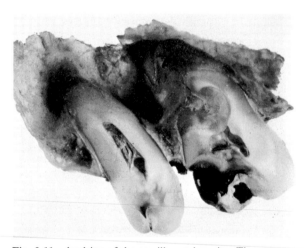

Fig. 9.11 Avulsion of the maxillary tuberosity. The specimen has been sectioned to show the antrum extending deeply between the roots of the teeth.

Mandibular third molars

When these teeth are unable to erupt into a normal position they may either (a) remain buried and asymptomatic or (b) erupt sufficiently to become exposed in the mouth and be the source of a variety of complications.

Asymptomatic third molars

Mere impaction of a third molar is *not* in itself an indication for its removal. Extraction should only be considered if impaction gives rise to any of the complications described below and there is evidence of irreversible disease. There is also little evidence for the benefit of removal of third molars solely to prevent or relieve overcrowding of anterior teeth.

A follow-up study on 11 598 patients with 3702 impacted but asymptomatic third molars which had remained untreated for an average period of 27 years showed that the only significant complications were the development of dentigerous cysts in 0.8%, periodontal ligament damage and bone loss distal to the second molar in 4.5%, or pressure resorption of the latter in 4.8%. There was no major increase in complications with increasing age. By contrast, 8.8% of 636 treated patients had complications, including one fracture of the mandible, as a result of the extractions.

Not surprisingly, therefore, extraction of third molars, often without any real justification, is one of the more common causes of medicolegal claims.

Complications from misplaced third molars

Most complications result from partial eruption and infection but include the following.

1. *Pain.* Pain is the result of infection after the gum overlying the tooth has been penetrated. Though it is said that pain from a completely buried tooth can arise as a result of pressure as it tries to erupt (particularly when obstructed by a second molar), there is little evidence that this is the case.

2. *Infection.* When eruption is incomplete, part of the crown of the tooth remains covered by a flap of gum. Infection under this gum flap

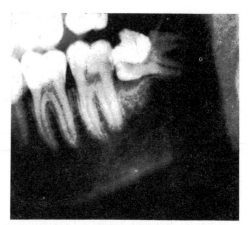

Fig. 9.12 A mismanaged, impacted third molar. The radiograph shows some of the problems that may be caused by these teeth. The third molar is in a mesioangular position and fairly superficially placed, i.e. access is good. Caries has almost destroyed the crown of the third molar and has attacked the distal surface of the second molar. The distal root of the third molar is rather sharply curved and the tooth would have to be removed by cutting off the fragile crown and taking out the roots separately.

(pericoronitis) is common and is the main cause of pain from lower third molars.

When pericoronitis develops and it is clear that the tooth is unable to erupt fully it should be extracted, but only after the acute infection has been overcome.

3. *Caries.* The filling of an incompletely erupted tooth is pointless unless the tooth is going to come into a functional position. A carious wisdom tooth should therefore be extracted before the crown is seriously damaged or periapical infection develops.

4. *Damage to the second molar.* The second molar may be tilted or become resorbed as a result of pressure on it by the tooth behind. A stagnation area forms between the two teeth, sometimes causing a deep pocket on, or caries of, the distal surface of the second molar.

5. *Cyst formation.* The crown of a third molar may become surrounded by a dentigerous cyst and the tooth displaced downward or backwards. A periodontal cyst on a first or second molar can also involve a buried third molar in a somewhat similar fashion. Occasionally a third molar may become involved in an ameloblastoma.

6. *Eruption under a denture.* A buried wisdom tooth may occasionally erupt very late in life after

all the other teeth have been lost. This may cause pain and infection under a denture.

Misplaced, healthy third molars do *NOT* cause temporomandibular joint pain.

Acute pericoronitis

Incomplete eruption of a wisdom tooth produces a large stagnation area, which can easily become infected through the opening, causing pericoronitis. The trouble is caused or made worse by the following factors:

1. *Impaction of food and plaque accumulation under the gum flap*
2. *Biting on the gum flap by an upper tooth*
3. *Ulcerative gingivitis*
4. *Diminished resistance.*

Although pericoronitis can be an acute and severe infection its microbial causes have not been defined. However, it is likely that several of the many pathogens of dental plaque, particularly anaerobes, can be causative.

Clinical features. Young adults are affected. The main symptoms are soreness and tenderness around the partially erupted tooth. Pain, swelling and difficulty in opening the mouth quickly follow. The regional lymph nodes are enlarged, there may be slight fever and, in severe cases, suppuration and abscess formation. The swelling and difficulty in opening the mouth may be severe enough to prevent examination of the area.

Management. The mouth should be cleaned and food debris removed from under the gum flap by irrigation. A radiograph must be taken to show the position of the affected tooth, its relationship to the second molar, and any other complicating factors.

Frequent use of hot mouth rinses alone often relieves the trouble but there may be recurrences until the stagnation area is removed. This may happen naturally by further eruption or by extraction of the tooth after the infection has been overcome.

If radiographs show that the third molar is badly misplaced or impacted or carious, it should be extracted after the inflammation has subsided.

When an upper tooth is biting on the flap it is often preferable to extract it, especially if the lower tooth is ultimately going to be removed. If, however, there are strong reasons for retaining the upper tooth, then the cusps should be ground away sufficiently to prevent it from continuing to traumatise the flap. Trichloracetic acid used very sparingly on cotton wool pledget, followed by glycerine, is often useful to reduce the operculum.

In mild cases it may be enough for the patient to keep the mouth clean and to use hot mouth rinses whenever symptoms in the affected area develop until the condition rights itself.

Metronidazole or penicillin or both should be given in exceptionally severe cases where malaise and lymphadenopathy are associated.

Spread of infection (cellulitis or osteomyelitis) may follow extraction of the tooth while infection is still acute and is a possible but rare complication.

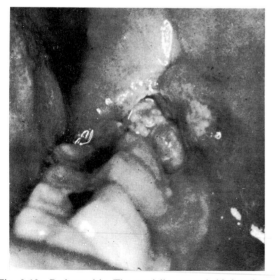

Fig. 9.13 Pericoronitis. The partially erupted third molar is covered by bacterial debris (plaque), and the inflamed, swollen soft tissues bulge up around it, further increasing stagnation.

Extraction of misplaced third molars

The difficulties and planning depend on factors which include the following.

1. *State of eruption*. The tooth may be covered by soft tissue alone or may be embedded in bone. The thickness and density of the overlying bone

must be determined by intraoral and lateral radiographs.

2. *Position.* The diagram shows the usual types of misplacement. Mesio-angular impaction is most common. The tooth may also be displaced buccally or lingually so that an occlusal view is necessary. This also shows whether the crown of the third molar is locked under the curve of the distal surface of the second molar's crown. The relationship of the tooth to the inferior dental nerve should also be assessed.

3. *Accessibility.* The distance between the second molar and the ramus is in effect the space in which the operation must be carried out.

4. *Form of the roots.* The roots of third molars are often more or less conical, but if curved and their direction unfavourable the operation is more difficult.

5. *Condition of the crown.* Caries or, rarely, resorption of the crown may cause it to break off during the operation, leaving inaccessible roots.

6. *The overlying soft tissues.* Pericoronitis prohibits operation, as discussed earlier.

7. *Condition of the second molar.* If caries, extensive restorations, resorption of or pocketing behind the distal surface have seriously damaged the second molar, its removal is often preferable, particularly if this is going to provide space for the wisdom tooth to erupt.

8. *Thickness of the mandible.* A thin mandible, in an older patient who is edentulous apart from the buried wisdom tooth, may fracture at oper-

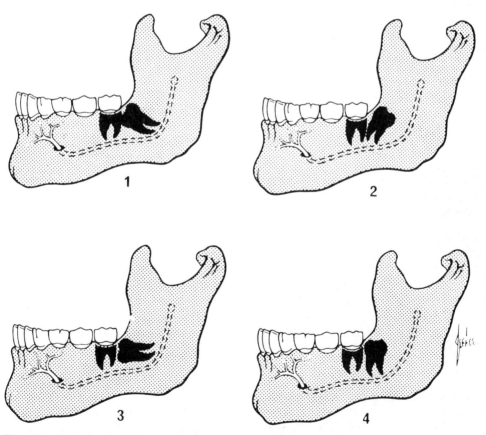

Fig. 9.14 Positions of misplaced third molars. The commonest positions are (1) mesio-angular, (2) disto-angular, (3) horizontal and (4) vertical. Other positions, such as inversion, are rare. In addition to the displacement of the tooth's axis in the vertical plane, it may be placed buccally or lingually, and superficially or deeply in relation to the other teeth.

ation. Apart from making sure that the tooth is removed with minimal stress on the weakened jaw, splints should be prepared beforehand.

9. *Disorders of bone.* Neoplasms or osteodystrophies which will further complicate the operation are rare but are usually quite unsuspected until shown by radiographs.

General principles of operation. Simple mesio-angular impactions are usually dealt with under local anaesthesia and often respond easily to the application of an elevator. If a little more force is applied to an elevator giving great leverage, a broken tooth or a fractured jaw can result.

When the operation is more difficult, particularly if it involves removal of considerable amounts of overlying bone, endotracheal anaesthesia in the operating theatre is usually preferable.

An adequate flap must be made to expose the bone and sufficient bone removed to give good access to the tooth. This may allow it to be moved with an elevator. Care must be taken not to damage the inferior dental or lingual nerves, and the soft tissues must be protected. In favourable cases the tooth may be removed whole. Alternatively the tooth may have to be divided and removed in parts.

It is worth repeating that mismanagement in extracting third molars is one of the most common sources of medicolegal claims.

Maxillary canines

The permanent canine develops on the palatal aspect of its predecessor and is usually displaced in this direction. A palatally placed canine commonly lies almost horizontally and obliquely with its roots over the premolars and molars. Less often the canine is placed buccally to the arch and may be vertical or oblique in direction.

Complications of malposition

Though canines are the most frequently misplaced teeth in the upper jaw, lower third molars are more than twice as often affected. Misplaced upper canines are also much less common causes of trouble than the lower wisdom tooth, particularly as they are not subject to pericoronitis.

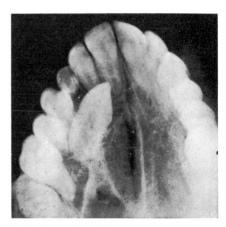

Fig. 9.15 A misplaced maxillary canine. This is the position in which an upper canine is most often misplaced, lying almost horizontally in the palate with its root in relation to the premolars. The deciduous canine has been retained and remains in position.

The main complications from malposition of an upper canine are:

1. Orthodontic problems
2. Cyst formation
3. Resorption of the canine or adjacent teeth.

Orthodontic aspects. Development of the normal form of the upper dental arch is dependent on the presence of the canine, and its absence detracts from the patient's appearance. It is therefore desirable to bring this tooth into a normal position, though this is often difficult and may be impossible. It is often also difficult to determine exactly the position of a misplaced canine, and radiographs must include lateral and occlusal views.

If the canine is misplaced labially there is usually a good chance of bringing it into the arch, provided that space can be made for it. Treatment should be begun at the earliest opportunity.

In some cases a palatally placed canine may be brought into position by traction. The crown is exposed surgically, and elastic bands anchored to an orthodontic appliance are fixed to it.

It usually takes about a year for a canine to be brought into position in this way, and during this period the patient has to wear an appliance.

When orthodontic treatment is not feasible, for instance because the canine lies too far away or at such an angle that it cannot be brought into normal occlusion, then it can be moved surgically. This means extracting the tooth from its palatal position, raising a buccal flap and transplanting it into a prepared, artificial socket.

With this type of treatment, success depends on avoiding any damage to, or treatment of, the canine root and preserving the vitality of such tissue as covers it. Surprisingly a new socket wall and apparently normal periodontal tissues form. In many cases, the non-vital pulp requires endodontic treatment. Less often, and for unknown reasons, there may be mild or severe resorption.

The 2-year success rate for autogenous tooth transplantation appears to be about 70%. If there is no deterioration after 2 years, then there is probably a good chance that the tissues can remain healthy.

In cases where there is no room (or room cannot be readily made) for the canine to erupt into, the buried tooth (in the absence of complications) is best left alone. When there is no space available, there is no justification for extracting a first premolar merely to make room for the canine.

Cyst formation. A dentigerous cyst may involve a buried canine. The cyst is dealt with in the usual way and the tooth can sometimes be brought into a functional position.

Very occasionally cysts involving buried canines may not become apparent until very late in life and are one of the rarer causes of swellings under dentures.

Resorption. A buried canine, particularly if it is pressing against the root of an adjacent tooth, may lead to resorption of either or both, especially if the tooth is left in position for a long period.

SUGGESTED FURTHER READING

Ah Pin P J 1987 The use of intraligamentary injections in haemophiliacs. Br Dent J 162: 151–152

Benoliel R, Leviner F, Txukert 1986 Dental treatment for the patient on anticoagulant therapy: Prothrombin time value—what difference does it make? Oral Surg, Oral Med, Oral Pathol 62: 149–151

Caplin R L 1989 Oral surgery: assessment and treatment. Brit Dent J 166: 128–131

Caplin R L 1989 Oral surgery: problems. Brit Dent J 166: 171–177

Hasson D M, Poole A E, de la Fuente B, Hoyer L W 1986 The dental management of patients with spontaneous acquired factor VIII inhibitors. JADA 131: 633–636

Krekmanov L, Nordenram A 1986 Postoperative complications after removal of mandibular third molars. Effects of penicillin V and chlorhexidine. Int J Oral Maxillofac Surg 15: 25–59

Leading Article 1987 Oral anticoagulant control. Lancet 2: 488–489

Lysell L, Rohlin M 1988 A study of indications used for removal of the mandibular third molar. Int J Oral Maxillofac Surg 17: 161–164

Monsour P A, Kruger B J, Harden P A 1986 Prevalence and detection of patients with bleeding disorders. Aust Dent J 31: 104–110

Pogrel M A 1987 Evaluation of over 400 autogenous tooth transplants. J Oral Maxillofac Surg 45: 205–211

Schwartz O, Frederiksen K, Klausen B 1987 Allotransplantation of human teeth. A retrospective study of 73 transplantations over a period of 28 years. Int J Oral Maxillofac Surg 16: 285–301

Scully C, Cawson R A 1991 Medical problems in dentistry, 3rd edn. Wright, Bristol

Shankar S, Lee R 1984 DDAVP and tranexamic acid for dental extractions in a haemophiliac. Br Dent J 156: 450–453

Shepherd J P, Shore C J C 1987 Oral surgery in general practice: techniques and scope. Dental Update June: 217–223

Sindet-Pedersen S, Stenbjerg S 1986 Effect of local antifibrinolytic treatment with tranexamic acid in haemophiliacs undergoing oral surgery. J Oral Maxillofac Surg 44: 703–706

Van Wovern N, Nielsen H O 1989 The fate of impacted lower third molars after the age of 20. Int J Oral Maxillofac Surg 18: 277–280

10. Cysts of the jaws

Cysts are pathological, fluid-filled cavities lined (in most cases) by epithelium. They are the most common cause of chronic swellings of the jaws.

Cysts are more common in the jaws than in any other bone because of the many rests of epithelium remaining in the tissues after dental development. Cysts formed from epithelium remaining after tooth formation (odontogenic cysts) account for all but a few cysts of the jaws. By far the most common is the periodontal cyst (dental cyst) which forms at or near the apex of a dead tooth as a consequence of periapical inflammation.

Classification

Many classifications of cysts have been devised, but these are largely an academic exercise. In the first place these classifications cannot have any fundamental basis since the precise pathogenesis of many of these lesions is unknown. In the second place the management of cysts is rarely affected by these ideas.

Cysts of the jaws originate in three main ways, they may be

1. *Developmental.* This group comprises most of the non-inflammatory cysts of the jaws, particularly the dentigerous and primordial cysts.
2. *Inflammatory.* These are the common periodontal cysts.
3. *Neoplastic.* A few cysts arise within neoplasms, particularly ameloblastomas, but only occasionally become clinically apparent as such.

The main types of cyst are therefore as follows, but radicular, periodontal cysts will be discussed first since they are the most common and, in that respect, the most important.

- *Cysts with epithelial lining*
  1. Odontogenic cysts
     a. Radicular—periodontal (apical, lateral, or residual)

b. Coronal: (i) dentigerous, (ii) eruption (soft-tissue cyst)

c. Cysts unrelated to a tooth
—Odontogenic keratocysts
—Calcifying odontogenic cyst

d. Cysts within neoplasms—ameloblastoma

2. Non-odontogenic cysts (so-called fissural cysts)
— Nasopalatine and median palatine
— Nasolabial

3. Cysts of doubtful origin
— Globulomaxillary

● *Cysts without epithelial lining (pseudocysts)*

—Solitary (simple) bone cyst

—Aneurysmal bone cyst.

Odontogenic cysts (not surprisingly) affect the tooth-bearing region of the jaws. Non-odontogenic cysts are all developmental in origin, and most of them form in the region of the anterior maxilla.

Relative frequency of different types of cyst

Several large series of cysts have been published, and there is a moderate degree of agreement as follows:

Periodontal 65 to 70%
Dentigerous 15 to 18%
Keratocysts   3 to 5%
Nasopalatine 2 to 5%

Mechanisms of cyst formation

The main factors responsible for cyst development appear, in varying degree, to be:

1. Proliferation of the epithelial lining and of the connective tissue capsule.
2. Accumulation of fluid within the cyst.
3. Resorption of the surrounding bone and new bone formation.

Epithelial proliferation

In case of periodontal cysts, infection from the pulp chamber is the source of irritation causing proliferation of the epithelial rests of Malassez. That irritation from the infected pulp chamber is the main stimulus to formation of these cysts is shown by the fact that small periodontal cysts (up to 1 or 2 cm diameter) regress without surgical treatment once infection has been eliminated from the root canal. On the other hand large cysts (residual cysts) occasionally remain after extraction of the tooth from which they originated. However, the epithelium of these cysts may gradually degenerate.

Hydrostatic effects of cyst fluids

The fact that radicular and many other types of cyst tend to assume a balloon-like form (wherever the local anatomy permits) strongly suggests that internal pressure is a factor in their growth. The hydrostatic pressure within cysts is about 70 cm of water and therefore higher than the capillary blood pressure.

Early experiments showed that cyst fluids contained mainly low-molecular-weight proteins. It was suggested therefore that the cyst wall acted as a semi-permeable membrane and prevented the entry of high-molecular-weight proteins from the serum and that osmotic tension was the main factor in cyst expansion.

More recent experiments, by contrast, have shown that cyst fluid is largely inflammatory exudate and contains high concentrations of proteins, some of high molecular weight.

Other components of cyst fluid are cholesterol, the breakdown products of erythrocytes, inflammatory cells, exfoliated epithelial cells, and fibrin. These findings are consistent with the usual presence of an inflammatory cellular exudate in cyst walls.

It appears therefore that the cyst wall does not act entirely as a simple semi-permeable membrane; low-molecular-weight proteins are present in similar concentrations to those in the plasma, while high-molecular-weight proteins are present in lesser amounts. The capillaries in the cyst wall are more permeable as a result of inflammation and contribute varying amounts of immunoglobulins and other proteins. The net effect is that pressure is created by osmotic tension within the cyst cavity.

The growth of keratocysts seems to depend on different mechanisms. In some, keratin formation is so active that this semi-solid material fills the cyst cavity and osmotic tension presumably therefore does not contribute to the cyst's expansion. Other primordial cysts produce little keratin or may be entirely fluid filled. Nevertheless, whatever their contents, primordial cysts tend not to show the expansive growth typical of other cysts, but rather to extend finger-like projections into the surrounding cancellous bone.

Bone resorbing factors

Experimentally, cyst tissues in culture have been shown to release bone-resorbing factors. These are predominantly prostaglandins E2 and E3. It is suggested that different cysts and tumours differ in the quantities of prostaglandins produced but it is uncertain whether, if this is so, it affects the mode of growth of the cyst. The mechanism of prostaglandin production is unknown.

There is also some evidence that collagenase is present in the walls of keratocysts, but its contribution to cyst growth is also unknown.

Common features of cysts

Most cysts of the jaw behave similarly and are usually characterised by slow expansive growth. They differ mainly in their relationship to a tooth, and the radiological features are usually a fair guide as to the nature of the cyst. Even when it is not possible to decide the nature of a cyst, this rarely affects treatment. It is, however, particularly important to distinguish cysts arising within an ameloblastoma from true cysts. These occasionally have identical radiological appearances, and diagnosis ultimately depends on the histopathology.

PERIODONTAL (RADICULAR) CYSTS

Pathology

All stages can be seen from a periapical granuloma containing a few strands of proliferating epithelium to an enlarging cyst with a hyperplastic epithelial lining and dense inflammatory infiltrate.

These cysts are the result of irritation originating in an infected root canal, chronic inflammatory

periapical changes and proliferation of the epithelial roots of Malassez. If, as mentioned earlier, the infection is eliminated by effective root canal treatment then young cysts regress and disappear without surgical intervention.

The epithelial lining

The lining is derived from the epithelial rests of Malassez, which give rise to a stratified squamous epithelial lining of varying thickness, though in some cases the lining is incomplete. Early, active proliferation of the lining epithelium is associated with inflammation, and in this phase of growth the epithelium may be thick, irregular and hyperplastic or show a net-like appearance, forming rings and arcades. There is a heavy associated infiltration by chronic inflammatory cells.

Though the epithelium is stratified squamous in type, it is not well formed and does not show a defined basal cell layer.

The cyst capsule and wall

The cyst capsule consists of collagenous fibrous connective tissue. During active growth the capsule is vascular and shows a moderately heavy inflammatory infiltrate adjacent to the proliferating epithelium.

Plasma cells are often prominent or the predominant type of cell, and this suggests antibody production against irritant products leaking through the apex of the tooth. In larger, more mature cysts the epithelial lining becomes flattened and inflammatory cells become progressively fewer.

Round the periphery of the capsule of the developing cyst there is osteoblastic activity and resorption of the bone which forms the cyst wall. Beyond the zone of resorption there is usually active replacement of bone. The net consequence is that the cyst expands but retains a bony wall, even after it has extended beyond the normal bony contours. This bony wall nevertheless becomes progressively thinner since repair is slower than resorption, until it forms a mere eggshell, then ultimately disappears altogether and the cyst starts to distend the soft tissues. Longstanding cysts are typically characterised by a thin flattened epithelial

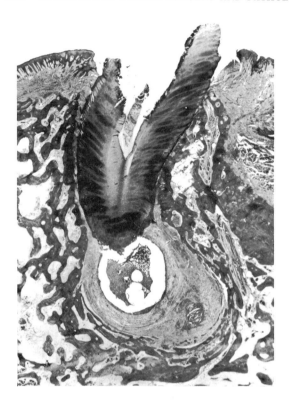

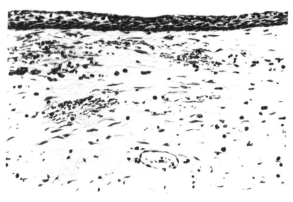

Left **Fig. 10.1** A developing dental cyst. This is in effect a large periapical granuloma in which an epithelium-lined cavity has formed. There is a thick fibrous capsule infiltrated by chronic inflammatory cells and containing a group of clefts. The alveolar bone has been resorbed and remodelled to accommodate the slowly expanding swelling (× 7).

Above **Fig. 10.2** The lining of a mature cyst. The epithelium forms a thin layer of flattened cells. The capsule consists of connective tissue with few inflammatory cells (× 130).

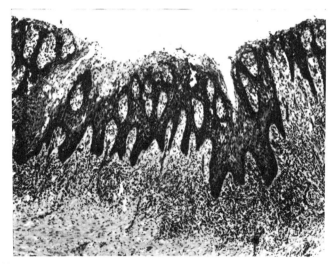

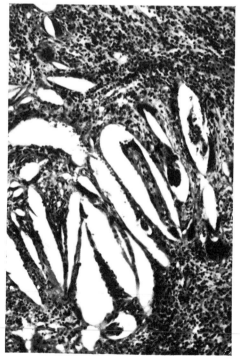

Above **Fig. 10.3** The lining of a developing cyst. The epithelium is thick and hyperplastic with deep downgrowths into the underlying connective tissue which is heavily infiltrated with chronic inflammatory cells (× 40).

Right **Fig. 10.4** Clefts in a cyst wall. These are left by cholesterol crystals, dissolved out during the preparation. The smaller clefts can be seen to be within giant cells, the cytoplasm of which has been stretched out around them (× 100).

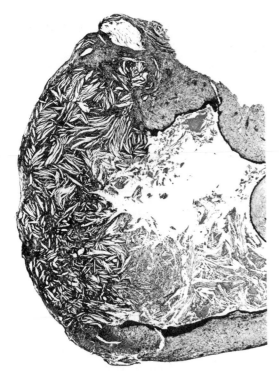

Fig. 10.5 Clefts in a cyst wall. This shows the relationship of the clefts to the cyst. The clefts are formed in the fibrous wall. The epithelium overlying this focus has broken down and the cholesterol leaks into the cyst contents. The remainder of the lining is a flattened layer of squamous epithelium (× 14).

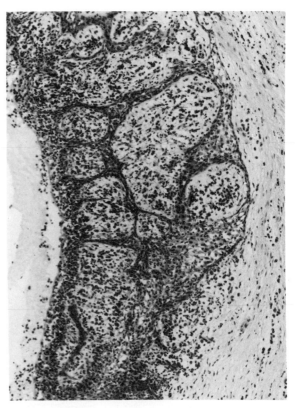

Fig. 10.6 Dental cyst. The formation of these arcades of slender strands of epithelium interspersed with scattered inflammatory cells is typical of many periodontal cysts.

lining, a thick fibrous wall and minimal inflammatory infiltrate.

Clefts

Within the cyst capsule there are often areas split up by fine needle-shaped spaces or clefts. These spaces are left by cholesterol dissolved out during preparation for sectioning. The smaller clefts are enclosed within the cytoplasm of foreign body giant cells, and extravasated red cells and blood pigment are associated. Such clefts are often seen in other parts of the body where there has been haemorrhage and breakdown of blood cells. Clefts may also be seen extending into the cyst contents but are formed in the cyst wall.

Cyst fluid

The fluid is usually watery and opalescent or sometimes thicker, more viscid and yellowish. Cholesterol crystals may be seen and give it a shimmering appearance. A smear of this fluid may show the characteristic notched cholesterol crystals under the microscope. In a section of a cyst the protein content of the fluid is usually seen as amorphous eosinophilic material, often containing broken-down leucocytes and cells distended with fat globules.

Clinical features

Periodontal cysts are the most common cause of major, chronic swellings and the most common type of cyst of the jaws. They are rarely seen before the age of 10 and are most frequent between the ages of 20 and 60. They are more common in men than women, roughly in the proportion of 3 to 2. More than three times as many cysts affect the maxilla as the mandible.

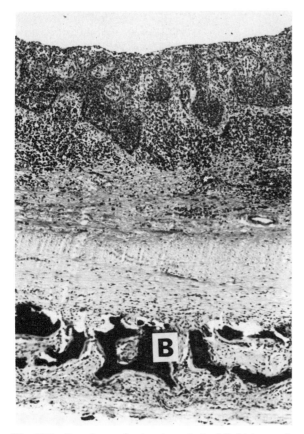

Fig. 10.7 Dental cyst. Section through the full thickness of a cyst wall shows (from top to bottom) the epithelial lining, fibrous wall with the inflammatory infiltrate immediately beneath the epithelium and the bony wall (B). The cyst has expanded out through the cortex of the jaw and the bone in this case is reparative in character and clinically would be no more than eggshell thickness.

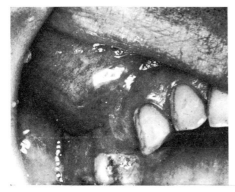

Fig. 10.8 A periodontal cyst. The cyst is bulging out through the buccal surface of the alveolus. The bony wall of the cyst has become progressively thinned until there is only a fibrous covering on this aspect.

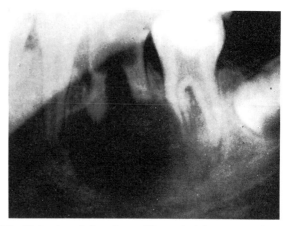

Fig. 10.9 A periodontal cyst. The typical features are the rounded and sharply defined area of radiolucency and the dead tooth from which the cyst has arisen.

The vast majority of periodontal cysts, like other cysts of the jaws, if uncomplicated, cause slowly progressive painless swellings. There are no symptoms until they become large enough to be conspicuous. If infection enters, the swelling becomes painful and may rapidly increase in size, partly due to inflammatory oedema at the periphery.

The swelling is rounded and at first hard. Later, when the bone has been reduced to eggshell thickness, a crackling sensation may be felt on pressure. Finally part of the wall is resorbed entirely away, leaving a soft fluctuant swelling, bluish in colour, beneath the mucous membrane.

The dead tooth from which the cyst has originated is (by definition) present, and its relationship to the cyst will be apparent in a radiograph.

Residual cysts

The dead tooth from which a periapical cyst has arisen may be extracted but the cyst can persist. Cysts of the jaws in older persons are usually of this kind, and residual cysts are one of the most common causes of swelling of the edentulous jaw.

Residual cysts may cause trouble by interfering with the fit of dentures, but there is some evidence that residual cysts may slowly regress spontaneously. This is suggested by the progressive thinning or even disappearance of their lining.

Lateral periodontal cysts

Lateral cysts are even less common. They form at the side of the tooth as a result of the opening of a lateral branch of the root canal. On rare occasions the tooth is vital and it appears that cyst formation has been the result of inflammation in an adjacent gingival pocket.

Radiological features

A cyst appears as a rounded, clearly radiolucent area with a sharply defined outline. There is sometimes a condensed radiopaque periphery or 'cortex'. This is present only if growth is very slow and is usually therefore only seen in older patients.

The dead tooth from which the cyst has arisen can be seen and often has a large carious cavity. Adjacent teeth usually remain vital but may be tilted or displaced a little or occasionally become slightly mobile.

Very large cysts in the maxilla may extend in any available direction and become irregular in shape.

Infection of a cyst causes the outline to become hazy as a result of increased vascularity and resorption of the surrounding bone.

Differential diagnosis

Circumscribed areas of radiolucency in the jaws may be caused by the following:

1. Anatomical structures such as the maxillary antrum and foramina
2. Cysts of other types and pseudocysts
3. Neoplasms, particularly ameloblastoma
4. Giant cell granuloma of the jaws
5. Hyperparathyroidism
6. Cherubism.

A periodontal cyst is usually readily recognised, from its clinical and radiographic features. When examined histologically, the lining of simple stratified squamous epithelium with an inflammatory infiltrate confirms the diagnosis.

The next most commonly seen type of cyst is the dentigerous cyst which is distinguished by the presence of a tooth whose crown is surrounded by the cyst.

Aspiration. The cystic nature of a radiolucent area can be confirmed by aspirating its contents by a needle inserted through the wall under aseptic conditions. The presence of fluid does not distinguish one cyst from another or a cystic neoplasm from a true cyst. The presence of cholesterol crystals is not of diagnostic importance.

Neoplasms. Benign (odontogenic) tumours or occasionally an ameloblastoma may appear radiologically as a simple cyst. For diagnosis it is essential that the whole of the cyst lining be available for examination, since part of the lining, even though of neoplastic origin, may appear as a thin layer of flattened stratified squamous epithelium like that of a simple cyst.

Resorption of the apices of adjacent teeth is suggestive of a neoplasm rather than a cyst but is not diagnostic in itself.

Rarely a secondary tumour of the jaw may cause a sharply defined area of radiolucency. More often it causes a lesion with a hazy outline and irregular shape. Tumours also tend to be painful and to grow more rapidly than cysts. Nevertheless it may be difficult or impossible to distinguish them from an infected cyst in radiographs, but at operation the solid nature of a tumour will be obvious and histological examination will confirm the diagnosis.

Treatment of cysts

Enucleation and primary closure

This is the usual mode of treatment and in the vast majority of cases is completely satisfactory.

Only the affected (dead) tooth need be extracted or may be root filled and preserved.

Access is made by raising a mucoperiosteal flap over the cyst and opening a window of adequate size in the overlying bone. The cyst wall is then carefully separated from the bone and the entire structure removed intact. The cyst lining should be sent complete in fixative for histological examination.

The edges of the bone cavity are smoothed off and free bleeding stopped by application of dry swabs. The cavity is irrigated to wash away debris.

The mucoperiosteal flap is replaced and sutured in position. The sutures should be left for at least 10 days.

Advantages and disadvantages of enucleation

Advantages are that

1. The cavity usually heals without complications and little aftercare is necessary
2. The complete lining is available for examination to confirm that it is a cyst and that no neoplasm is present.

There is sometimes misapprehension that enucleation of a cyst is to prevent neoplastic change in the lining. This is not a practical consideration, as discussed later.

Possible disadvantages of enucleation include the following.

1. The clot filling the cavity may become infected. This is exceedingly rare.
2. Incomplete removal of the lining may lead to recurrence. Keratocysts may recur for this reason, but recurrence of the periodontal cysts is remarkably rare.
3. Serious haemorrhage, either primary or secondary, may follow, but, with care, rarely happens.
4. Damage to the apices of vital teeth. Adjacent teeth may project into a cyst cavity and be covered only by the cyst lining, removal of which may damage the blood supply to the teeth and cause their death.
5. Damage to the inferior dental nerve.
6. The antrum may be opened if an attempt is made to enucleate a large cyst of the maxilla.
7. The jaw may fracture if an exceptionally large mandibular cyst is enucleated.

Generally speaking, enucleation is a completely satisfactory form of treatment and in skilled hands can be applied even to very large cysts. There are few contraindications and these are not often absolute.

Contraindications to enucleation

These include:

1. *Very large cysts*, particularly of the mandible. Removal of sufficient bone may so weaken the jaw that there is a danger of fracture. Under these circumstances the cyst can be decompressed by temporary marsupialisation. When adequate new bone has formed, the cyst can be enucleated.
2. *Dentigerous cysts*. Occasionally the enclosed tooth is needed and would erupt if allowed to. Marsupialisation may allow this to happen.

Marsupialisation

The extent of the cyst must be estimated as accurately as possible using correctly angled radiographs. With these as a guide the cyst is opened by reflecting a mucoperiosteal flap, and a window made as large as the anatomy of the area allows but not such as to invite the risk of fracture. The cyst fluid is washed out and the cyst lining sutured to the mucous membrane at the margins of the orifice. The object is to produce a self-cleansing cavity which becomes in effect an invagination of the oral cavity. The cavity is initially packed with ribbon gauze soaked in acriflavine emulsion or a temporary plug of gutta percha can be made. The sutures and pack are removed after a week and a permanent plug or extension to a denture is made for the same purpose. Once the cavity has filled up from the base and sides sufficiently to become self-cleansing the plug can be removed. The cavity usually becomes closed by regrowth of the surrounding tissue and restoration of the normal contour of the part. The operation has disadvantages, as follows.

1. The orifice may close and the cyst reform.
2. The epithelial lining of the cyst may be friable or incomplete and cannot be sutured to the margins of the opening.
3. The patient has to be provided with a syringe and must wash out the cavity after meals.
4. Several visits are necessary to assess repair of the cavity and to decide when the plug can be removed.
5. The complete lining is not available for histological examination.

Marsupialisation has largely become obsolete, and its main application is for temporary decompression of exceptionally large cysts.

DENTIGEROUS CYSTS

A dentigerous cyst surrounds the crown of a tooth and is an enlargement of the follicle, hence the alternative name *follicular cyst*. The cyst is attached to the neck of the tooth, prevents its eruption and may displace it for a considerable distance.

Dentigerous cysts account for 15–17% of all cysts of the jaws and are second in frequency only to periodontal cysts, which preponderate in the ratio of at least 4 to 1.

Pathogenesis and pathology

The main way in which dentigerous cysts arise seems to be as a result of cystic change in the remains of the enamel organ after enamel formation is complete. The attachment of the cyst lining at or near the amelocemental junction suggests that this is probably the case, and specimens are occasionally found where the division between the remnants of the internal enamel epithelium covering the enamel and the external enamel epithelium forming the greater part of the cyst lining can be seen at the attachment of the cyst to the neck of

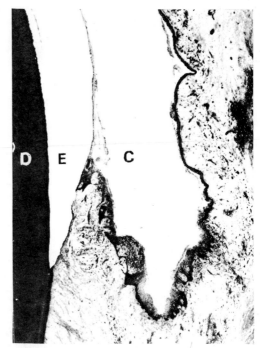

Fig. 10.11 Dentigerous cyst. The probable mode of origin is shows. To the left is the dentine (D). E is the enamel space left after decalcification and is separated from the cyst cavity (C) by a thin layer left by the inner enamel epithelium. The cyst itself appears to have formed as a result of accumulation of fluid between the inner and outer enamel epithelium and by continued proliferation of the latter to form the cyst lining which joins the tooth at the epithelial attachment (× 15)

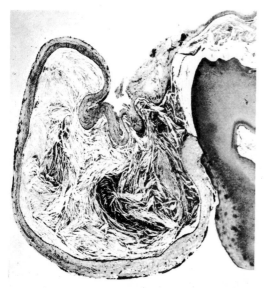

Fig. 10.10 Dentigerous cyst. The cyst surrounds the crown of this molar and the wall is attached to its neck. There is a uniform, thin epithelial lining with minimal inflammatory changes. Clefts in the amorphous contents are from a focus elsewhere in the cyst wall (× 5).

the tooth. Though such a cyst appears to form between the layers of the reduced enamel epithelium, the layer which remains attached to the surface of the enamel is usually of negligible thickness and hence the enamel is in virtually direct contact with the cyst contents. The cyst lining originates from the major part of the reduced enamel epithelium, and progressive growth of the cyst leads to dilatation of the dental follicle.

The cause of the development of dentigerous cysts is not known. However, there is a strong association between failure of eruption of teeth and formation of dentigerous cysts. This is not merely that a dentigerous cyst may prevent a tooth from erupting, but dentigerous cysts predominantly affect teeth which are particularly prone to failure of eruption: namely, maxillary canines and mandibular third molars in particular.

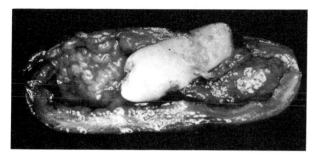

Fig. 10.12   An enucleated dentigerous cyst. The tooth lies with its crown within the cyst cavity and with the cyst wall attached round its neck. The fibrous wall of the cyst is thick and has shelled out cleanly from the surrounding tissues.

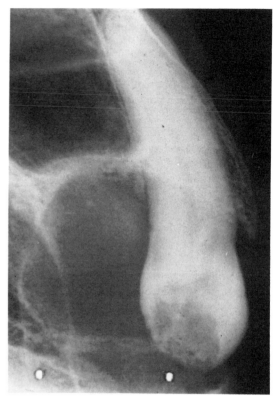

Fig. 10.14   Dentigerous cyst. The crown of this buried canine within the cyst shows resorption. This is only seen in long-neglected cysts, as in this otherwise edentulous patient.

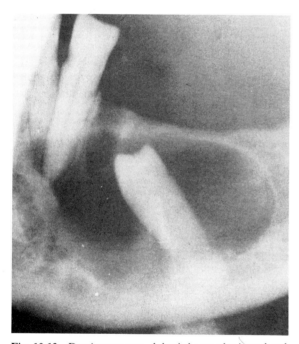

Fig. 10.13   Dentigerous cyst. A buried premolar is enclosed within the cyst but the cyst wall (in spite of radiographic appearances) is attached round the neck of the tooth as in the previous pictures.

The lining of dentigerous cysts typically consists of flattened stratified epithelial cells. This epithelium may occasionally keratinise, but this is regarded as a metaplastic change. Mucous cells are often present in the lining.

The structure of the cyst wall is similar to that of periodontal cysts, but inflammatory changes are typically absent.

Clinical features

Dentigerous cysts are more than twice as common in males as females.

Dentigerous cysts are uncommon in the first decade of life and are most often found between the ages of 20 and 50.

Like other cysts, uncomplicated dentigerous cysts cause no symptoms until the swelling becomes noticeable. A dentigerous cyst may however be detected by chance in radiographs or when the cause is sought for a missing tooth. Infection of a dentigerous cyst causes the usual symptoms of pain and increased swelling.

Radiological features

The appearance is that of a well-defined cyst containing the crown of a tooth displaced from its normal position. The cavity is rounded and

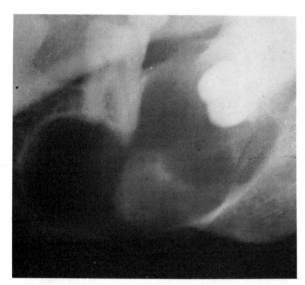

Fig. 10.15 Dentigerous cyst. The cyst has developed round the crown of the buried third molar (right) but has extended forward to involve the roots of a vital second molar. It should not, however, be confused with a periodontal cyst arising from the latter.

unilocular. Occasionally there may be pseudo-loculation as a result of trabeculation or ridging of the bony wall. The slow, regular growth of these cysts results in a sclerotic bony outline and a well-defined cortex in most cases. The affected tooth is often displaced a considerable distance, and a third molar for instance may be pushed to the lower border of the mandible. Occasionally the tooth within a dentigerous cyst is a supernumerary tooth.

A dentigerous cyst may be readily differentiated from a periodontal cyst by the features described. Rarely, however, a keratocyst may envelop the crown of the tooth, as may an ameloblastoma, and either of these may produce an appearance exactly simulating a dentigerous cyst. The diagnosis ultimately therefore depends on histological examination.

Management

Once the diagnosis is established it may occasionally be preferable to marsupialise a dentigerous cyst and allow the tooth to erupt. This is only feasible if the tooth is in a favourable pos-ition and there is space available. Alternatively the tooth can be transplanted to the alveolar ridge or extracted, as appropriate, and the cyst enucleated.

ERUPTION CYST

An eruption cyst occasionally forms in the gum overlying a tooth about to erupt. Strictly speaking an eruption cyst is a soft-tissue cyst but probably arises from enamel organ epithelium after enamel formation is complete and is, in effect, a superficial dentigerous cyst.

Clinical features

Eruption cysts affect children and involve deciduous teeth or permanent molars, that is to say teeth having no predecessors. They are uncommon and probably account for fewer than 1% of cysts.

The cyst lies superficially in the gum overlying the unerupted tooth and appears as a soft, rounded, bluish swelling.

Management

The tissue overlying the crown of the tooth may be removed to allow the tooth to erupt, but it is

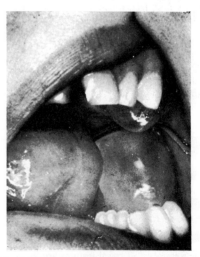

Fig. 10.16 An eruption cyst. The thin-walled, bluish swelling over an upper molar has prevented it from erupting. A mirror placed below the eruption cyst shows its extent and appearance.

probable that many eruption cysts burst spontaneously and never come to surgery.

ODONTOGENIC KERATOCYSTS

Though these cysts are uncommon, accounting for perhaps 4–8% of odontogenic cysts, the are important because of their peculiar mode of growth and because of their strong tendency—unlike other cysts—to recur after removal.

The term *odontogenic keratocyst* has caused a good deal of confusion in that it was originally applied to any cyst of the jaw which showed keratinisation of the epithelial lining. However some keratocysts, though they have a characteristic type of epithelial lining, fail to form significant amounts of keratin, while other types of cyst can show metaplastic keratinisation. Nevertheless the term odontogenic keratocyst is often

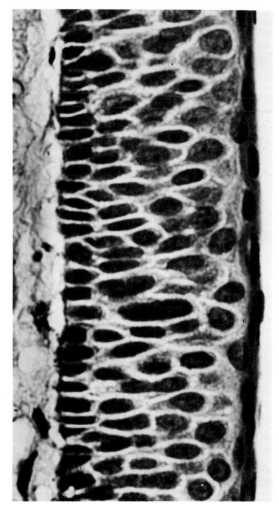

Fig. 10.18 Keratocyst, parakeratotic type. A higher-power view shows the characteristic feature of these cysts, namely the uniform thickness of the epithelium, well-defined basal cell layer, a thin layer of parakeratin and absence of any inflammatory infiltrate.

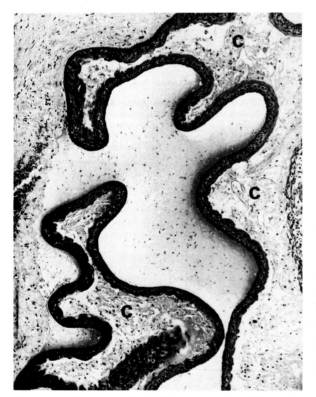

Fig. 10.17 Keratocyst. Typical features are the well-formed epithelium of uniform thickness and its tortuous infolding. The space in the centre has been formed by separation of the epithelium from the connective tissue (a common finding in keratocysts). The cyst cavity itself (C) is indicated.

used exclusively for primordial cysts. Two types are recognised: namely, parakeratotic and orthokeratotic, as discussed later.

Pathogenesis and pathology

It seems likely that keratocysts arise from any of the primordial tissues: that is, the dental lamina or its remains or, as originally believed, from the enamel organ before tooth formation. If this is so, it is difficult to reconcile the frequent appearance of primordial cysts in middle age unless the cyst

This feature of more active mural growth and active epithelial proliferation is probably a factor determining the frequency with which keratocysts recur.

Pathology

Two types are recognised: namely, parakeratotic and orthokeratotic. Important differences are that (a) parakeratotic cysts are more common and may account for up to 85% of keratocysts, (b) orthokeratotic cysts affect women three times as frequently as men, (c) orthokeratotic cysts are typically monolocular and may appear to be dentigerous, and (d) parakeratotic cysts are more aggressive and likely to recur.

The cyst wall is thin and usually much folded. The features of the lining of keratocysts are characteristic and as follows.

1. The epithelium forms a layer of uniform thickness, typically about 7 to 10 cells thick without rete ridges.
2. The lining consists of well-formed stratified squamous epithelium, with a clearly defined basal layer of taller cells, particularly in the parakeratotic variant.
3. Keratin formation is variable. It may be slight and parakeratotic or abundant and orthokeratotic.
4. Keratin formation varies from a thin eosinophilic layer of pre-keratin to abundant orthokeratin formation which fills the cyst cavity with semi-solid material. When there is keratinisation there is a well-defined granular cell layer.
5. The fibrous wall is thin.
6. Inflammatory cells are typically absent or scanty.

Mode of growth

Keratocysts differ from other cysts in that growth of the wall is more prominent than expansion of the cyst cavity, and, as discussed earlier, they tend to extend by fingerlike processes along the lines of least resistance: namely, the cancellous spaces. Hence these cysts may be a considerable size before they expand the jaw and become clinically

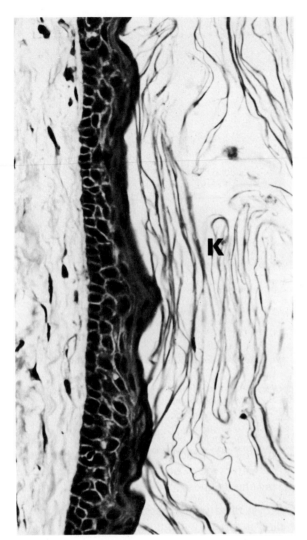

Fig. 10.19 Keratocyst, orthokeratotic type. The epithelium is similar to that in the previous specimen, but in this case there is considerable keratin formation (K) filling the cyst cavity.

growth is quite remarkably slow. The aetiology of keratocysts is therefore speculative.

Radioactive labelling techniques have been used to estimate the mitotic activity of the epithelium of keratocysts, and it is suggested that in spite of their slow growth the lining may be proliferating more actively than buccal mucous membrane. The bulk of evidence therefore suggests that mural growth is the major factor involved in the enlargement of primordial cysts rather than the osmotic pressure exerted by the cyst's contents.

apparent, but to accommodate this overgrowth the cyst lining becomes much folded.

Clinical features

Keratocysts are uncommon and probably account for about 5% of jaw cysts. As with other jaw cysts, they are more common in men than in women.

Most series have recorded a peak incidence in the second and third decades but other large series have shown peaks between the fifth and seventh decades.

Clinically keratocysts are essentially similar to other cysts of the jaws. They are symptomless until the bone is expanded or they become infected. The main difference is that expansion of the jaw is much less than would be expected from the extent of the cyst. Hence clinical signs often fail to appear until the cyst is well advanced, and occasionally extensive cysts are found by chance on routine radiographs.

The mandible is usually affected. The site of at least 50% of keratocysts is the angle of the mandible extending for variable distances into the ramus and forwards into the body. Extension of the cavity up the ramus even to the neck of the condyle is characteristic.

Radiological features

Keratocysts appear as well-defined radiolucent areas, either more or less rounded with a scalloped margin or multiloculated and simulating an ameloblastoma. The bony wall appears as a sharply demarcated cortex.

Rarely, as mentioned earlier, a primordial cyst may extend to envelop an unerupted tooth and similate a dentigerous cyst. As they enlarge, keratocysts tend to displace the roots of adjacent teeth. When, however, a keratocyst presents the characteristic multiloculated radiological appearance it may be almost impossible to differentiate from an ameloblastoma. The final diagnosis depends on the histopathology.

Management

It is preferable to confirm the diagnosis before operation, both because there may be doubt as to

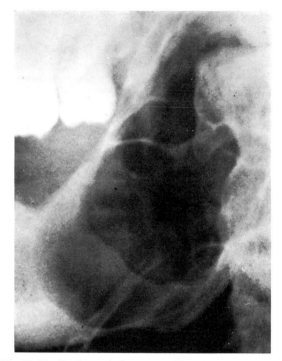

Fig. 10.20 Parakeratotic keratocyst. The characteristic appearance is that of a multilocular cyst involving the ramus with the third molar absent.

whether the lesion is an ameloblastoma and also because of the problem of dealing satisfactorily with keratocysts. The following may assist in making the diagnosis.

1. A cyst filled with keratin and having no cyst fluid is virtually diagnostic. Squames in the cyst fluid are strongly *suggestive* of a primordial cyst but are not in themselves diagnostic as other cysts can form keratin and, very rarely, a carcinoma with cystic change may shed squames into its interior.
2. Electrophoretic studies have shown that keratinising cysts have a very low soluble protein content in the cyst fluid, and a protein level of less than 4 G/dl suggests a primordial cyst.
3. Biopsy, however, provides the most reliable and often the quickest confirmation of the nature of the lesion.

Once the diagnosis of keratocyst has been confirmed, treatment should be by complete enucleation. This is usually difficult as the lining is friable (particularly if inflammation has become superimposed) but treatment should be thorough, even aggressive, to try to be certain that every fragment of cyst lining has been removed.

Recurrence

One of the most important clinical features of the keratocyst, particularly the parakeratotic variant, is its strong tendency to recur after treatment. Recurrence rates of up to 60% have been reported, but a variety of factors, particularly the standard of surgical treatment, have affected these rates.

The reasons for the strong tendency of keratocysts to recur are not clear but several features may contribute. (1) Their linings are thin and fragile and, particularly when the cysts are large, are very difficult to enucleate intact. (2) Extensions of the cyst into cancellous bones increases the difficulty of removal of the lining. (3) They may have satellite daughter cysts in their periphery and these may be left behind after enucleation of the main cyst. (4) Evidence that the epithelial lining of keratocysts shows more vigorous proliferative activity than that of other cyst linings suggests that if a few epithelial cells remain then they can readily form another cyst after enucleation of the main lesion. (5) If, as seems likely, they develop from remnants of dental lamina then, in a susceptible patient, other remnants of dental lamina could contribute to the formation of another cyst which appears as a recurrence. The fact that recurrences have been reported up to 40 years after the original operation suggests that new lesions of this sort develop.

The time of recurrence is very variable. It is often within the first 5 years but may sometimes be many years after treatment.

Though vigorous treatment is likely to reduce the risk of recurrence, there is no absolute certainty of a complete cure, and patients should be followed up with regular radiological examinations at intervals.

The syndrome of multiple jaw cysts, skeletal anomalies and multiple basal cell carcinomas

This syndrome, often called the Gorlin Goltz syndrome, is not excessively rare and is inherited as an autosomal dominant trait.

The salient features are as follows:

1. Multiple keratocysts of the jaws
2. Multiple basal cell carcinomas of the skin sometimes developing early in life
3. Skeletal anomalies (usually of a minor nature) such as bifid ribs and abnormalities of the vertebrae
4. Characteristic facies with frontal and temporoparietal bossing and a broad root to the nose
5. Intracranial anomalies frequently include a characteristic lamellar calcification of the falx cerebri and an abnormally shaped sella turcica.

A great variety of other findings have been reported, and the effects on the patient depend on the predominant manifestation. Thus in some cases there are innumerable basal cell carcinomas which can be disfiguring or troublesome in other ways. Though termed 'naevoid' these tumours differ from typical basal carcinomas only in their early onset.

Other patients have a great many jaw cysts, necessitating repeated operations.

The importance of this syndrome, from the dental viewpoint, is to warn the patient of the likelihood of development of further cysts which must be dealt with by orthodox means as they arise. If neglected these cysts can cause any of the complications of other jaw cysts.

Structurally the cysts are usually indistinguishable from other keratocysts and, like the latter, are more common in the body or ramus of the mandible.

Calcifying odontogenic cyst

The calcifying odontogenic cyst is a rarity and, though recognised in the jaws only in 1962, its cutaneous counterpart (benign calcifying epithelioma of Malherbe) was described in 1880. However, it is probable that this lesion is a cystic neoplasm, and solid variants are also seen.

The cyst lining consists of epithelium, often with palisading of the basal cells which may resemble ameloblasts. The most striking feature is areas of abnormal keratinisation producing swollen cells whose outlines and nuclei become progressively paler (ghost cells) and eventually disappear to leave hyaline masses. The extent of this change may be such as to fill the cyst cavity. The ghost cells typically calcify in patchy fashion. (see Figs 10.21 and 10.22).

Clinically there is no special age, sex, or site predilection. The cyst may be intraosseous or merely indent the jaw. Otherwise the behaviour is similar to that of other cysts.

On radiographs, flecks of calcification may be seen within the area of radiolucency.

Enucleation is usually effective.

NASOPALATINE AND RELATED CYSTS

Nasopalatine cysts are uncommon. They form in

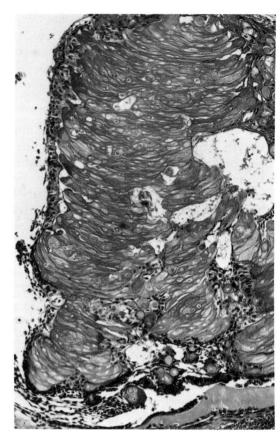

Fig. 10.22 Calcifying odontogenic cyst. In another part of the specimen there is extensive abnormal keratinisation forming a mass of ghost cells where the original epithelial cell membranes and traces of the nuclei are still apparent.

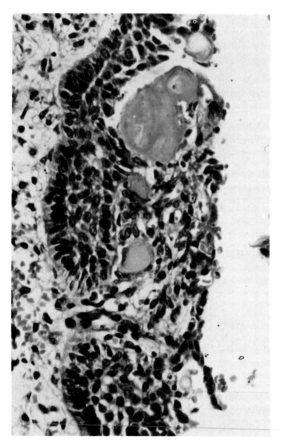

Fig. 10.21 Calcifying odontogenic cyst. The ameloblast-like basal cells can be seen. In addition there is a small patch of abnormal keratinisation (K).

the midline of the anterior part of the maxilla. The nasopalatine incisive canal cyst, median palatine cyst, palatine papilla and median alveolar cysts are probably all variants of the same lesion, varying slightly in position in relation to the postulated line of the incisive canal.

Pathogenesis

Incisive canal cysts arise from the epithelium of the nasopalatine ducts in the incisive canal. In man vestiges of a primitive organ of smell in the incisive canal can be found in the form of incomplete epithelium-lined ducts, cords of epithelial cells, or merely epithelial rests.

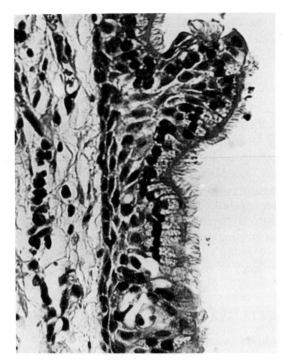

Fig. 10.23 Nasopalatine cyst. The lining, in part at least, may consist of respiratory (cilated columnar) epithelium as here.

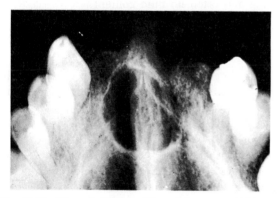

Fig. 10.24 Nasopalatine cyst. The usual appearance is a rounded or pear-shaped area of radiolucency, mainly in the midline.

Histopathology

The epithelial lining of these cysts is usually either stratified squamous epithelium or ciliated columnar (respiratory) epithelium or both together. A few scattered chronic inflammatory cells are often seen beneath the epithelium in some parts of the cyst wall but are not a prominent feature. Mucous glands are often also present in the wall.

An unusual feature is the frequent presence of neurovascular bundles in the wall. These are the long spheno-palatine nerve and vessels which pass through the incisive canal and are often removed with the cyst.

Clinical features

The cyst is slow-growing and resembles other cysts of the jaws clinically, apart from its site. Occasionally they cause intermittent discharge with a salty taste. If allowed to grow sufficiently large, nasopalatine cysts may produce a swelling in the midline of the anterior part of the palate, particularly when superficial (the so-called palatine papilla cyst).

Radiological examination shows a rounded, ovoid or occasionally heart-shaped radiolucent area with a well-defined often sclerotic margin in the anterior part of the midline of the maxilla. These cysts are usually symmetrical but may be slightly larger to one side.

The anterior palatine fossa must be distinguished from a small nasopalatine cyst. The maximum size of a normal fossa is up to 6 or 7 mm.

Treatment

The cyst should be enucleated and recurrence is then unlikely.

Globulomaxillary cyst

This exceedingly rare cyst has been traditionally ascribed to proliferation of sequestered epithelium along the line of fusion of embryonic processes. It is now accepted that this view of embryological development is incorrect and there is no evidence that epithelium becomes buried in this fashion.

It appears that most so-called globulomaxillary cysts are in fact odontogenic.

Nasolabial cyst

This exceedingly rare lesion is a soft-tissue cyst. It forms outside the bone, deep to the nasolabial fold. The aetiology is unknown. These cysts are usually lined by pseudo-stratified columnar epithelium with or without some stratified columnar epithelium in addition. If allowed to grow sufficiently large, the cyst produces a swelling of the upper lip and distorts the nostril. Treatment is usually by simple excision but occasionally may be complicated if the cyst has perforated the nasal mucosa and discharged into the nose.

OTHER RARE TYPES OF CYSTS

Gingival cysts

Dental lamina cyst of the newborn (Bohn's nodules)

Up to 80% of newborn infants have small nodules or cysts in the gingivae, due to proliferation of the epithelial rests of Serres or of non-odontogenic epithelium (Epstein's pearls). These may enlarge sufficiently to appear as creamy-coloured swellings a few millimetres in diameter, but they rupture and resolve spontaneously in a matter of months.

Gingival cysts of adults

Gingival cysts are exceedingly rare. They usually form after the age of approximately 40. Clinically they form dome-shaped swellings less than 1 cm in diameter and sometimes erode the underlying bone. They are lined by very thin flat, stratified squamous epithelium and may contain fluid or layers of keratin.

Lateral periodontal cysts

These rare intraosseous cysts form beside a vital tooth. They are usually seen by chance in routine radiographs and resemble other odontogenic cysts apart from their position beside a tooth, near the crest of the ridge. They cause no symptoms unless they erode through the bone to extend into the gingiva.

Microscopically the lining is squamous or cuboidal epithelium, frequently only one or two cells thick, but sometimes with focal thickening. Some of the cells may have clear cytoplasm and resemble those seen in the dental lamina.

The cyst should be enucleated and the related tooth can be retained if healthy.

Botryoid odontogenic cyst

The botryoid odontogenic cyst is regarded as a multilocular variant of, and even more rare than, the lateral periodontal cyst. It typically affects the mandibular premolar to canine region in adults over 50. Microscopically it is multilocular with fine fibrous septa. The lining consists of flattened non-keratinised epithelium interspersed with clear, glycogen-containing cells and sporadic bud-like proliferations protruding into the cyst cavity.

It should be enucleated if necessary and has no tendency to recur.

CYSTS WITHOUT EPITHELIAL LINING

Solitary (simple) bone cyst

This rare lesion used to be called a 'traumatic' or 'haemorrhagic' bone cyst, though without any obvious justification, or alternatively a 'simple' bone cyst. It is a bone cavity but has no epithelial lining and often no fluid content.

Pathogenesis

The pathogenesis of solitary bone cysts is quite unknown but it has been suggested in the past that these cysts are the result of injury to, and haemorrhage within, the bone of the jaw. This was then supposed to be followed by a failure of organisation of the clot and of repair of the bone. There is, however, no evidence that a blow insufficient to cause a fracture can cause extensive bleeding within the bone nor, if there were such intrabony bleeding, that the consequence would be anything other than normal repair. Moreover, bone cavities filled with blood form in the jaws as a consequence of enucleation of true cysts, but solitary bone cysts do not arise as a result of this bleeding. In addition a common form of treatment for solitary bone cysts is to open them and to allow bleeding into the cavity. Normal healing then follows. It seems hardly likely that intrabony haemorrhage can both cause and cure these lesions.

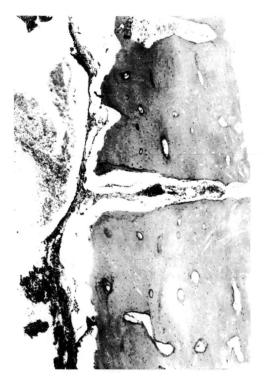

Fig. 10.25 Solitary ('haemorrhagic') bone cyst. The cyst has a rough bony wall lined by a thin layer of fibrous tissue. Epithelium is entirely absent; in some cases even the fibrous lining is lacking (× 45).

It is obvious, therefore, that there has been much futile speculation about these lesions and their cause remains unknown.

Histopathology

The cavity has a rough bony wall and such lining as there may be is of thin connective tissue or there may be only a few red cells, blood pigment or giant cells adhering to the surface of the bone.

There are often no cyst contents but there may sometimes be a little fluid.

Clinical features

Solitary bone cysts are mostly seen in teenagers, and are rare after the age of 25. The mandible is mainly affected. Females are affected more often than males in a ratio of about 3 to 2. They form painless swellings or are fortuitous radiographic findings.

Radiological features

These cavities form rounded, radiolucent areas which generally tend to be less sharply defined than odontogenic cysts, and have two characteristic features:

1. The area of radiolucency is typically much larger than would be expected from the size of the swelling
2. The cavity arches up between the roots of the teeth and may as a consequence be first seen on a bite-wing radiograph.

Management

Solitary bone cysts are not seen in older patients, and in those that have refused surgery it is apparent that these lesions resolve spontaneously. It may be necessary, however, to open the cavity if only to confirm the diagnosis. The characteristic lack of cyst fluid and the unlined bony wall are usually enough to provide a diagnosis, but it is preferable if possible to remove some of the connective tissue lining for this purpose. Opening of the cavity is followed by healing, probably as a result of bleeding. Or it may be that this represents the natural regression of the lesion.

Aneurysmal bone cyst

This lesion barely deserves more than a mention as it hardly ever affects the jaw.

Nothing is known of the aetiology or pathogenesis and the most likely possibility is that the aneurysmal bone cyst is a vascular malformation.

Pathology. The aneurysmal bone cyst is in no sense a cyst except in its radiographic appearance. Histologically there is a highly cellular mass of blood-filled spaces which has been likened to a blood-filled sponge. The extreme cellularity, mitotic activity and frequent presence of giant cells may, however, lead to confusion with a sarcoma. It is essential that this mistake should not be made and the patient subjected, as a consequence, to unnecessarily radical and possibly hazardous treatment.

Clinical features. Most patients are between 10 and 20 years of age, and there appears to be no strong predilection for either sex. The mandible is usually affected.

The main manifestation is usually a painless swelling and a radiolucent area, which may be balloon-like or occasionally show a suggestion of trabeculation or loculation.

Treatment consists of thorough curettage which may, however, need to be repeated, as the lesion occasionally recurs.

Cysts within neoplasms

Cysts frequently form within ameloblastomas but are usually microscopic. In a few cases such a cyst may expand faster (presumably by the effect of hydrostatic pressure) than the tumour grows and, as a result, envelops the tumour. In some cases the gross specimen therefore appears to be a cyst while the tumour is represented by no more than mural thickenings. Once fluid has accumulated within such cysts the epithelial lining becomes flattened and may be indistinguishable from that of a simple cyst histologically. Radiologically too, an ameloblastoma may sometimes exactly simulate a dental or dentigerous cyst. It is not surprising therefore that the idea has got around that neoplasms can arise within cyst linings.

Though this is not a common cause of confusion, it makes it important to enucleate cysts completely. This makes the whole lining available for examination to exclude the possibility that the cyst contains any neoplastic tissue.

Neoplastic change within cysts

The possibility exists that neoplasms, either ameloblastomas or carcinomas, can arise from the epithelial lining of cysts.

There is scant evidence that ameloblastomas arise in this way, and the idea has almost certainly grown up as a result of incorrect radiological interpretation or faulty histological diagnosis, as explained earlier.

With regard to carcinomatous change in relation to cysts it is important to exclude other possibilities before such a diagnosis is made. Since cysts of the jaws are common it is not unlikely that a neoplasm might develop coincidentally nearby

and grow until it involves and fuses with the cyst wall.

In spite of the difficulties in being certain of the origin of a carcinoma within a cyst lining, there are a few well-authenticated cases, but it is an exceedingly rare phenomenon.

CYSTS OF THE SOFT TISSUES

The main varieties of cysts of the soft tissues are as follows:

1. Sublingual dermoid
2. Mucous cyst (mucocoele)
3. Ranula.

The common mucous cyst (extravasation or retention cyst) and the ranula originate in minor salivary glands (Ch. 17). Cysts arising from the soft tissues mainly affect the lips, floor of the mouth and the cheeks. They can readily be distinguished from cysts of the jaws which have extended into the soft tissues after the bony shell has been destroyed. Such cysts appear then as soft bluish swellings, arising from a broad base on the jaw.

Sublingual dermoid

These cysts probably form as a result of some abnormality of development of the branchial arches or pharyngeal pouches.

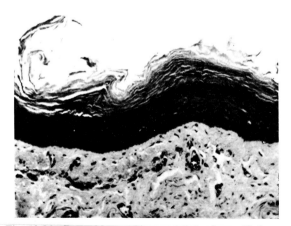

Fig. 10.26 Dermoid cyst. The usual lining is stratified squamous epithelium often actively keratinising and filling the cyst with semi-solid keratinous material (× 100).

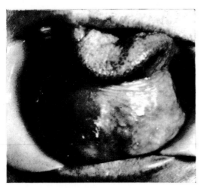

Fig. 10.27 Sublingual dermoid cyst. This is an unusually large specimen but appears even larger because the patient is raising and protruding her tongue. This cyst, unlike a ranula, can be seen to have a thick wall having arisen from the deeper tissues of the floor of the mouth.

The histopathology is variable. The lining of *epidermoid* cysts is keratinising stratified squamous epithelium alone. Desquamated keratin may fill the cyst cavity, giving it a semi-solid consistency. Less often, cysts also have dermal appendages in the wall and are then referred to as *dermoid* cysts. Still others are lined in part by keratinising stratified squamous epithelium and in part by respiratory (ciliated columnar stratified) epithelium.

Clinical features

Dermoid cysts develop between the hyoid and jaw or may form immediately beneath the tongue. They are sometimes filled with semi-solid keratinous material giving them a putty-like consistency. A sublingual dermoid is more deeply placed than a ranula; the latter is obviously superficial, having a thin wall and a bluish appearance. A dermoid causes no symptoms until large enough to interfere with speech or eating. Nevertheless a surprisingly large swelling can be accommodated in the floor of the mouth without disability and can be completely concealed by the tongue in its normal resting position.

Treatment consists of dissecting out the cyst.

SUGGESTED FURTHER READING

Cawson R A, Eveson J W 1987 Oral pathology and diagnosis. William Heinemann Medical Books, London and Gower Medical Publishing, London

Dayan D, Buchner A, Gorsky M, Harel-Raviv M 1988 The peripheral odontogenic keratocyst. Int J Oral Maxillofac Surg 17: 81–83

Forssell K, Forssell H, Happonnen R P, Neva M 1988 Simple bone cyst. Review of the literature and analysis of 23 cases. Int J Oral Maxillofac Surg 17: 21–24

Forssell K, Forssell H, Kahnberg K-E 1988 Recurrence of keratocysts. A long-term follow-up study. Int J Oral Maxillofac Surg 17: 25–28

Gorlin R J 1987 Nevoid basal-cell carcinoma syndrome. Medicine 55: 98–113

Haring J I, Van Dis M L 1988 Odontogenic keratocysts: A clinical, radiographic and histopathologic study. Oral Surg, Oral Med, Oral Pathol 66: 145–153

Hoffman S, Jacoway J R, Krolls S O 1987 Intraosseous and parosteal tumors of the jaws. Fascicle 24. Armed Forces Institute of Pathology, Washington

Macdonald A W, Fletcher A 1989 Expression of cytokeratin in the epithelium of dentigerous and odontogenic keratocysts: an aid to diagnosis. J Clin Pathol 42: 736–739

Matthews J B, Mason G I, Browne R M 1988 Epithelial markers and proliferating cells in odontogenic jaw cysts. J Pathol 156: 283–290

Meghji S, Harvey W, Marris 1989 Interleukin 1-like activity in cystic lesions of the jaws. Br J Oral Maxillofac Surg 27: 1–11

Partridge M, Towers J F 1987 The primordial (odontogenic keratocyst) its tumour-like characteristics and behaviour. Brit J Oral Maxillofac Surg 25: 271–279

Waldron C A 1988 Odontogenic tumors and selected jaw cysts. In: Gnepp D R (ed) Pathology of the head and neck. Churchill Livingstone, New York

Woolgar J A, Rippin J W, Browne R M 1987 A comparative histological study of odontogenic keratocysts in basal cell naevus syndrome and control patients. J Oral Pathol 16: 75–80

11. Tumours and tumour-like lesions of the jaws

Odontogenic tumours
Ameloblastoma
Malignant ameloblastoma and ameloblastic carcinoma
Adenomatoid odontogenic tumour
Calcifying epithelial odontogenic tumour
Clear cell odontogenic tumour
Calcifying odontogenic cyst
Squamous odontogenic tumour
Ameloblastic fibroma
Odontogenic myxoma
Odontogenic fibroma
Cemental tumours and dysplasias
Cementoblastoma
Cementifying fibroma
Periapical cemental dysplasia
Odontomas
Compound odontoma
Complex odontoma

Other types of odontomas
Non-odontogenic tumours
Osteoma and other bony overgrowths
Osteochondroma
Ossifying fibroma
Chondroma
Giant-cell granuloma of the jaws
Haemangioma of bone
Melanotic neuroectodermal tumour of infancy
Malignant tumours of bone
Osteosarcoma
Chondroma and chondrosarcoma
Ewings's sarcoma
Multiple myeloma
Amyloidosis
Langerhans' cell histiocytosis
Secondary tumours—carcinoma

ODONTOGENIC TUMOURS

Odontogenic tissues, both ectodermal and mesenchymal, can give rise to true neoplasms and also to hamartomas (odontomas).

Odontogenic tumours are all rare, but the ameloblastoma is the most common neoplasm of the jaws.

Ameloblastoma

The ameloblastoma is a tumour of odontogenic epithelium, which typically produces the appearance of a multilocular cyst on radiographs. It is slowly invasive locally, but otherwise benign.

Most ameloblastomas are first recognised between the ages of 40 and 50. They are rare in children and old people. 80% form in the mandible; of these, 70% develop in the posterior molar region, and often involve the ramus. They are symptomless until the swelling becomes notice-

able. If neglected, the tumour can perforate the bone and spread into the soft tissues, making subsequent excision difficult.

Radiological features

Radiographically ameloblastomas typically form rounded, well-defined, cyst-like, radiolucent areas with well-defined margins. The most readily recognised pattern is that of a multilocular cyst. Lingual expansion may sometimes be seen in an occlusal radiograph, but is not pathognomonic of ameloblastoma.

Other variants are a honeycomb pattern of radiolucency, a single well-defined cavity indistinguishable from a radicular or, rarely, a dentigerous cyst. However, differentiation from non-neoplastic cysts and other tumours or tumour-like lesions of the jaws alone is not possible by radiography alone.

247

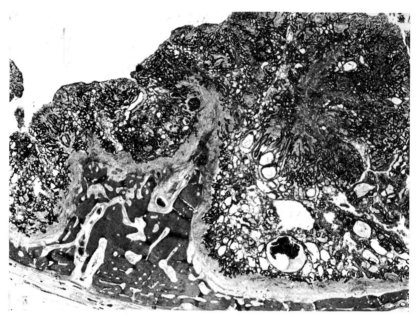

Fig. 11.1 Ameloblastoma. Processes of darkly-staining tumour cells are extending in all directions; there are many small cystic spaces and the edge of a larger one can be seen. The tumour is separated from the bone by a well-defined zone of connective tissue; nevertheless the tumour cells are pushing forward into the connective tissue and bone has been extensively resorbed ($\times$ 10).

Subtypes

Microscopically, several subtypes have been described and some of these variations may be seen within limited areas of a single tumour.

The follicular type forms the most readily recognisable pattern with islands and trabeculae of epithelial cells in a connective tissue stroma. These epithelial processes consist of a well-organised single layer of tall, columnar, ameloblast-like cells which have nuclei at the opposite pole to the basement membrane, and surround a core of loosely arranged polyhedral or angular cells, resembling stellate reticulum. In other specimens, or other parts of the same tumour, the peripheral cells may be cut obliquely or be more cuboidal and resemble basal cells.

Cyst formation is common and varies from microcysts within a predominantly solid tumour, to a cyst which has enveloped the main tumour mass. Cysts may develop either within the epithelial islands or result from cystic degeneration of the connective tissue stroma.

When a cystic area of an ameloblastoma envelops the remainder of the tumour, the neoplastic epithelial lining of the cyst often becomes flattened and resembles that of a non-neoplastic cyst. Biopsy of the cyst wall alone may, therefore, lead to its being misdiagnosed as a simple cyst.

The plexiform type of ameloblastoma consists mainly of thin trabeculae of small, darkly staining epithelial cells in a sparsely cellular connective tissue stroma.

In the acanthomatous type of ameloblastoma there is squamous metaplasia of the central core of epithelium which otherwise, resembles the more common follicular type.

Basal cell ameloblastomas consist of more darkly staining cells predominantly in a trabecular pattern with little evidence of palisading at the periphery. They have been mistaken for basal cell carcinomas.

Granular cell ameloblastomas are rare. They usually resemble the more common follicular type, but the epithelium, particularly in the central areas of the tumour islands, forms sheets of large eosinophilic granular cells.

These variations in the histological configuration do not seem to affect the tumour's behaviour but

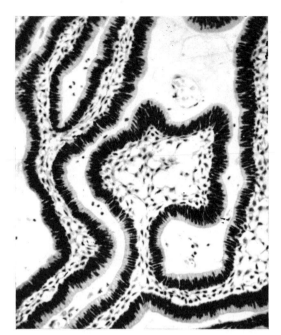

Fig. 11.2 Ameloblastoma, follicular type. Section of a typical tumour at greater magnification shows the highly characteristic tall, columnar cells with basally placed nuclei (resembling the black and white keys of a piano) radially arranged around a core of loosely arranged, rather stellate cells separated by fluid. The epithelial cells are supported by a vascular connective tissue stroma (× 220).

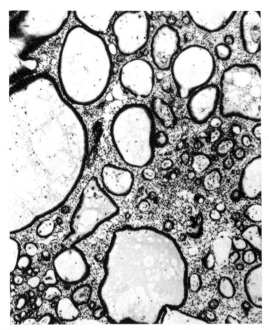

Fig. 11.3 Ameloblastoma; stromal cysts. These are formed by breakdown of the connective tissue stroma, leaving only the epithelial cells surrounding the cyst cavities.

it has been suggested that the granular cell type is more likely than other types to recur.

Clinical features. Ameloblastomas are usually first recognised between the ages of forty and fifty, and rarely seen in children or old people. The mandible is involved in 80%; usually in the posterior of the molar region. They are symptomless until the swelling becomes noticeable. If neglected, the tumour can perforate the bone and, ultimately, spread into the soft tissues making subsequent excision difficult.

Radiographically, ameloblastomas typically form rounded, radiolucent areas with well-defined margins. The most readily recognised appearance is that of a multilocular cyst. Other variants are a honeycomb pattern or a single well-defined cavity indistinguishable from a radicular cyst. Lingual expansion may sometimes be apparent on an occlusal radiograph, but is not pathognomonic of ameloblastoma.

Management

The diagnosis must be confirmed by biopsy. Treatment is by wide excision, preferably taking up to 2 cm of apparently normal bone around the margin. Complete excision will produce a cure but anything less is followed by recurrence.

Complete excision of a large ameloblastoma may mean total resection of the jaw and bone grafting. It is preferable therefore to avoid so extensive an operation whenever possible by leaving the lower border of the jaw intact and extending the resection subperiosteally. Bony repair can then take place and a good deal of the jaw reforms. The tumour penetrates cancellous bone more readily than compact and the lower border may be uninvolved. If tumour is left behind recurrence follows but this may take several years and regular radiographic follow-up should be carried out. A further limited operation can then be carried out to remove the recurrence. This approach is generally less unpleasant for the patient, who must be warned of the necessity of regular follow-up and, possibly, of a further operation.

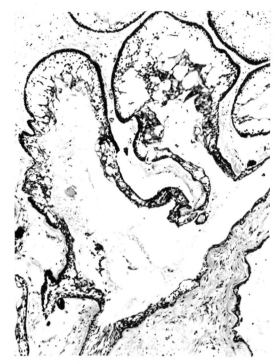

Fig. 11.4 Cyst formation in ameloblastoma. The many small epithelial cysts are coalescing to form larger cysts, at first irregular in shape. As fluid accumulates, the cyst lining becomes flattened, resembling that of simple cysts.

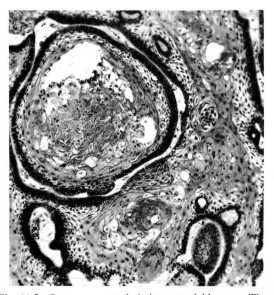

Fig. 11.5 Squamous metaplasia in an ameloblastoma. The outer cells of the tumour processes are the same as those seen in the earlier pictures but the central cells have reverted to a squamous type.

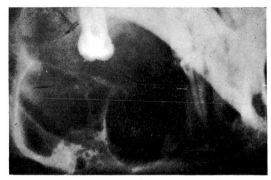

Fig. 11.6 Ameloblastoma. The typical radiological appearance of an ameloblastoma is a multilocular cyst or multiple cyst cavities of different sizes as shown here.

Malignant ameloblastoma and ameloblastic carcinoma

Both of these are exceptionally rare tumours and are little more than pathological curiosities—though not to the patient of course.

Malignant ameloblastoma is a histologically typical ameloblastoma, which, nevertheless has given rise to pulmonary metastases which have retained the same microscopic appearances as the primary. Few of the reported cases have been authenticated, and some, at least, have resulted from aspiration implantation. If so, local excision of the secondary deposit should be curative.

Ameloblastic carcinoma is a tumour which has the microscopic features, initially, of an ameloblastoma, but loses differentiation and behaves in a malignant fashion: namely, spreading to lymph nodes or beyond. In the later stages the microscopic appearances become similar to a squamous cell carcinoma. Rarely the progressive loss of differentiation can be seen in successive specimens from the same patient and confirms the diagnosis.

The treatment is that of an intraosseous carcinoma and if, in addition, metastases are already present, the prognosis is correspondingly poor.

Adenomatoid odontogenic tumour

This uncommon lesion, previously known as adenoameloblastoma, is completely benign, and probably a hamartoma. It is neither invasive like an ameloblastoma nor has it any glandular component.

Clinically, adenomatoid odontogenic tumour is found either in late adolescence or young adults. Females are more frequently affected in the ratio of 2 to 1. The tumour is most frequently found in the anterior maxilla and forms a very slow-growing swelling or may be noticed by chance on a radiograph. The latter frequently simulates a dental or dentigerous cyst. Most specimens are only a few centimetres in diameter.

Microscopically, there is a well-defined capsule which encloses whorls and strands of epithelium, among which are microcysts, resembling ducts cut in cross section and lined by columnar cells similar to ameloblasts. These microcysts may contain some homogeneous eosinophilic material. They have led to the tumours being called adenomatoid—they are not ducts and are never seen cut longitudinally. Fragments of amorphous or crystalline calcification may also be seen among the sheets of epithelial cells.

These lesions shell out readily, and enucleation seems to be curative.

Calcifying epithelial odontogenic tumour

This rare tumour, with bizarre microscopic features, is more simply termed a Pindborg tumour, after its discoverer, or CEOT. Though rare, it is important, particularly because it has been mistaken for a poorly differentiated carcinoma.

Clinically adults are mainly affected at an average age of about 40. The typical site is the posterior body of the mandible, which is twice as frequently involved as the maxilla. Symptoms are usually lacking until a swelling becomes apparent.

Radiographs show a translucent area with poorly defined margins and, usually, increasing calcification and radiopacities within the tumour as it matures.

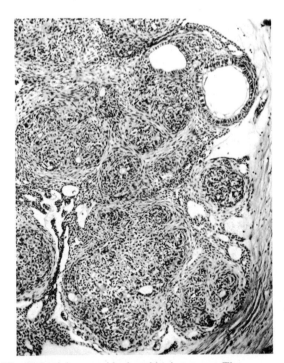

Fig. 11.7 Adenomatoid odontoblastic tumour. The epithelial cells form compact whorls, and among them are several rounded cysts lined by columnar cells. The tumour is surrounded by a fibrous capsule. The tumour was removed from a boy of 16, and appears on radiographs as a dentigerous cyst (× 55).

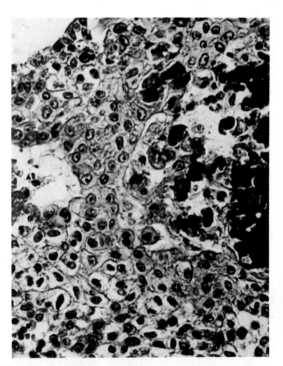

Fig. 11.8 Calcifying epithelial odontogenic tumour. The epithelial cells with their sharply defined cell membranes resembling squamous epithelium show enlarged nuclei with prominent nucleoli. The appearance therefore closely resembles squamous cell carcinoma. The dark amorphous material near the bottom of the picture is a focus of calcification typical of these tumours.

Microscopically CEOT consists of sheets or strands of epithelial wells in a connective tissue stroma. The epithelial cells are roughly polyhedral and typically have distinct outlines and inter-cellular bridges. Gross variation in nuclear size, including giant nuclei and multinucleated cells, is frequently striking. These nuclei are usually hyperchromatic and, though mitoses are rare, produce an alarming resemblance to a poorly differentiated carcinoma. However, unlike most carcinomas, an inflammatory reaction is typically absent.

Within the tumour, there are typically homogeneous hyaline areas, with the staining characteristics of amyloid, which may calcify. These calcifications form concentric masses in and around degenerating epithelial cells and may form large masses.

Calcifying epithelial odontogenic tumours are not encapsulated, are locally invasive and their behaviour seems to be similar to that of ameloblastomas.

Diagnosis depends on histological examination. It is particularly important to distinguish this pleomorphic tumour from a poorly differentiated carcinoma, as the treatment and prognosis are widely different.

Complete excision of the tumour with a border of normal bone appears to be curative. If excision is inadequate, recurrence follows.

Clear cell odontogenic tumour

This rare neoplasm has features in common with the Pindborg tumour but affects elderly patients (60 to 74 years). It causes expansion of the jaw and a ragged area of radiolucency.

Microscopically the tumour is poorly circumscribed and consists of uniform-sized clear cells with a central nucleus and a well-defined cell membrane. They form large sheets, interrupted by strands of fibrous tissue, in which there is no inflammatory infiltrate. The epithelial cells mostly have a clear cytoplasm but some contain glycogen. There may also be smaller, dense areas of small basaloid epithelial cells with scanty cytoplasm. There may be some nuclear pleomorphism but few mitoses. Important differences from CEOT are the lesser degree of nuclear pleomorphism and the lack of calcifications or amyloid-like material. However, it is even more important to distinguish a clear cell odontogenic tumour from a metastasis from a renal cell carcinoma.

Wide excision appears to be effective, and no recurrences have been seen in short periods of follow up.

Calcifying odontogenic cyst (Gorlin cyst)

The calcifying odontogenic cyst is rare and, despite its name, can also be solid and is almost certainly a benign neoplasm (see also p. 239).

Clinically, almost any age and either jaw can be affected. The site is most often anterior to the first molar but occasionally it is the gingival mucosa and the underlying bone is merely indented. On radiographs, the appearance is usually that of cyst but it may be multilocular or contain flecks of calcification. Occasionally roots of adjacent teeth are eroded.

Microscopically the lining of any cystic areas consists of squamous epithelium with cuboidal or ameloblast-like basal cells. This epithelium is sometimes thick and can contain areas resembling stellate reticulum. Solid variants of this tumour may therefore appear similar to an ameloblastoma. However, the most conspicuous feature is abnormal keratinisation producing areas of swollen, eosinophilic cells which become progressively paler, leaving only their outlines (ghost cells), and which eventually disappear to leave hyaline masses. The ghost cells typically calcify in patchy fashion, and where this keratin-like material comes into contact with connective tissue it excites a foreign body reaction.

Approximately 10% of calcifying odontogenic cysts are associated with odontomas or other odontogenic tumours (see Figs 10.21 & 10.22).

The behaviour of a calcifying odontogenic cyst is similar to that of a non-neoplastic cyst, and overlying bone is only occasionally eroded. However, it is capable of continued growth and can recur after incomplete removal.

Squamous odontogenic tumour

This rare tumour mainly affects young adults and involves the alveolar process of either jaw, close to the roots of erupted teeth. Radiographically therefore, the squamous odontogenic tumour can mimic severe bone loss from periodontitis or produce a cyst-like area.

Microscopically, circumscribed, rounded, or more irregular islands of squamous epithelium are set in a fibrous stroma. Foci of keratin or parakeratin may form in the epithelium, which may also contain laminated calcifications or globular eosinophilic structures.

This tumour appears to be benign, though there may occasionally be invasion of adjacent structures by maxillary lesions. However, curettage and extraction of any teeth involved appears usually to be effective.

Ameloblastic fibroma

This tumour, though rare, is important in the differential diagnosis of ameloblastoma.

Clinically, ameloblastic fibromas, unlike most ameloblastomas, are usually seen in young adults or adolescents, but it may appear very similar radiographically, namely as a multi- or unilocular cyst in the posterior body of the mandible. Ameloblastic fibromas are also slow-growing and usually asymptomatic, but eventually expand the jaw.

Microscopically both the epithelium and connective tissue are neoplastic. The epithelium consists of ameloblast-like or more cuboidal cells surrounding others resembling stellate reticulum or more compact epithelium. The epithelium is sharply circumscribed by a basal membrane and forms islands; strands or mushroom-like proliferations in a loose but cellular, fibromyxoid connective tissue, which resembles the immature dentine papilla.

An ameloblastic fibroma may rarely be combined with mixed calcifying dental tissues (ameloblastic fibro-odontoma), and radiographs typically show the densely opaque dental tissues in the otherwise radiolucent area.

The ameloblastic fibroma and fibro-odontoma are benign: they do not infiltrate bone and they separate readily from their bony walls. Conservative resection is effective, but, if incomplete, recurrence follows.

Ameloblastic sarcoma (ameloblastic fibrosarcoma)

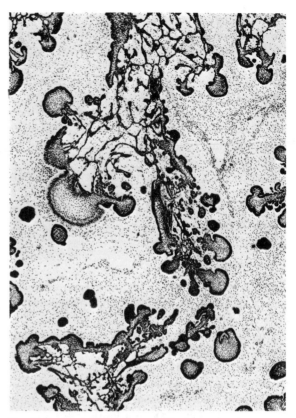

Fig. 11.9 Ameloblastic fibroma. The appearance is somewhat similar to that of ameloblastoma but the pattern of epithelial proliferation is different and the connective tissue component resembles the undifferentiated mesenchyme of the dentine papilla (× 20).

is the exceedingly rare malignant counterpart of ameloblastic fibroma and behaves accordingly.

Odontogenic myxoma

The odontogenic myxoma is peculiar to the jaws and consists of dental mesenchyme.

Clinically, young people are predominantly affected. The tumour gives rise to a fusiform swelling and an area of radiolucency with scalloped margins or a soap bubble pattern which may be similar to that of an ameloblastoma.

Microscopically myxomas consist of scanty spindle-shaped or angular cells with long, fine, anastomosing processes, distributed in loose mucoid material. A few collagen fibres may also be present, and there may be small, scattered epithelial rests. The margins of the tumour are ill-defined and peripheral bone is progressively resorbed.

Myxomas are benign, but can infiltrate widely. Recurrence and persistence even after several operations is well recognised. Wide excision is therefore desirable, but, in spite of vigorous treatment, some tumours persist, and have been described over 30 years after the original operations. By this time they appear inactive and are symptomless.

Rare variants with a more cellular and pleomorphic microscopic picture may be categorised as myxosarcomas but appear to have little or no potential for metastasis.

Odontogenic fibroma

The odontogenic origin of this rare endosteal tumour is suggested by its site and the presence of epithelial rests.

Clinically, odontogenic fibroma more frequently affects the mandible. It forms a slowly growing mass and usually remains unrecognised until it expands the jaw or is found by chance in a radiograph, where it appears as a sharply defined, rounded area of lucency in a tooth-bearing area.

Microscopically the odontogenic fibroma consists of spindle-shaped fibroblasts and bundles of

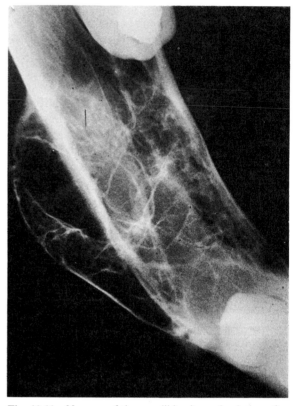

Fig. 11.11 Myxoma of the mandible. An occlusal view of the jaw of the same patient as in Fig. 11.10 but showing even better the finely trabeculated, soap-bubble appearance and expansion of the jaw. Evidence of residual tumour was still present after 35 years in spite of vigorous treatment, both surgery and radiotherapy, in its earlier stages.

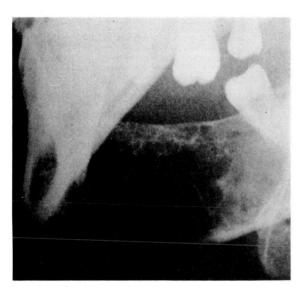

Fig. 11.10 Myxoma of the mandible.

whorled collagen fibres, and contains islands of epithelium resembling the rests of Malassez.

The odontogenic fibroma does not infiltrate or adhere to the surrounding bone and will shell out from its surroundings.

CEMENTAL TUMOURS AND DYSPLASIAS

Cemental tumours and dysplasias are characterised by continued proliferation of cementum, but form a group which lack consistently definable characteristics and as a consequence have suffered changes in terminology. Diagnosis depends on the clinical, radiographic and microscopic picture. Four main types are usually described but all are rare.

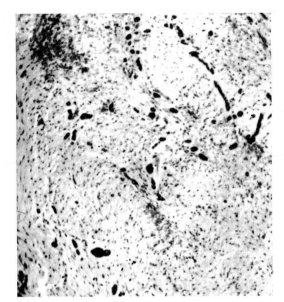

Fig. 11.12 Odontogenic fibroma. This rare tumour consists of proliferating fibrous tissue containing epithelial rests resembling those of the periodontal membrane.

Cementoblastoma

Cementoblastoma is a benign neoplasm which forms a mass of cementum-like tissue as an irregular or rounded mass attached to the root of a tooth.

Clinically cementoblastomas are mainly seen in young adults, particularly males, typically below the age of 25. They are usually slow-growing and most frequently arise from a mandibular first molar. The jaw is not usually expanded, but occasionally cementoblastoma can produce gross bony swelling and pain.

Radiographically there is typically a rounded radiopaque mass, with a thin radiolucent margin, attached to the roots of a tooth. The mass is sometimes irregular in shape and mottled in texture. Resorption of the roots of the originating tooth is common, but it remains vital.

Microscopically the mass consists of cementum which often contains many reversal lines, resembling Paget's disease. Cells are enclosed within the cementum, and in the irregular spaces are many osteoclasts and osteoblast-like cells. The cellular appearance may sometimes appear so active as to be mistaken for an osteosarcoma. At the periphery there is a broad zone of unmineralised tissue, and

the mass is surrounded by a connective tissue capsule.

These appearances are essentially the same as those of an osteoblastoma, a rare bone tumour, and they are only distinguishable by the cementoblastoma's relationship to a tooth.

Cementoblastomas are benign, and, if completely excised and the tooth extracted, there should be no recurrence. Incomplete removal leads to continued growth.

Cementifying fibroma

This lesion is typically seen in patients between 30 and 40 and in females approximately twice as frequently as males. It usually forms round the roots of the mandibular premolars or molars, and radiographically the lesion appears as a well-circumscribed area of radiolucency which may contain flecks of calcification. It gradually becomes more densely calcified and may expand the lower border of the mandible or extend up into the ramus.

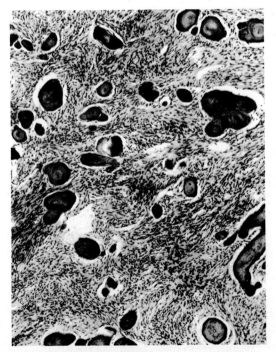

Fig. 11.13 Cementifying fibroma. The tumour is cellular, consisting of great numbers of fibroblast-like cells surrounding rounded calcified nodules. These progressively increase in size and fuse together to form large masses.

Microscopically, cementifying fibroma consists of a rounded mass of cellular, fibrous connective tissue, which contains heavily calcified nodules resembling the cementicles sometimes seen in the periodontal ligament. However, the calcifications may have no clear resemblance to cementum, and osteoid or bone may be associated. These nodules gradually grow, fuse to become lobulated and ultimately form a dense mass. A capsule may be discernible. The histological and radiographic appearances are therefore dependent on the stage of development, and they may be indistinguishable from those of an ossifying fibroma.

Though previously classified as a benign tumour, cementifying fibroma, once fully calcified, does not seem to progress and is a cemental dysplasia. Small lesions may be readily enucleated but large specimens can cause considerable distortion of the jaw and require local resection and, sometimes, bone-grafting.

Periapical cemental dysplasia

Periapical cemental dysplasia affects women (particularly the middle-aged) more than 10 times as

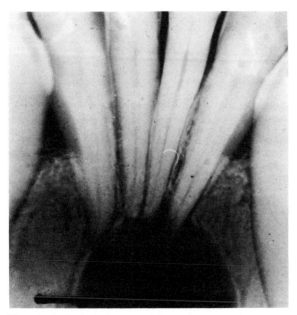

Fig. 11.14 Periapical cemental dysplasia. An exceptionally large example simulating a cyst in its early stages before calcification. The teeth were vital.

frequently as men, and is also more common in blacks. It most frequently affects the mandibular incisor region, but can affect several sites or be generalised. It is asymptomatic but can be seen in radiographs in its early stages, as rounded radiolucent areas related to the apices of the teeth. They simulate periapical granulomas but the related teeth are vital. Later, increasing calcification, starting centrally, causes the masses to become densely radiopaque, but all stages of development may be seen in multiple lesions.

Microscopically these lesions resemble cementifying fibromas and consist, in their early stages, of cellular fibrous tissue containing foci of cementum-like tissue. Progressive calcification leads to the formation of a solid, bone-like mass.

Once early lesions have been distinguished from periapical granulomas by dental investigation, further treatment is unnecessary, as the disorder does not progress.

Gigantiform cementoma (florid cemento-osseous dysplasia)

This is probably a florid form of periapical cemental dysplasia and affects a similar group of persons. The sclerotic masses are frequently symmetrical and may involve all four quadrants. They are asymptomatic unless they become infected, but can expand the jaw. Radiologically, gigantiform cementoma appears as radiopaque, somewhat irregular masses without a radiolucent border and in the past has been interpreted as chronic osteomyelitis or even Paget's disease.

Microscopically the appearances are generally similar to periapical cemental dysplasia.

Treatment is not indicated except rarely for cosmetic reasons or if the mass becomes infected, in which case it may have to be excised entirely to allow the infection to resolve.

ODONTOMAS (odontomes)

Odontomas are developmental malformations (hamartomas), not neoplasms, of dental tissues. Like teeth, once fully calcified, they do not develop further. Even when the morphology is grossly distorted (as in complex odontomas), the

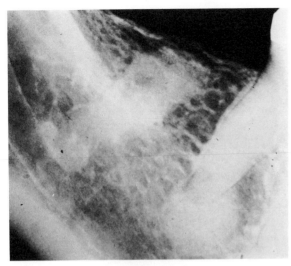

Fig. 11.15 Gigantiform cementoma. This shows some of the dense radiopaque apical masses without a radiolucent border, typical of this lesion. The patient was middle-aged and similar masses were distributed symmetrically on the opposite side of the mandible.

pulp, dentine, enamel and cementum are in normal anatomical relationships with one another, and also, like teeth, odontomas tend to erupt.

Odontomas affect the maxilla slightly more frequently than the mandible and are often detected in early adolescence in routine radiographs.

When odontomas have erupted, infection develops in one of the many stagnation areas, and abscess formation commonly follows. In other cases, odontomas displace teeth or block their eruption or become involved in cyst formation.

Compound odontomas

These consist of many separate, small, tooth-like structures (denticles), possibly produced by localised, multiple budding-off from the dental lamina and formation of many tooth germs.

The denticles are embedded in fibrous connective tissue, and have a fibrous capsule. Inflammatory or cystic changes may involve the mass.

Clinically a compound odontoma usually forms in the anterior part of the jaws and gives rise to a painless swelling. The denticles may be seen radiologically as separate calcified bodies.

The mass should be enucleated as a potential obstruction to tooth eruption.

Complex odontoma

Complex odontomas consist of an irregular mass of hard and soft dental tissues, having no morphological resemblance to a tooth and frequently forming a cauliflower-like mass.

Clinically, complex odontomas are usually seen in young persons, but may escape diagnosis until late in life. Typically a hard painless swelling is present, but the mass may start to erupt and infection follows. The mass may also undergo cystic change or resorption.

Radiologically, when calcification is complete, an irregular radiopaque mass is seen containing areas of densely radiopaque enamel. Should the mass become infected, the calcified tissues may be mistaken for a sequestrum or an area of sclerotic bone.

Histologically, the mass consists of all the dental tissues in a disordered arrangement, but frequently with a radial pattern. The pulp is usually finely branched so that the mass is perforated, like a sponge, by small vascular channels.

The mass should be removed by as conservative surgery as possible.

Other types of odontomas

In the past, complex classifications have been devised to include such developmental anomalies as *dilated, gestant (invaginated)* and *geminated* odontomas. These abnormalities are, in part, obviously tooth-like. Dilated and gestant odontomas arise by invagination of cells of the enamel organ or of the epithelial sheath of Hertwig, which actively proliferate until they expand the developing tooth. Gestant odontomas range in severity from a cingular pit in an otherwise normal upper lateral incisor to the so-called *dens in dente*.

The geminated odontoma is most common in the incisor region. The pulp-chambers may be entirely separate, joined in the middle of the tooth, or branched with the pulp-chambers of separate crowns sharing a common root canal.

The crowns may be entirely separate or divided

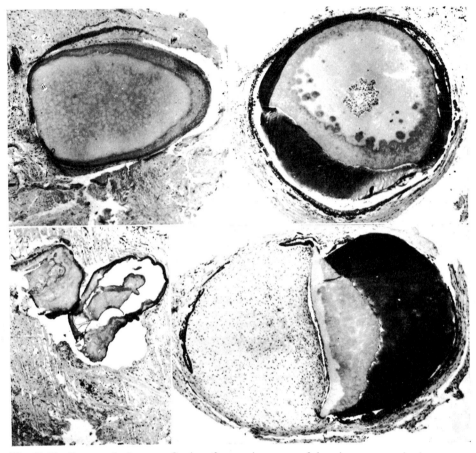

Fig. 11.16 Compound odontoma. Sections from various areas of the odontoma seen in the radiograph shown in Fig. 11.17, show denticles of dentine and enamel cut in various planes, and more irregular calcified tissues, within a connective tissue capsule (× 30).

only by a shallow groove. The roots may be single or double.

These malformed teeth should be removed before they obstruct the eruption of other teeth or become infected, or for cosmetic reasons.

Enamel pearls are uncommon, minor abnormalities, which are formed on otherwise normal teeth by displaced ameloblasts below the amelocemental junction.

Enamel pearls may consist only of a nodule of enamel attached to the dentine, or may have a core of dentine containing a horn of pulp. The pearls are usually round, a few millimetres in diameter, and often form at the bifurcation of upper permanent molar roots. They may cause a stagnation area at the gingival margin, but, if they contain

pulp, this will be exposed when the pearl is removed.

Dentinoma. Calcified masses called 'dentinomas' have rarely been described. However, there is justifiable doubt about their nature since dentine forms only under the inductive effect of ameloblasts. The existence of 'pure' dentinomas therefore seems unlikely.

Combined forms and malignant odontogenic tumours

Exceedingly rarely odontomas and odontogenic tumours are combined. The main example is the odontoameloblastoma which consists of an ameloblastoma associated with a composite odon-

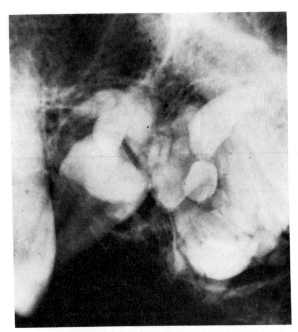

Fig. 11.17 Compound odontoma. The mass consists of many denticles which overlap each other in the radiograph but nevertheless may be just visible as individual tooth-like structures.

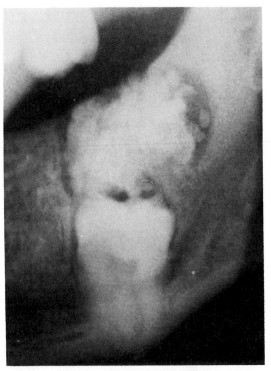

Fig. 11.18 Complex odontoma. In this radiograph the odontoma overlies the crown of a buried molar and shows the typical dense amorphous area of radiopacity.

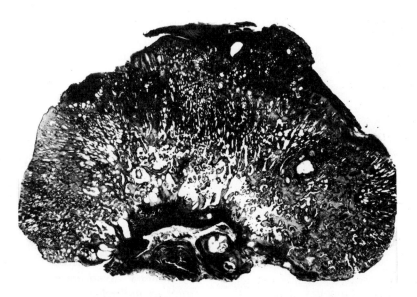

Fig. 11.19 Complex odontoma. The specimen consists of a cauliflower-like mass of dentine, enamel and cementum penetrated by fine divisions of a much-branched pulp (× 4).

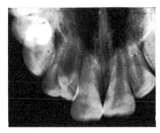

Fig. 11.20 A geminated odontoma. The lateral incisor tissue has been doubled and the teeth are united along their whole length.

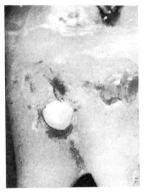

Fig. 11.21 An enamel pearl. A rounded nodule of ectopic enamel is seen in the usual position for these malformations, i.e. at the bifurcation of the roots of a molar.

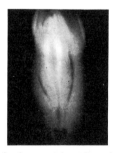

Fig. 11.22 Dens in dente; an invaginated odontome. Ameloblasts have been invaginated, forming a pocket of enamel continuous with the surface enamel within the tooth; dentine has been formed on the invaginated enamel. The pulp chamber can be seen on either side of the invagination.

toma. The behaviour of such lesions is that of the neoplastic component.

Malignant odontogenic tumours such as the malignant ameloblastoma and the ameloblastic fibrosarcoma also exist. However, they are so rare

that they are little more than pathological curiosities—but not to the patient.

NON-ODONTOGENIC TUMOURS

Many of these tumours are considerably more common in other parts of the skeleton but include the following:

Osteoma and other bony overgrowths

True tumours consisting of bone (either compact or cancellous) are occasionally seen, but localised overgrowths of bone (exostoses) are more common. They consist of lamellae of compact bone, but large specimens may have a core of cancellous bone. Small exostoses may form irregularly on the surface of the alveolar processes and specific variants are *torus palatinus* or *torus mandibularis*. They differ from other exostoses only in that they develop in characteristic sites and are symmetrical.

Torus palatinus. The common site is towards the posterior of the mid-line of the hard palate, and the swelling is rounded and symmetrical, sometimes with a mid-line groove. It is not usually noticed until middle age and, if it interferes with the fitting of a denture, should be removed.

Tori mandibularis. These form on the lingual aspect of the mandible opposite the mental foramen. They are typically bilateral, forming hard, rounded swellings. Their behaviour and management is the same as that of torus palatinus.

Compact and cancellous osteoma

Compact osteomas consist of lamellae of bone, sometimes in layers like an onion but not in Haversian systems. This dense bone contains occasional vascular spaces, and grows very slowly.

Cancellous osteomas consist of slender trabeculae of bone, with interstitial marrow spaces and a lamellated cortex.

Osteomas should be excised only if they become large enough to cause symptoms or make the fitting of a denture difficult.

Gardner's syndrome. Gardner's syndrome comprises multiple osteomas of the jaws, polyposis coli with a high malignant potential, and often other abnormalities such as dental defects and

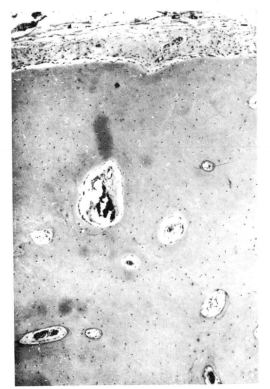

Fig. 11.23 Compact osteoma. Dense bone is laid down in lamellae with occasional vascular spaces, but there is no attempt to form Haversian systems (× 45).

epidermal cysts or fibromas. It is inherited as an autosomal dominant trait but penetrance is weak.

Osteochondroma (cartilage-capped osteoma)

This bony overgrowth grows by ossification beneath a cartilaginous cap. Nearly 95% of cases arise from the region of the coronoid or condylar process and form a hard bony protuberance which can interfere with joint function. The cartilaginous cap may not be visible in radiographs. Almost any age can be affected.

Microscopically the lesion is subperiosteal and has a cap of hyaline cartilage where the cartilage cells are sometimes regularly aligned or irregular and contain minute foci of ossification. As age increases, the mass consists increasingly of bone which is usually mostly cancellous.

These tumours are benign and usually cease to grow after skeletal maturation. Removal is therefore curative.

Ossifying (cementifying) fibroma

The essential features are the same as those of the cementifying fibroma described earlier (see also Fig. 11.13).

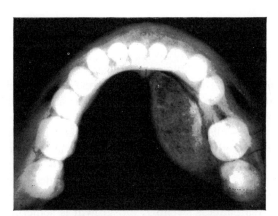

Fig. 11.24 Cancellous osteoma of the mandible. The tumour has arisen from a relatively narrow base on the lingual aspect of the molars but has been moulded forward during formation by pressure of the tongue. The trabecular pattern of the cancellous bone can be seen. Torus mandibularis arises further forward on the jaw and forms a smaller swelling arising from a broad base and is bilateral.

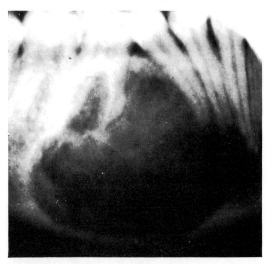

Fig. 11.25 Ossifying (cementifying) fibroma. The tumour forms a characteristic rounded circumscribed area, cloudily radiolucent in its earlier stages. It is slow-growing, as can be seen by the displacement of the teeth.

Chondroma

Chondromas of the jaws are exceedingly rare and cannot be reliably distinguished, except by their behaviour, from chondrosarcomas, which are discussed below.

Giant-cell granuloma of the jaws

Central giant-cell granulomas of the jaws are, as their behaviour indicates, hyperplastic rather than neoplastic. The giant-cell tumour (osteoclastoma), by contrast, is an aggressive neoplasm which chiefly affects the limbs but virtually never the jaws.

Pathogenesis. The earlier name 'giant-cell reparative granuloma' derives from the irrational idea (also applied to solitary bone cysts) that it was a reaction to trauma which caused intramedullary haemorrhage. No evidence supports this idea, and giant-cell hyperplasia does not follow bleeding into

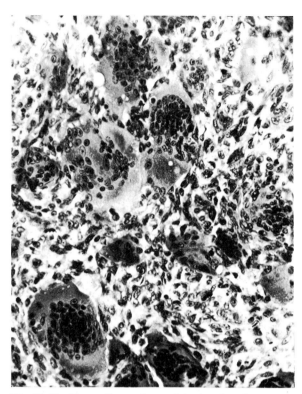

Fig. 11.27   Giant-cell granuloma of the jaw. In other areas there may be many large multinucleate cells among plump spindle cells. A biopsy under the circumstances may be indistinguishable from an osteoclastoma or hyperparathyroidism (× 270).

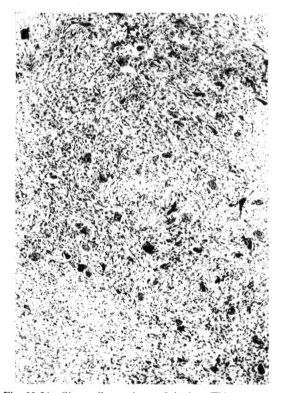

Fig. 11.26   Giant-cell granuloma of the jaw. This tumour-like lesion consists of foci of smallish multinucleate cells in a predominantly connective-tissue mass (× 70).

bone after a fracture or enucleation of a cyst. Moreover, these lesions are locally destructive rather than 'reparative'.

Giant-cell granuloma is probably a developmental disorder, and similar collections of giant cells can be seen in fibrous dysplasia and related conditions.

Giant-cell granuloma is usually seen in young people under 20, and in females twice as frequently as males. The mandible, anterior to the first molars, where the teeth have had deciduous predecessors, is the usual site. There is frequently only a painless swelling, but growth is sometimes rapid. Radiographs show a rounded cyst-like area of radiolucency, often with a suggestion of loculation or a soap bubble appearance. The roots of teeth can be displaced or, less frequently, resorbed, and the mass can occasionally break

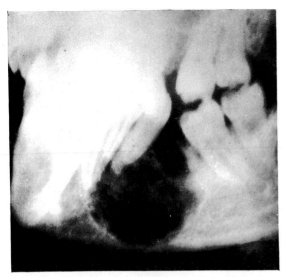

Fig. 11.28 Giant-cell granuloma of the jaw. The 'tumour' forms a radiolucent area somewhat cystic in appearance and with a suggestion of loculation. The premolar in immediate relation to the lesion has been pushed aside but there has also been resorption of the root.

through the bone, particularly of the alveolar ridge, to produce a purplish soft-tissue swelling.

Microscopically, giant-cell granuloma forms a lobulated mass of proliferating vascular connective tissue packed with giant cells (osteoclasts). Signs of bleeding into the mass and deposits of haemosiderin are frequently seen. Fibroblastic proliferation or prominent osteoid and bone formation, particularly near the periphery, are probably signs of retrogression.

There are no changes in blood chemistry, but the histological features are indistinguishable from other disorders, including the following.

1. *Hyperparathyroidism*. This causes raised serum, calcium and alkaline phosphatase levels and multifocal bone lesions.
2. *Fibrous dysplasia*. A limited biopsy may show foci of giant cells but the radiographic and histological features, and behaviour are distinctive.
3. *Cherubism*. Microscopically this may be indistinguishable from giant-cell granuloma, but lesions are typically symmetrical, particularly near the angles of the mandible and sometimes in the maxilla also.

4. *Giant-cell tumour (osteoclastoma)* affects long bones and is aggressive. This is typically indicated by atypia of the stromal spindle cells, and if atypia is present then the possibility of a true neoplasm must be considered. Repeated recurrence after surgery would be confirmatory.
5. *Aneurysmal bone cysts* may contain many giant cells but consist predominantly of multiple blood-filled spaces.

Curettage of giant-cell granulomas is adequate and wide excision unnecessary; small fragments that may be left behind seem to cause little trouble, rarely require further treatment and may resolve spontaneously. Rarely, recurrence follows incomplete removal and a further limited operation becomes necessary.

Haemangioma of bone

Haemangiomas are rare tumours of bone, but a relatively high proportion are in the mandible and particularly in women. Clinically haemangiomas of bone cause progressive painless swellings which, when the overlying bone is resorbed, may become pulsatile. Teeth may be loosened and there may be bleeding, particularly from the gingival margins if involved by the tumour.

Radiographically there is a rounded or pseudo-loculated radiolucent area with ill-defined margins and often a soap bubble appearance.

Microscopically, haemangiomas of bone are essentially similar to those in soft tissue (Ch. 17). They are usually cavernous, but there is also an arteriovenous type (fast-flow angiomas) which have large feeder arteries and, as a consequence, tend to be rapidly expanding and likely to bleed severely if opened.

An intraosseous haemangioma may not be suspected if there are no clinical signs suggestive of a vascular lesion. Opening an haemangioma or extracting a related tooth can sometimes therefore release torrents of blood, but, in other cases, surprisingly little.

However, once the diagnosis has been made, wide en bloc resection is the only practical way of dealing with the problem, but if there are identifiable feeder vessels then selective arterial embolisation makes surgical management considerably safer.

Melanotic neuroectodermal tumour of infancy
(progonoma)

This rare tumour, which arises from the neural crest, may appear in the first year of life in the anterior maxilla. It is usually painless, and slowly expansive, but occasionally grows rapidly and appears to be aggressive. Radiographically there is an area of bone destruction, frequently with a ragged margin, and displacement of the developing teeth. However, the lesion is benign. *Microscopically* the tumour consists of pigmented and non-pigmented cells in a fibrous stroma. The pigmented cells have large pale nuclei and are filled with coarse melanin-containing cytoplasmic granules. They are either arranged in solid groups or line small spaces. The non-pigmented cells have large, densely hyperchromatic nuclei and form small groups, either in the stroma or in the spaces lined by the pigmented cells.

The tumour is non-encapsulated but usually separates easily from the bone at operation. Conservative treatment is usually curative but, even when excision is incomplete, recurrence is rare. Irradiation is contraindicated.

MALIGNANT TUMOURS OF BONE

Osteosarcoma

Osteosarcoma is highly malignant and the most common *primary* neoplasm of bone, but overall is rare, especially in the jaws.

Osteosarcomas rarely have identifiable aetiological factors but a few develop late in life after irradiation or Paget's disease of bone, but the latter type virtually never affects jaws.

Osteosarcoma of the jaws is typically seen between the ages of 30 and 40. Males are slightly more frequently affected, and the body of the mandible is a common site.

There is typically a firm swelling which grows noticeably in a few months and becomes painful. Teeth may be loosened and there may be paraesthesia or loss of sensation in the mental nerve area. Metastases to the lungs may develop early. The

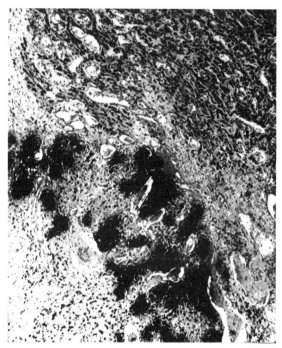

Fig. 11.29 Osteosarcoma. The section is of part of the tumour shown in the next pictures. There are islets of osteoid tissue formed by the sarcoma cells which can be seen throughout the section; they are darkly staining and angular in shape, resembling osteoblasts. Among the tumour cells are many large vascular spaces; the growth readily spreads by the bloodstream to reach the lungs ($\times$ 125)

radiological features are variable but irregular bone destruction usually predominates over bone formation. Bone formation in a soft-tissue mass is highly characteristic of osteosarcoma. A sun-ray appearance at the surface or Codman's triangles at the margins, due to lifting of the periosteum and new bone formation, are rarely seen and are not specific to osteosarcoma. Radiographs of the chest should also be taken, as secondary deposits may be already present.

Microscopy. Osteosarcomas originate from bone cells which are very variable in appearance and have wide potentialities. The neoplastic osteoblasts are variable in size and shape, they may be small and angular or large and hyperchromatic; mitoses may be prominent, particularly in the more highly cellular areas of the tumour. Giant cells may be conspicuous, but many cells are nondescript in appearance. The amount of bone formation may be small but osteoid formation is the main criterion

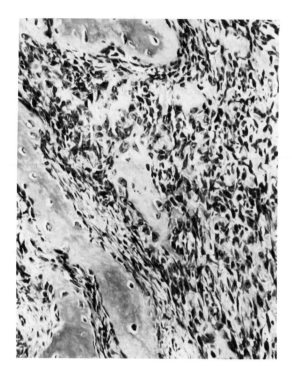

Fig. 11.30 Osteosarcoma. Higher-power view showing the densely crowded, heavily staining malignant osteoblasts clustered round irregular foci of tumour bone formation.

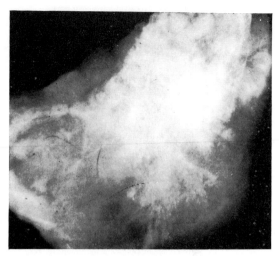

Fig. 11.31 Osteosarcoma. A radiograph of the jaw removed from the same patient shows the entirely irregular picture of bone destruction and of new bone formation completely replacing the normal structure.

of diagnosis; this also may be scanty. Cartilage and fibrous tissue are usually also present and sometimes predominate but sometimes only in part of the tumour. A small biopsy may, therefore, show only a single tissue, such as cartilage, and can lead to a mistaken diagnosis.

Osteosarcoma of the jaws is rapidly invasive and the treatment is early radical excision by mandibulectomy or maxillectomy together with wide excision of any soft-tissue extensions of the tumour. This may be combined with radiotherapy and/or chemotherapy.

The prognosis depends mainly on the extent of the tumour at operation and deteriorates with spread to the soft tissues, to lymph nodes (in about 10% of cases), or to the base of the skull. In approximately 50%, there is local recurrence within a year of treatment. The prognosis then deteriorates sharply. The 5-year survival rate may range from 40% for tumours less than 5 cm in diameter to zero for tumours over 15 cm. Chondroblastic or fibroblastic variants have a

slightly better prognosis than the more common osteoblastic type.

Chondroma and chondrosarcoma

A chondroma is particularly rare in the jaws and far more frequently found (though still rare) in the nasal cavity, and hence it can occasionally be found in the maxilla. Clinically, true chondromas are small and likely to be no more than chance findings. *Microscopically* chondromas consist of hyaline cartilage, but the cells are irregular in size and distribution. Calcification or ossification may develop. However, it is difficult to differentiate chondromas from well-differentiated chondrosarcomas, and it has been reported that 20% of chondrosarcomas in the maxillofacial area were originally thought to be chondromas.

Treatment is by excision, including a wide margin of normal tissue, because of the difficulty in distinguishing benign from malignant tumours and the fact that chondrosarcomas in the maxillofacial region are considerably more frequent than chondromas.

Chondrosarcoma

Chondrosarcomas of the jaws affect adults at an

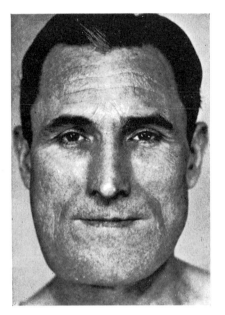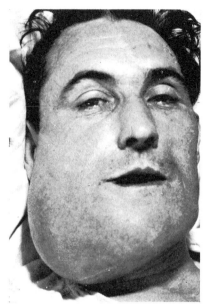

Fig. 11.32 Osteosarcoma. The pictures show the progress of the tumour over a period of three months. The patient died with metastases in the lungs, about a month after the second picture was taken.

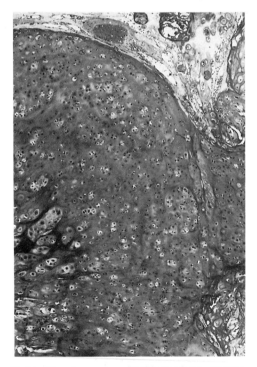

Fig. 11.33 Chondrosarcoma. In this specimen, tumour cartilage is readily recognisable and its maligant nature is indicated by the multinucleate chondrocytes with prominent nucleoli.

average age of about 45. The anterior maxilla is the site in 60% of cases.

Pain, swelling or loosening of teeth associated with a radiolucent area are typical features. The radiolucency can be well or poorly circumscribed, or may appear multilocular. Calcifications are frequently present and may be widespread and dense.

Microscopically the cartilage in jaw tumours is usually comparatively well formed or, less often, poorly differentiated and myxoid. The chondrocytes are pleomorphic, may be binucleate and may show mitotic activity.

Maxillofacial chondrosarcomas are aggressive, and the main cause of death is local recurrence or persistent tumour. Fewer than 10% of these tumours metastasise, but the lungs or other bones are the usual sites of distant spread.

Chondrosarcomas must be widely excised as early as possible, but this can be difficult in the maxillofacial region. Inadequate excision usually leads to recurrences beyond the original site and deterioration of the prognosis. The response to radiotherapy is usually poor.

Mesenchymal chondrosarcoma is an uncommon but highly malignant variant. It is a highly cellular tumour in which there are only small foci of tissue recognisable as poorly formed cartilage, and it is sometimes very vascular.

Ewing's sarcoma

Ewing's sarcoma is rare but, when it affects the head and neck region, has a strong predilection for the body of the mandible.

Clinically patients are usually children or young adults. Typical symptoms are bone swelling and often pain, progressing over a period of months. Teeth may loosen and the overlying mucosa ulcerate. Fever, leukocytosis, a raised ESR and anaemia may be associated and indicate a poor prognosis.

Microscopically Ewing's sarcoma cells appear similar to lymphocytes but are about twice the size and, by immunocytochemistry, stain for neural markers. These cells have a darkly staining nucleus, surrounded by a rim of cytoplasm, which is typically vacuolated and stains for glycogen, and they are in diffuse sheets or loose lobules, separated by septa.

Distant spread is usually to the lungs and other bones, and Ewing's sarcoma in the jaws may therefore be a metastasis from another bone. Lymph nodes are involved in a minority.

Currently the initial treatment is wide excision or, if not possible, megavoltage irradiation. Combination chemotherapy should also be given and appears to have improved the survival rate but increases the risk of lymphoid tumours later.

Multiple myeloma

Multiple myeloma is a neoplasm of plasma cells which produce a monoclonal immunoglobulin and also cause multiple foci of bone destruction, bone pain and tenderness. Rarely a jaw lesion or a complication such as oral amyloidosis may produce the first symptoms. Proliferation of myeloma cells in the marrow frequently causes anaemia and sometimes thrombocytopenia, or infections may result from depressed production of normal immunoglobulins. Occasionally myeloma is detected before symptoms appear, by the chance finding, in a routine examination, of a greatly raised ESR as a result of the overproduction of immunoglobulin (usually IgG) which appears as a monoclonal spike on electrophoresis and confirms the diagnosis.

Skeletal radiographs typically show multiple punched-out areas of radiolucency, particularly in the vault of the skull. *Microscopically* myeloma appears as sheets of neoplastic plasma cells which may be well or poorly differentiated, and diagnosis depends on marrow biopsy and serum electrophoresis.

Light chain overproduction, demonstrable by serum electrophoresis, is common and leads to Bence-Jones proteinuria and often amyloidosis.

There is frequently an initial response to treatment with combination chemotherapy, but less than 20% of patients survive for 5 or more years. Dental treatment may be complicated by anaemia, haemorrhagic tendencies, or increased susceptibility to infection.

Solitary (extramedullary) plasmacytoma

Approximately 80% of these rare tumours form in the soft tissues of the head and neck region. Multiple myeloma develops in up to 50% of patients, usually within 2 years.

Solitary plasmacytoma of bone occasionally develops in the jaw but has a significantly better prognosis than soft-tissue plasmacytoma. Bone pain, tenderness, or a swelling and a sharply defined area of radiolucency are typical features. Treatment is by radiotherapy. Over 65% of patients survive for 10 or more years, but the majority eventually develop multiple myeloma.

Microscopically the appearances of solitary and multiple myeloma are the same.

Amyloidosis

Amyloidosis is the deposition in the tissues of an abnormal protein with characteristic staining properties. It can result from overproduction of immunoglobulin light chains, usually by multiple myeloma. In over 20% of such cases, amyloid is deposited in the mouth, particularly the tongue, to cause macroglossia or localised swellings, particularly of the gingivae. Macroglossia due to amyloid can be so gross as to protrude from the mouth. Purpura and anaemia may be associated.

Microscopically amyloid appears as weakly eosinophilic, hyaline homogeneous material. It is typically perivascular and stains with Congo red, which also shows a characteristic apple green birefringence under polarised light. There is also positive fluorescence with thioflavine T and a characteristic fibrillary structure by electron microscopy.

Widespread amyloidosis can cause renal failure or myeloma, when it is the primary cause, and is fatal, but progress of the disease may be delayed by chemotherapy.

Langerhans' cell histiocytosis (histiocytosis x)

Langerhans' cells are dendritic, macrophage-like cells within epithelia; they act as antigen-presenting cells but rarely give rise to bone tumours. Three forms may be recognised:

1. Solitary eosinophilic granuloma
2. Multifocal eosinophilic granuloma (including Hand–Schuller–Christian disease)
3. Letterer Siwe syndrome.

In these tumours, both the surface markers of Langerhans' cells and, by electron microscopy, the characteristic Birbeck granules may be recognisable.

Solitary eosinophilic granuloma

Solitary eosinophilic granuloma mainly affects adults. When it involves the jaw, it causes localised bone destruction with swelling and often pain. Occasionally there is gross periodontal destruction exposing the roots of the teeth. A rounded area of radiolucency with indistinct margins and an appearance of teeth 'floating in air' are typical.

Microscopically there are varying proportions of histiocytes and eosinophils, sometimes with other types of granulocytes. The histiocytes have pale, vesiculated and often lobulated nuclei, and weakly eosinophilic cytoplasm. The response to local resection is often good.

Multifocal eosinophilic granuloma

Patients may be adolescents or children. The jaws,

skull, axial skeleton and femora, and also sometimes the viscera (hepato-splenomegaly) or the skin may be involved in multifocal disease. Hand–Schuller–Christian disease comprises exophthalmos, diabetes insipidus and lytic skull lesions, but this triad is present only in a minority.

Letterer Siwe disease

This is an aggressive form of histiocytosis which affects infants or young children, with involvement of skin, viscera and bones.

Progression, to widespread disease and, frequently, a rapidly fatal outcome despite treatment by such means as irradiation and/or chemotherapy is to be expected.

Overall, the behaviour of Langerhans' cell histiocytosis is unpredictable, but the younger the patient and the greater the number of organ systems affected, the worse the prognosis.

Secondary tumours—carcinoma

Carcinomas of the bronchus, breast or prostate are common tumours and the most common sources

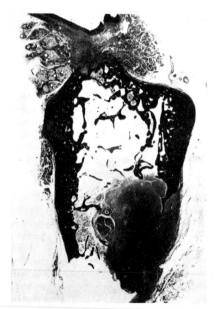

Fig. 11.34 Secondary carcinoma of the jaw. Section across the mandible shows a deposit of carcinoma cells that has destroyed the lingual plate of bone and is extending into the medulla around the inferior dental nerve (3 ×).

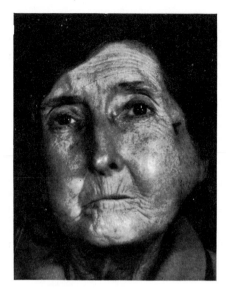

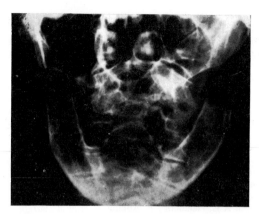

Fig. 11.36 Secondary carcinoma, A radiograph of the same patient showing that the left ramus has been virtually destroyed by the tumour deposit. (From *Dent Pract* 1959, **IX**: 240.)

Fig. 11.35 Secondary carcinoma of the mandible. The swelling developed in the ramus quite suddenly in an apparently fit patient. Investigations showed a deposit of a poorly differentiated carcinoma in the jaw, and signs of a bronchial carcinoma.

of metastases, which reach the jaw by the bloodstream. Carcinomas of the thyroid or kidney can also metastasise to the jaws.

Rarely a malignant deposit in the jaw causes the first symptoms and can lead to diagnosis of the primary. More often the growth has been treated a year or more previously. In either case a metastasis in the jaw is indicative of life-threatening disease.

Patients are usually middle-aged or elderly. Common symptoms are pain or swelling of the jaw, and there may be paraesthesia or anaesthesia of the lip.

There is typically an area of radiolucency with a hazy outline which sometimes simulates an infected cyst or may be quite irregular and simulate osteomyelitis. Sometimes the entire mandible may

have a moth-eaten appearance. By contrast bone sclerosis is a typical result of prostatic carcinoma.

Microscopically, secondary deposits are usually adenocarcinomas but depend on the nature of the primary growth. Bone destruction by osteoclasts near the periphery of the deposit is the most common effect, but bone sclerosis can result, particularly from metastases from the prostate.

If biopsy of the jaw lesion confirms the diagnosis, a careful history, especially of previous operations, should be taken. General and blood examinations and a skeletal survey will show how extensive the disease is.

The primary growth should be treated if this is still feasible, and, in the case of the breast and prostate, hormone therapy may cause secondary deposits to regress for a time. In most cases bony metastases imply that palliative treatment is the best that can be achieved. Irradiation may sometimes make the lesion in the jaw regress for a time and decrease pain.

SUGGESTED FURTHER READING

Bacchini P, Marchetti C, Mancini L et al 1982 Ewing's sarcoma of the mandible and maxilla. Oral Surg, Oral Med, Oral Pathol 61: 278–283

Brahim J S, Katz R W, Roberts M W 1988 Non-Hodgkin's lymphoma of the hard palate mucosa and buccal gingiva associated with AIDS. J Oral Maxillofac Surg 46: 328–330

Cawson R A 1987 Oral pathology—colour aids in dentistry. Churchill Livingstone, Edinburgh

Cawson R A, Eveson J W 1987 Oral pathology and diagnosis. William Heinemann Medical Books, London and Gower Medical Publishing, London

Forbes G, Earnest F, Jackson I T et al 1986 Therapeutic embolization angiography for extra-axial lesions in the head. Mayo Clin Proc 61: 427–441

Frame J W, Putnam G, Wake M J C, Rolfe E B 1987 Therapeutic embolisation of vascular lesions in the maxillofacial region. Br J Oral Maxillofac Surg 25: 181–194

Garrington G E, Collet W K 1988 Chondrosarcoma. I A selected literature review. J Oral Pathol 17: 1–11

Garrington G E, Collet W K 1988 Chondrosarcoma. II Chondrosarcoma of the jaws: analysis of 37 cases. J Oral Pathol 17: 12–20

Hashimoto Y, Matsuhiro K, Nagaki M, Tanioka H 1989 Therapeutic embolization for vascular lesions of the head and neck. Int J Oral Maxillofac Surg 18: 47–49

Hoffman S, Jacoway J R, Krolls S O 1987 Intraosseous and parosteal tumors of the jaws. Fascicle 24. Armed Forces Institute of Pathology, Washington

Hough A J, Page D L 1989 Perspectives on cartilaginous tumours. Human Pathol 20: 927–929

Howell R E, Handlers J P, Abrams A M et al 1987 Extranodal oral lymphoma. Part II Relationship between clinical features and the Lukes-Collins classification of 34 cases. Oral Surg, Oral Med, Oral Pathol 64: 597–602

Kaban L B, Mulliken J B 1986 Vascular anomalies of the maxillofacial region. J Oral Maxillofac Surg 44: 203–213

Keller E E, Gunderson L L 1987 Bone disease metastatic to the jaws. J Am Dent Assoc 115: 697–701

Lambertenghi-Deliliers G, Bruno E, Cortelezzo A et al 1988 Incidence of jaw lesions in 193 patients with multiple myeloma. Oral Surg, Oral Med, Oral Pathol 65: 533–537

Millar B G, Browne R M, Flood T R 1990 Juxtacortical osteosarcoma of the jaws. Br J Oral Maxillofac Surg 28: 73–79

Nicopoulou-Karayianni K, Mombelli A, Lang N P 1989 Diagnostic problems of periodontitis-like lesions caused by eosinophilic granuloma. J Clin Periodontol 16: 505–509

Persky M S 1986 Congenital vascular lesions of the head and neck. Laryngoscope 96: 1002–1015

Ryan R F, Eisenstadt S, Shambaugh E M 1986 Osteogenic sarcoma of the mandible: A plea for radical initial surgery. Plastic Reconstr Surg 78: 41–44

Wei-Yung Y, Guang-Sheng M, Merrill R G, Sperry D W 1989 Central hemangioma of the jaws. J Oral Maxillofac Surg 47: 1154–1160

Wood R E, Nortje C J, Hesseling P, Grotepass F 1990 Ewing's tumor of the jaw. Oral Surg, Oral Med, Oral Pathol 69: 120–127

12. Genetic, metabolic and other non-neoplastic diseases of bone

GENETIC DISEASES OF BONE

Osteogenesis imperfecta

Osteogenesis imperfecta is an hereditary disorder, usually transmitted as an autosomal dominant, in which the bones are poorly formed and fragile. The osteoblasts fail to form bone in adequate amounts, as a result of an underlying defect of biosynthesis which leads to decreased formation of type I collagen, but there are at least 5 subtypes of this disease.

The bones are thin and lack the usual cortex of compact bone, but development of the epiphyseal cartilages is unimpaired and bones can grow to their normal length. Weakness of the bones leads to multiple fractures and distortion.

The most severe cases (Type II) usually die at birth or soon after; mild cases (Type V) may have little disability. In the common (Type I) form, the many fractures can cause severe deformities. The sclera of the eyes also appear blue (their thinness allows the pigment layer to be seen through them), deafness also develops and dentinogenesis imperfecta is sometimes associated.

There is no effective treatment, it is essential to protect the child as far as possible from the slightest injury and to minimise deformity by attending to fractures as they happen. Care must be taken during dental extractions, but fractures of the jaws are uncommon in this disease. (See also Ch. 2.)

Osteopetrosis—marble bone disease

Osteopetrosis is a rare genetic disease characterised by solidification of the bones, which become dense but brittle. The essential defect appears to be inactivity of the osteoclasts and absence of normal modelling resorption; the medullary cavities are not formed, and the epiphyseal ends of the bones are club-shaped. Because of the absence of marrow space in the bones, the liver and spleen take over blood-cell formation, but anaemia is common. Osteomyelitis is a recognised complication. (Fig. 12.2).

There is no effective treatment.

Achondroplasia

Achondroplasia is the most common type of genetic skeletal disorder and produces short-limbed dwarfs who often become circus clowns.

The essential defect is failure of normal proliferation of cartilage in the epiphyses and in the base of the skull. The limbs are therefore ex-

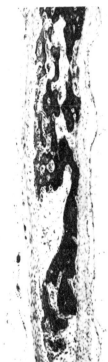

Fig. 12.1 Osteogenesis imperfecta. A section from the vault of the skull of a stillborn infant with osteogenesis imperfecta shows that the bone is small in amount, primitive (woven) in character, contains many osteoclasts and there is no attempt at differentiation into cortical plates with a medullary space (× 45).

cessively short in relation to the trunk, and the head, which is normal in size, appears disproportionately large. Defective growth at the base of the skull causes the middle third of the face to be retrusive and the profile to be concave. The mandible is often protrusive, and as a result of the disparity of growth of the jaws, there is usually severe malocclusion. There is no effective treatment for the skeletal defects but the occlusion may be improved by orthodontic treatment.

Cleidocranial dysplasia

This rare familial disorder is characterised by defective formation of the clavicles, delayed closure of the fontanelles and retrusion of the maxilla. The partial or complete absence of clavicles allows the patient to bring the shoulders together in front of the chest.

This disorder is one of the few recognisable causes of delayed eruption of the permanent dentition. The permanent teeth may remain embedded in the jaw until late in life. The dental features are described in Chapter 2.

Cherubism

This disease is inherited as an autosomal dominant trait. Like fibrous dysplasia the histological appearances vary with the maturity of the lesion. The important differences from fibrous dysplasia are that the lesions are symmetrically distributed and, microscopically, consist predominantly of giant cells. Boys are predominantly affected. Swellings appear at the age of 2 to 4 years, and affect the lower jaw in the region of the angles; the maxillae are also involved in severe cases.

Growth is rapid for a few years, then slows down until puberty is reached. There is then slow regression until by middle age normal facial contour may be restored, though radiolucent areas may persist longer.

Clinically the lesions cause fullness of the cheeks, and in severe cases the maxillary swellings cause the eyes to appear turned upwards, producing the characteristic cherubic appearance. There is no pain or tenderness, but the regional lymph nodes may be enlarged (Fig. 12.5).

The radiological features are well-defined, apparently multilocular, radiolucent areas with a thin expanded cortex. Teeth are often displaced or buried.

Microscopically the lesion consists of multilocular giant cells and resembles a giant cell granuloma or hyperparathyroidism. With the passage of time, giant cells become fewer and there is bony repair of the defect.

Management

Because of the natural regression of the disease in most cases, treatment can usually be avoided. Should disfigurement be severe the lesions appear to respond to curettage or to paring down of excessive tissue.

Hypophosphatasia

Hypophosphatasia is an uncommon recessive genetic disorder. The early-onset type causes

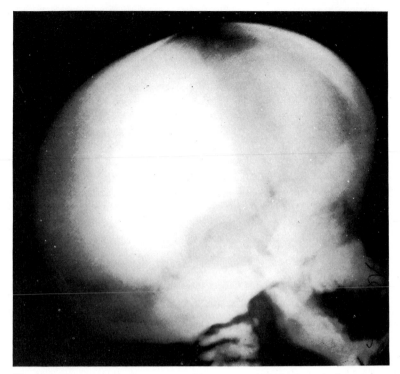

Fig. 12.2 Osteopetrosis. In contrast with osteogenesis imperfecta the bone is excessively thick and dense as a result of defective resorption.

rickets-like skeletal disease with defective mineralisation. Defective cementogenesis results in premature loss of teeth, and this is sometimes the only sign of the disease (Ch. 6). The plasma alkaline phosphatase levels are low but urinary phosphoethanolamine excretion is increased.

Late onset hypophosphatasia is sometimes a dominant trait, and its main manifestation is fragility of the bones.

Sickle cell anaemia and thalassaemia major

These diseases, particularly thalassaemia, can cause bony malformations of the maxillofacial region as a result of extramedullary erythropoiesis (Ch. 20).

METABOLIC BONE DISEASE

Rickets

In children defective absorption of calcium due to deficiency of vitamin D causes rickets. The essen-

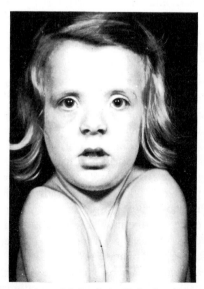

Fig. 12.3 Cleidocranial dysplasia. Defective development of the clavicles allows this abnormal mobility of the shoulders. Other members of the family were also affected.

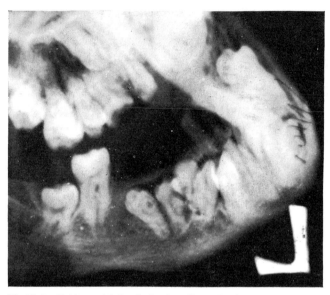

Fig.12.4 Cleidocranial dysplasia. A radiograph of the jaw of the father of the patient in the previous picture. There are many additional teeth but widespread failure of eruption. The intraoral appearances are shown in Fig. 2.5.

tial feature of rickets is defective calcification and development of the skeleton.

Rickets is now rare but immigrant children in the North of Britain are particularly likely to be affected. The main reasons appear to be lack of sunlight (vitamin D is synthesised in the skin in strong sunlight), a high-carbohydrate diet and possibly also the use of wholemeal flour (as in chupattis) containing factors which may impair calcium absorption.

Disorders of calcium and phosphorus metabolism may also result from chronic renal disease (either hereditary or inflammatory) in which excretion of these minerals is abnormal. These diseases ('renal rickets') may therefore cause similar defects of development of bone.

Pathology

Throughout the bone but especially at the ends of the shafts trabeculae formed before the onset of the disease become surrounded by newly formed, uncalcified osteoid matrix.

In the zone of provisional calcification mineralisation of cartilage fails to take place, and the

cartilage cells continue to proliferate, until the epiphyseal plate becomes greatly thickened, wide and highly cellular. Blood vessels invade and branch irregularly among the proliferating cartilage cells, and are accompanied by connective tissue which further disorganises the epiphysis.

Clinical features

The onset of rickets is usually in infancy. The main defects are broadening of the growing ends of bones, due to the epiphyseal defects (shown as prominent costochondrial junctions—the 'rickety rosary'), and bending of the weakened bones. Typical changes in the skull are wide fontanelles, bossing of the frontal and parietal eminences and thinning of the back of the skull. Radiographs show the wide, thick epiphyses and deformities.

There are usually normal serum calcium but low phosphorus levels, or either may be depressed. The alkaline phosphatase level is raised.

Dental changes. There is evidence that the teeth have a priority over the skeleton for minerals, and dental defects rarely result from rickets.

Hypocalcification of dentine, with a wide band

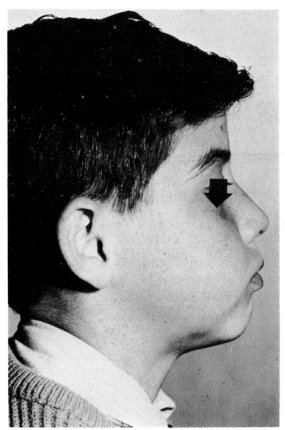

Fig. 12.5 Cherubism. The typical 'cherubic' bulging of the cheeks can be seen.

of predentine and excessive interglobular spaces, has been described in cases of renal rickets and in exceptionally severe nutritional rickets. Eruption of the teeth may be delayed.

Rachitic children are not abnormally susceptible to dental caries, and 'shortage of calcium' as a cause of dental caries is a lay superstition.

Treatment. The essential measure is to give vitamin D, the equivalent of 2000 to 3000 i.u. daily, and to make sure that the diet is adequate in other respects. Orthopaedic treatment may be needed to correct deformities.

Scurvy

Scurvy causes defective formation of collagen and osteoid matrix; such matrix as forms is well calcified. Infantile scurvy, with skeletal defects, is of little more than historical interest in Britain but has been described, for instance, in an infant whose mother had eccentric ideas about diet.

The amount of osteoid matrix formed is small but highly calcified so that the ends of the long bones are sharply defined radiologically. Weakness of the connective tissue and the haemorrhagic tendency (purpura) cause detachment of the periosteum by bleeding and bone pain. The haematoma becomes calcified as shown in the radiograph (Fig. 12.8).

Hyperparathyroidism

Primary hyperparathyroidism is uncommon but is usually caused by hyperplasia or adenoma of the parathyroids. The effect of increased secretion of parathormone (PTH) is to mobilise calcium and raise the plasma calcium level.

Pathology

Calcium can be removed from the skeleton by macrophages or osteoclasts. The main effects are thinning of bone trabeculae, subperiosteal resorption of the bone of the fingers and resorption of the terminal phalangeal tufts. In severe cases, foci of osteoclasts resorb and replace bone and can be seen on radiographs as radiolucent cyst-like areas (osteitis fibrosa cystica) often with a multiloculated appearance.

Histologically these foci of osteoclasts are indistinguishable from giant-cell granulomas of the jaws (Ch. 11). Unlike the latter, however, there are characteristic changes in the blood chemistry and sometimes multifocal involvement of other bones. Occasionally the bone lesions cause pathological fractures (Fig. 12.9).

The increased excretion of calcium leads ultimately to renal calcinosis or stone formation and renal damage. Other clinical features also result from the hypercalcaemia.

Blood chemistry examination is essential in patients found to have giant-cell lesions of the jaws, especially adults of middle age or over. Characteristic findings in hyperparathyroidism are:

1. Raised plasma calcium (2.8 mmol/l or more)

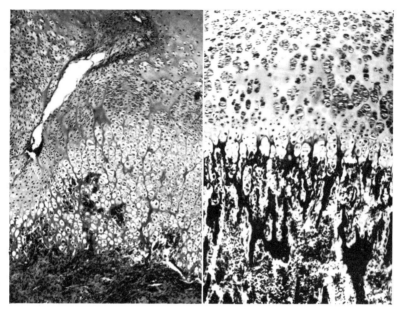

Fig. 12.6 Rickets. The specimen on the left is from a child of 14 months with rickets due to chronic renal disease. The epiphyseal cartilage shows irregular overgrowth of cartilage cells and absence of calcification; a layer of vascular connective tissue is starting to invade the cartilage. In the normal epiphyseal cartilage of a newborn infant (right) the columns of cartilage are short and regular; immediately below them is the zone of provisional calcification with darkly-staining trabeculae of calcified osteoid (× 72).

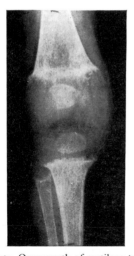

Fig. 12.7 Rickets. Overgrowth of cartilage (as shown in the section above) causes the epiphyseal plate to be broad, thick and irregular, and the ends of the bone become splayed. The growing end of the bone is ill-defined and calcification defective.

2. Low plasma phosphorus (less than 0.8 mmol/l)
3. Raised plasma parathyroid hormone levels
4. Raised plasma alkaline phosphatase (over 100 u/l).

Clinical features

Primary hyperparathyroidism is most common in post-menopausal women.

The clinical picture of the disease has changed in recent years, and the most common symptoms result from renal damage which leads to hypertension or other cardiovascular disease. Peptic ulcer symptoms or mere malaise are also common. Bone disease is now rarely evident but small lesions may be detectable radiographically. Among dental patients a cyst-like swelling of the jaw with the histological features of a giant-cell lesion is the

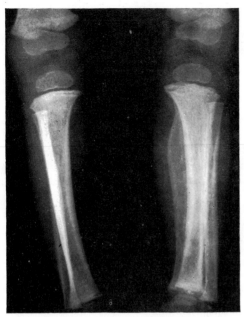

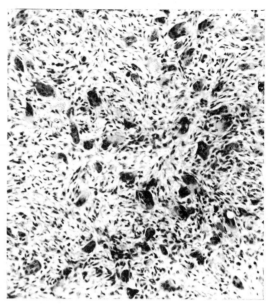

Fig. 12.8   Scurvy. In contrast to rickets calcification is unimpeded and there is a thick layer of calcified cartilage at the end of the bone. Osteoid formation on the other hand is reduced, so that little bone can be formed. The attachment of the periosteum to the bone is weak, so that it is easily separated; there may be haemorrhage beneath it (as here) due to scorbutic purpura, and this becomes calcified.

Fig. 12.9   Hyperparathyroidism. Biopsy of the 'cystic' area of the jaw seen in the next picture shows proliferating connective tissue and giant cells, i.e. the same picture as a giant-cell granuloma of the jaw but in this case there were multiple skeletal lesions and the serum calcium was raised (× 130).

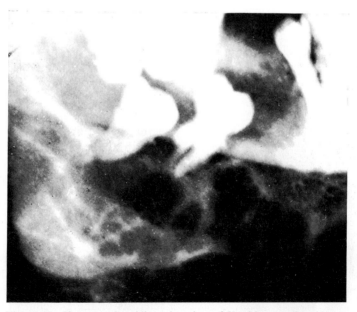

Fig. 12.10   Hyperparathyroidism. A patient of 51 with a parathyroid adenoma. There is an area of bone destruction simulating a multilocular cyst but filled with the tissue shown in the section.

usual way by which hyperparathyroidism is detected. It is essential not to miss this diagnosis, because of the probability of progress to irreversible renal damage in the absence of treatment. The possibility of secondary hyperparathyroidism (see below) should also be excluded. In primary hyperparathyroidism surgical removal of the parathyroids is curative.

Secondary hyperparathyroidism

Secondary hyperparathyroidism results from prolonged stimulation of the parathyroids by a persistently depressed plasma calcium. The most common cause is chronic renal failure.

Secondary hyperparathyroidism is now more frequently a cause of osteolytic bone lesions than is primary and shows the same histological picture of osteoclastic proliferation. Such lesions may also be a sign of rejection of a renal transplant.

The essential measure is to treat the renal failure if possible. Bone lesions may respond to oral administration of vitamin D, the metabolism of which is abnormal as a result of the renal disease. If the hypocalcaemia is of very long standing, parathyroid hyperplasia may be irreversible (so-

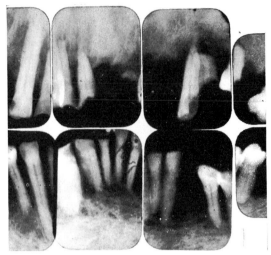

Fig. 12.12 Hyperparathyroidism. There is general softening of the bone shadow and in places complete loss of the normal trabecular pattern or 'ground glass' appearance, but there are no localised foci of resorption as in the previous case. In comparison with the rarified bone the teeth appear excessively dense and all trace of the lamina dura of the sockets is lost.

called tertiary hyperparathyroidism) and need to be treated by parathyroidectomy.

Gigantism and Acromegaly

Overproduction of pituitary growth hormone, usually by an adenoma, before the epiphyses fuse, gives rise to overgrowth of the whole skeleton (gigantism). After fusion of the epiphyses, overproduction of growth hormone gives rise to acromegaly. The main features are continued growth at the mandibular condyle, causing gross prognathism, macroglossia, thickening of the facial soft tissues and overgrowth of the hands and feet. (See also Ch. 20.)

Fluorosis

Excessive amounts of fluorides in the drinking water, as in certain parts of Northern India, cause severe mottling of the teeth (Ch. 2) and also sclerosis of the skeleton. The intervertebral ligaments and insertions of muscles calcify, causing stiffness, particularly of the back, and pain. His-

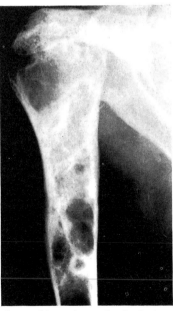

Fig. 12.11 Areas of bone destruction in the humerus similar to those in the jaw were present in the same patient.

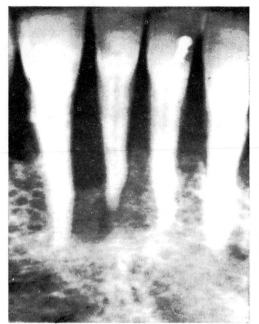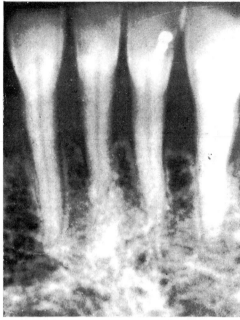

Fig. 12.13 Hyperparathyroidism. An area of bone destruction is present in relation to the lower incisors but in this case the lamina dura of the other teeth is unaffected. On the right is shown repair of the defect with restoration of the normal bony pattern as a result of removal of the parathyroid tumour. (Radiographs kindly lent by Mr A. J. Bridge and Dr F. L. Ingram.)

tologically the bone changes are somewhat similar to those of Paget's disease.

BONE DISEASES OF UNKNOWN CAUSE

Paget's disease of bone—osteitis deformans

Paget's disease is of unknown cause; it affects patients past middle age most severely. In severe form it is easily recognised. The main features are an enlarged head, thickening of the bones, which bend under stress, and tenderness or aching pain.

Pathology

In Paget's disease bone resorption and replacement becomes rapid, irregular, exaggerated and purposeless.

One or many bones may be affected, and though the process does not go on in a uniform fashion the result is thickening of affected bones without localised swellings.

In general, the early stages are characterised by bone resorption and later stages by sclerosis, but since closely adjacent parts of the bone may show different stages of the disorder a common result is patchy areas of osteoporosis and of sclerosis. The process of destruction and new bone formation may alternate rapidly, and the change in the activity of the bone is marked by blue staining reversal lines. The pattern of reversal lines characteristically produces a mosaic appearance of the bone.

The main histological changes are the mosaic pattern of reversal lines, many osteoblasts and osteoclasts (often abnormally large), fibrosis of the marrow spaces and increased vascularity.

In the late stages affected bones are thick, the cortex and medulla are obliterated and the whole bone is spongy in texture.

Clinical features

Patients are usually elderly when seen and males

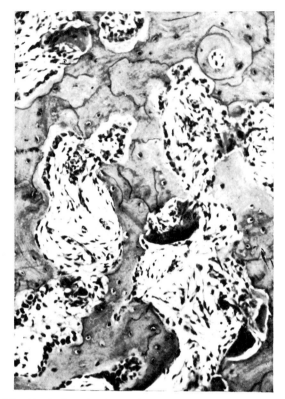

Fig. 12.14 Paget's disease of bone. There is a well-marked mosaic pattern of the bone due to repeated alternation of resorption and apposition. The marrow has been replaced by fibrous tissue and there are many osteoblasts and osteoclasts lining the surface of the bone (× 100).

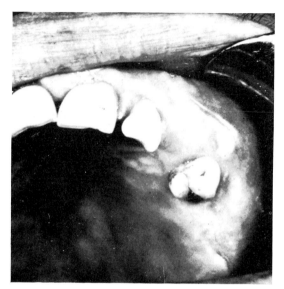

Fig. 12.15 Paget's disease of the maxilla. The great broadening and deepening of the alveolar process are characteristic.

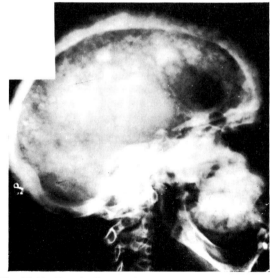

Fig. 12.16 Paget's disease of the skull and maxilla. The thickening of the bone and the irregular areas of sclerosis and resorption, which give it a fluffy appearance, are in striking contrast to the unaffected mandible.

are more frequently affected. It is estimated that 3% of people over 40 are affected, but clinically obvious cases are much less common.

Bones most frequently affected are sacrum, spine, skull, femora and pelvis. The disease may be widespread and is usually symmetrical, but sometimes a single bone is affected. Severe and almost intractable bone pain can be a feature.

The vault of the skull is more often affected than the facial skeleton, and the maxilla much more frequently than the mandible. When the jaws are affected the alveolar process becomes symmetrically and grossly enlarged. There may also be gross and irregular hypercementosis of the teeth, which may become fused to sclerotic areas of the bone. Attempts to extract affected teeth may fail completely or succeed only by tearing away a large mass of bone. Severe bleeding or osteomyelitis of an ischaemic bone mass may follow.

The main radiological features are decreased density of the bone in the early stages and sclerosis in the later stages. These changes are patchily distributed and the loss of normal trabeculation causes the bone to have a characteristic 'cotton-wool' appearance.

Chemical investigation is an important aid to diagnosis. Serum calcium and phosphorus levels are usually normal, but the alkaline phosphatase level is high and may reach 700 u/l.

The development of osteosarcoma is a recognised but rare complication of Paget's disease and virtually never affects the joints. Many patients live to an advanced age in spite of their disabilities.

Treatment is with calcitonin or diphosphonates (such as sodium etidronate) or both. Calcitonins, such as salcatonin, have to be given by injection and are more effective for reducing bone pain and osteolysis, but can cause nausea and an unpleaseant taste. Calcitonin is also given preoperatively to reduce bleeding from the highly vascular bone and may help to relieve neurological complications. Diphosphonates can be given orally and depress turnover by slowing both the dissolution and growth of hydroxyapatite crystals.

FIBRO-OSSEOUS LESIONS

This term is frequently used for disorders ranging from fibrous dysplasia to the circumscribed lesions of ossifying or cementifying fibroma and the cemental dysplasias (Ch. 11). In broad terms their essential feature is tumour-like growth in early life but spontaneous arrest and increasing ossification, roughly coinciding with skeletal maturation. In this difficult area the diagnosis depends as much on the clinical and radiographic as the microscopic findings.

Fibrous dysplasia

Monostotic fibrous dysplasia is characterised by a swelling caused by a poorly circumscribed area of fibro-osseous proliferation. This starts in childhood but typically undergoes increasing ossification and arrest in adulthood. The jaws, particularly the maxillae, are the most frequent sites in the head and neck region. Males and females are almost equally frequently affected.

Clinically monostotic fibrous dysplasia is mainly seen in young persons, usually in their 20s, as a painless, smoothly rounded swelling usually of the maxilla. The mass may become large enough to

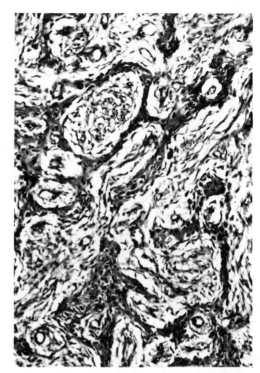

Fig. 12.17 Fibrous dysplasia. There is a pattern of thin trabeculae of cellular (woven) bone in a matrix of connective tissue. The picture is suggestive of osteogenic activity. Appearances change considerably before becoming stabilised by the laying down of lamellar bone usually later on in adult life ($\times$ 120).

disturb function and cause malocclusion by displacing teeth.

Polyostotic fibrous dysplasia is rare and characterised by histologically similar lesions in several bones, skin pigmentation and endocrine abnormalities. Females are affected in the ratio of 3 to 1. Polyostotic fibrous dysplasia, skin pigmentation and sexual precocity is termed Albright's syndrome.

Polyostotic fibrous dysplasia involves the head and neck region in up to 50% of cases. A jaw lesion may then be the most conspicuous feature and the patient may appear to have monostotic disease. In a young girl, in particular, a search for other skeletal lesions and pigmentation may therefore be indicated. Skin pigmentation consists of brownish macules which frequently overlie affected bones and particularly the back of the neck, trunk, buttocks, or thighs, but are hardly ever on the oral mucosa.

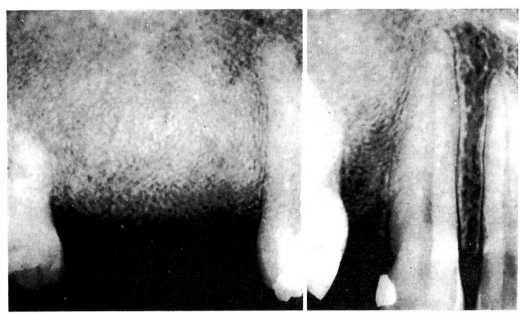

Fig. 12.18 Fibrous dysplasia. This is a well-established lesion with considerable new bone formation. A finger-print pattern has been produced by the fine regular trabeculae of new bone as shown in the section. The lesion has produced a rounded swelling and merges imperceptibly with the surrounding normal tissue.

Radiographically there is typically an area of reduced radiopacity, with a fine orange-peel texture which merges imperceptibly with the surrounding normal bone and which may have an eggshell thin cortex of expanded bone. The appearances vary, particularly with the degree of ossification. Predominantly fibrous lesions may appear cyst-like, while heavily ossified lesions may have a patchily sclerotic appearance.

Microscopically the mass typically consists of loose cellular fibrous tissue containing slender trabeculae of woven bone of variable shape which merge imperceptibly into the surrounding bone.

Osteoblasts are scattered throughout the substance of the trabeculae rather than surrounding them. Some lamellar bone or calcified spherules and occasional loose foci of giant cells can also be seen.

The different patterns of bone formation do not seem to be related to any differences in behaviour of these lesions.

Progress and treatment. The disease is (by definition) self-limiting, but grossly disfiguring lesions may need to be excised. This should be delayed if possible until the lesion has become inactive. There is also a small risk of sarcomatous change, particularly in the polyostotic variant.

SUGGESTED FURTHER READING

Cannell H 1988 The development of oral and facial signs in B-thalassaemia major. Br Dent J 164: 50–51
Cantrill J A, Anderson D C 1990 Treatment of Paget's disease of bone. Clin Endocrinol 32: 507–518
Cawson R A 1987 Oral pathology—colour aids in dentistry. Churchill Livingstone, Edinburgh
Cawson R A, Eveson J W 1987 Oral pathology and diagnosis. William Heinemann Medical Books, London and Gower Medical Publishing, London
Cole W G, Jaenisch R, Bateman J F 1989 New insights into the molecular pathology of osteogenesis imperfecta. Quarterly J Med 70: 1–4

Geist J R, Katz J O 1990 The frequency and distribution of idiopathic osteosclerosis. Oral Surg, Oral Med, Oral Pathol 69: 388–393
Muller H, Slootweg P J 1981 Maxillofacial deformities in neurofibromatosis. J Maxillofac Surg 9: 89–95
Sciubba J J, Younai F 1989 Ossifying fibroma of the mandible and maxilla: review of 18 cases. J Oral Pathol Med 18: 315–321
Waldron C A 1985 Fibro-osseous lesions of the jaws. J Oral Maxillofac Surg 43: 249–262
Younai F, Eisenbud L, Sciubba J J 1988 Osteopetrosis: A case report including gross and microscopic findings in the mandible at autopsy. Oral Surg, Oral Med, Oral Pathol 65: 214–221

13. Fractures of the jaws and facial skeleton

Fractures of the jaws and related bones range from minor fractures of the alveolar process to severely destructive injuries of the facial skeleton. The latter—often caused by road accidents or, increasingly now, as a result of assault—can present an immediate threat to life, be associated with brain damage or severe injuries to other parts and may need, as a consequence, to be managed by experts in several different specialties. Fractures of the mandible, by contrast, are often isolated injuries. These fractures are common and their management is in many cases fairly straightforward.

The healing of fractures

The main stages in the healing of fractures are:

1. Haematoma formation
2. Organisation of the clot
3. Provisional callus formation
4. Definitive callus formation.

Finally, if the fragments have been correctly aligned and immobilised, the normal contour of the bone is restored.

Haematoma formation

Vessels of the broken bone and torn soft tissues bleed freely to form a bulky clot between the bone-ends. The clot spreads into the adjacent muscles and fascia, and the periosteum is distended. This fibrin network is the scaffolding in which repair takes place. The clot is weak and delicate but its size ensures that a large mass of tissue can form to support the broken bone until there is firm union.

Damage to the tissues provokes a mild inflammatory reaction even in the absence of infection. Phagocytes remove necrotic debris. Osteoclasts resorb bone spicules and jagged edges of the broken bone.

Organisation

The scavenging phase lasts a few days and is immediately followed by the ingrowth of fibroblasts and vascular endothelial cells, to form granulation tissue (capillary buds and fibroblasts). Macrophages also infiltrate the area. Fibroblasts lay down collagen fibres between the bone-ends until these become joined by young vascular fibrous tissue. This process should be well under way within a week, and the haematoma is usually fully organised after about 10 to 14 days.

Though the fracture is by then repaired with cellular tissue, it is vulnerable. Movement of the bone-ends damages the delicate connective tissue and tears the young blood vessels. This may lead to failure of bone formation.

Provisional callus

Up to this stage there is no apparent difference between the healing of a fracture and of a soft-tissue injury. Thereafter normal healing of the fracture is characterised by deposition of osteoid as a result of differentiation of the fibroblasts. These secrete a translucent ground substance between the collagen fibres to form osteoid fibres. Progressive precipitation of mineral salts in the osteoid tissue forms woven bone, so called because of the intertwining pattern of fibre bundles in its matrix. The osteoblasts formed by the differentiation of fibroblasts are angular in shape and border the surface of the trabeculae of woven bone.

The trabeculae of woven bone join the bone ends, block the medulla and form a spindle-shaped mass ensheathing the area of the fracture. This provisional callus is poorly calcified and not visible in radiographs at first. As time goes on, increasing amounts of mineral salts are deposited and the callus becomes progressively more dense and radiopaque.

In the early inflammatory phase the local reaction within the tissue is acid (the acid tide); this presumably helps to bring calcium into solution locally after the resorption of bone fragments by the osteoclasts. Later the local pH rises (the alkaline tide) and may enable the alkaline phosphatase to produce a local supersaturation of phosphate and precipitation of calcium and phosphate in the osteoid.

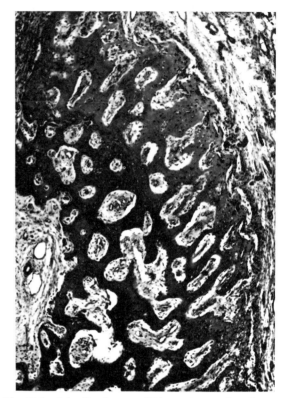

Fig. 13.1 A healing fracture. This specimen, taken 6 weeks after the accident, shows primary bony callus consisting of cellular, woven bone forming a rounded mass round the original cortex ($\times$ 35).

A minority of fibroblasts differentiate into chondroblasts and lay down islands of hyaline cartilage which also rapidly become calcified. Thus the provisional hard callus which joins the bone-ends consists of both woven bone and calcified cartilage. If, however, immobilisation of the bone-ends is poor, more cartilage is formed.

The role of the periosteum in the formation of the callus is by reversion to its fetal state after the injury. This is characterised by the proliferation of the osteoprogenitor cells (osteoblasts and osteoclasts) from the deep surface of the membrane.

Adequate amounts of provisional callus should be formed by about 3 weeks, and a fracture of the jaw usually shows clinical evidence of union after 3 to 4 weeks. At this stage the provisional callus is not readily visible on radiographs and, in any event, does not form to a significant extent in mandibular fractures as compared with the long bones.

Definitive callus formation

This final stage of healing of the fracture is characterised by progressive strengthening of the callus and remodelling activity.

Osteoclasts actively resorb the woven bone and calcified cartilage to enable blood vessels and osteoblasts to grow into the area of resorption. The blood vessels are surrounded by osteoblasts which lay down bone in concentric lamellae to form the basic haversian system of lamellar bone. This bone is formed in thick trabeculae laid down in relation to lines of stress. The callus is progressively strengthened in this way.

The compact cortical bone is reformed by the replacement of the irregular woven bone by haversian systems forming massive seams arranged to form a plate-like structure. The internal callus is resorbed and replaced by thin trabeculae of cancellous bone in a net-like arrangement to contain the fatty or haemopoietic marrow.

The external callus which ensheathed the fracture and formed the characteristic fusiform swelling is removed entirely and ultimately leaves a smooth outer surface to reconstitute the original form of the bone. This process may take many months or even years to complete; there is also constant remodelling of this lamellar bone in response to stress.

Bone grafting

Bone grafting is rarely needed after fractures of the jaw, but may be necessary when there has been gross loss of tissue caused, for example, by a gunshot wound. Grafts for the mandible are usually autogenous (from the same patient), and a piece of the iliac crest, or less frequently a rib is convenient. Homografts (from other individuals) may rarely be used, and under certain circumstances even heterografts (from other species of animal) may be considered.

In all bone grafts the cellular elements are destroyed by the loss of blood supply, but in the case of homografts and heterografts there is also a graft rejection reaction. The grafted bone is therefore inert, but usually provides good support for the fracture and may provide some degree of internal fixation. The bone of the graft forms a framework through which granulation tissue grows.

When the graft has vascularised it is progressively removed by osteoclastic action and provides a local source of bone salts. After the graft has been resorbed it is replaced by bone-forming granulation tissue which lays down woven, then lamellar bone in a process essentially similar to that in a healing fracture. Grafts are not therefore incorporated into the bone where they are placed but, in addition to their function in supporting the bone-ends, provide a framework for, and to initiate the process of, new bone formation to fill the gap.

Grafts may also be made up of fragments of cancellous bone or bone chips. These provide no support of the engrafted area but their large surface area allows more rapid ingrowth of granulation tissue and more rapid replacement by new bone. A combination of a corticocancellous strut to provide support and internal fixation, and cancellous bone chips to allow rapid regeneration of new bone, is often the best method of replacing an extensive bone defect.

FRACTURES OF THE JAWS—SPECIAL FEATURES

The same general principles apply to the management of fractures of the jaws as to fractures of other bones, but there are certain special features which must be taken into consideration. These include the following.

1. *Involvement of airway*. The jaws surround the upper end of the airway, and respiratory obstruction is a special danger of fractures of the jaws.

If the anterior part of the mandible is fragmented the attachments of the genial muscles are lost and the tongue, having no firm anterior fixation, can fall backwards to block the oral airway. The nasal airway may also be blocked by a blood clot from fractures of the nasal bones and septum, inhaled teeth, or by the maxilla being pushed downwards and backwards toward the pharynx.

The first step in dealing with severe fractures of the jaws is, therefore, to make sure that the patient does not asphyxiate from any of these causes.

2. *Access of cutaneous infection*. The overlying skin is loose, and fractures of the jaws (apart from those such as gunshot wounds which cause

gross tissue damage) are seldom open to the external surface and infection from the skin. The blood supply to the soft tissues and periosteum is good, and healing of fractures of the jaw is normally rapid.

3. *Exposure to saliva*. On its oral surfaces the jaw is covered by a thin adherent mucoperiosteum which often tears, opening the fracture to the oral fluids. Infection from saliva is resisted well, as might be expected from the readiness with which extraction wounds normally heal.

4. *Teeth in the fracture line*. When there is a tooth in the fracture line, organisms from the gingival margin or a periodontal pocket can infect the fracture. If the blood supply to the pulp is cut off, the pulp dies and forms a nidus of infected necrotic matter in the fracture. It may be necessary, therefore, to extract teeth in the fracture line.

5. *Areas of weakness of the jaw*. The presence of teeth, particularly the root of the lower canine or an unerupted third molar, weakens the jaw, and a fracture line often passes through the periodontal membrane. Other areas of weakness are governed by the surgical anatomy of the jaws, as discussed later.

6. *Muscular displacement of fractures*. The position and direction of the fracture line in relation to the muscle attachments determine whether the fragments are displaced away from each other or pulled together. The general direction of pull of the muscles is such that the anterior part of the body of the mandible is displaced downwards and backwards and the posterior part upwards and medially.

7. *Restoration of occlusion and immobilisation.* When teeth are present, alignment of the bony fragments must be such as to restore occlusion precisely. The teeth, however, provide a means by which this can be done and are often invaluable for immobilising a fracture. Immobilisation of fractures of the jaws is usually therefore by quite different methods from those used for other bones.

8. *Complications of fractures of the upper jaws.* The upper jaw is a strongly attached bone forming part of the face and continuous with the cranium and base of the skull. Injuries to the upper jaw vary from minor fractures of the alveolar process to widespread fragmentation and displacement of the facial skeleton, opening and infection of the paranasal sinuses, destruction of part of the orbital walls and opening of the anterior cranial fossa. These injuries can endanger life, affect sight and cause gross disfigurement. Once the patient's life is out of danger, therefore, the main aim is to restore the facial appearance. To this end the dental surgeon makes an essential contribution.

FRACTURES OF THE MANDIBLE

The common causes of fractures of the lower jaw in peacetime are road accidents, fights and falls, and, occasionally, dental extractions.

The mandible is prominent and is more often fractured than the much more strongly supported middle third of the face. Fractures of the mandible are often unassociated with injuries elsewhere, and their general management is correspondingly more straightforward.

Surgical anatomy

The mandible is mobile but its mobility is limited and it is strongly supported by the masticatory muscles. In addition to the masticatory muscles there are the important anterior attachments of the muscles of the base of the tongue and of the hyoid. The body of the mandible is roughly oval in cross section and forms a strong arch. The ramus, by contrast, is thin and blade-like. At the posterior part of the body of the mandible, the masseter and temporalis muscles are inserted and extend further forward than the insertion of the medial pterygoid. These factors help determine the frequency and direction of mandibular fractures near the junction between body and ramus when there is a blow on the chin, directed obliquely backwards.

Other sites of weakness are on either side of the mental prominence, the deep-rooted canine teeth. An unerupted or partially erupted third molar further weakens the region of the angle of the mandible.

The neck of the condylar process is particularly weak. However, the condylar neck, by readily fracturing under a strong force, protects the condylar head from being displaced through the roof of the glenoid fossa.

Direction of displacement of fragments

The effects of the various muscle attachments on displacing fractures of the mandible is discussed in relation to fractures in specific sites.

Clinical features

The main features of a fracture of the jaw are a history of an injury followed by pain, swelling and deformity (particularly malocclusion) and abnormal mobility, unless the fracture is minor and self-stabilising.

If the injuries have been more severe, as in a road accident, damage to the skull, cervical spine or chest must first be excluded and obstruction to the airway prevented. The face and mouth must be cleaned, and dried blood and clot removed. Extraoral and intraoral examination, under anaesthesia if appropriate, can then be carried out by inspection and palpation.

The main clinical features of fractures of the mandible alone are as follows.

1. *Pain.* Pain is most severe when the patient tries to move the jaw or when it is being examined. There is tenderness over the region of the fracture. Pain is relieved by fixation of the fragments.
2. *Bleeding.* There is usually bleeding into the mouth from the torn mucoperiosteum. The skin is usually unbroken, but there may be bruising.
3. *Swelling.* Swelling is caused by haemorrhage and oedema of the soft tissues. Swelling may be so gross after severe injuries as to disguise the underlying bony damage.
4. *Paraesthesia or anaesthesia* of the lip can follow stretching of the inferior dental nerve.
5. *Loosening of teeth.* This is a result either of their being involved in the fracture line or a fracture of the alveolar process.
6. *Disturbance of occlusion.* This is often the most obvious intraoral sign of fracture of the jaw, particularly when there is a step deformity of the occlusion. It is important to make certain that some pre-existing abnormality, such as a crossed bite or Class III dental relationship, is not mistaken for the effect of an injury.

7. *Abnormal mobility.* The fragments are mobile unless impacted into each other. One fragment of the mandible is usually pulled askew by unbalanced action of the muscles.

Tests for abnormal mobility must be carried out gently. The ramus is steadied by holding it between the fingers and thumb of one hand, the fingers being placed along the posterior border within the mouth. The anterior fragment is held with the other hand, with the thumb on the lower border externally and the fingers intraorally on the occlusal surface of the teeth.

Crepitus is another sign, but should not be elicited deliberately.

Failure of transmitted movement is another aspect of abnormal mobility and is apparent, for example, when the neck of the condyle is fractured. The head of the condyle can be palpated through the skin of the preauricular region or, better, through the anterior wall of the external auditory meatus with the tip of the finger. In such a case, movement of the head of the condyle cannot be detected when the remainder of the mandible moves in the normal way.

Radiographic examination

Radiographs are essential for the following purposes:

1. To confirm the presence of the fracture
2. To determine the direction of the fracture line
3. To determine the severity of bony damage
4. To determine the relationship of teeth to the fracture line
5. To detect fractures in other parts of the bone.

The classical radiological sign of a fracture is interruption of continuity of the bone by a radiolucent line. Care must, however, be taken to avoid mistaking the radiolucent line of the pharynx or other structures crossing the jaw for a fracture. If the bone-ends overlap, there is usually a radiopaque line.

Radiographs should usually be taken from at least two viewpoints at right-angles to one another, but the most useful is a panoramic radiograph. This shows the whole of the jaw from condyle to condyle in a single view and can be done quickly, simply and with minimal disturbance of the patient. Any associated disease, such as a cyst, is also shown. The region of the symphysis, however, may be poorly defined.

In the absence of panoramic facilities, oblique lateral views should be taken. These show the area from the premolars to the condyle and should be centred on the probable area of the fracture. Both sides of the jaw should be taken. These must always be supplemented with a postero-anterior view. This shows the whole of the mandible, but the condylar heads are often hidden by the zygomatic bone and mastoid process. The incisor region is obscured by superimposition of the cervical vertebrae.

The occlusal view shows the direction of the fracture line in the horizontal plane and any fracture in the region of the symphysis.

Intraoral films are useful mainly for showing bony detail, particulary the relationship of a tooth to the fracture line.

Sites of fracture of the mandible

The angle is one of the most common sites. If the fracture line runs downwards and forwards, the muscles attached to the ramus pull the posterior fragment against the anterior fragment, preventing displacement, and the fracture is said to be *horizontally favourable*. If, on the other hand, the fracture line runs downwards and backwards there is nothing to stop the posterior fragment from being pulled upwards, and the fracture is said to be *horizontally unfavourable*. A short posterior fragment is difficult to control unless it carries a tooth.

If the fracture line runs backwards and medially so that the fragments tend to be impacted into each other, medial displacement of the posterior fragment is prevented. This is said to be *vertically favourable*. When the fracture line runs backwards and laterally the fracture is unstable and *vertically unfavourable*.

Somewhat confusingly the terms 'horizontal' and 'vertical' used in this way refer to the direction from which the displacement is *viewed*: that is, from the side or from above, respectively.

The neck of the condyle. There is sometimes little displacement if the periosteum remains intact but the external pterygoid attached to the head of the condyle exerts a strong force which usually displaces the detached fragment forwards and medially. The effect of displacement of the head of the condyle is to shorten the effective length of the ramus. The results are that the posterior teeth meet prematurely on the affected side and the chin deviates in the same direction.

The fractured end of the condylar neck can lacerate the anterior wall of the auditory meatus and cause bleeding from the ear. This must be distinguished from a fracture involving the middle cranial fossa, when blood mixed with CSF can escape.

The condyles of both sides may be fractured, for example, by a fall onto the point of the chin. This causes premature contact of the posterior teeth on both sides and an anterior open bite. Injuries of this type causing bilateral condylar neck fractures often also cause an oblique fracture of the symphysis. Surprisingly such fractures can be completely missed until the patient complains—occasionally much later—that the teeth do not 'meet properly'.

The body of the mandible. A common site is the canine region because this long root weakens the bone. The same factors determine whether the fracture is stable as in the region of the angle, except that the mylohyoid opposes the upward pull of muscles attached to the ramus. If there are bilateral fractures in the canine regions the central fragment tends to be displaced backwards by muscle pull, and control of the tongue may be lost.

The symphysis. Fractures through the symphysis are uncommon. They are stable if the fracture line runs directly antero-posteriorly, since the muscles tend to pull the fragments medially and together. If the fracture line is oblique, there are strong forces causing the fragments to override one another.

The ramus. These fractures are uncommon because of the protection by the thick investing muscles. They are stable because the fragments tend to be impacted together by the combined pull of the muscles.

Principles of management

General considerations

If there have been severe injuries the first essentials are to *make sure that the patient has a clear*

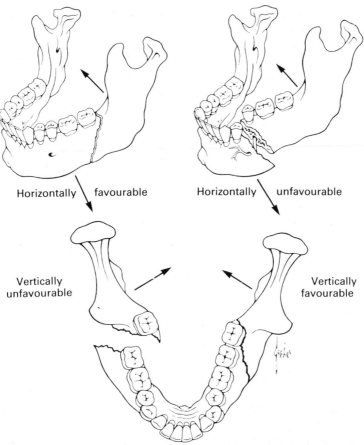

Fig. 13.2 Displacement of the posterior fragment in mandibular fractures. Displacement is determined by the direction of the fracture lines and classified according to the direction from which the fracture is viewed. When viewed from the side ('horizontally') the fragments may either be pulled together by the muscles and the fracture is then Horizontally favourable (HF), or the posterior fragment may be displaced upwards and it is then Horizontally unfavourable (HU). When viewed from vertically above, the fragments may either be pulled together (Vertically favourable, VF) or the posterior fragment may be displaced medially and the fracture is Vertically unfavourable (VU). In practice, combinations of these types of displacement are found. The arrows show the main direction of the pull of the muscles.

airway, to deal with haemorrhage and, if necessary, to treat shock.

The posture is of paramount importance. If the patient is conscious, a sitting position with the head held well forwards is permissible. If the patient feels faint, or is semi-conscious, he should be put in the usual postoperative recovery position, that is turned to one side with the trachea inclined downwards so that the tongue tends to fall forward. This facilitates drainage of blood and saliva. Suction, if available, is most useful. *On no account should the patient be allowed to lie on his back.*

Once first-aid measures have been carried out, clot and debris can be removed and the wound examined. The injury to the jaw should be examined in as much detail as possible and the fracture immobilised temporarily if movements of the jaw are causing pain. This is rarely necessary.

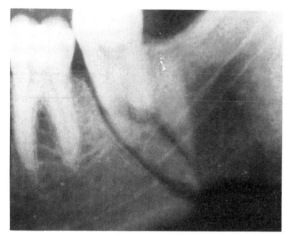

Fig. 13.3 Fracture of the body of the mandible. The radiograph shows the typical appearance of a simple fracture. The fracture is unstable and the posterior fragment displaced upwards (horizontally unfavourable). The fracture could be immobilised using the teeth remaining in the posterior fragment. Unfortunately the fracture lines involve the periodontal tissues, and strict precautions would have to be taken to prevent spread of infection into the bone.

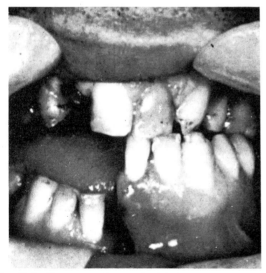

Fig. 13.4 Fracture at the symphysis. There is gross vertical displacement of the right fragment as a result of a second fracture on this side at the angle. The patient incidentally also has pitting hypoplasia of the incisal third of the enamel.

Many patients, particularly as a result of fights, have one or more fractures of the lower jaw but no other significant injury. Under these circumstances treatment can be started immediately.

The aims of definitive treatment are:

1. *Reduce* displacement to restore normal occlusion
2. *Immobilise* the fragments rigidly until the bone unites.

Steps must be taken to prevent infection and to ensure that the patient can be fed in spite of fixation of the jaw.

If the fracture is open to infection from the mouth or skin, or there is a tooth (which needs to be retained) in the fracture line, it is common practice to give an antibiotic such as 600 mg of penicillin, by mouth if possible, prophylactically and to continue it 6-hourly for 4 or 5 days.

Teeth involved in the fracture line

A tooth can be a source of infection if the socket is in the fracture line. Before the era of antibiotics such teeth had usually to be extracted because of the danger of osteomyelitis; but this is not often necessary now. Radiographs of the fracture should be examined closely to determine which tooth is affected.

If teeth are so loose as to be useless for fixation, or if their vitality is in doubt, they should be extracted. On the other hand, a single tooth in an otherwise edentulous posterior fragment is valuable as a means of control and may justifiably be retained until callus formation has begun. A buried tooth in the fracture line should also be left alone; any attempt to remove it causes additional trauma and bone destruction.

Reduction of fractures

The method by which the fragments are brought into correct alignment depends primarily upon whether there is a sufficient number of firmly attached teeth in each fragment with which to control the bone.

Broadly speaking, reduction of fractures of the jaws can be carried out in the following ways according to the complexity of the case, the facilities available and the state of the patient.

1. Manual reduction with the aid of an analgesic such as pethidine or nalbuphine, together

with diazepam or midazolam if necessary, or under regional analgesia

2. Slow elastic traction applied to splints on the teeth or jaws
3. Manual reduction under general (endotracheal) anaesthesia
4. Open operation under general (endotracheal) anaesthesia.

Immobilisation of fractures of the mandible

Interdental eyelet wiring. When there are sufficient firm teeth of good shape in each fragment it is usually possible to wire them together and to teeth of the opposite jaw. This is an effective means of immobilisation which restores occlusion exactly, since the occlusal surfaces of the teeth are brought together. It requires minimal facilities.

A batch of eyelet wires, and lengths of straight (tie) wires are prepared beforehand. The ends of the eyelet wire are passed between and around pairs of teeth, one end being passed through the eyelet and twisted tightly with the other end. The eyelets are then joined to the teeth in the opposite jaw by the straight (tie) wires passed through the eyelets.

Interdental wires can also be attached to pre-formed arch bars to give additional rigidity, if for example there are some mobile or missing teeth. Wiring is overall probably the most useful method of mandibular fixation in that it can be done immediately and requires no laboratory facilities.

Cast metal cap-splints. When the teeth are too few, too badly distributed or too unsatisfactory in shape interdental wiring, for-cast cap-splints cemented to the teeth can be used to immobilise the jaws with complete stability for as long as necessary.

Impressions are taken and the models set up on an articulator. At the fracture line the model is cut to allow 'reduction' on the articulator and restoration of normal occlusion. The locking plates and locking bar assembly traversing the fracture site can then be accurately positioned. This laboratory work greatly reduces the time spent in the theatre. The splints are cemented to the teeth pre-operatively.

The splints on each fragment are then fixed together by locking plates and connecting bars

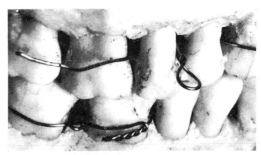

Fig. 13.5 Interdental eyelet wiring. In the upper jaw the eyelet has been formed and passed between the premolars, while the ends are still free. In the lower jaw the wire has been completed by passing one free end through the eyelet, drawing the wire up tightly round the teeth and twisting the ends firmly together.

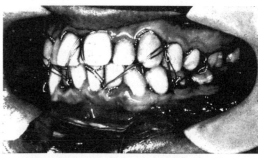

Fig. 13.6 Interdental eyelet wiring. The eyelet wires have been completed, the fracture has been reduced and the tie wires have been passed through the eyelets and tightened. The ligatures are arranged at an angle to each other to give a cross-bracing effect.

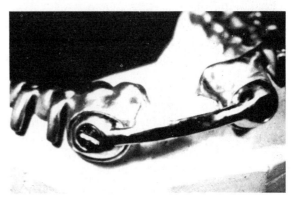

Fig. 13.7 Cast metal splints. The splints cover the entire crowns of the teeth, forming a rigid and firmly attached structure. The locking bar bridges the fracture line and enables the fragments to be fixed firmly and accurately together after reduction. The hooks cast into the buccal aspects of the splint are used to attach ligaments to a similar splint on the upper arch so that the mandibular fracture is also supported by the upper jaw and independent movement is impossible.

screwed to each splint after reduction of the displacement, and the upper and lower splints are joined by elastic bands.

The thickness of metal interposed between the occlusal surfaces of the teeth tends to produce a slight error of occlusion, but this can usually be overcome by selective grinding of interfering cusps after removal of the splints.

The main limitation of this method of immobilisation is the facilities and skills needed for the laboratory work, and the time required. Wherever possible, wiring is probably therefore generally used.

Immobilisation of the edentulous mandible

Fractures of the edentulous mandible are generally closed (without tearing of the mucoperiosteum) and unite without difficulty. If there is no serious displacement, the patient may be made comfortable by a simple supporting bandage round the jaw, thickly padded with cotton wool.

More severe or unstable fractures may be immobilised by means of *Gunning-type splints*. Gunning-type splints are essentially denture baseplates made from impressions of the patient's mouth, and they simply rest on the mucous membrane. The fracture can be immobilised only by stabilising the splint over the underlying bone. A wire is therefore drawn round the splint and through the alveolar bone of the upper jaw (peralveolar wiring) on each side. Though the wire passes from the oral cavity into the bone, infection is uncommon if the operation is carefully carried out. In the case of the lower jaw the wire is passed round the body of the bone (circumferential wiring).

This method is suitable (i) for cases where the fracture line is sufficiently far forward to be well within the denture-bearing area and (ii) for more posterior fractures which can be stabilised with little displacement when the rest of the jaw is immobilised.

The short edentulous posterior fragment. When the posterior fragment is edentulous but the fracture line is favourable, it is sufficient to immobilise the jaws in one of the ways already mentioned, and no direct fixation of the posterior fragment is necessary.

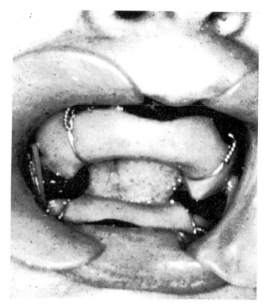

Fig. 13.8 Immobilisation of the edentulous mandible. Acrylic base plates are lined with gutta percha for accurate and comfortable adaptation to the alveolar ridges. Stainless steel wires are passed through the base of the alveolar process on either side of the upper jaw, and round the base plates (peralveolar wiring); wires are also passed round the body of the mandible (circumferential wiring), to attach the splints firmly to the jaws. The bite is adjusted to the correct height by means of composition placed in the molar region. The mandible is immobilised to the upper jaw by elastic or wire ligatures attached to hooks embedded in the acrylic plates. The space between the base plates in front allows the patient to be fed easily.

This method is often satisfactory even when the fracture line appears unfavourable. Slight upward displacement of a short posterior fragment does not necessarily have any serious or even noticeable consequences and is usually preferable to the use of direct fixation by pins or wires.

If the posterior fragment is long enough, upward displacement may be prevented by a saddle extension lined with gutta percha, fixed to a splint on the anterior fragment, and bearing on the mucous membrane behind.

Transosseous wiring

Fractures which remain uncontrollable after reduction may be immobilised by wiring the fragments together across the fracture line. Transosseous wiring may be carried out intraorally using holes drilled through the alveolar bone on either side of the fracture line (upper border wiring), or extraorally, through a submandibular incision using holes drilled through the basal bone (lower border wiring). This is an effective method for these difficult fractures, but, if the fracture is seriously infected from the mouth, osteomyelitis, sequestration of bone, sloughing of the wires and loss of control of the fracture may follow.

In addition to transosseous wiring, it is usually necessary to immobilise the whole jaw as well, by one of the methods already described, to get sufficient stability.

Bone plating

Bone plates may consist of vitallium strips about 2–3 cm long with four holes. The bone is exposed by an external approach and holes drilled into it on either side of the fracture line. The plate is then fixed with vitallium screws.

Bone plates are preferably malleable, such as Champy plates or, better, of titanium mesh (T mesh). Titanium mesh is more readily adaptable to surfaces curved in more than one plane than other bone plates and is not springy. The plates are fixed to the bone with screws.

Bone plating is increasingly widely used for immobilisation of fractures of the mandible and even of the maxilla. The advantages of plating are that it is very rigid and immobilisation of the jaw is often unnecessary. This simplifies the general management of the patient but is particularly useful when the neck of the condyle is also fractured and early movement is necessary. No laboratory facilities are needed.

The disadvantages are that a general anaesthetic is needed and a scar is left on the face.

Pin fixation to extraoral appliances

Heavy (3 mm diameter) stainless steel screw pins are inserted, generally in pairs, into the fragments. The pins pass through the skin and attach to a metal frame strong enough to hold the fragments of bone in place.

However, it is difficult to make the pins and extraoral fixation rigid enough to resist the pull

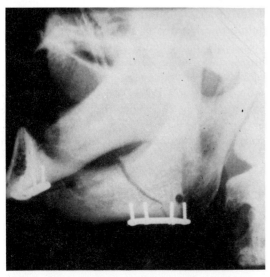

Fig. 13.9 Bone plating. A vitallium strip has been screwed to the lower border of the mandible to immobilise a horizontally unfavourable fragment. A similar plate controls a fracture on the opposite side of the jaw.

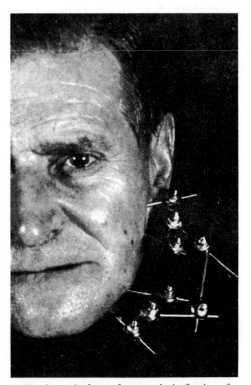

Fig. 13.10 An early form of extraoral pin fixation of a fracture which shows the essential principles. The patient is edentulous and has a fracture at the angle controlled by a pair of pins in each fragment.

of the muscles, and the pins may loosen in the bone. Infection may also track inwards to the bone. The appliance attached to the side of the patient's face is awkward and prominent; it is easily damaged and the patient may have difficulty in finding a comfortable position for sleeping.

Transosseous wiring is usually more simple and satisfactory. Pin fixation is, as a result, rarely used for civilian injuries, but mainly for gunshot wounds where there has been loss of bone. It can also occasionally be used when infection of the fracture line prevents direct wiring.

Fractures of the neck of the condyle

The condylar neck is inaccessible from the mouth, and displacement of the head of the condyle causes dislocation of the temporomandibular joint. The displaced condylar head almost invariably unites with the rest of the mandible but, in spite of malunion of the fragments causing malalignment of the joint surfaces, the temporomandibular joint retains good function. However, most cases heal with good function without operative interference.

Types and effects of condylar fracture

Most fractures are through the neck of the condyle. In the mildest cases there is no displacement and the bones remain in normal relationship. Alternatively the upper fragment may become angulated or displaced medially. In the most severe cases the joint is dislocated.

Angulation or displacement of the condyle shortens the height of the ramus, and the jaw deviates to the affected side. If both condyles are fractured, the shortening on both sides causes the posterior teeth to meet prematurely, resulting in an anterior open bite.

Fracture of the condyle may be seen in an orthopantomogram or an oblique lateral radiograph, but a postero-anterior view of the skull and temporomandibular joint views may also be needed. Fractures in other parts of the jaw should also be looked for.

Unilateral fractures. To relieve pain and to prevent deviation the jaws can be wired together for 7 days, but this is rarely necessary and active movements should be encouraged from the start.

There may be temporary deviation of the jaw on closure, due to muscle spasm, but this soon wears off, and the patient learns to adopt a new pattern of neuromuscular coordination which ensures correct centric relationship. Deviation of the chin towards the affected side when opening the mouth tends to persist but is of no significance.

Prolonged immobilisation of the jaw (for more than 10 days) should not be used for unilateral fractures. The results are no better, and in some cases the condyle unites in a bad position; only limited movement of the mandible is then possible. If deviation of the jaw persists, cap splints carrying a guiding flange can be fitted. These flanges prevent the patient from closing the mouth unless centric occlusion is achieved by muscular effort.

Bilateral fractures. These require immobilisation for up to 3 to 4 weeks otherwise the retroposed position and open-bite persist. In severe cases, over-distraction of the rami is necessary by interposing blocks 2–3 mm thick between the last upper and lower molar teeth and using elastic traction anteriorly. Final function is often surprisingly good, although lateral excursion and maximum opening are generally restricted to some extent. As previously mentioned, care should be taken to exclude a parasymphyseal fracture which, if present, should be reduced and immobilised.

Intracapsular comminuted fractures, especially in children, frequently result in bony ankylosis unless active movements are maintained. Bilateral injuries, and injuries of this type in patients with prolonged unconsciousness, have a poor prognosis. Condylectomy and other surgical procedures for reconstruction of the joint are generally required eventually.

Surgical exploration and reduction of fractures involving the temporomandibular joint is *very rarely justifiable* as an immediate procedure.

Complications of fractures of the mandible

The main complications are as follows:

1. *Infection*
2. *Delayed union or non-union*
3. *Malunion and deformity*
4. *Disorders of occlusion*

5. *Impaired function of the temporomandibular joint*
6. *Anaesthesia of the lower lip.*

With modern methods of management these complications are uncommon.

Infection

Apart from delaying healing, infection can constitute a problem in itself since spreading osteomyelitis can follow introduction of infection, especially from the skin. This is surprisingly uncommon, especially now that antibiotics are used prophylactically. Infection is more common in fractures of the jaw after radiation therapy of the mouth and in immunodeficient patients.

Delayed union or non-union

The main causes are as follows.

Infection. This may be the result of direct infection of the haematoma from the mouth, but this is rare. In the case of a gunshot wound there may be infection from the exterior or there may be a foreign body in the wound. Penicillin should be given prophylactically and continued as long as necessary (for 4 to 5 days at least), assuming that sensitivity tests do not show the organism to be resistant and that the patient is not allergic.

Teeth in the fracture line. Infection from the gingival margin may enter along the torn periodontal membrane. In other cases death of the pulp may follow damage to the apical vessels, and provide a nidus of necrotic and infected material within the fracture. These teeth should be extracted before infection can become established unless retention of the tooth is essential for control of one of the fragments. Antibiotic cover may then be necessary.

Poor immobilisation is an important cause of delayed union. Movement between the fragments may prevent ossification and cause fibrous tissue to form between the bone ends. If this happens a false joint forms and bony union fails to develop.

Wide separation of fragments is likely only to result from loss of tissue caused by a gunshot wound or if there is complete failure of reduction with one fragment grossly displaced. Where there is severe bone loss, grafting is necessary.

Interposition of soft tissue or foreign bodies. This is rare except in the case of severe injuries.

Diseases of bone. Malignant tumours, osteodystrophies, or irradiation damage to the bone are *rare* complications interfering with repair.

Systemic disorders. In the elderly, healing is somewhat delayed. Atherosclerosis may reduce the central blood supply of the mandible, which then depends increasingly upon the periosteal circulation. Fractures of the edentulous atrophic mandible in the elderly may fail to unite for this reason.

Specific diseases such as syphilis, tuberculosis, scurvy, or uraemia are so rare as hardly to be of practical importance.

Corticosteroid treatment may delay healing by impairing protein synthesis or may promote infection.

Management of delayed union. Where there is some local cause such as an infected tooth in the fracture line, this should be removed. Immobilisation should be checked and replaced or modified if not firm. These measures may be adequate but, should they fail, the fracture should be exposed, the bone-ends freshened and the jaw immobilised again.

In general, fractures of the jaws promptly treated by modern methods providing effective immobilisation are rarely affected by complications. Inadequate immobilisation and infection are the most important causes of failure but prevention is easier than cure.

Malunion and deformity

Should reduction have been imperfect the fragments unite in an abnormal position causing deformity. Usually, remodelling of the bone will progressively obliterate the defect and eventually restore a fairly normal contour. This is especially the case in children with a high osteogenic potential and remodelling capacity of the periosteum.

Disorders of occlusion

This may be minor when a consequence of inaccurately fitting cap splints or severe when due to malunion. Probably the most common cause of severe malocclusion is an unnoticed and neglected

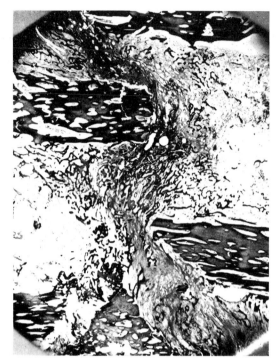

Fig. 13.11 Malunion of a fracture. The bone-ends have been displaced in relation to each other, the connective tissue fibres of the callus have become reorientated and stream across the ends of the fragments instead of along the line of the bones. Trabeculae of bone (hard callus) have formed mainly in the direction of the connective tissue fibres, across the medullary cavity and to a lesser extent between the bone-ends.

fracture of both condylar necks following a fall onto the chin and leaving an anterior open bite.

Minor defects of occlusion can be dealt with by selective grinding. Severe cases usually require selective extractions.

Impaired function of the temporomandibular joint

This may result from unnoticed bilateral condylar neck fractures leaving an anterior open bite and restricted movement. Persistent deviation on closure is generally attributable to a malunited unilateral condylar fracture.

Limitation of movement may also result from prolonged immobilisation when there are associated fractures of other parts of the jaw.

The most important measure is prevention, making sure that movement is normal at an early stage and that the joint is kept mobile. For this purpose plating of associated mandibular fractures is valuable.

Chronic pain from arthritis following damage to the temporomandibular joint due to a fracture is uncommon but may be important not only clinically but also from a medicolegal standpoint.

Anaesthesia of the lower lip

The inferior dental nerve may be stretched or compressed or fibres torn or severed in fractures of the body of the mandible. The degree and duration of anaesthesia is proportional to the severity of the injury to the nerve. Mild injury is followed by full recovery within 1 or 2 months. Severe injuries may not heal for 18 months and be associated with dysaesthesia. Thereafter, recovery is unlikely.

FRACTURES OF THE FACIAL SKELETON

Fractures of the maxilla and related bones are less common than those of the mandible, but because they are often the result of a severe blow to the face, particularly in road accidents, tend to have more serious effects. The dura can be torn, with the risk of intracranial infection, sight may be impaired, or disagreeable sensory loss can be caused. But most important is the immediate *threat to the airway*. The ease with which the airway can be obstructed in this type of injury means that the patient can die within a few minutes if this problem is not dealt with immediately.

In addition to measures already described for fractures of the mandible, the value of early endotracheal intubation with a *cuffed* tube by a skilled anaesthetist must be emphasised. Effective suction is also necessary, and this not only maintains the airway but also prevents aspiration of blood.

Fractures of the upper jaw may be broadly divided into: (1) affecting only the alveolar process; (2) affecting the facial skeleton.

Fractures of the facial skeleton may involve many bones, including the maxilla, but, apart from gunshot wounds, the injury always tends to crush and flatten the face. Gross disfigurement may result from ineffective treatment, and the orbits, the cranial cavity and the nasal sinuses may be severely damaged.

Fractures of the mandible are often unassociated with fractures of the remainder of the facial skeleton or with injuries elsewhere. Fractures of the mid-facial skeleton, by contrast, being the result of more severe trauma, are often associated with fractures of the lower jaw. The management of the latter is essentially along the same principles as outlined earlier but modified as necessary by the nature of any injuries elsewhere.

Structural considerations

Understanding the main types of fracture of the maxilla and their effects may be made easier by consideration of the construction of the facial skeleton.

Together the maxillae are roughly triangular in shape when viewed from the front. The alveolar process forms the base, the nasal cavity fills the centre, the antra fill the lateral parts, and the roof of the antrum on each side forms the greater part of the floor of the orbits.

The maxillae are joined at their apex to the frontal bone and, between the eyes, the maxillae are joined to the ethmoids, the roof of which is the cribriform plate in the centre of the anterior cranial fossa.

On each side the maxillae are joined to the zygomatic bones which form the lateral parts of face. Posteriorly, the maxillae are unsupported except by the slender pterygoid processes of the sphenoid on either side of the wide posterior nasal openings. Posterolaterally, in the floor of the orbit the maxilla is separated from the greater wing of the sphenoid by the inferior orbital fissure.

The zygomatic bones form the lateral, and part of the inferior, margins of the orbit. The broadest part of the body of the zygomatic bone is attached to the maxilla below the orbit. The frontal process has a slender attachment to the edge of the wing of the sphenoid in the lateral wall of the orbit, and to the frontal bone at its apex. Posteriorly the temporal process joins the delicate zygomatic process of the temporal bone to form the zygomatic arch. The zygomatic bone is otherwise unsupported from behind.

Directions of the main fracture lines

Most injuries to the upper jaw and face are directly or obliquely from in front and drive a greater or lesser part of the face backwards. The structure of the facial skeleton is not buttressed against frontal force, and it is common for the whole middle third of the face (from orbits to upper teeth) to be sheared from, and driven downwards and backwards along, the sloping cranial base.

The lines of fracture of the maxilla follow the lines of weakness of the facial skeleton. The alveolar process and palate are supported only by the walls of the antrum which are attached to a limited part of the denture-bearing area, more than half of which lies under the nasal cavity. A blow to the front of the mouth centred on the upper lip can therefore shear the alveolar bone from the rest of the maxilla and drive it backwards (Guérin's fracture or Le Fort's type I[*]).

A severe blow in the centre of the face can separate the maxilla from its attachments just above the nasal aperture. The fracture passes along the inferomedial margin of the orbit near the sutures with the zygomatic bone, through the lateral walls of the antrum, and through the pterygoid plates behind. In this way a pyramidal fragment comprising virtually the whole of the maxilla below the zygomatic bones is driven backwards (Le Fort's type II).

A heavy blow by a broad object can drive backwards the whole of the face below the frontal bones. A line passing downwards and backwards from the fronto-maxillary suture through the paper-thin walls of the ethmoid and the necks of the pterygoid processes forms a line of weakness along which the maxilla can be sheared from the base of the skull. Laterally, the maxillae are separated from the skull by the inferior orbital fissures, and are supported only by the zygomatic bones which are also weakly supported from behind. The result of such an injury is a high fracture line through the root of the nose, comminuting the ethmoids and breaking the necks of the pterygoid plates. The fracture line includes the inferior orbital fissures and disrupts the attachments of the zygomatic bones through the edge of

---

[*] Réné le Fort: French orthopaedic surgeon (1869–1951).

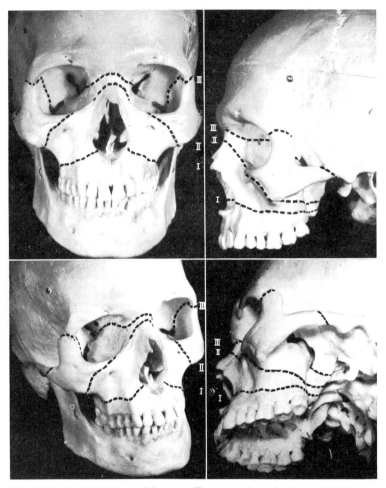

Fig. 13.12 Le Fort's lines of fracture. The approximate levels at which the bones of the facial skeleton tend to fracture in different types of injury are shown. It can be seen how the high-level, suprazygomatic fracture (type III) involves the inferior orbital fissure, the lateral wall of the orbit, the zygomatic arch and the pterygoid plates so that the whole of the middle third of the face can be detached from the cranial base and driven backwards and downwards. The oblique views show how the inferior orbital fissure is continuous with the sphenopalatine fissure, forming a natural line of weakness. In practice these main lines of fracture often tend to be complicated by comminution of the fragments making a more irregular pattern.

the wing of the sphenoid and near the fronto-zygomatic suture. In addition the zygomatic arch is also broken near its thinnest part. The facial skeleton is therefore driven downwards and backwards, and the main fragment includes the floor of the orbits. This high-level suprazygomatic fracture is Le Fort's type III.

Fractures of the zygomatic arch

In addition to fractures of the main part of the face (the central middle third), the zygomatic bone may be driven inwards by an oblique blow. The severity of the injury may vary from fracture of the arch alone, with little displacement, to a severe injury which comminutes the lateral wall of the maxillary antrum and the floor of the orbit. The coronoid process of the mandible, caught between the depressed zygoma and the side of the skull, may also be fractured or impede the movements of the mandible.

Other fractures of the facial skeleton

Other injuries to the face are fractures of the nasal bones (an occupational disease in boxers), and fractures of the many other smaller bones which help to form the structure of the face and which are involved in the more major injuries to the maxilla just described.

Classification

Bearing in mind that the precise course of the fracture lines varies in individual patients due to variations in the exact cause of the injury, fractures of the maxilla follow the lines suggested above and are governed by the structural weakness of the facial skeleton and by the direction of the force supplied. These injuries may be classified as follows:

1. **Fractures of the alveolar process**
2. **Fractures of the central middle third of the face**
   a. — Bilateral detachment of the alveolar process and palate
      Low-level subzygomatic fracture of Guérin (Le Fort type I)
   b. — Pyramidal, subzygomatic fracture of the maxilla (Le Fort type II)
   c. — Fracture of central and lateral parts of the face
      High-level suprazygomatic fracture (Le Fort type III)
3. **Fractures of the zygomatic bone and arch**
   a. With minimal displacement and associated injury
   b. With damage to the lateral antral wall and floor of the orbit
4. **Fractures of the nasal bones.**

Note: Fractures of the Le Fort type may be associated with a paramedian split of the palate just to one side of the septum. Fractures can

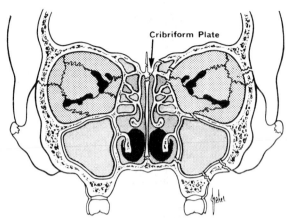

Fig. 13.13 A coronal section of the middle third of the facial skeleton. The bony structure is mainly arranged to withstand the vertical stresses of mastication; the centre section (consisting of the nasal cavity and ethmoids) is delicate. It can be seen that in a Le Fort type I (Guerin's) fracture, detachment of the whole alveolar process must also involve the floor of the antra and the nasal cavity. The line of a high-level, Le Fort type III fracture is largely determined by the line of weakness formed by the inferior orbital fissures and the fragile ethmoid; the cribriform plate immediately above may be fractured, opening the anterior cranial fossa.

sometimes be unilateral or may be at one level on one side and at a different level on the opposite side.

The purpose of the classification is broadly to relate the main types of injury to their management.

Fractures of the alveolar process alone can be stabilised by intraoral methods. Fractures of the central middle third of the face are the most serious; the antra are usually involved and there may be more widespread damage. Fixation must be by extraoral methods or internal wire suspension in most cases, but unilateral fractures can be immobilised by intraoral splints. Fractures of the zygoma are usually depressed and must be elevated. Fractures of the nasal bones will not be discussed further here.

General clinical aspects

Fractures affecting the middle third of the face range from minor fractures of the alveolar process to severe injuries affecting the whole of the middle and lower thirds of the face. The clinical features can therefore include the following.

1. *Blockage of the airway.* This is by far the most important complication of fractures of the facial skeleton. It is not an invariable consequence but, when it happens, can cause death of the patient, either within a few minutes of the injury or later—even during transport or examination of the patient—if mishandled.

    The airway may be blocked by blood clot, or the maxillary fragment may be driven downwards and backwards, forcing the soft palate and the dorsum of the tongue together against the posterior wall of the pharynx.

2. *Oedema of the face.* Oedema is often gross, causing ballooning of the features, and then disguises the extent of the underlying injury.

3. *Ecchymoses.* Circumorbital and subconjunctival bleeding produce the picture shown in Fig. 13.14 and are particularly characteristic of Le Fort II or III fractures. Ecchymoses develop later than the initial oedema. Subconjunctival haemorrhage extends over the white of the eye to the edge of the cornea, producing the characteristic red eye appearance.

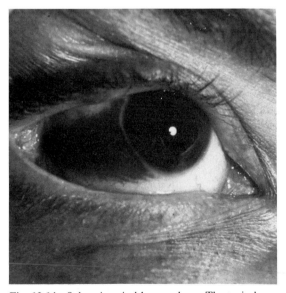

Fig. 13.14 Subconjunctival haemorrhage. The typical bleeding producing the red eye of a Le Fort II or III fracture can be seen.

4. *Bleeding.* Initial bleeding from the nose and into the nasopharynx tends to stop quite quickly of its own accord.

5. *Mobility of the upper jaw.* Mobility varies according to the nature of the fractures, as discussed in more detail below.

6. *Disturbance of occlusion.* This is usually shown by premature contact of the last molars, gagging the bite open. This also produces the characteristic lengthening of the face, though this too may be disguised by the general oedema.

Clinical features of the main types of fractures of the facial skeleton

A variety of permutations and combinations of fractures is possible, especially in vehicle accidents where the victim can be tossed about and receive injuries from several directions in succession. They can be regarded as comprising the following main types, alone or together, and with or without fractures of the lower jaw.

The middle third of the face

Le Fort I fracture. Immediately after the injury, separation of the dento-alveolar segment may show little obvious abnormality, apart from mild bleeding from the nose and some disturbance of occlusion.

Le Fort II and III fractures. Extension of the fractures into the orbital area with fracture of the nasal bones and sometimes of the ethmoid and zygomatic bones produces an alarming picture due to the swelling and bruising. When this has happened the main features seen are those described earlier, namely oedema of the face (especially round the eyelids); bleeding from the nose and into the nasopharynx; mobility of the upper jaw and disturbance of occlusion, usually premature contact of the last molars gagging the bite open. Circumorbital and subconjunctival ecchymoses develop later.

The features of a patient with a middle third fracture are therefore ballooning of the face, bulging of the eyelids and a livid colour due to the combination of oedema and extravasation of blood. Midfacial fractures should always be suspected

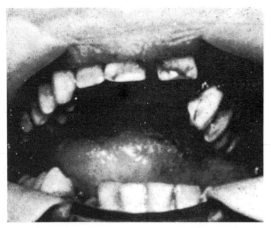

Fig. 13.15 Unilateral fracture of the maxilla. The fragment is displaced medially, and fractures of the left zygomatic bone and mandible are also present. After reduction, fixation was by intraoral means using cast cap-splints and locking bars.

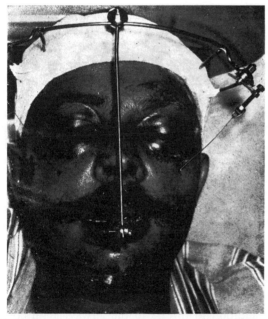

Fig. 13.16 A fracture of the middle third of the face and craniomaxillary fixation. The patient has a Le Fort type II fracture with displacement of the left zygomatic bone. The fractures have been reduced but the characteristic gross oedema of the face and ecchymosis round the eyes is still present. The fracture of the maxilla has been immobilised by extraoral fixation to a plaster head-cap and by wires passing through the cheek and attached to the upper splint.

whenever this picture is seen, so that the possible complications should be looked for and dealt with.

The zygomatico-maxillary complex. Immediately after the injury there is obvious depression of the cheek (the zygomatic prominence).

Bleeding and oedema soon follow, filling and masking the depression. When this has happened the main features suggesting this type of injury are a history of a blow to the upper part of the face, followed by bleeding from the nose on that side and often limitation of movement of the mandible. There is often paraesthesia of the infraorbital nerve supplying the greater part of the cheek, side of the nose and upper lip. The associated teeth and gingival tissues may also be affected.

The nasal bones and naso-ethmoidal complex. The bridge of the nose is flattened distorted laterally, and there is bleeding and aspiration of blood, with obstruction of the airway constituting an important hazard.

History

Information should be obtained from witnesses or the patient if he is able to speak. Some assessment of the nature of the accident is helpful as a guide to the type and severity of injuries to be expected. Nevertheless, serious effects such as intracranial haemorrhage can follow relatively trivial accidents. It is important to know whether there has been any loss of consciousness or of memory of the period just before or after the injury, as these are indications of cerebral damage.

Pain in any part of the body should be asked about and an attempt made to find out whether the patient is receiving any drugs for systemic disease, or is allergic to penicillin. It is useful to know when the patient last had food and whether he has been drinking.

Initial examination and primary care

A preliminary examination of the patient when first seen is necessary to get some idea of the extent of the injuries and, if necessary, to institute primary care to maintain life. More precise assessment depends on hospital facilities and use of radiographs.

The following are the most important requirements:

1. Ensure a clear airway
2. Look for and control bleeding, whether intra- or extracranial
3. Look for other injuries, particularly to the cervical spine, thorax and abdomen
4. Look for fractures of other bones
5. Look for leakage of cerebrospinal fluid
6. Look for injuries to the eyes
7. Establish a neurological baseline for future reference.

The most urgent and important of these is *attention to the airway*. One thing that must *not* be done is to give the patient a narcotic analgesic such as morphine or pentazocine, as explained later.

Preservation of the airway

It is important to emphasise again the need to maintain the patient's airway and prevent aspiration. Patients with maxillofacial injuries alone do not die from hypovolemic shock unless a major vessel is severed, but many arrive dead at hospital as a result of airway obstruction. Danger signs are cyanosis of the lips or tongue and violent attempts at respiration against the obstruction.

The main measures are as follows.

1. The patient should be turned onto his side and the trachea preferably tilted downwards by a support beneath the chest. However, great care must be taken if there is any possibility that there has been a spinal injury. If allowed to lie on his back, the tongue can fall backwards and foreign bodies can impact against the pharyngeal wall.

2. Rarely, the upper jaw may be driven downwards and backwards, pushing the soft palate and dorsum of the tongue together against the pharyngeal wall. This, together with oedema and bleeding, is an acute and severe threat to the airway.

In this unusual but dangerous situation immediate disimpaction is necessary. This is done by steadying the head with one hand on the forehead, while the fingers of the other hand are hooked up behind the soft palate and the fragments distracted by firm traction forwards and upwards.

3. Foreign bodies, including loose teeth, dentures, or large clots of blood, should be removed. In the first instance this must be done with the finger and gauze swabs to sweep away mucus and blood. A sucker with a soft tube is more effective and should be used as soon as it is available. Traction may be needed to pull the tongue forwards. If a tongue stitch is used it should be inserted transversely as far back as possible, *not* through the tip of the tongue.

4. Intubation. Initially a nasopharyngeal tube passed to a point just beyond the free edge of the soft palate is a useful safety measure as long as the lumen can be kept clear. This involves constant aspiration to remove blood and mucus, which usually accumulate rapidly.

The ideal is to pass a cuffed endotracheal tube as soon as possible; this effectively maintains the airway, eliminates the risk of aspiration of blood into the lungs and also allows aspiration of the bronchial tree.

Tracheostomy is rarely necessary except as a last resort in an emergency.

Shock

Hypovolemic shock is unlikely to be the result of maxillofacial injury alone, but is usually a warning that there are severe injuries elsewhere, particularly in the thorax or abdomen. The alarming appearance of severe maxillofacial injuries often distracts attention from the possibility of injuries elsewhere and causes failure to assess the patient's general state. Obviously it is essential not to overlook such possibilities as other head injuries, fractured cervical vertebrae, a stoved-in chest, bleeding into the thorax, or rupture of the liver or spleen.

Complications associated with severe maxillofacial injuries

In addition to threats to the airway, a variety of complications should be looked for if not immediately obvious. These include the following.

1. *Loss of consciousness*. The damage to the facial skeleton often absorbs most of the force of the injury and there is not necessarily any disturbance of cerebral function. If cerebral function is dis-

turbed it may range from temporary loss of consciousness (concussion) to severe and permanent cerebral damage. Expert neurosurgical assessment is usually essential.

2. *Opening of the antra*. Fractures of the middle third and most fractures of the zygomatic bone disrupt the antral walls and expose the antra to infection from the nasal aspect, but the mucosa over the lateral walls generally remains intact. Antral infection is, however, surprisingly rare.

3. *Displacement of the eye*. Double vision may be caused by damage to the supporting ligaments of the eye and the extraocular muscles or their nerve supply.

4. *Opening the cranial cavity*. A high-level fracture of the middle third may fracture the cribriform plate of the ethmoid and tear the overlying dura. Cerebrospinal fluid escapes from the nose, and infection can enter the cranial cavity to cause meningitis.

5. *Damage to cranial nerves*. The infra-orbital nerves may be damaged in zygomatic complex or Le Fort type II and III fractures, leaving an area of anaesthesia of the upper lip. Any of the superior dental nerves may also be injured but the region of anaesthesia within the mouth is easily overlooked.

Anosmia is caused by tearing the olfactory fibres which pass through the cribriform plate in the roof of the nasal cavity and is a complication which is not usually noticed till later.

In addition to the loss of the sense of smell, much of the sense of taste is lost. Anosmia is a permanent and serious handicap which should be tested for after a fracture of the middle third of the face, but, in the early stages, blood clot may produce a false positive result.

Summary

The essential aspects of primary care discussed above can be summarised in two useful mnemonics.

Immediate dangers:

A Airway
B Bleeding (either extracranial or intracranial)
C Control of the tongue
D Derangement of occlusion
E Eyes. Ears. Escape of CSF
F Fractures elsewhere
G General injuries.

Immediate management must form a logical PATTERN, and this provides the basis for the second mnemonic, as follows:

P Posture
A Aspiration
T Tongue traction
T Tubes (oral, nasopharyngeal, or endotracheal)
E Examination in detail
R Reassurance
N Notification of specialist services.

Assessment of extraoral injuries

One misleading aspect of severe injuries to the facial skeleton, especially of the middle third, is the minimal degree of soft-tissue wounding. If, however, the patient has gross swelling (ballooning) of the features, oedema of the eyelids and circumorbital ecchymosis followed by subconjunctival bleeding, he must be assumed to have a Le Fort type II or III fracture. In most such patients the soft-tissue wounds are limited to sites where the soft tissues have been rolled over sharp margins of bone, particularly the bridge of the nose and the superior orbital margin. Lip laceration from contact with teeth or dentures is usually also present, but this may be the only soft tissue injury in a patient in whom the mandible, maxilla, zygomatic bones or orbital floors and ethmoids have been grossly fractured and displaced.

If the cranial cavity is opened, both blood and CSF can leak from the nose, but cannot be distinguished from each other. Later, after the blood has clotted, the CSF continues to flow and is seen especially when the patient is in a sitting position. If the patient is lying down, the CSF may be unnoticed as it passes down the nasopharynx, though the patient may sometimes be aware of a salty taste. CSF can be identified by electrophoresis and its glucose content.

Gross oedema makes examination of the eyes difficult, but it is essential to assess reflex responses. If any damage is found, an ophthalmologist's help is essential.

Soft-tissue wounds

The nature, extent and depth of soft-tissue wounds must be assessed and foreign bodies removed.

The vascularity of the facial tissues ensures that they survive extraordinarily well, and every fragment possible should be conserved.

Palpation

Palpation should start at the outer aspect of the superior orbital margin and follow round the orbital rim. Defects should be looked for, particularly at the frontozygomatic suture and the inferior orbital margin.

The nasal bones and the region of the frontal sinus should be checked and the zygomatic prominences and arches compared. Differences in contour can often be seen more easily when standing above the patient and looking downwards over the face.

Palpation of the mandible should start at the condyles, pass along the back of the rami and along the lower border of the body to the symphysis.

Intraoral assessment

Through-and-through wounds, which often affect the sulcus, should be looked for. The soft tissues can be rolled backwards over the mental prominence, producing partial 'degloving'.

Penetrating wounds, and lacerations involving the tongue and fauces present a particular danger, in that swelling after surgical débridement and closure can endanger the airway. In such cases, if the jaws have to be immobilised, an elective tracheostomy must be considered.

Separation of the two maxillae by a paramedian split of the palate may be concealed by adherent clot. This may be seen when the clot is swabbed away, or it may be detected by gentle springing apart of the two halves of the upper jaw.

Detachment of the upper jaw from the remainder of the facial skeleton may result in impaction or a loose floating fragment. Many fractures are overlooked because the mucoperiosteum is intact and penetrating wounds of the sulcus are rare.

Because of the anatomical considerations discussed earlier, a forceful blow to the centre of the face results in a tilting downwards and backwards of the upper jaw. This in turn leads to bilateral gagging on the maxillary molars and an anterior open bite.

These effects are essentially similar to those which follow bilateral condylar fractures, and if both types of fracture coexist then the displacement is made more severe. Apart from the obvious evidence of facial injury, the main difference between the effects of this type of fracture of the middle third and those of condylar fractures alone is in the mobility of the upper jaw.

The downward and backward displacement of the middle third leads to the characteristic dish-face deformity which becomes obvious only after oedema has subsided.

When testing for mobility of the maxilla, care should be taken to prevent a false impression being given by the free movement of the skull beneath the scalp. One hand should therefore be placed with the palm on the forehead and the index finger and thumb on either side of the bridge of the nose. The incisor teeth and alveolar bone can then be grasped with the thumb and first two fingers of the other hand, and an attempt can be made to move the fragments between the two hands.

A useful sign characteristic of a fracture through the antrum is percussion of the premolar or molar teeth with a metal instrument. When the antrum is normal and intact, percussion gives a clear resonant sound, but a fracture through the antrum produces a 'cracked teacup' sound.

Radiological examination

The complexity of the facial skeleton is such that middle third fractures are frequently difficult to see in radiographs. Where there is any doubt, the clinical findings are more important than uninformative radiographs. A variety of views may have to be taken, but overall the most useful are the 10° and 30° occipitomental, and the standard lateral skull film. However, additional views, such as a coronal section tomograph for Le Fort III fractures, may be necessary.

A brow-up, lateral view with the patient lying supine is also useful. It may show fluid levels in the sinuses.

The middle third of the facial skeleton is best seen in occipitomental view. For this purpose the patient is prone and the tube centred over the external occipital protuberance, while the point of the chin and nose are placed on the film. This projection shows the outlines of the main facial bones and the antra with the minimum of overlap of other bones. It is essential both for diagnostic and medicolegal purposes to take routine skull films. A true lateral view of the skull and facial bones, including the cervical spine, is also useful.

Other views, such as panoramic for mandibular fractures, may also be necessary, but in the first instance it is desirable not to disturb the patient excessively. If a paramedian split of the upper jaw is suspected, an occlusal film should be taken.

Chest radiographs may also be needed if there is any possibility of aspiration of teeth or other foreign bodies.

Records

With all maxillofacial injuries it is essential to keep accurate, detailed records of the nature of the injuries and the methods of treatment and results. The requirements of the police, in the case of injuries resulting from assaults, and the possibility of claims by the victim against the assailant or even against the dental surgeon if the patient feels that the injury has been mismanaged, are some of the important reasons for keeping as detailed records as possible.

Treatment

Once an adequate airway has been ensured, and intracranial or other serious injuries have been dealt with, the maxillofacial damage can be attended to. This consists of soft-tissue repair following reduction and immobilisation of the fractures.

Soft-tissue repair

The facial tissues are highly vascular, and healing is good. As much tissue as possible should be preserved and only minimal débridement need be carried out in most cases. Nevertheless it is essential that great care is taken in cleansing the wound and thoroughly removing particles of dirt and debris. If this is not done, ugly tattooing remains and is difficult to remove later.

Wounds are closed after minimal trimming of the margins to ensure a uniform edge at right angles to the surface and which is undermined sufficiently to permit closure without tension. Deep catgut sutures should be used to approximate the tissues to prevent distortion of the margins and the skin is closed with fine interrupted silk sutures. Skin loss requires replacement by grafting or the use of flaps. It is, however, a fundamental principle that reduction and fixation of the fractures of the facial skeleton must form the basic foundation and precede closure of the soft tissues.

Reduction

Fractures of the maxilla and adjacent bones may be reduced instrumentally, by elastic or weight traction or, in the case of the zygomatic bone, by elevation through a skin or mucosal incision.

For the majority of maxillofacial injuries, general anaesthesia, given by endotracheal tube, is the method of choice.

Immobilisation

Immobilisation of the mobile fragments produced by a fracture of the middle third of the face is difficult because of the lack of a suitable stable base to which they can be anchored. As a consequence a wide variety of methods and apparatus has been devised. Only the basic principles and methods of this specialised subject are therefore discussed here.

Intraoral fixation. This is applicable only to unilateral fractures, namely fractures of part of the alveolar process or of one half of the maxilla. Using metal cap-splints on the teeth, the mobile fragment is joined to the fixed part of the maxilla by means of locking plates. Alternatively an arch bar may be employed.

Extraoral fixation. This method is applicable to all bilateral fractures of the maxilla but is decreasingly used now. For example, the vault of the skull can be used for anchorage by means of a closely fitting plaster head cap. The upper teeth are covered by a cap-splint incorporating a double-screw locking plate base in the incisor region. Upper cap-splints are connected to a framework

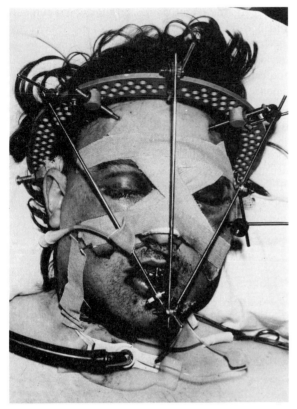

Fig. 13.17 Multiple fractures of the facial skeleton causing a Le Fort II type injury of the upper jaw. The fractured nasal bones have been immobilised with plaster of Paris covered by adhesive strapping, the fracture of the left zygomatic bone stabilised by pin fixation, and a fracture at the right angle of the mandible aligned by transosseous wiring. A halo frame of the Royal Berkshire Hospital type has been secured to the outer table of the skull with screw pins to provide craniomaxillary fixation, via triple rods and universal joints, to a projecting bar screwed onto the upper cast silver cap splint. Note the tracheostomy, and the vacuum drainage tube from the right angle of the mandible. (By courtesy of Mr J. Bowerman.)

embedded in the plaster head cap by an anterior projecting bar secured to the locking plate base and fixed to a vertical rod connected in turn to the framework by universal joints.

This method has been widely used, and effectively, in the past for all types of bilateral fractures of the maxilla and is relatively simple to carry out. Its disadvantages are that (1) fixation is not rigid, due to movement of the scalp on the cranium, (2) the skull is inaccessible should neurosurgery be need and (3) the arrangement of bars in front of the jaw is awkward and can easily be damaged.

The plaster head cap has been replaced in many hospitals by the halo frame. The latter encircles the head and is secured to the outer table of the cranium by four short rods which just engage the cortex but do not penetrate into the diploë. This provides a rigid base to which the upper splint can be connected by one or more vertical rods and universal joints in the manner previously described.

Alternatively, a Levant frame can be used in which pins are inserted supraorbitally and the frame attached to bars joined to upper cap splints.

With such methods it is important to have primary fixation to the upper teeth to enable the lower teeth to be easily separated from the upper in an emergency threatening the airway.

Bone plating

The disadvantages of extraoral fixation are such that, wherever possible, bone plating is used. Titanium mesh can be adapted to irregular bone surfaces and provides firmer immobilisation than wiring or external rods fixed to a head frame.

Internal wiring

In these methods subcutaneous wires are connected indirectly to the teeth below and to some stable part of the facial skeleton above the fracture lines. This method overcomes most of the disadvantages of extraoral fixation and avoids the need for maxillofacial technical laboratory services. Theoretically the wires passing through the mouth or nasal cavity could be a source of infection of the deeper tissues but this can be prevented by use of antibiotics.

Circumzygomatic, frontal and mandibular wiring are most commonly used. To improve stability, the upper and lower teeth may be wired to arch bars, the upper and lower arch bars wired together, and the lower arch bar fixed to the mandible by circumferential wiring. The suspension wires are attached to the lower arch bar so that the fractured region is sandwiched between the lower jaw and the intact facial skeleton above the fracture line.

A disadvantage is that the pull of the suspension wires is directed unfavourably in a slightly posterior direction. However, provided that the

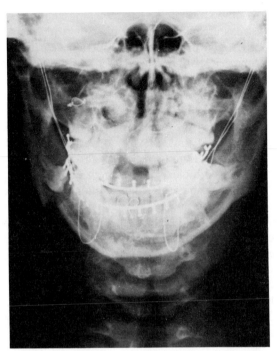

Fig. 13.18 Fixation by internal skeletal wiring. The upper and lower jaws have been wired together using arch bars. There is also circumferential wiring round the mandible and suspension wires attached to the lower arch bar. The posterior fragment on the right side of the mandible contains an unerupted molar and remains displaced. Improvement in the position of the latter would need intraosseous wiring, and the buried tooth would probably need to be removed if this did not excessively weaken the mandible.

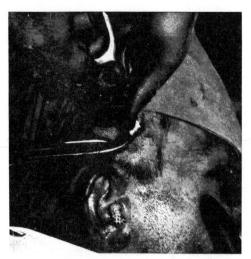

Fig. 13.19 Elevation of the zygomatic bone. A Bristow's elevator has been passed through an incision in the temporal fascia, and the fragment is being repositioned by gentle upward and outward pressure. The position of the fragment is checked by the fingers of the assistant seen in the bottom right-hand corner of the picture.

mandibular condyles are intact, and there is a good incisal overlap and cuspal interdigitation, the maxilla will not relapse posteriorly.

Fractures of the zygomatic bone or arch

Fractures of the zygomatic bone are depressed fractures which flatten the cheek. A severe injury can impact the zygomatic bone into the lateral wall of the antrum; the floor or lateral wall of the orbit may then be comminuted and there may be diplopia. Fractures of the zygomatic arch, alone, cause depression of the side of the face and, often, severe limitation of movement of the mandible by pressing on the coronoid process.

Diplopia is mainly caused either by displacement of the frontal process of the zygomatic bone, to which the suspensory ligament of the eye is attached, so that the eye drops; or by fibrous adhesions between the fascia or capsule surrounding the globe, the inferior rectus and oblique muscles, and the periorbital fat which has herniated through a defect in the orbital floor. Diplopia is one of the most serious complications of a fracture of the zygomatic bone. The patient's ocular coordination should therefore be carefully tested throughout the entire range of movement.

Treatment

A fracture of the zygomatic bone should be treated early, (within 10 days of the injury) as fibrous union is rapid. The main principles are to elevate the zygomatic bone and, if necessary, support the orbital floor from below. Elevation is carried out by the Gillies' approach through an incision in the temporal fossa situated within the hair-line and passing through the skin and temporal fascia. An elevator is passed down over the surface of the temporal muscle until it is beneath the zygomatic bone which is then lifted outwards and upwards. The fragments are usually stable and normally require no additional fixation. If, however, the zygomaticofrontal suture is widely separated, direct interosseous wiring may be necessary to join the fragments and to restore the margins of the orbit.

In cases where the orbital floor is comminuted but the fragments are still attached to the periosteum, the antrum may be packed with gauze soaked in Whitehead's varnish, via a Caldwell-Luc approach, to give support from below. The pack is removed after 2 to 3 weeks.

Fractures of the orbital floor with loss of bone require restoration of continuity by the insertion of either an autograft from the ilium, a homograft of lyophilised dura mata, or an allelograft such as dacron-reinforced silastic sheet. The approach is via a subperiosteal dissection through an incision just below the lower eyelid.

Pain

Pain is rarely a problem with maxillofacial injuries. In any case, whatever the cause of the pain, *morphine is absolutely contraindicated* as accurate assessment of eye signs is essential in the detection and evaluation of intracranial damage. Morphine causes constriction of the pupil and hence conceals pupillary signs. Morphine also depresses respiration and the cough reflex. Other narcotic analgesics, including pentazocine, have similar disadvantages.

Most neurosurgeons therefore forbid the use of any analgesic or sedative until intracranial injury or bleeding can be excluded.

Immobilisation is the most satisfactory means of managing pain from facial fractures. Control of pain from any other part of the body is the responsibility of the surgeon concerned.

Antibiotic prophylaxis

Antibiotics are frequently given to lessen the risk of infection complicating facial fractures, but objective studies of their effectiveness are scanty. It is doubtful whether they have any significant value, and they may even increase the risk of resistant infections. Nevertheless it is common practice to give penicillin (600 mg i.m.) for 5 days as a precaution.

In some sites such as the zygoma and maxilla, infections are so uncommon that the usefulness of antimicrobial prophylaxis cannot be evaluated.

However, antibiotic prophylaxis is particularly important when there are complex open injuries such as gunshot wounds, poor dental health, or when open reduction is carried out. In such cases, an infection rate greater than 40% has been reported, and this may be greatly reduced by perioperative administration of antibiotics such as ampicillin with cloxacillin in high dosage. If there is gross contamination then tetanus immunisation may also be necessary.

If there is CSF leakage it is probably advisable to give an antimicrobial that reaches the CSF to lessen the risk of meningitis from nasal bacteria such as meningococci or staphylococci. Co-trimoxazole can be given, but many strains of these bacteria are now resistant. Rifampicin (20 mg/kg) is more effective against such bacteria and is possibly a better alternative.

Management of complications

Where modern facilities for early treatment exist, infection and malunion are rare unless there has been gross loss of, or damage to, tissue, particularly after gunshot wounds. Even in these cases remarkable improvements can be made by the use of skin and bone grafts and, if necessary, prostheses.

Fractures involving the cranial cavity

The escape of CSF only becomes apparent after the blood has started to clot, allowing clear CSF to be seen, but escape of CSF from the nose can be entirely masked when the patient is lying down. CSF rhinorrhoea usually stops spontaneously after a few days, particularly if there has been early immobilisation of the middle third.

Some neurosurgeons recommend repair of the torn dura in all cases where there is leakage of CSF, as late meningitis may develop in up to 20% of cases after apparent spontaneous healing. However, this may apply mainly to cases sent to neurosurgical units as a result of fractures of the *upper* third of the face and tearing of the frontal dura. In any case, if CSF rhinorrhoea persists for

10 days or more a neurosurgical opinion should be sought, as repair of the dural tear is likely to be necessary.

Diplopia

It is difficult to examine the eyes in the early stages because of oedema, but if there is any doubt about function an ophthalmologist's opinion should be sought.

Diplopia is a serious and incapacitating complication and may be caused by damage to the supporting ligaments of the eye, the intraocular muscles or to their nerve supply.

Double vision may be present immediately after the injury as a result of haemorrhage and effusion around the eye affecting the extraocular muscles. This is temporary and affects all directions of gaze.

Damage to the insertion of the suspensory ligament of the eye (to the frontal process of the zygomatic bone) causes diplopia which persists after the initial effusion has subsided and is permanent if untreated. Later, fibrous adhesions form between the orbital periosteum and the fascial coverings of the eye and limit its movements.

Blowout fractures of the orbital floor are important to look for. Such fractures are the consequence of a blow on the globe of the eye by an object, such as a tennis or squash ball, which is slightly larger than the orbital diameter. The globe of the eye may remain intact, as may the rim of the orbit, but the violent impact forces the globe backwards and compresses the periorbital fat within the conical orbital cavity. The compressed fat bursts the thin floor into the antrum.

The eye, which is initially proptosed by haemorrhage, subsequently remains displaced backwards (enophthalmos) by this loss of periorbital fat. In addition, fibrosis develops round the fat and often involves the inferior oblique and inferior rectus muscles which, as a consequence, become bound to the bony defect below. Upward rotation of the eye is thus very limited and there is severe diplopia.

This type of injury is accompanied by circumorbital and subconjunctival ecchymoses which disguise the enophthalmos. In addition, if there is no loss of continuity of the orbital margins, there are no obvious palpable or radiological abnormalities. The defect can best be seen in tomograms in the coronal plane or in xeroradiographs, but the appearance of the so-called 'hanging drop' sign suspended from the roof of the antrum in the standard occipitomental radiograph should arouse suspicion.

Injuries to cranial nerves

Injury to the olfactory nerve, causing anosmia, is permanent and causes significant disability. Sensory loss, from damage to the infraorbital nerve for example, usually recovers, though the period is very variable. Failure of recovery after about 18 months suggests that there will be permanent loss. During this healing period there should be no attempt to explore the area surgically, as more harm than good is usually done.

Damage to the optic nerve with partial or complete loss of sight, as a result of maxillofacial fractures, is rare.

Damage to the IIIrd, IVth and VIth nerves and ophthalmic division of the Vth nerve, which pass through the superior orbital fissure, can result in the *superior orbital fissure syndrome*. This comprises, in complete cases:

1. Proptosis due to oedema and loss of tone of the extraocular muscles

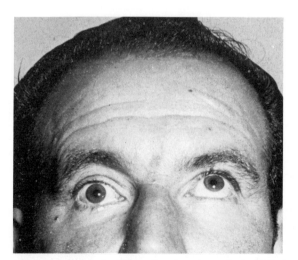

Fig. 13.20 Diplopia. The patient is trying to look upwards, but as a result of IIIrd nerve damage there is loss of vertical movement of the right eye, which remains staring ahead.

2. Ptosis of the upper lid, due to damage to the oculomotor (IIIrd) nerve
3. Fixed dilated pupil, due to damage to the parasympathetic supply
4. Limited eye movements, due to damage to the IIIrd, IVth and VIth nerves
5. Sensory loss in the area of the ophthalmic division of trigeminal nerve.

Damage to the trigeminal nerve is uncommon but is then usually extracranial as in the case of fracture of the mandible, as mentioned earlier. However, the ophthalmic division of V may be damaged in the superior orbital fissure syndrome.

SUGGESTED FURTHER READING

Adi M, Ogden G R, Chisholm D M 1990 An analysis of mandibular fractures in Dundee, Scotland (1977–1985). Br J Oral Maxillofac Surg 26: 194–199

Ching M, Hase M P 1987 Comparison of panoramic and standard radiographic radiation exposures in the diagnosis of mandibular fractures. Med J Aust 147: 226–229

Chole R A, Yee J 1987 Antibiotic prophylaxis for facial fractures. Arch Otolaryngol Head Neck Surg 113: 1055–1057

Klotch D W, Bilger J R 1987 Plate fixation for open mandibular fractures. Laryngoscope 95: 1374–1377

Langdon J D 1986 Current thinking in oral and maxillofacial surgery. Dental Update Jan/Feb: 29–37

Laskin D M, Best A M 1988 Current trends in the treatment of maxillofacial injuries in the United States. J Oral Maxillofac Surg 45: 595–602

Lindqvist C, Sorsa S, Hyrkas T, Santavirta S 1986 Maxillofacial fractures sustained in bicycle accidents. Int J Oral Maxillofac Surg 15: 12–18

Shepherd J P 1989 Surgical, socio-economic and forensic aspects of assault: a review. Br J Oral Maxillofac Surg 27: 89–98

Shetty V, Freymiller E 1989 Teeth in the line of fracture: a review. J Oral Maxillofac Surg 47: 1303–1306

Wiederhold W C, Melton L J, Annegers J F et al 1989 Short term outcome of skull fracture: a population-based study of survival and neurological complications. Neurology 39: 96–102

14. Disorders of the temporomandibular joints and periarticular tissues

Disorders of the temporomandibular joint may cause limitation of movement of the jaw, pain, or clicking sounds; various combinations of these symptoms are often associated.

Limitation of movement

Inability to open the mouth fully is usually temporary, and often called *trismus*; occasionally it may be more persistent, and causes include the following.

1. *Infection and inflammation in or near the joint.* The main cause is acute pericoronitis. Rare causes include suppurative arthritis, osteomyelitis or cellulitis.
2. *Mandibular block injections.* These may cause irritation of the tissues round the joint and oedema, either because of irritation by the local anaesthetic solution or because of introduction of infection. Occasionally limitation of movement may be more persistent, due to organisation of a haematoma caused by the injection. Forced opening under general anaesthesia may then be necessary.
3. *Buried wisdom teeth.* Pericoronitis of a partly erupted third molar is common, but there is no way by which a completely unerupted and uninfected tooth can affect movement of the jaw.
4. *Injuries.* Fracture of the necks of the condyles or dislocation, if untreated, cause an anterior open bite or fixation in the open position, respectively.
5. *Tetanus and tetany.* These are rare causes of spasm which may involve the masticatory muscles. Nevertheless, though rare, it is important to exclude tetanus because of its high mortality. This possibility should be considered whenever a patient develops acute severe limitation of movement of the jaw without local cause.
6. *Temporomandibular pain dysfunction syndrome.* Pain dysfunction syndrome is one of the more common causes of temporary limitation of movement of the temporomandibular joint as discussed later.

Management

In all these conditions the essential treatment is to relieve the underlying disorder.

Permanent limitation of movement

Extra-articular causes

1. **Fibrosis**. Fibrosis of the tissues near or around the joint is the only important cause and may be due to (a) deep burns of the face; (b) therapeutic irradiation.

Irradiation. The penetrating powers of modern sources such as cobalt isotopes or linear accelerators are such that high doses can damage tissues intervening between the surface and the neoplasm, but without a superficial burn. Radiation involving the region of the masticatory muscles, for the treatment of a maxillary tumour for instance, can lead to fibrosis of muscle and fibrous adhesions to the surrounding fascial layers, producing a fixed mass bound to the jaw. When this happens there is severe limitation of opening the mouth or complete ankylosis. Treatment is difficult and may involve the division of muscle attachments from the jaw or section of the angle or body of the mandible to produce a false joint.

2. **Oral submucous fibrosis**. This condition is relatively common in the Indian sub-continent and is seen in Britain only among immigrants. It is characterised by progressive fibrosis, particularly of the buccal but also of palatal and other oral mucous membranes, associated with atrophy of the overlying epithelium and loss of underlying muscle. The thickened layer of dense collagenous connective tissue eventually becomes so board-like that it may become virtually impossible to indent the buccal mucosa with the finger tip. In severe cases the patient may be able only to open the mouth less than a centimetre and depends ultimately on a fluid diet.

There is no specific treatment, and in severe cases plastic surgery may be necessary.

3. **Systemic disease**. The connective tissue disease, systemic sclerosis (Ch. 20) can cause fixation of the jaw by dense periarticular fibrosis.

Intra-articular causes

1. **Congenital**. This is probably due to injury to the joint at birth.

2. **Trauma**. Intracapsular fracture of the neck of the condyle disorganises the joint and causes bleeding followed by fibrosis. Usually, however, an effective false joint forms and function is little impaired.

3. **Acute pyogenic arthritis**. This is exceedingly rare but, if it should develop and be treated ineffectively, complete fixation (ankylosis) of the joint follows.

4. **Juvenile arthritis**. Some of the variants of juvenile arthritis are more severe and disabling

than adult rheumatoid arthritis and have been reported to lead to ankylosis of the temporomandibular joint. This may be preventable with modern treatment.

Adult rheumatoid arthritis or osteoarthritis are not causes of ankylosis of the temporomandibular joint.

5. **Tumours and other abnormalities of the condyle**. Osteomas, chondromas, or hyperplasia of the condyle are exceedingly rare causes of limitation or loss of movement of the jaw.

Management

When the joint becomes fixed by fibrous adhesions it may be possible to cut these at open operation. If this fails or if there is bony ankylosis, a false joint can sometimes be made by excising the condyle and interposing soft tissue. Alternatively, a wedge resection near the angle may be used for the same purpose.

Dislocation of the jaw

The temporomandibular joint may become fixed in the open position by dislocation; this is due to forcible opening of the mouth by a blow on the jaw, or as a result of dental extractions under general anaesthesia. In the latter case, the condition should be noticed immediately. It must be corrected before the patient recovers consciousness, by pressing downwards and backwards on the lower posterior teeth.

Occasionally the dislocation remains unnoticed and, surprisingly, a patient may tolerate the disability and discomfort for weeks or even months. In these cases effusion into the joint, following the injury, becomes organised, forming fibrous adhesions. When this has happened manual reduction becomes impossible and open operation, to divide adhesions, must be carried out.

Recurrent dislocation

Recurrent dislocation of the temporomandibular joint is a rarity but may be caused by, and is sometimes a typical feature of, some of the heritable disorders of collagen formation, notably Ehlers Danlos (often unsuspected in mild form or called

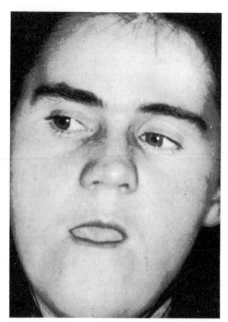

Fig. 14.1 Long-standing dislocation of the jaw: The teeth had been extracted about a month previously: in spite of the patient's inability to close her mouth and the distorted appearance, the dislocation remained unrecognised.

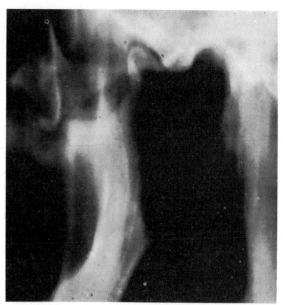

Fig. 14.3 Dislocation of the jaw. Radiographs of the temporomandibular joints of the same patient show complete dislocation of the condyle in the front of the eminentia articularis.
(Illustrations 14.1 to 14.3 by courtesy of Prof. I. Curson and British Dental Journal (1959) 107: 351.)

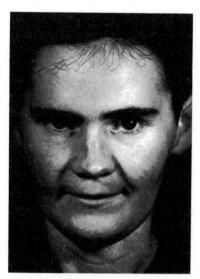

Fig. 14.2 Reduction of the dislocation (done by open operation because of development of fibrous adhesions) restores the patient's normal appearance and movements of the jaw.

'double jointedness') and Marfan's syndromes. In such cases some form of arthroplasty may be needed to improve the stability of the joint.

Tardive dyskinesia

This term describes involuntary, disfiguring grimacing as a result of movements of the jaw and face. It is a late ('tardive') complication of giving phenothiazines, particularly for psychoses. Metoclopramide, which has phenothiazine-like actions, can cause persistent trismus. There is no reliably effective treatment.

PAIN IN OR AROUND THE JOINT

The main causes are as follows.

1. *Injury*. Dislocation or fractures of the neck of the condyle can cause pain of varying degrees of severity, but, surprisingly often, fractures in this region pass unnoticed.
2. *Infection and inflammation*. Acute pyogenic arthritis and osteomyelitis are exceedingly rare. Lyme disease of the temporomandibular joint has also been reported.
3. *Rheumatoid arthritis*. The temporomandibular joints tend to be much less severely affected than others.

4. *Pain of vascular origin.* Temporal arteritis is the main cause by producing ischaemia and pain in the masticatory muscles.
5. *Muscle spasm.* The main cause and one of the most common causes of pain in the region of the temporomandibular joint is so-called pain dysfunction syndrome.
6. *Salivary gland disease.* Painful conditions of the parotids (inflammatory or neoplastic) can cause pain in this region.

Pain dysfunction syndrome

Pain dysfunction syndrome predominantly affects young women and is characterised by pain, clicking sounds from the joint, or limitation of movement.

Aetiology

The female to male preponderance is nearly 4 to 1. Most patients are between 20 and 40, older people are rarely affected. There is no evidence that the disease is progressive and goes on to produce permanent changes, or that there is disease of the joint itself. The condition is probably self-limiting, but may be sufficiently troublesome to justify treatment.

Abnormalities of occlusion are often blamed for this disorder, such as lack of posterior occlusal support from loss of molar teeth, though there is no evidence that they are a cause or even that these abnormalities are more common in this syndrome than in normal persons. In spite of the problems created by dentures, for instance, edentulous patients seem rarely, if ever, to be affected.

Trauma, particularly minor injuries such as may be caused by violent yawning, laughing, or dental treatment, is occasionally a possible factor but the evidence does not seem strong.

It may be noted that in the USA, temporomandibular joint disorders are frequently investigated and treated with a degree of enthusiasm that would be unusual in Britain. For example, methods of investigation in the USA now range from conventional radiography to magnetic resonance imaging and liquid crystal thermography. Cynics might suggest that one reason for this degree of concern about comparatively trivial complaints might be related to the financial incentives involved.

Nevertheless concern about the confusion surrounding the nature of this disorder, the profusion of names for it, the multiplicity of treatments that have been devised and the increasing amount of related litigation has led the American Dental Association to try to reach a consensus, particularly on its management. Illustrative of some of the difficulties in identifying the disorder was the finding that its prevalence reported in different surveys ranged from 12% to 86% of adults.

Among the few matters on which there was general agreement were that research had failed to implicate occlusion in the aetiology and that treatment should, initially at least, be conservative. These measures could include counselling, habit management, physical therapy, bite appliances, short-term analgesics and biofeedback therapy. There was no agreement on any indications for more active intervention such as surgery or 'occlusal therapy'. In fact, it was agreed that psychosocial stress was a major factor in the aetiology and that there was a strong placebo effect in every type of treatment.

To summarise, it is clear that pain dysfunction syndrome is a condition of dubious aetiology and typically affects only a restricted group of the population. It is self-limiting and there is no known pathology of the joint. It does not go on to permanent damage or degenerative arthritis later in life, and elderly patients are remarkably free from symptoms from this joint. Defective neuromuscular coordination, causing areas of spasm of the masticatory muscles, appears to be the basic cause of the symptoms.

Clinical features

The onset is gradual in most cases, but a few patients ascribe the onset to violent yawning, laughing, or some similar incident.

Pain is usually one-sided and is rarely severe; it is typically a dull ache made worse by mastication. The condylar region is the main site, and pain is typically felt in front of the ear. In some cases pain is felt lower down over the ramus, occasionally at the angle of the jaw and, more rarely still, other sites nearby.

There is often also limitation of opening, or 'locking' of the jaw in the open or closed position. The joint may be tender on palpation, and a clicking sound, when the mouth is opened or closed, is common.

Defects of occlusion can often be found as they can in any other patients.

Investigation

It should be appreciated that, in view of the absence of objective signs, diagnosis is largely by exclusion. It is essential therefore to exclude organic causes (most of which have been enumerated above but are rarely found) of pain or limitation of movement of this joint.

As in all cases of pain in the region of the jaws, careful examination must be made for referred pain due to pulpitis.

Rheumatoid arthritis should be excluded by general examination if necessary but is unlikely to be a cause of such symptoms. The temporomandibular joint should be palpated for tenderness or swelling which, if present, suggest organic disease.

Movements of the head of the condyle can be felt through the overlying skin or with the finger in the auditory meatus. With practice, abnormal excursions or asymmetrical movement of the condyles, or crepitus, may be detected.

Lateral radiographs of the joints should be taken with the jaw in the open and closed positions to make sure that movements are not excessive in either direction and are equal on both sides. The main value of radiographs, however, is to exclude organic disease shown by such changes as the presence of fluid (causing an increase in the size of the joint space) or damage or deformity of the joint surfaces.

Trigeminal neuralgia should be suspected in patients of middle age or over (particularly when the pain is severe) since it can be occasionally triggered by movement of the jaw. If an attack comes on while the patient is in the surgery and the patient is obviously suffering agonising pain which may bring tears to their eyes, then this excludes the diagnosis of temporomandibular arthrosis. Treatment too can cause confusion, in that trigeminal neuralgia is subject to spontaneous remissions, and if a remission follows the fitting of an appliance then the wrong conclusions can be drawn.

Some still carry out detailed occlusal analysis but, as indicated earlier, the most practical approach is to fit an acrylic overlay appliance covering the occlusal surfaces of the teeth. This allows free occlusion without cuspal interference and also tends to relieve abnormal grinding habits. This simple measure alone is usually surprisingly effective.

Management

Management may be considered under four main headings. These are:

1. Reassurance
2. Bite appliances
3. Habit management and physical therapy.
4. Analgesics.

Many other forms of treatment (sufficient in fact, to fill large text-books) have been recommended, but this is merely another reflection of how little is known about this disorder.

Reassurance and counselling. Once the diagnosis has been established, it is important to reassure a patient that there is no serious disease and that the symptoms, though troublesome at the moment, are likely to subside of their own accord after a time.

Reassurance alone is sometimes effective; nothing else need then be done. It may also be helpful to give diazepam 2 mg three times a day as an initial dose but progressively increased until it has the desired result without undue drowsiness as a side effect. This should not be continued for more than 2 weeks. There is, as always, wide individual variation in patients' response. Some claim that diazepam alone is often adequate treatment. Apart from its tranquilising effects diazepam is a mild muscle relaxant which can only be helpful.

Bite appliances. In very many cases the disorder can be dealt with effectively by the fitting of an acrylic overlay appliance covering by the fitting of an acrylic overlay appliance covering the occlusal surfaces of the teeth. This allows free occlusion without cuspal interference and tends to relieve abnormal grinding habits. It is not uncommon for these patients to have severe overclosure with a deep anterior overbite. This also can be managed by means of an appliance, using an anterior bite plane which will allow further eruption of the posterior teeth.

The appliance should be worn day and night in severe cases and may have to be replaced or built up as necessary, as it wears down during use. The appliance should be firmly fitting and retained by means of cribs. Patients usually accommodate quickly to the wearing of these appliances which, after a day or so, interfere little with speech or mastication. In many cases the relief of pain or other symptoms is a strong impetus to continue wearing the appliance.

Overall, the use of these types of appliances is probably the most satisfactory form of treatment for this disorder. It is usually effective and is much less time-consuming than other methods. If necessary diazepam can also be given, particularly in the early stages.

Habit management and physical therapy. Abnormal biting habits should be identified and controlled. Faulty neuromuscular control should be dealt with by exercises to correct faulty patterns of neuromuscular activity as shown by such abnormalities as deviations on closure.

Analgesics. Short-term use of anti-inflammatory analgesics may be additionally helpful.

'Costen's syndrome'

This syndrome was said to comprise headache, ear symptoms (tinnitus or deafness) and burning pain in the tongue and throat. These symptoms were ascribed to overclosure causing excessive backward movement of the head of the condyle. This syndrome does not exist.

Temporal arteritis

Temporal arteritis occasionally causes ischaemic pain in the masticatory muscles in elderly patients and should be considered in patients over middle age who complain of pain on mastication (see Ch. 18).

Osteoarthritis

Osteoarthritis is traditionally regarded as a wear and tear disease predominantly, therefore, affecting the elderly. However, it appears that it is a metabolic defect of articular cartilage, characterised by increased hydration and decreased content of many essential glycosaminoglycans and proteoglycans. Damage to the defective articular cartilage may be worsened by physical stresses, and inflammatory mediators are released. Hence pain is greatest in heavily stressed joints such as the hips in overweight persons. By contrast there can be gross osteoarthritis and distortion of the joints of the hands but there may be no pain.

The temporomandibular joint, like virtually any other joint, can be affected by osteoarthritis in the elderly, but like other lightly stressed joints, symptoms may be minimal or absent and the disease only found by chance by radiography. In the absence of symptoms, treatment is not indicated, but in the rare cases where pain is associated, anti-inflammatory analgesics may be required.

In young persons osteoarthritis of the temporomandibular joint alone has been described, but in the absence of more widespread involvement is likely to be some other undefined disorder.

Rheumatoid arthritis

This common disease is characterised by chronic inflammation affecting many joints, with pain, progressive limitation of movement and varying degrees of constitutional upset.

Rheumatoid arthritis is the only important inflammatory disease of the temporomandibular joint. Nevertheless it is rarely a cause of significant TMJ symptoms.

Clinical features

Women are mainly affected, particularly in the third and fourth decades. Loss of weight, malaise and depression are common. The smaller joints are mainly affected (particularly those of the hands), and the distribution tends to be symmetrical (Ch. 20).

The main symptoms when the temporomandibular joint is involved are crepitus and limitation of movement, but pain itself is surprisingly uncommon. The temporomandibular joints are never involved alone, and the other affected joints usually dominate the picture.

Thus in one study of 100 patients with rheumatoid arthritis sufficiently severe for them to attend a rheumatology centre, 71% showed clinical abnormalities of the temporomandibular joints (compared with 41% for controls), while 79% showed radiological abnormalities compared with 34% for controls. In spite of the fact that these were middle-aged patients with long-standing disease, pain was *not* significantly more common than in control patients. The main clinical abnormalities were limitation of opening, or crepitus, both of which were considerably more common than in other patients.

The main radiological features of rheumatoid arthritis are reduced mobility, surface and pocket erosions of the bone and flattening of the joint surfaces.

Generally speaking, therefore, rheumatoid arthritis, which is a common disease, frequently affects, but is not an important cause of temporomandibular joint pain.

Management

The diagnosis must be made on the clinical and radiological features and laboratory investigations.

Treatment is predominantly with anti-inflammatory analgesics.

A complication affecting a minority of patients with rheumatoid arthritis is Sjögren's syndrome and this may itself cause pain in the parotids which may *occasionally* be severe enough to cause confusion with temporomandibular joint pain.

Lyme disease

Lyme disease is a recently described but rare cause of temporomandibular joint pain. This infection may respond to tetracycline or other antibiotics (Ch. 8).

SUGGESTED FURTHER READING

Baum J 1990 Arthritis in children. Med Int 74: 3080–3084

Cawson R A, Eveson J W 1987 Oral pathology and diagnosis. William Heinemann Medical Books, London and Gower Medical Publishing, London

Clark G T, Seligman D A, Solberg W K, Pullinger A G 1989 Guidelines for the examination and diagnosis of temporomandibular disorders. J Craniomandib Disord Facial Oral Pain 3: 7–14

Donlon W C, Moon K L 1987 Comparison of magnetic resonance imaging, arthroscopy and clinical and surgical findings in temporomandibular joint internal derangements. Oral Surg, Oral Med, Oral Pathol 54: 2–5

Eriksson L, Westesson P-L 1985 Long-term evaluation of meniscectomy of the temporomandibular joint. J Oral Maxillofac Surg 47: 1048–1052

Hamerman D 1989 The biology of osteoarthritis 1989 New Engl J Med 320: 1322–1330

Harinstein D, Buckingham R S, Braun T et al 1988 Systemic joint laxity (the hypermobility syndrome) is associated with temporomandibular joint dysfunction. Arthritis Rheumat 31: 1259–1254

Harris R J 1988 Lyme disease involving the temporomandibular joint. J Oral Maxillofac Surg 46: 78–79

Helmy E S, Bays R A, Sharawy M M 1989 Histopathological study of human TMJ perforated discs with emphasis on synovial membrane response. J Oral Maxillofac Surg 47: 1048–1052

Katzberg R W 1989 Temporomandibular joint imaging. Radiology 170: 297–307

Kirk W S 1989 Diagnosing disk dysfunction and tissue changes in the temporomandibular joint with magnetic resonance imaging. JADA 119: 527–530

Larheim T A, Bjornland T 1989 Arthrographic findings in the temporomandibular joint in patients with rheumatic disease. J Oral Maxillofac Surg 47: 780–784

Lundh H, Westesson P-L 1989 Long-term follow-up after occlusal treatment to correct abnormal temporomandibular joint disk position. Oral Surg, Oral Med, Oral Pathol 67: 2–10

MacFarlane D 1990 Rheumatoid arthritis. Med Int 74: 3067–3072

McCain J P, de la Rue H, Le Blanc W G 1989 Correlation of clinical, radiographic and arthroscopic findings in internal derangements of the TMJ. J Oral Maxillofac Surg 47: 913–921

Mayne R 1989 Cartilage collagens. What is their function and are they involved in articular disease? Arthritis Rheumat 32: 241–246

Ohrbach R, Gross R 1989 Summary of the Workshop on Temporomandibular Joint Disorders sponsored by the American Dental Association. J Periodontal 60: 222–224

Quemar J C, Bernard A M, Akoka S et al 1989 Magnetic resonance imaging of the TMJ; identification of anatomic elements by controlled movement and application to normal and pathologic clinical situations. J Craniomandib Disord Facial Oral Pain 3: 30–24

Raveh J, Vuillemin T, Ladrach K, Sutter F 1989 Temporomandibular joint ankylosis: surgical treatment and long-term results. J Oral Maxillofacial Surg 47: 900–906

Ross R D, Williams R B, DiCosimo C J, Williams S V 1987 Gout and pseudogout of the temporomandibular joint. Oral Surg, Oral Med, Oral Pathol 63: 551–554

Tolvanen M, Oikarinen V J, Wolf J 1988 A 30-year follow-up study of temporomandibular joint meniscectomies: a report on five patients. Br J Oral Maxillofac Surg 26: 311–316

Wilkes C H 1989 Internal derangements of the temporomandibular joint. Arch Otolaryngol Head Neck Surg 115: 469–477

15. Stomatitis and related diseases

Stomatitis
Primary herpetic stomatitis
Herpes labialis
Hand, foot and mouth disease
Herpes zoster of the trigeminal nerve
Candida albicans infections
Clinical types of candidosis
Thrush
Chronic hyperplastic candidosis
Angular stomatitis
Denture stomatitis
Other causes of stomatitis
Secondary syphilis
The acute specific fevers
Stomatitis of unknown cause
Recurrent aphthae

Behçet's syndrome
Lichen planus
Pemphigus vulgaris
Mucous membrane pemphigoid
'Desquamative gingivitis'
Acute erythema multiforme
Other mucocutaneous disease
'Allergic' stomatitis
Fordyce's spots
Oral reactions to drugs
Isolated mucosal ulcers
Traumatic ulceration
Tuberculosis
Syphilis
Tongue disorders
Sore tongue and glossitis

Ulceration of the mouth may primarily affect the gingivae (acute ulcerative gingivitis), may be due to disease affecting the oral mucosa generally (stomatitis), or be a solitary lesion in an otherwise healthy mucosa, due, for instance, to local injury.

Stomatitis

The oral mucous membrane is an epithelial surface like the skin, and the many kinds of stomatitis are diseases that can affect both skin and mucous membranes. The main types are as follows.

1. *Infective stomatitis*
   a. *Viral infections*
      — Herpes simplex
      — Herpes zoster of the trigeminal area
      — Hand, foot and mouth disease
      — The acute specific fevers
   b. *Bacterial and mycotic infections*
      — Thrush and other *Candida albicans* infections
      — Secondary syphilis

2. *Non-infective stomatitis*
   —Recurrent aphthae
   —Lichen planus
   —Pemphigus vulgaris
   —Mucous membrane pemphigoid
   —Other mucocutaneous diseases
3. *Drug-associated stomatitis*
   —Local reactions
   —Systemically mediated reactions
4. *Isolated mucosal ulcers*. A solitary lesion may develop in an otherwise healthy mucous membrane; the causative factor is often local injury, or irritation such as the site of inoculation of a microorganism. The main examples are:
   —Trauma
   —Tuberculosis
   —Primary syphilis
   —Carcinoma (Ch. 16)
5. *Disorders of the tongue*. The tongue may be involved in stomatitis or may be the site of an isolated lesion such as a traumatic ulcer,

but in addition there are a few disorders peculiar to the tongue. These are:
— Glossitis
— Geographical tongue
— Furred tongue
— Black hairy tongue
— Median rhomboid glossitis.

These categories of mucosal lesions are somewhat arbitrary and, clinically at least, there is some overlap between them. Lichen planus and chronic candidosis can, for instance, produce leukoplakia-like lesions, while syphilis can produce an isolated lesion or generalised stomatitis according to its stage. However, it is important to try to clarify the distinctions between the main clinical groups of mucosal disease.

Primary herpetic stomatitis

The usual cause is herpes simplex virus Type 1. The primary infection is often in infancy or childhood and is an acute stomatitis characterised by painful ulcers preceded by vesicles.

After the primary infection there may be recurrent infections but these take a different form, *herpes labialis*.

Epidemiology

Transmission of herpes is by close contact such as from labial lesions. Occasionally, small outbreaks affect groups of children living closely together.

In countries with large, poor, urban communities with a low standard of living, up to 90% develop positive antibody titres to herpes during early childhood. In London, by contrast, the incidence of positive titres among 5 to 10 year olds has fallen from 60% in 1949 to 40% in 1969 and this trend is almost certainly continuing. Most recently a large study in Michigan of several hundred dental students and also staff showed positive antibody titres in only 25%.

Herpetic stomatitis is therefore increasingly seen in adolescents and adults and less often in young children.

Immunodeficiency, such as that arising from HIV infection, is a strong predisposing factor.

Pathology

The earliest recognisable lesion is the vesicle. It is sharply defined and intraepithelial. Its roof is several cells thick and, as a consequence, relatively strong. Intact vesicles are often therefore seen in the mouth.

In the floor of the vesicle, viral-infected epithelial cells can be seen. In smears, these cells have pleomorphic nuclei and are swollen and pale with the chromatin distributed as a thin rim round the periphery (ballooning degeneration). Giant cells containing many of these swollen nuclei form by incomplete division of the cytoplasm.

After the rupture of the vesicle there is a brief pre-ulcerative stage where the epithelium is intact, but in a restricted area shows extensive viral damage almost throughout the thickness of the epithelium.

Finally, the infected and dying cells are shed, leaving a sharply defined ulcer with inflammatory changes in the base.

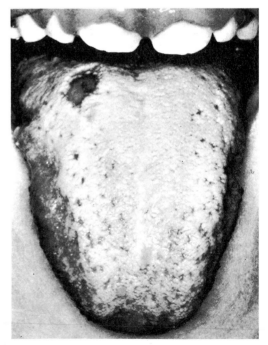

Fig. 15.1 Herpetic stomatitis. There are the characteristic red and swollen gingivae and an ulcer on the dorsum of the tongue; the latter is heavily furred in keeping with the febrile systemic upset.

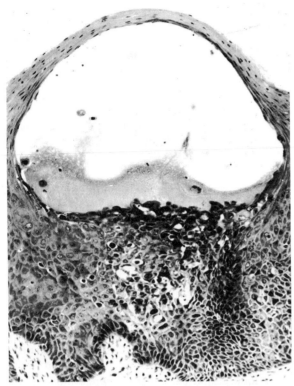

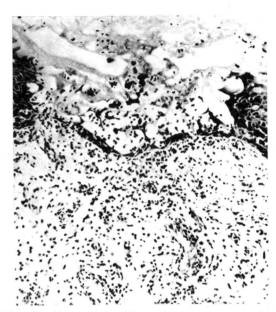

Fig. 15.3 Herpetic ulcer. The vesicle has ruptured, and destruction of the epithelium extends to the basement membrane. Infected cells are escaping from the floor of the ulcer (× 125).

Fig. 15.2 Herpetic vesicle. The vesicle is formed by accumulation of fluid within the prickle cell layer. The virus-infected cells, identifiable by their enlarged nuclei, can be seen in the floor of the vesicle and a few are floating freely in the vesicular fluid (× 125).

Clinical features

Herpetic stomatitis can be seen in infants, adolescents, or adults. The vesicles are distributed sparsely or densely on any part of the oral mucous membrane, but the hard palate and dorsum of the tongue are characteristic sites. The vesicles are circular, dome-shaped and usually 2–3 mm in diameter. Recently ruptured vesicles leave circular, sharply defined, yellowish, coin-shaped lesions and are followed by development of the ulcers. These are also circular, sharply defined, shallow with a yellowish or greyish floor and a red margin. The ulcers are painful and may interfere with eating and cause salivation.

The gingival margins are usually swollen and red, particularly in children. The regional lymph nodes are enlarged and tender. There is often fever and systemic upset, sometimes severe.

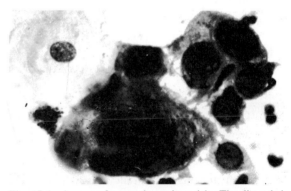

Fig. 15.4 A smear from an herpetic vesicle. The distended, degenerating nuclei of the epithelial cells are clustered together, forming giant cells with oedematous cytoplasm. A normal squamous cell is present on the left; the size and the chromatin pattern of the nucleus can be compared with those of the abnormal cells (× 600)

The oral lesions usually clear up within a week to 10 days but malaise may continue for a considerable time afterwards, and an adult may not recover fully for several weeks.

Herpetic stomatitis is contagious, and contact can lead to a finger infection, herpetic whitlow, in

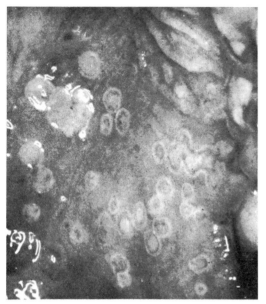

Fig. 15.5 Herpetic stomatitis. A group of recently ruptured vesicles are on the hard palate, a characteristic site. The individual lesions are of remarkably uniform size but several have coalesced to form larger irregular ulcers.

dental staff. Occasionally patients, in turn, have become infected from this source.

Herpetic stomatitis is common in AIDS or its prodromes, and in immunosuppressed patients.

Diagnosis

The characteristic clinical features which lead to the diagnosis are: (i) well-defined vesicles succeeded by ulcers; (ii) the involvement of any area of the oral mucous membrane; (iii) enlarged and tender lymph nodes, and usually febrile systemic upset.

The diagnosis may be confirmed by taking direct smears from an early lesion when viral-damaged nuclei showing ballooning degeneration or multinuleate cells should be found.

A rising titre of antibodies reaching a high level after 2 to 3 weeks provides absolute confirmation of the diagnosis.

Differential diagnosis

1. **Teething**. An infant who develops an acutely sore mouth during the course of eruption of the teeth usually has herpetic stomatitis. Acute generalised soreness of the mouth, especially associated with enlarged regional lymph nodes, is not the result of eruption of the teeth.

2. **Ulcerative gingivitis**. The ulcers of herpetic stomatitis may sometimes affect the tips of the interdental papillae and may as a consequence be mistaken for acute ulcerative gingivitis. However, the presence of vesicles and ulcers in other parts of the mouth together with the enlarged and tender cervical lymph nodes and systemic upset readily distinguish the two conditions. So-called Vincent's in children is almost invariably herpetic stomatitis. Acute ulcerative gingivitis is not seen in children in Britain.

3. **Herpes zoster**. The restricted distribution of the lesions and the symptoms are quite different, as discussed later. In zoster the first symptom is pain, not soreness, may resemble toothache, and usually precedes the appearance of the lesions.

4. **Recurrent aphthae**. The individual ulcers may closely resemble those of herpetic stomatitis, and there is usually a history of recurrent ulcers for a long period beforehand, there is no systemic upset and the regional lymph nodes are rarely enlarged. Vesicles are never seen, and the hard palate, dorsum of the tongue, and gingival margins are typically spared.

5. **Hand, foot and mouth disease**. In the vast majority of cases this is a much milder infection. Usually there are only one or two small scattered ulcers in the mouth and intact vesicles are rarely if ever seen. The regional lymph nodes are not involved, there is no associated gingivitis, and in addition the characteristic lesions may be found on the extremities.

Treatment

Acyclovir is a potent antiherpetic drug with low toxicity. Its effectiveness is shown by the fact that it is life-saving in herpetic encephalitis or disseminated infection. Acyclovir suspension used as a rinse and then swallowed should accelerate healing of herpetic stomatitis in severe cases and should be given as early as possible.

In AIDS or other immunodeficient patients, systemic acyclovir (tablets or intravenous injection) is advised.

Idoxuridine, an early antiherpetic agent is of questionable effectiveness.

In mild cases, tetracycline suspension as a mouthwash to be rinsed round the mouth several times a day may relieve pain and possibly hasten healing by reducing secondary infection.

Patients who are febrile should preferably be kept in bed and given a soft diet. Young infants readily become dehydrated during the painful stomatitis and may require rehydration.

Herpes labialis

After the primary infection the virus persists in latent form in the trigeminal ganglia and is reactivated by various factors. Neutralising antibodies are produced in response to the primary infection but they do not protect against recurrences.

20–30% of patients may be subject to recurrent infections. These recurrences are not within the mouth (except on exceedingly rare occasions) but affect the area around the lips. The lesions are familiarly known as *cold sores* or *fever blisters*. Recurrences of herpes labialis are precipitated by disturbances such as the common cold, fevers (particularly lobar pneumonia), exposure to sunshine, menstruation, emotional upsets, local irritation and probably other factors.

Clinical changes follow a consistent course. There are pricking or burning sensations in the site of the attack, which becomes red. This is followed within an hour or two by vesicles which often enlarge, coalesce and weep exudate. After 2

to 3 days the vesicles rupture, the raw area crusts over, but new vesicles may appear for a day or two.

The vesicles usually form in clusters at points along the mucocutaneous junction between the skin and the lip but may also spread to the upper lip below the nostrils.

The vesicles scab over and usually heal without scarring. The whole cycle may take up to ten days.

Treatment

Treatment with acyclovir cream should start as soon as the premonitory pricking or burning sensations are felt. However, viral damage is rapid, and this treatment may only slightly shorten the illness.

Hand, foot and mouth disease

This is a common mild viral infection often producing minor epidemics among school children. It is characterised by ulceration of the mouth and a vesicular rash on the extremities.

Hand, foot and mouth disease must be distinguished from foot and mouth disease of cattle, a rhinovirus infection, which rarely affects humans.

Pathology

Hand, foot and mouth disease is caused by strains of Coxsackie A virus. It is highly infectious

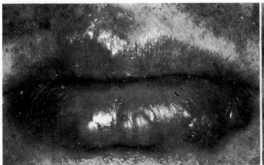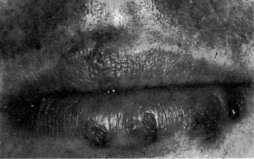

Fig. 15.6 Herpes labialis. The lesion is the same i.e. groups of vesicles, as in the primary infection but affecting the margins of the lips (left). Rupture of the vesicles leaves the typical crusted ulcers or 'cold sores' (rights).

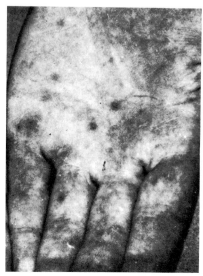

Fig. 15.7 Hand, foot and mouth disease. The rash consists of vesicles or bullae on the extremities; in this patient, a dental student, they consisted of small deep seated vesicles surrounded by erythema. The oral lesions resembled those of herpetic stomatitis.

and the incubation period is between 3 and 10 days. Microscopically there is viral damage of the epithelium, followed by vesiculation and ulceration.

Clinical features

The stomatitis consists of small scattered ulcers which are much less painful than those of herpes simplex. Vesicles are rarely seen, and the gingivae are not affected. The regional lymph nodes are rarely enlarged, and systemic upset is mild or absent.

The rash consists of vesicles, which are sometimes deep seated, or occasionally bullae, mainly seen around the base of the phalanges of the hands or feet but any part of the limbs may be affected. The rash is often the most noticeable feature, and in some cases the mouth or extremities alone may be affected. Many patients therefore go to their doctor rather than to a dentist.

The stomatitis and rash usually clear up within a week.

The main features differentiating this disease from herpetic stomatitis are that in hand, foot and mouth disease there are (a) usually reports of several cases, (b) signs and symptoms are mild, and (c) a characteristic rash affects the extremities.

There is no specific treatment, and it is hardly needed.

Herpes zoster of the trigeminal nerve

Zoster (shingles) is a viral infection characterised by pain, a vesicular rash and stomatitis in the area of distribution of a sensory nerve.

Pathology

The varicella zoster virus (VZV) causes chickenpox in the non-immune (mainly children), while zoster appears to be a reactivation of the latent virus and thus comparable with herpes labialis. Unlike the latter, however, there is usually only a single episode of zoster.

In a minority the appearance of zoster is an indication of an underlying immunologic defect, and is a recognised early manifestation of HIV infection, Hodgkin's disease, or (less often) other tumours.

The zoster virus produces similar epithelial lesions to those of herpes simplex, but in addition causes acute inflammation of the posterior root ganglion of affected nerves. This can cause severe pain and sometimes persistent disturbance of sensation in the affected area.

Clinical features

Herpes zoster usually affects adults, often of middle age or over. The first sign is pain and irritation or tenderness in the skin area corresponding to the nerves affected. Malaise and fever usually also develop. The pain may be severe and sometimes completely indistinguishable from toothache by the patient.

After a few days vesicles appear on one side of the face and within the mouth up to the midline. The regional lymph nodes are enlarged and tender. The pain continues until the lesions crust over and start to heal. This acute phase usually lasts about a week. Secondary infection may cause suppuration and scarring of the skin.

The fact that patients are often unable to distinguish the pain of trigeminal zoster from toothache

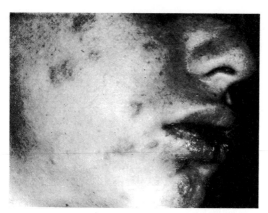

Fig. 15.8

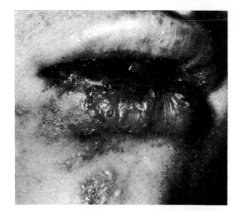

Fig. 15.9

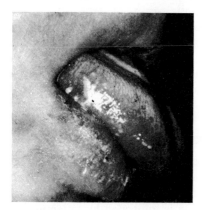

Fig. 15.10

Figs 15.8, 15.9 and 15.10 Herpes zoster of the trigeminal nerve. The distribution of the lesions is within the area of the 2nd and 3rd division; both skin and oral mucous membrane are affected; the lesions stop sharply at the midline and consist of groups of thin-walled vesicles. On the skin the ruptured vesicles crust over and in the mouth form shallow ulcers. There was severe pain and the patient was febrile and unwell.

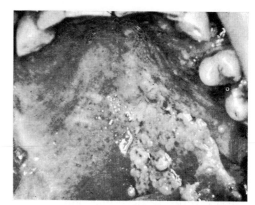

Fig. 15.11 Herpes zoster. A severe attack in an older person shows confluent lesions on the hard and soft palate of one side.

has often led to a demand for a tooth to be extracted. When this is done the rash follows in the normal course of events and this has given rise to the myth that dental extractions can precipitate facial zoster.

Characteristic features which distinguish herpes zoster from herpes simplex and other types of stomatitis are:

1. Severe pain (usually) preceding the rash
2. Facial rash accompanying the stomatitis and
3. Localisation of the lesions to one side and within the distribution of the second and third divisions of the trigeminal nerve.

Management

Oral acyclovir (200 mg, 8 times daily, usually for 5 days) should be given at the earliest possible moment. Analgesics should also be given. In severe cases, intravenous acyclovir is required as zoster in an elderly patient can cause a debilitating illness. Intravenous acyclovir should also be given to immunodeficient patients, especially those with AIDS—in whom herpes zoster is potentially lethal.

Post-herpetic neuralgia

This complication mainly affects the elderly. The pain can be almost as severe as trigeminal neuralgia, but is persistent rather than paroxysmal and does not respond to carbamazepine. Very early high-dose acyclovir has been reported to reduce the risk of this complication. Otherwise analgesics may be of some help, or transcutaneous electrical stimulation may be effective, but there is no consistently reliable treatment.

CANDIDA ALBICANS INFECTIONS (CANDIDOSIS)

The best known type of candidal infection is thrush, but both acute and chronic forms of infections are seen, and the mouth is one of the most commonly affected sites.

In addition to superficial infections *Candida albicans* can also cause systemic infections. These are uncommon but severe and often fatal. They are of particular importance because of their frequency as a complication of immunosuppressive or cytotoxic treatment or of cardiac surgery and other invasive procedures.

Mycology

Candida albicans is a yeast-like fungus which is strongly Gram-positive. It exists as yeast cells which reproduce by budding but, in the tissues especially, forms hyphae which invade the epithelial cells. These Gram-positive hyphae can be seen, often in large numbers, in direct smears from lesions such as thrush and also in sections of infected tissues.

Candida albicans is found as a commensal in up to 40% of normal mouths. The fungus is capable of causing disease in patients whose resistance is diminished. Local factors, such as the wearing of dentures and smoking, help to promote the infection. In addition there are patients who are susceptible to persistent candidal infections who remain in otherwise good health and where the factors determining their susceptibility to this infection are less clear.

Candida albicans is resistant to the commonly used antibacterial antibiotics, and broad-spectrum antibiotics in particular, such as tetracycline, may promote candidal infection.

Clinical types of candidosis

Candida albicans infections of the mucous membrane are characterised by plaque formation due to epithelial proliferation. The main forms, which are distinct both clinically and histologically, are:

1. *Acute oral candidosis.* Thrush.
2. *Chronic oral candidosis.* Chronic hyperplastic candidosis (candidal leukoplakia (see Ch. 16).
3. *Denture-associated candidosis.* Denture stomatitis.
4. *Angular stomatitis* (angular cheilitis). This lesion is common to, and can be seen in association with, any type of oral candidosis. In clinical practice it is most commonly associated with denture stomatitis. It has been shown, however, that angular stomatitis can be caused by other organisms than *Candida albicans*, as discussed later.

Thrush

Thrush, an acute infection by *Candida albicans*, is characterised by soft creamy-yellow patches which form on the surface of the oral mucous membrane.

Aetiological factors

These include
1. Altered physiology—infancy and pregnancy
2. Antibiotic treatment (especially tetracyclines)
3. Immunosuppressive treatment
4. Natural immune defects; congenital or the result of disease particularly AIDS
5. Unknown factors (some apparently healthy adults).

Pathology

The patches of thrush are produced by invasion of the surface by *Candida albicans* and proliferation of superficial epithelium, forming a thick plaque. The plaque is infiltrated by inflammatory oedema and leucocytes which separate the epithelial cells from one another (Fig. 15.13). As a result of this fluid and cellular infiltrate, the plaque is soft, friable and easily rubbed off the underlying mucous membrane. The deeper epithelium is hyperplastic and inflammatory cells infiltrate the connective tissue.

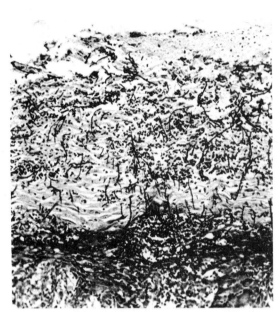

Fig. 15.12 Thrush. The plaque (the clinical white patch) consists of epithelial cells invaded by hyphae of *Candida albicans*, seen as darkly staining threads. The epithelium is infiltrated by inflammatory cells and oedema, most intense at the junction with the deeper epithelium (× 125).

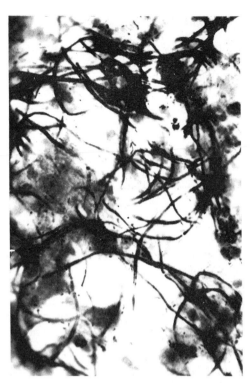

Fig. 15.14 Direct smear from thrush. The tangled mass of Gram-positive hyphae of *Candida albicans* is diagnostic. A few yeast cells may be present as well, but it is the large number of hyphae which is important.

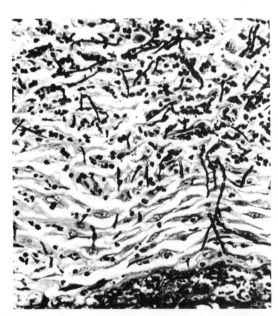

Fig. 15.13 Thrush. At higher power the components of the plaque can be clearly seen, viz. proliferating epithelium, fungal hyphae and inflammatory cells. The epithelium cells are separated by inflammatory oedema, making it clear why the plaque is so soft and friable (× 300).

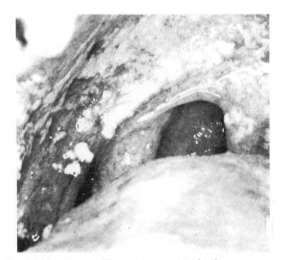

Fig. 15.15 Thrush. The lesions consist of soft, creamy patches lying superficially on an erythematous mucosa. On the palate the patches are becoming confluent.

Clinical features

The superficial plaques of thrush are soft and creamy-yellow, and are seen in such sites as the buccal mucous membrane or soft palate. The lesions vary from small flecks to confluent plaques covering a wide area.

One of the most characteristic features of the plaques of thrush is that they can be rubbed off, leaving a red area of mucosa. Symptoms are usually slight and include such complaints as dryness or roughness of the mucosa. Extension of the infection into the pharynx may cause a sore throat.

Thrush is one of the most common early manifestations of AIDS.

The diagnosis is readily confirmed by a smear from one of these patches. This shows great numbers of Gram-positive candidal hyphae and detached epithelial cells. The mere presence of yeast forms or a few hyphae is not diagnostic.

Acute antibiotic stomatitis

This may follow the use of antibiotics topically in the mouth or prolonged heavy doses of broad-spectrum drugs such as tetracycline.

It is characterised by a red, oedematous and sore mucous membrane, often with angular stomatitis.

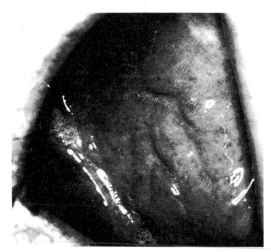

Fig. 15.16 Antibiotic stomatitis. The mucosa is red, swollen with oedema, and sore. Flecks of thrush can often be found in protected situations, and angular stomatitis is often also present (see also Fig. 15.52).

Flecks of thrush may be obvious or may only be found in protected situations such as the upper buccal sulcus.

In the past this reaction was thought to be either hypersensitivity to penicillin or vitamin B deficiency induced by interference by the antibiotic with the gut flora. There is no evidence that either is the case. *Candida albicans* can be isolated, and the condition responds rapidly to anti-candidal treatment.

Acute antibiotic stomatitis is much less commonly seen now, because of greater restraint in the use of antibiotics.

Management

Thrush was described in the 19th century as 'a disease of the diseased'. This has been abundantly confirmed by its frequent association with AIDS. When an apparently healthy patient is affected, therefore, the possibility of immunodeficiency should be considered, and latent systemic disease must be excluded by physical and laboratory examination. Haematological investigation, particularly for iron deficiency, is also important. When no underlying cause can be found, thrush responds to the use of nystatin lozenges (500 units each) allowed to dissolve in the mouth 3 times a day. Amphotericin lozenges are also effective. Thrush in infants may be treated by dropping a suspension of nystatin or amphotericin into the mouth.

In the case of a seriously ill patient, such as those with HIV infection, more potent antifungals such as ketoconazole are indicated.

Acute antibiotic stomatitis usually resolves when the antibiotic is stopped. If, however, it persists or antibiotic treatment has to be continued, nystatin or amphotericin should be used.

Chronic hyperplastic candidosis (Candidal leukoplakia)

See Chapter 16.

Angular stomatitis

Angular stomatitis is a recognised sign of iron deficiency anaemia but can be associated with any

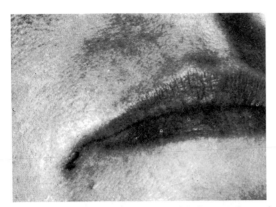

Fig. 15.17 Angular stomatitis. The epithelium at the angle of the mouth has broken down and there is an inflamed linear lesion covered by a crust but liable to bleed if stretched. The patient, though a young woman, was edentulous and had denture stomatitis. It can be seen that there are no folds at the angle of the mouth; the primary reservoir of infection is under the upper denture. The lesions cleared up with the topical antifungal treatment.

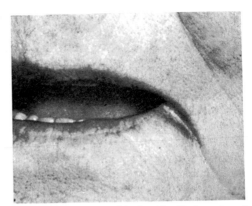

Fig. 15.18 Angular stomatitis. In this elderly patient there is a deep fold at the angle of the mouth. This does not in itself cause trouble but, should it become infected by *Candida albicans* from denture stomatitis, inflammation can spread along the length of the fold.

type of candidal infection of the mouth and is the only feature common to all types of oral candidosis.

Among dental patients angular stomatitis is most often associated with denture stomatitis but in all patients where candidosis is the cause of angular stomatitis the reservoir of infection is in the mouth and it is the intraoral infection that needs to be treated.

Angular stomatitis has also been shown in some patients to be staphylococcal or to be a mixed infection, hence bacteriological examination by a swab of the infected area is necessary. Angular stomatitis as an isolated lesion with an otherwise normal mouth seems to be more often due to staphylococci, which are probably carried in the nasal cavity. Angular stomatitis associated with denture stomatitis is usually candidal in nature.

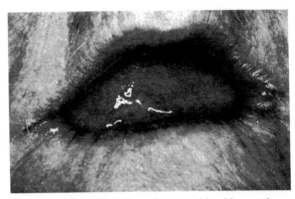

Fig. 15.19 Treatment of angular stomatitis with nystatin. In this elderly lady there are moderately severe lesions in the folds at the angles of the mouth, especially on the left where there has been some inflammatory thickening. Severe denture stomatitis was present.

Clinical features

Angular stomatitis varies from mere reddening at the angles of the mouth to ulcerated and crusted fissures. It is common in older patients who have full upper and lower dentures. Many of these patients have, as a result of age changes in the face, deep folds at the angles of the mouth. Infec-

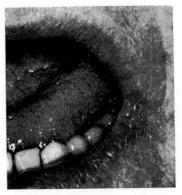

Fig. 15.20 The same patient after a course of nystatin lozenges shows complete healing and abolition of inflammatory changes.

tion and inflammation can spread along these skin creases and therefore become more extensive and conspicuous. The legend has therefore grown up that deep folds at the angles of the mouth are due to an 'overclosed bite' and that these cause angular stomatitis. There is *no* evidence that this is the case, and casual observation of denture patients will show that sagging of the facial tissues and, usually, a skin crease at the angles of the mouth is an almost invariable accompaniment of ageing, whether or not the patient is wearing dentures. These skin creases are not inflamed except in a small minority of patients. By contrast younger patients, including children, who develop intraoral candidosis frequently develop angular stomatitis even though they have no skin crease at the angles of the mouth.

Management

Bacteriological investigation should be carried out. When, as is usually the case, there is intraoral candidosis it is essential to eliminate this source of infection, as discussed below. Local applications of antifungal or other drugs to the angle of the mouth are then unnecessary and have at best a temporary effect as a result of reinfection by the saliva.

In staphylococcal infections an effective drug is fucidin ointment, but it may be necessary also to try and eliminate nasal carriage by treating the nasal cavity similarly.

When there are mixed staphylococcal and candidal infections, both need to be treated. Miconazole, like other imidazoles, has antibacterial as well as antifungal activity and may be effective.

When deep folds are present at the angles of the mouth, dentures with inadequate vertical dimension should obviously be corrected. Much more often the vertical dimension is adequate and cannot be changed.

Riboflavin deficiency can also cause angular stomatitis but is hardly ever seen in this country except rarely in patients with malabsorption syndrome. The commonly seen cases of angular stomatitis do not therefore benefit from being given B group vitamins.

Denture stomatitis

Denture stomatitis is an iatrogenic disease, in that its development is dependent on the prolonged occlusion of the oral mucous membrane by a close-fitting denture. Enclosure of mucous membrane

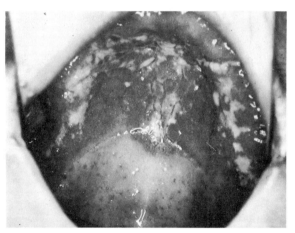

Fig. 15.21 Denture stomatitis. The clear demarcation between the erythema of the denture-bearing area and the pallor of the palate behind the post dam line is clearly seen. The white areas are plaques of thrush also localised to the denture-bearing area. The patient was iron and folate deficient; the candidal infection could be controlled only by remedying these deficiencies.

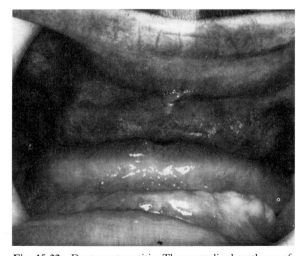

Fig. 15.22 Denture stomatitis. The generalised erythema of the upper denture-bearing area is in striking contrast to the normal lower ridge. A smear from the palatal mucosa showed hyphae of *Candida albicans*, and culture was also positive.

by the denture provides a protected environment which favours growth of this fungus. Any irritant metabolic products produced by the organism are also kept in close contact with the mucous membrane by this means. It is perhaps more surprising that so many patients can wear a denture, literally day and night, for periods of 20 or more years without ill-effects.

Some experimental work has suggested that acrylic dentures themselves favour the growth of *Candida albicans* and that the fungus may grow in the surface of the denture in microscopic pores or irregularities rather than on the oral mucous membrane itself. Smears taken from either the denture or the denture-bearing mucous membrane sometimes show long coiled masses of candidal hyphae, suggesting that the organism proliferates in the interface between denture and mucous membrane.

Denture stomatitis is virtually only seen under an upper denture and, because the lower denture usually fits very much less closely, is continually being lifted by the muscles of mastication and allows a free flow of saliva between the denture and the denture-bearing area.

Clinical features

Denture stomatitis is usually symptomless, and the alternative name 'denture sore mouth' is inappropriate. The feature which often draws attention to denture stomatitis is associated angular stomatitis.

The characteristic appearance of denture stomatitis is an area of bright, uniform erythema exactly corresponding to, and precisely limited by, the upper denture-bearing area. A sharp line of demarcation between the redness of denture stomatitis and normal mucosal pallor is seen at the posterior border of the denture. In more severe cases there is oedema of the upper denture-bearing mucosa and the palate is indented along the line of the posterior border of the denture.

Smears from the palate show hyphae of *Candida albicans*. Culture is also positive.

Angular stomatitis is often associated but is remittant and may not be present when the patient is first seen. A history of cracks or sores at the angle of the mouth should therefore be enquired into. A deep fold at the angles of the mouth (as mentioned earlier) caused by sagging of the facial muscles after middle age is often also present but it is not an essential predisposing factor.

A few of these patients are suffering from iron deficiency and this should be investigated, especially when angular stomatitis is present.

Denture stomatitis is sometimes said to be due to denture 'trauma' or to hypersensitivity to denture base material. There is no evidence for these ideas or that denture materials such as polymethylmethacrylate can produce a contact hypersensitivity reaction in the mouth. Positive patch tests on the skin reported in the past have been due to faulty testing procedure.

Management

Vigorous antifungal treatment should be given. The patient should stop wearing the denture (except for social occasions) to allow the drug access to the infected area, and suck nystatin lozenges (3 a day for 2 weeks). Alternatively, or in addition, miconazole gel can be applied to the denture while it is being worn. The denture should be kept scrupulously clean by scrubbing the fitting surface with a hard brush and soap and water. The denture should be kept in an antiseptic such as 1% sodium hypochlorite and should not be worn at night.

Any underlying disorder such as iron deficiency must be treated. Occasionally such treatment is followed by clearance of the candidal infection without any direct antifungal measures.

OTHER CAUSES OF STOMATITIS

Secondary syphilis

In the secondary stage of syphilis there is sometimes stomatitis associated with a rash, enlarged lymph nodes, and fever, as discussed later.

The acute specific fevers

The fevers which cause a vesicular rash (smallpox and chickenpox) cause the same lesions in the mouth, especially when infection is severe.

In the prodromal stage of measles, Koplik's spots may be seen on the buccal mucosa and are pathognomonic of the disease. They consist of tiny white spots on a bright red base. These acute fevers are rarely seen in dentistry.

Palatal petechiae or ulceration, involving the fauces especially, are sometimes a feature of glandular fever and are associated with the characteristic and usually widespread glandular enlargement.

STOMATITIS OF UNKNOWN CAUSE

Recurrent aphthae (aphthous stomatitis)

Recurrent aphthae constitute the most common oral mucosal disease and affect approximately 10% of the population, but many cases are so mild as to give rise to no complaint.

Etiology

Any theories as to etiology have to explain the following characteristic features of the disease:

1. Most patients are otherwise healthy
2. An onset frequently in childhood, a peak in adolescence or early adult life
3. Its self-limiting nature in most cases
4. Intermittent attacks at variable but sometimes fairly regular intervals.

That speculation about the cause of recurrent aphthae has continued for at least half a century, and the variety of current theories, are indicative of how little is known. However, the main factors thought to contribute to the etiology include the following:

1. Genetic predisposition
2. Trauma
3. Infections
4. Immunological abnormalities
5. Gastrointestinal diseases
6. Haematological deficiencies
7. Hormonal factors
8. Stress.

1. Genetic factors. There is some evidence for a genetic predisposition to aphthae. The family history is sometimes positive and the disease appears to affect identical twins more frequently than non-identical. However, this appears only to apply to a minority of patients. A variety of HLA associations have been reported but no one haplotype seems to be consistently associated. In the possibly related Behcet's syndrome (discussed below) the evidence for a genetic predisposition is much stronger.

2. Trauma. Some patients think that the ulcers result from trauma because the early symptoms simulate pricking of the mucosa by (for instance) a toothbrush bristle. Trauma may dictate the site of ulcers in patients who already have the disorder, but most aphthae are in relatively protected sites. It is noteworthy that the masticatory mucosa is generally spared.

3. Infections. There is no evidence that aphthae are directly due to any microbes, and there is scanty evidence that cross-reacting antigens from streptococci or L-forms play any significant role. The hypothesis that there may be defective immunoregulation by herpes or other viruses is unproven.

4. Immunological abnormalities. Since the etiology of recurrent aphthae is unknown there is a facile tendency to label them as 'autoimmune'. As a consequence a great variety of immunological abnormalities have been reported. However, there have been almost as many contrary findings and no convincing theory of immunopathogenesis that takes into account the clinical features. It is also possible that the immunological abnormalities are as much a consequence of the ulcers as the cause.

Evidence of an association with atopic (IgE mediated) disease is unconfirmed. Circulating antibodies to crude extracts of fetal oral mucosa have been reported, but their titre is unrelated to the severity of the disease and in many patients there are no significant changes in immunoglobulin levels. Antibody-dependent cytotoxic mechanisms have been postulated but not convincingly demonstrated.

The histological features of aphthae (as discussed below) have also been invoked to support hypotheses that the disease is either an immune complex-mediated (type III) or a cell-mediated (type IV) reaction according to taste. However, later workers have failed to confirm the presence of circulating immune complexes, and in any case the significance of such complexes, which are sometimes detectable in the absence of disease, is notoriously difficult to interpret.

Reduced circulating, helper/suppressor T lymphocyte ratios have been reported but other workers have found no difference between active and remittant phases of the disorder.

Recurrent aphthae also lack virtually all features and any association with typical autoimmune diseases (Ch. 20). They also fail to respond reliably to immunosuppressive drugs and may become more severe in the immune deficiency state induced by HIV.

5. Gastrointestinal disease. Though these ulcers were at one time known as 'dyspeptic ulcers' they are only rarely associated with gastrointestinal disease and, when they are, it is usually because of a deficiency, particularly of vitamin B12 or folate secondary to malabsorption. An association with coeliac disease (sometimes asymptomatic) has been found in approximately 5% of patients with aphthae, but it is likely that a secondary haematinic deficiency, particularly folate deficiency, is the main factor.

6. Haematological deficiency states. Deficiencies of vitamin B12, folate, or iron have been reported in up to 20% of patients with aphthae. Such deficiencies are probably more frequent in patients whose aphthae start or worsen in middle age or later. In many such patients, the deficiency is latent, the haemoglobin is within normal limits, and the main sign is abnormalities of erythrocyte morphology. In patients who thus prove to be vitamin B12 or folate deficient, remedying the deficiency can cause dramatically rapid resolution of the ulcers.

7. Hormonal factors. In a few women, aphthae are associated with the stressful luteal phase of the menstrual cycle, but there is no strong evidence that hormone treatment is reliably effective.

8. 'Stress'. Some patients relate exacerbations of ulceration to times of stress, and some studies have reported a correlation. However, stress is notoriously difficult to quantify, and the most recent study has found no correlation.

In brief, therefore, the etiology of recurrent aphthae is unclear. There is no evidence that they are a form of autoimmune disease in any accepted sense, and it is uncertain whether many of the reported immunological abnormalities are cause or effect. However, in a minority of patients there is a clear association with haematological deficiencies. The latter in turn may be secondary to small-intestine disease or other cause of malabsorption.

Clinical features

Females are not significantly more frequently affected than males. The onset is frequently in childhood or adolescence and may reach a peak in early adult life or a little later, then gradually wanes. Recurrent aphthae are rare in the elderly and the edentulous. However, older persons may be affected if a haematological deficiency develops. The great majority of patients are clerical, semiprofessional, or professional workers and are total non-smokers. Occasionally the onset of aphthae is dated from when smoking was given up.

The usual history is of painful ulcers recurring at intervals of approximately 3 to 4 weeks or, less often, are continuously present. Unpredictable remissions of several months may be noted. Individual minor aphthae persist for 7 to 10 days then heal without scarring.

With few exceptions aphthae affect only the nonkeratinised mucosa such as the buccal mucosa, sulcuses, or lateral borders of the tongue.

Ulcers are of three clinically distinguishable types, as follows.

1. *Minor aphthae* are the common type, are usually shallow, rounded, 5 to 7 mm across, with an erythematous margin and yellowish floor. More severe inflammatory oedema may occasionally raise the margins and cause the ulcer to appear cratered. One or several ulcers at varying stages of development may be present.

2. *Herpetiform aphthae* are uncommon. They are 1–2 mm across but are so numerous as often to be uncountable and can coalesce to form larger more irregular ulcers. Their borders are less sharply defined than those of minor aphthae and there is widespread bright erythema round them.

3. *Major aphthae* are also uncommon. The ulcers are frequently several centimetres across and sometimes so deeply destructive as to mimic a carcinoma. They persist for several months, so that new ulcers appear before earlier ones have healed. Unlike minor aphthae the masticatory mucosa

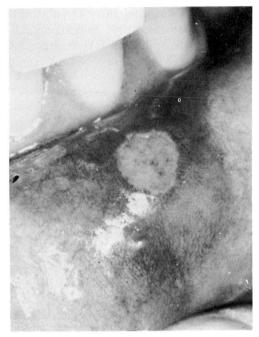

Fig. 15.23 Aphthous stomatitis. This typical rounded ulcer has sharply defined margins, a pale floor and surrounding erythema.

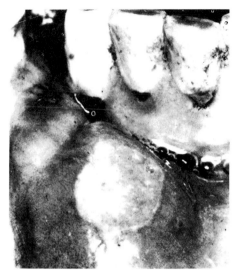

Fig. 15.25 Major aphthae. In this rare severe form of recurrent aphthae the ulcers are usually over 1 cm in diameter as here and each usually persists for several months.

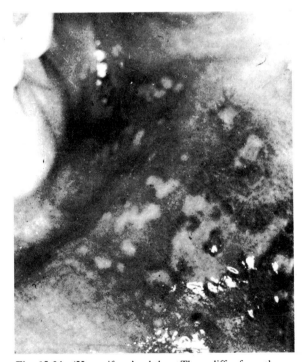

Fig. 15.24 'Herpetiform' aphthae. These differ from the commoner type of recurrent aphthae seen in Fig. 15.23. They are much more numerous and shallower; the ulcers are either small or coalesce to form large irregular lesions. The widespread erythema is also characteristic.

such as the dorsum of the tongue or occasionally the gingivae are involved. Healing in the most severe cases leaves visible scarring. The pain that such large ulcers inevitably cause can interfere with eating, but many that suffer from them do not lose weight or deteriorate in health. However, major aphthae are sometimes a feature of AIDS and add to such patients' burdens.

Microscopically there is said to be initial lymphocytic infiltration followed by destruction of the epithelium and infiltration of the tissues by neutrophils. Mononuclear cells may also surround blood vessels (perivascular cuffing). These changes are said to be consistent with either type III or IV reactions, but vasculitis is more frequently described than seen. The appearances overall can hardly be said to be anything other than nonspecific, and biopsy is of no value in the diagnosis of recurrent aphthae and is only of value in the case of major aphthae to exclude more dangerous diseases.

Diagnosis and management

The most important feature is the history of recurrences of self-healing ulcers at more or less regular intervals often for a period of months or years. The only other disease with this history is Behçet's

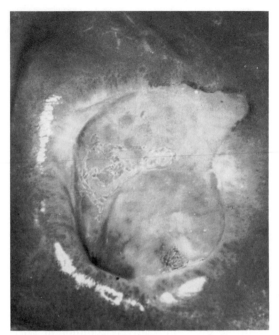

Fig. 15.26 Major aphthae. The same lesion as in the previous picture, 6 weeks later, showing fibrosis beginning to draw the edges downward. The ulcer took more than 3 months to heal and left an obvious scar.

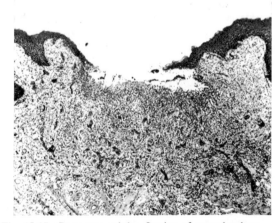

Fig. 15.27 Recurrent aphtha. Section of an early ulcer showing the break in the epithelium, the inflammatory cells in the floor and the inflammatory changes more deeply where dilated vessels can be seen ($\times$ 45).

syndrome. In many cases, increasing frequency of ulcers brings the patient to seek treatment. Otherwise most patients appear well, but haematological investigation is particularly important in older patients, as mentioned earlier. Routine blood indices are informative, and usually the most important finding is an abnormal mean corpuscular volume (MCV). If macro- or microcytosis is present then further investigation is necessary to find and remedy the cause. Treatment of vitamin B12 deficiency (usually pernicious anaemia) or folate deficiency is sometimes sufficient to control or abolish aphthae.

Apart from the minority with underlying systemic disease, treatment of recurrent aphthae is empirical and palliative only. Despite reports of the effectiveness of a variety of agents, even those reported to be effective on the basis of apparently adequately controlled trials, none can be confidently relied upon to have the desired effect. It is important therefore to emphasise to patients that the trouble cannot be cured but can usually be alleviated and that it is virtually certain to resolve sooner or later of its own accord.

Corticosteroids. Some patients get relief from the use of Corlan (hydrocortisone hemisuccinate 2.5 mg) pellets allowed to dissolve in the mouth 3 times a day. There is no reason to suppose that corticosteroids hasten the healing of ulcers once formed, hence the most rational form of treatment is for the patient to take these pellets continuously (whether or not ulcers are present) to enable the corticosteroid to act in the very early stages of ulcer formation before the patient is aware of them. This form of treatment is only applicable to those who have frequent ulcers (at 2- or 3-week intervals or more frequently). Such a regime should be tried for 2 months then stopped for a month to assess whether there has been any improvement and whether there is any deterioration without treatment.

Triamcinolone dental paste is a corticosteroid in a vehicle which sticks to the moist mucosa. When correctly applied the vehicle absorbs moisture and forms an adhesive gel which can remain in place for one or several hours but it is exceedingly difficult to apply a fragment of this paste to the ulcer and then to get it to adhere effectively. It is only of use when a patient has infrequent ulcers, when the ulcers tend to be mainly in the front of the mouth and in patients dextrous enough to be able to follow the instructions.

This gel should form a protective layer over the ulcer to help make it comfortable. In addition the corticosteroid is slowly released and (it is hoped) has an anti-inflammatory action.

Systemic effects of topical corticosteroids. Topically applied corticosteroids, particularly when used in large quantities on the skin, can have detectable and sometimes severe effects on adrenal function. There is no evidence, however, that the topical corticosteroids at present available for use in the mouth depress adrenal function. Even continuous use of Corlan pellets, as described above, is acceptable, but interruption to assess the effect of treatment can also be regarded as a safety measure.

Tetracycline mouth rinses. There is no obvious rationale for this treatment, but controlled trials both in Britain and the USA have shown that tetracycline rinses significantly reduce both the frequency and severity of aphthae. The tetracycline may be used in combination with an antifungal agent (Mysteclin syrup) in patients who are susceptible to superinfection by *Candida albicans*. This is a convenient and pleasant-flavoured preparation. Otherwise tetracycline mixture can be used (250 mg of tetracycline in 10 ml of fluid). This should be held in the mouth for 2 to 3 minutes 3 times daily as soon as it seems likely to the patient that a crop of ulcers is developing. Some patients feel it helpful to use the mouth bath regularly for 3 days each week if they have frequent ulcers.

Chlorhexidine. A 0.2% solution has also been used as a mouth rinse for aphthae. Used 3 times daily after meals and held in the mouth for a period of at least 1 minute, it has been shown to reduce the duration and discomfort of aphthous stomatitis to some degree. Zinc sulphate or zinc chloride solutions may also have a slight beneficial effect.

Topical salicylate preparations. Salicylates have an anti-inflammatory action and also have local effects. Preparations of choline salicylate in a gel can be applied to aphthae. These preparations, which are available over the counter, are thought to be helpful by some patients with mild aphthous stomatitis.

Treatment of major aphthae

Major aphthae present a special problem because of their painfulness and persistence. Isolated major aphthae are as difficult to treat as those associated with Behçet's syndrome or with HIV infection. Treatments that have been reported to be effective include thalidomide, azathioprine, cyclosporin, colchicine and dapsone. All of these are toxic in varying degrees, and their use is rarely justified for major aphthae in otherwise healthy persons who are not made desperate by their oral ulcers.

Behçet's syndrome

Behçet's syndrome comprises oral aphthae, genital ulceration and ocular lesions, particularly uveitis. It is a multisystem disease and, in addition to mucocutaneous and ocular, arthritic and neurological types are recognised. The central nervous system is involved in up to 25% of patients and this is potentially lethal. Thrombophlebitis is also a recognised but overall less common manifestation.

Behçet's syndrome is rare in Britain and most parts of the USA but relatively common in Turkey (Behçet was a Turk) and so common in Japan that its prevalence in the individual prefectures has been mapped. This racial distribution suggests a strong genetic component, and there appears to be an association of HLA B12 with the mucocutaneous type, HLA B5 with the ocular, and HLA B27 with the arthritic type.

The oral aphthae of Behçet's syndrome are not distinguishable from those described earlier; they are the most consistently found feature and are frequently the first manifestation. As a result Behçet's syndrome should be considered in the differential diagnosis of aphthous stomatitis. The frequency of other manifestations is highly variable. As a result there are no absolute criteria or reliable tests for the diagnosis of Behçet's syndrome.

Because arthritis is a common minor manifestation, Behçet's syndrome is frequently classified with the rheumatic (connective tissue) diseases. However, unlike the latter, males are predominantly affected.

Lichen planus

Lichen planus is a common chronic inflammatory disease of skin and mucous membranes. It mainly affects patients of middle age or over, especially women.

Aetiology

In spite of histological changes which may be highly characteristic and specific, the aetiology of lichen planus remains problematical.

Immunological mechanisms have (of course) been suggested, particularly in view of the predominantly lymphocytic infiltration. These suggest the possibility of immunological damage brought about by a cell-mediated immune reaction. This therefore remains a possibility, but tests of cellular immune responses to extracts of skin lesions of lichen planus have produced inconclusive results so far. Nor has it been possible to demonstrate humoral or lymphocytotoxic mechanisms. Progress in this field has been surprisingly slow.

The fact that a disease indistinguishable from lichen planus can be induced by certain drugs, notably gold and anti-malarial agents, remains unexplained.

Some studies have shown that lichen planus may be associated with an unusually high incidence of glucose intolerance or diabetes mellitus or, on the other hand, with rheumatoid arthritis. These observations have not been generally confirmed.

The long-held view that lichen planus is associated with emotional stress is difficult to evaluate or substantiate.

Lichen planus in graft-versus-host disease. Oral lichen planus is a virtually invariable feature of graft-versus-host disease (Ch. 20) and an early sign of this reaction.

Pathology

The lesions are of three types:

1. White lesions (striae)
2. Atrophic areas
3. Erosions.

These are distinct clinically and histologically.

The 'classical' features are characteristic and can be summarised as follows:

1. A saw-tooth profile of the rete ridges
2. Liquefaction degeneration of the basal cell layer
3. A band-like infiltrate of mononuclear cells which hugs the dermo-epidermal junction.

Striae show hyperkeratosis or parakeratosis, and the granular cell layer may be prominent. The rete pegs tend to be pointed and saw-tooth in shape. Along the junction between the epithelium and connective tissue there may be degeneration and liquefaction with beads of fluid accumulating along the basement membrane. The basal cell layer is not usually identifiable as such.

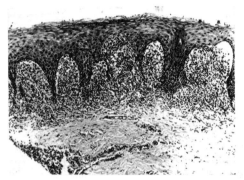

Fig. 15.28 Lichen planus. The characteristic features to be seen are the 'saw-tooth' form of the epithelial ridges ('rete pegs') and the compact band-like zone of chronic inflammatory cells having a clearly defined lower border but extending up close under the epithelium (× 50).

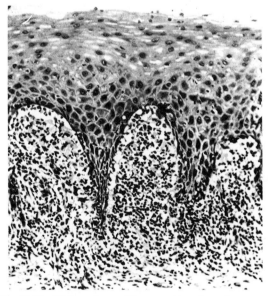

Fig. 15.29 Lichen planus. The rete ridges have the characteristic pointed (saw-tooth) outline. The liquefaction degeneration along the basal cell layer and lymphocytic infiltrate can also be seen.

In the connective tissue the infiltrate consists mainly of lymphocytes, close beneath the epithelium in a band-like distribution. These inflammatory cells form a compact zone which hugs the dermo-epidermal junction and has a well-defined lower border.

Atrophic lesions show severe thinning of the epithelium, but the inflammatory infiltrate often retains its characteristic distribution.

Erosions are characterised by destruction of the epithelium, leaving only the granulating connective tissue floor of the lesion.

Clinical features

Lichen planus is a chronic disease and is probably the only disease which can give rise to unrelieved soreness of the mouth for years on end. Such a history is uncommon now that more effective drugs are available. Adults, usually past middle age, are predominantly affected, though the disease is occasionally seen in young adults. Women account for at least 65% of the patients.

The lesions are characteristic both in their appearance and distribution, and both these factors should be taken into account in making the diagnosis.

Striae are characteristically sharply defined and form lacy, starry, or annular patterns. The striae may occasionally be interspersed with minute, white papules, or very rarely these may be the predominant pattern. Striae may not be palpable or may be felt to be rather stringy and firmer than the surrounding mucosa, with the texture of scar tissue.

Atrophic areas are often combined with the striae and present a picture of redness and thinning, but not ulceration.

Erosions are characterised by widespread, shallow irregular areas of total destruction of the epithelium. These also can be very persistent and may be covered by a smooth, slightly raised yellowish layer of fibrin. The margins may be slightly depressed due to progressive fibrosis and gradual healing at the periphery. Striae may radiate from the margins of these erosions.

Distribution. By far the most frequently affected are the buccal mucous membranes, particularly posteriorly, but the lesions may spread forward almost to the commissures. The next most common site is the tongue, either the edges or the lateral margins of the dorsum, or less frequently the centre of the dorsum. The lips, palate and gingivae may also be affected, but less often. The floor of the mouth seems hardly ever to be affected.

The lesions are very often symmetrical, often strikingly so. Rarely erosions may be the only sign or may long precede the appearance of the striae.

Symptoms are very variable. Striae alone may cause no symptoms and may only have been noticed by a dentist. In others the striae may cause a sensation of roughness or slight stiffness of the mucous membrane. Atrophic lesions are sore, and erosions usually cause more severe symptoms still and make eating difficult.

On the tongue the lesions frequently form a narrow whitish band of depapillation along each side of the dorsum, sometimes with elongated erosions in the centre of each band. Occasionally a dense snowy white (leukoplakia-like) plaque with irregular margins forms in the centre of the dorsum.

Skin lesions. Lichen planus is a common skin disease but dermal lesions are uncommon in those who complain of oral symptoms. The skin lesions characteristically form purplish papules, 2–3 mm across with a glistening surface marked by fine striae. These, however, can often only be seen with a magnifying glass. The lesions are usually irritating and their appearance may be altered by scratching. The lesions should be looked for on the flexor surface of the forearms and especially on the wrists.

Gingival lichen planus

Gingival involvement may be the predominant feature of lichen planus and needs to be distinguished from other forms of gingival disease. The most common type of lesion is atrophic: that is, the epithelium is thin (as seen histologically) and appears almost transparent, shiny, inflamed and smooth. Unlike marginal gingivitis, the inflamed area extends from the gingival margin to the reflection of the mucosa. Gingival lichen planus is often also patchily distributed and may involve the gum of only three or four teeth. Striae are not

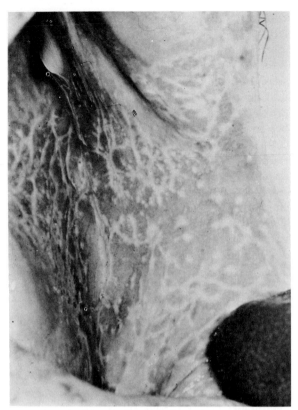

Fig. 15.30 Lichen planus. This is the most common site and type of lesion, i.e. a lacy network of whitish striae on the buccal mucous membrane. The lesions are usually symmetrically distributed.

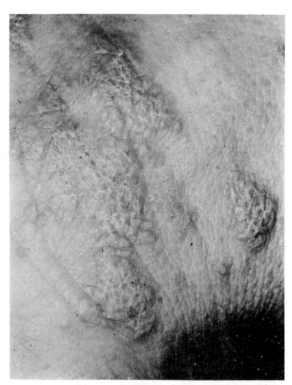

Fig. 15.32 Dermal lichen planus. This, the flexor surface of the wrists, is a characteristic site. The lesions consist of confluent papules with a pattern of minute white stria on their surface.

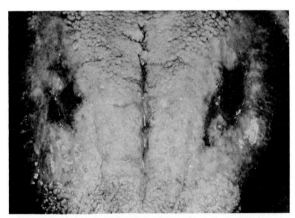

Fig. 15.31 Lichen planus of the tongue with typical bilateral distribution. Irregular erosions on each side are surrounded by proliferative white lesions.

often seen on the gingivae but may be present in another part of the mouth or absent altogether (see p. 125).

The soreness caused by these atrophic changes—often in the past labelled non-specifically as 'desquamative gingivitis'—makes brushing the teeth difficult. The accumulation of plaque and associated inflammatory changes seem to aggravate lichen planus and a vicious circle is set up. The contribution of local irritation to lichen planus is suggested by the fact that the lesion disappears when the teeth are extracted. Lichen planus of the denture-bearing area is virtually unknown.

Diagnosis

The diagnosis of lichen planus can usually be made on the history, the appearance of the lesions and their distribution. If there is any doubt a

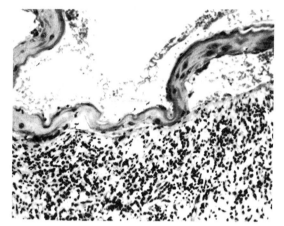

Fig. 15.33 Atrophic lichen planus. Compared with the lesions shown earlier the epithelium is severely thinned, being only a few cells thick; oedema at the junction with the dermis is tending to separate the epithelium (× 100).

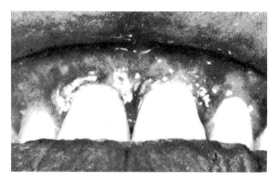

Fig. 15.34 Atrophic lichen planus. The thin epithelium seen in the section (Fig. 15.33) appears clinically almost transparent, shiny and inflamed. The typical reticular pattern of lichen planus was present on the buccal mucosa.

When the gingivae are mainly affected, as here, the appearance is often called 'desquamative gingivitis'.

biopsy should be taken, particularly when the striae are ill-defined. A streaky appearance is occasionally produced by dysplastic leukoplakias.

Management

In the past, oral lichen planus was virtually untreatable and the disease had to be allowed to take its course. Tetracycline mouth baths (used as described for recurrent aphthae) seem sometimes to be helpful in encouraging healing of erosions. Topical application of potent anti-inflammatory corticosteroids such as betamethasone valerate pellets has been shown to be highly effective in many cases, but an oral preparation is no longer available. Possible alternatives are to use similar corticosteroids (such as beclomethasone) from the aerosol inhalers used for the control of asthma. Approximately 6 puffs of such a preparation can be used to deliver a useful amount of the corticosteroid to an ulcer.

Potent corticosteroids used topically may occasionally promote thrush as a side effect. Triamcinolone dental paste applied to the lesions is an alternative but less effective form of treatment.

Gingival lichen planus is the most difficult to treat. The first essential is to maintain rigorous oral hygiene. Corticosteroids should be used in addition, as described above, and in this situation triamcinolone dental paste is often useful as it can readily be applied to the affected gingivae.

In exceptionally severe cases of lichen planus, if topical oral treatment fails, treatment with systemic corticosteroids is effective.

Pemphigus vulgaris

Pemphigus is a rare but serious disease characterised by formation of vesicles or bullae on skin and mucous membranes. It is usually fatal if untreated.

Aetiology and pathology

An immunopathogenesis can be more convincingly demonstrated in pemphigus vulgaris than in any other oral disease. The two main findings are, first, a raised titre of antibodies (predominantly IgG) to the intercellular substance of the epithelium and, second, antibodies demonstrable by immunofluorescence in the intercellular region of the epithelium. Electron microscopy has also shown that the antibody-binding site in pemphigus is the intercellular region of the epithelium, the site of the tissue damage.

The essential feature of the histopathology is that the epithelial cells lose their attachment to each other (acantholysis). The changes are intra-epithelial, take place initially just above the basal cell layer and are first seen as clefts within the epithelium. These splits widen until clinically visible vesicles or bullae form.

The epithelial cells which lose their attachments become rounded in shape and the cytoplasm contracts around the nucleus. Small groups of such rounded-up acantholytic cells can often be seen histologically in the contents of a vesicle or may be picked up in a smear from a recently ruptured vesicle.

Clinical features

Females, particularly between the ages of 40 and 60, are predominantly affected. The lesions may be seen first in the mouth but later involve the skin, particularly of the trunk.

The vesicles of pemphigus are fragile and not often seen intact in the mouth. A common appearance is therefore that of several small irregular erosions. These often have ragged edges and are superficial, painful and tender. A characteristic feature is that when the mucous membrane is gently stroked a vesicle or bulla may appear (Nikolsky's sign). If fluid is taken from a recently ruptured vesicle and a stained smear made, characteristic rounded acantholytic epithelial cells may be seen.

The progress of the disease is very variable. It may be fulminating in character with the rapid

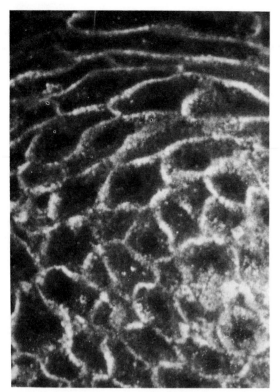

Fig. 15.35 Pemphigus vulgaris. Using anti-IgG conjugated with a fluorescent dye there is brilliant fluorescence along the line of the interepithelial attachments which is typical of this disease.

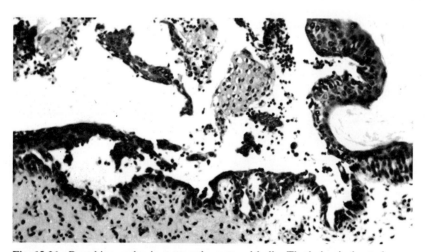

Fig. 15.36 Pemphigus vulgaris: a recently ruptured bulla. The lesion is due to loss of attachment of the epithelial cells to one another (acantholysis). The peculiar rounded appearance of the acantholytic cells can be seen and small groups of them are floating away together with inflammatory cells. It should also be noted that the bulla is intraepithelial i.e. entirely within the substance of the epithelium ($\times$ 100).

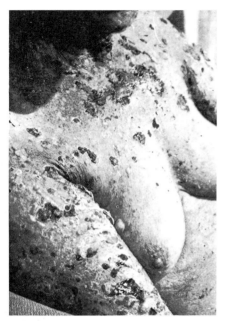

Fig. 15.37 Pemphigus vulgaris. The characteristic bullae often first appear in the mouth but soon spread over the skin, forming widespread moist or crusted lesions when they rupture.

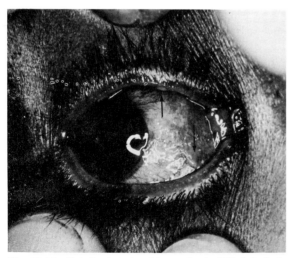

Fig. 15.38 Fulminating pemphigus vulgaris. This lady had oral lesions so severe and destructive that individual vesicles could not easily be seen. These ocular lesions developed within a few days. The arrows point to some of the smaller vesicles.

development of widespread ulceration of the mouth, spread to other sites such as the eye within a few days and very soon afterwards to the skin.

In other cases lesions may be localised to the mouth for months or longer before spreading to the skin.

Cutaneous involvement in pemphigus is characterised by vesicles or bullae varying from a few millimetres to a centimetre or so across. The bullae at first contain clear fluid which may then become purulent or haemorrhagic. Rupture of the vesicles leaves painful erosions, with ragged margins of loose epithelium, which gradually crust over.

As lesions spread over the body, loss of protein, fluid and electrolytes from the raw areas becomes severe and they readily become secondarily infected. Without treatment, death usually follows, but immunosuppressive drugs are life-saving in most cases.

Management

The severity of the disease is such that the diagnosis must be confirmed as early as possible. Biopsy is essential and the changes are sufficiently characteristic to make a diagnosis. Immunofluorescent studies should be confirmatory.

Once the diagnosis has been made the patient must be put on adequate immunosuppressive treatment. Systemic corticosteroids have been the main standby but have to be given in high dosage, and agents such as azathioprine have to be given to reduce side-effects. Treatment may have to be life-long, and this in itself can cause severe complications, particularly when corticosteroids are used.

Mucous membrane pemphigoid

Mucous membrane pemphigoid is an uncommon chronic disease causing bullae, painful erosions and scarring of mucous membranes. There can be serious complications such as blindness, but the disease is not fatal. Skin involvement is uncommon and often trivial.

Aetiology and pathology

The basic lesion is loss of attachment of the epithelium to the connective tissue and is therefore in the region of the basement membrane. The disease appears to be immunologically mediated, and the binding of immunoglobulin or more fre-

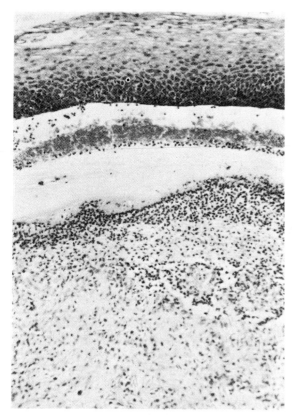

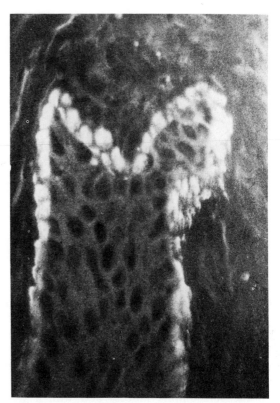

Fig. 15.39 Mucous membrane pemphigoid. The full thickness of the epithelium has separated cleanly from the underlying connective tissue in the formation of a fluid-filled bulla. An inflammatory infiltrate is present in the underlying connective tissue (× 100).

Fig. 15.40 Mucous membrane pemphigoid. Using conjugated anti-C3, brilliant immunofluorescence is seen along the line of the basement membrane.

quently of complement components along the basement membrane zone can often (but not invariably) be demonstrated. However, circulating autoantibodies are detectable only in a minority.

Histologically the lesions are characterised by separation of the full thickness of the epithelium from the connective tissue. Epithelium, though separated, remains for a time intact and forms the roof of a bulla. The floor of the bulla is formed by connective tissue alone, infiltrated with inflammatory cells, and the epithelial cells remain adherent to one another.

Clinical features

Women are mainly affected and are usually elderly. The mucous membrane of the mouth is

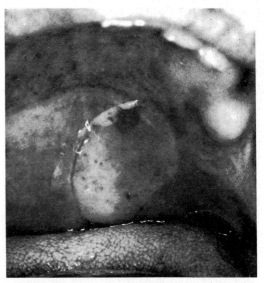

Fig. 15.41 Mucous membrane pemphigoid. A typical large, recently ruptured bulla on the soft palate of an elderly patient.

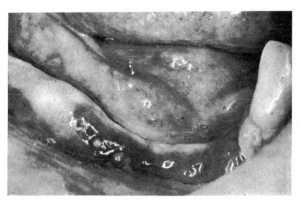

Fig. 15.42 Mucous membrane pemphigoid. A typical large erosion left by the rupture of a bulla is present on the ridge, and there are small lesions on the floor of the mouth.

often the first site. Other sites are the eyes or the mucous membranes of the nose, larynx, or oesophagus. The skin is rarely affected or to only a minor degree. Lesions are rarely widespread and progress is very slow.

In the mouth bullae form and can often be seen intact. When they rupture, raw areas are left level with the surrounding mucosa and with a well-defined margin. Individual erosions persist for some weeks then slowly heal with scarring in some sites. Further erosions may develop nearby and this process may persist for a year or more. Other mucous membranes may eventually be involved. In many patients the lesions may remain localised to the mouth for very long periods.

Diagnosis and management

The diagnosis can usually be confirmed by biopsy and immunofluorescence microscopy but it is essential to make sure that an intact vesicle or bulla is obtained. Nikolsky's sign may be positive as in pemphigus vulgaris, and a striking clinical finding is sometimes that the epithelium slides away underneath the edge of the knife when a biopsy is attempted.

When the diagnosis has been made, the patient should be referred for ocular examination for early changes in the eyes. These are the most troublesome complication in that scarring and fibrosis can lead to impaired sight or blindness. In other cases, but uncommonly, fibrosis can cause stenosis of the larynx or oesophagus.

When localised to the mouth, mucous membrane pemphigoid can often be effectively treated with topical corticosteroids. The disease may be controlled in this way for very long periods and this treatment is without side effects, as the doses involved are exceedingly small.

If there is any indication of spread of the disease, particularly to the eyes, systemic corticosteroids have to be given and are effective.

'Desquamative gingivitis'

The term desquamative gingivitis is a clinical description not a diagnosis. It is used for conditions in which the gingivae appear red or raw. Usually the whole of the attached gingiva of varying numbers of teeth is affected.

Lichen planus (as described earlier) is probably the most common cause and makes the gums look smooth, red and translucent due to the extreme thinness of the atrophic epithelium (see p. 340).

In older patients mucous membrane pemphigoid may affect the gingivae, and in this case the changes may be more severe with separation of the epithelium extending away from the tips of the interdental papillae. Pemphigus vulgaris is another possible cause.

In either case, the appearances are strikingly different from simple marginal gingivitis, but the diagnosis should preferably be confirmed by biopsy.

Acute erythema multiforme (Stevens–Johnson syndrome)

This is a disease of skin and mucous membranes but the mouth is probably invariably affected and is often the only site. Among patients coming to dental practice the oral features are the most prominent or the only ones present.

Aetiology and pathology

The cause is not clear and the disorder may be a reaction to a variety of causes.

Certain infections can precipitate the reaction, notably herpes or mycoplasmal pneumonia. Drugs, particularly sulphonamides and barbiturates, have been blamed but it is very rare to get a positive drug history. Even in cases where these drugs have been taken it is not always possible to exclude coincidence. In many patients no precipitating cause can be found.

In view of these possible precipitating factors the disease is (of course) regarded by some as being immunologically mediated, but no convincing mechanism has even been suggested.

The histological appearances are somewhat variable. Widespread necrosis of keratinocytes with eosinophilic colloid change in the superficial epithelium may be conspicuous. This is not specific but may progress to vesicle or bulla formation. However, subepithelial vesiculation is more frequent. Degenerative changes in the epithelium are associated with infiltration of inflammatory cells which also involve in the corium and occasionally have a perivascular distribution. Leakage of immunoglobulins from blood vessels has been reported, but vasculitis is not seen histologically.

Clinical features

Teenagers or young adults, particularly males, are predominantly affected.

In more severe cases the patient is acutely ill with fever and constitutional disturbance, and these prodromal symptoms may precede the appearance of the lesions by a few days. The most striking feature is often the grossly swollen, split, crusted and bleeding lips. Within the mouth there are usually widespread irregular erosions and widespread erythema.

The eyes are the next most frequently affected site, and conjunctivitis of variable severity may be seen. Dermal lesions may consist of widespread erythema alone or characteristic target lesions. These are red macules a centimetre or more in diameter with a bluish cyanotic centre. In severe cases the lesions are bullous. The attack usually lasts for 3 or 4 weeks with new crops of lesions developing over a period of about 10 days. Recurrences, usually at intervals of several months, for

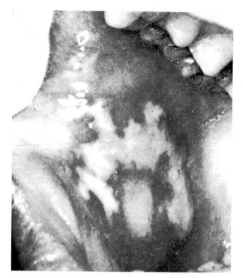

Fig. 15.43   Stevens–Johnson syndrome: acute erythema multiforme. The typical widespread ulceration following rupture of vesicles is seen in a young man in one of several attacks.

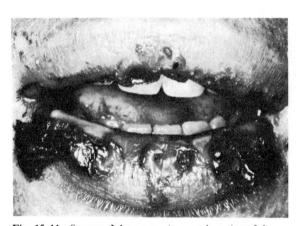

Fig. 15.44   Stevens–Johnson syndrome: ulceration of the vermilion border of the lip with bleeding, swelling and crusting is characteristic.

a year or two are characteristic and are sometimes increasingly severe.

In the most severe cases ocular damage may impair sight and occasionally cause blindness. Very rarely, renal damage can be fatal.

There is no specific treatment. Corticosteroids may give some symptomatic relief. Antibiotics are usually also given in severe cases with the idea of preventing secondary infection.

Other mucocutaneous diseases

Only the more important of the many diseases affecting the oral mucous membrane have been described. Others are only rarely seen. Nevertheless, some of them are serious and are indicators of severe underlying systemic disease such as lupus erythematosus (Ch. 20) for example.

If, therefore, stomatitis with unusual features is seen, and particularly if erosions, bullae, or desquamation are present, a serious attempt should be made to make a diagnosis by investigation of history, clinical features and biopsy. Alternatively the patient should be referred for an expert opinion. Particular attention should also be given to the medical and drug history, and whether there are any other mucous membranes affected or dermal lesions.

'Allergic' stomatitis

Many otherwise harmless substances coming into contact with the skin cause hypersensitisation in susceptible subjects. When this has happened further contact causes an inflammatory reaction. Examples are eczema or contact dermatitis caused by a wide variety of household and industrial materials.

Some mucous membranes such as the eyes can also become sensitised in this way, but the different parts of the body differ widely in their response. Sulphonamide ointments, for example, are highly sensitising to the skin but are widely used without trouble in the eyes.

The oral mucous membrane appears to show yet other differences and appears to be unable to mount reactions comparable with contact dermatitis, and there is no such condition as oral eczema.

Most so-called allergic reactions of the mouth are due to direct irritation by the substance. Even patients who are sensitised to a material such as nickel can tolerate it in the mouth; it may then cause a characteristic rash but not oral lesions. Amalgam restorations cause no trouble in patients sensitised to mercury, though the material should not be allowed to come into contact with the skin. Similar considerations apply to methylmethacry-

late. Those few people who are sensitised to the monomer can wear acrylic dentures with impunity. Inflammation under acrylic dentures, often in the past described as 'acrylic allergy' is usually candidal infection.

Authenticated cases of contact hypersensitisation of the oral mucous membrane are so few as to make it questionable whether the oral mucosa can mount this type of reaction. If it does so it must be phenomenally rare.

Fordyce's spots

Sebaceous glands may appear in the oral mucous membrane, particularly in older patients. These glands appear as scattered, creamy spots a few millimetres in diameter just beneath the epithelium. They are soft, symmetrically distributed and increase in number and size with age. The buccal mucous membrane is the main site but the lips are sometimes involved.

These glands are occasionally mistaken for disease but are a normal feature of the mucous membrane. If a patient notices these spots and is alarmed about them he can be reassured.

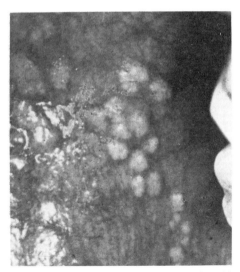

Fig. 15.45 Fordyce's granules. The creamy yellow lobules of sebaceous glands are slightly raised above the surrounding mucosal surface and, as age increases, become more numerous and widespread.

ORAL REACTIONS TO DRUGS

The mechanisms of reactions to drugs are often obscure, and the following classification is tentative.

1. Local reactions to drugs
   a. Chemical irritation
   b. Interference with the oral flora
2. Systemically mediated reactions
   a. Depression of marrow function
      —depressed white cell production
      —depressed red cell production
      —defects of haemostasis
   b. Depression of cell-mediated immunity
   c. Lichenoid reactions
   d. Erythema multiforme (Stevens–Johnson syndrome)
   e. Fixed drug eruptions
   f. Exfoliative dermatitis and stomatitis
3. Other effects
   a. Gingival hyperplasia
   b. Pigmentation
   c. Dry mouth.

Local reaction to drugs

Chemical burns. The best-known example is that of aspirin tablets held against the mucosa close to an aching tooth. This causes superficial necrosis and a white patch. When the irritant is removed the dead epithelium is shed and the mucosa heals. Other irritant chemicals are chromic acid, or phenol dropped on the mucosa.

Interference with the oral flora: superinfection. Prolonged topical use of antibiotics (particularly tetracycline) in the mouth kills off sensitive organisms and allows resistant ones, particularly *C. albicans*, to proliferate, causing thrush. In susceptible patients even 48 hours use of a topical antibiotic may precipitate candidal infection.

Systemically mediated reactions

Depression of marrow function. Few drugs significantly depress red cell production alone, though any drug which causes anaemia could in theory give rise to oral signs. The main example is prolonged use of phenytoin (for epilepsy) which, in susceptible patients, can occasionally cause folate deficiency and macrocytic anaemia. This in turn can produce severe aphthous stomatitis. This responds promptly when folate is given, and the blood picture returns to normal.

White cell production is depressed by a variety of drugs. Leucopenia may be severe enough to produce the clinical picture of agranulocytosis, with necrotising ulceration of the gums and throat which can go on to a severe prostrating illness and septicaemia, if untreated. Drugs which may have this effect include antibacterials, particularly co-trimoxazole, chloramphenicol, analgesics, particularly amidopyrine, phenothiazines and anti-thyroid agents.

When the main effect is on the granulocyte series, low-grade oral pathogens, particularly of the gingival margins, are able to overcome local resistance and produce necrotising ulceration.

Drugs may effect haemostastis and cause oral purpura (Ch. 20). Drug-induced purpura is often also an early sign of aplastic anaemia caused by drugs which depress marrow function, as indicated above. Purpura was often a sign of aplastic anaemia caused by chloramphenicol.

Purpura can produce severe spontaneous gingival bleeding or blood blisters and widespread submucosal ecchymosis.

Clotting function is impaired by other drugs, notably the anticoagulants such as the coumarins. In overdose these can cause severe bleeding after dental operations but do not otherwise cause abnormal oral signs.

Depression of cell-mediated immunity. This is common as a side-effect of such drugs as corticosteroids, particularly in patients having organ transplants or with immunologically mediated diseases.

Viral and fungal infections of the mouth are common in transplant patients and can be severe. Confluent vesiculation due to herpes may be clinically difficult to distinguish from the plaques of thrush. Both infections may be present together. Recurrences of childhood viral infections such as measles and chickenpox are also seen.

Herpes infections can be treated with acylovir, and candidal infections with antifungal drugs such as nystatin or amphotericin. Surprisingly perhaps, these infections rarely seem to become disseminated, and most patients seem to be able to overcome them without the immunosuppressive treatment being stopped.

Lichenoid reactions. Several drugs, notably gold and antimalarials (both used in the treatment of rheumatoid arthritis or other collagen diseases) and the antihypertensive agent methyldopa (Aldomet), can produce a disease indistinguishable from lichen planus, with characteristic oral signs. Though this is commonly assumed to be a hypersensitivity reaction there is little evidence as to how it is brought about.

Acute erythema multiforme (Stevens–Johnson syndrome). As mentioned earlier, this can produce striking oral signs, particularly grossly swollen, crusted and bleeding lips together with widespread erosive stomatitis. Though this is often thought to be a drug reaction, a positive history is not often obtained. The drugs most commonly associated with this reaction are long-acting sulphonamides and occasionally barbiturates, particularly phenobarbitone.

The mechanism of this reaction is also unknown, though again it is assumed to be immunologically mediated.

Fixed drug eruptions. These are characterised by sharply circumscribed skin lesions recurring in the same site or sites each time the drug is given. Many drugs are capable of causing this reaction, but phenolphthalein, a widely used component of purgative mixtures, is perhaps the best recognised and one of the more common causes. Involvement of the oral mucous membrane has been described but is exceedingly rare.

Exfoliative stomatitis and dermatitis. Exfoliative dermatitis is one of the most dangerous and severe types of reaction to drugs. Comparable changes to those on the skin may develop in the mouth and are seen as widespread erosions due to destruction of the epithelium. Occasionally the oral changes precede or may initially be more severe than the dermal changes, and these may cause the patient to seek an opinion for the extreme soreness of the mouth. Early diagnosis and treatment is important as the reaction can be lethal.

Metals are important causes. In the past these were the arsenicals and mercury, but gold is the only one at all widely used. Several other drugs, particularly phenylbutazone, the barbiturates and PAS have also been incriminated.

Healing of the oral lesions may leave behind a pattern of lichen planus.

Other drug effects

Gingival hyperplasia. This effect of phenytoin and other drugs, described in Chapter 6, is characterised by fibrous hyperplasias, particularly concentrated at the interdental papillae.

Oral pigmentation. In the past, heavy metals such as mercury, bismuth and lead caused deposits in the gingival sulcus due to the formation of sulphides by interaction with bacterial products in this situation. The blue lead line may be particularly sharply defined and indicate the level of the floor of the pocket. These effects are rarely seen now that mercury and bismuth are no longer used in medicine and lead is no longer a major industrial hazard. However, cisplatin, a cytotoxic drug, can cause a blue line.

Topical use of antibiotics and antiseptics may cause dark pigmentation, particularly of the dorsum of the tongue, probably due to overgrowth of pigment-forming bacteria.

Dry mouth is a relatively common side effect of drugs, particularly those with an atropine-like action, such as the tricyclic antidepressants which are widely used (Ch. 17).

General considerations

Oral reactions to drugs are not overall common; nevertheless they are of increasing importance as new varieties of drugs are introduced. These reactions may also be important because they may be an early sign of a dangerous or lethal reaction.

It should be remembered, however, that because a patient is taking a drug it is not necessarily the cause of any oral symptoms. Coincidence is often difficult to exclude, particularly with common oral conditions such as lichen planus. The problem is made more difficult by multiple drug treatment. In any case it is always important to get a detailed history of drugs being taken as this may have relevance to other aspects of dental treatment. An obvious example is a patient taking systemic corticosteroids who may have, as a consequence, oral candidal infection but at the same time is at risk when subjected to surgery under general anaesthesia.

ISOLATED MUCOSAL ULCERS

Traumatic ulceration

This is usually caused by a denture and is often in the buccal or lingual sulcus. The ulcer is tender, has a greyish or yellowish floor, and a red margin; there is no induration. A similar ulcer may be caused by the sharp edge of a broken-down tooth, in which case the tongue or cheek is usually affected.

Removal of the source of irritation allows the ulcer to heal within a matter of one or two days, and this confirms the diagnosis. If the ulcer persists or there is any other cause for suspicion, biopsy must be carried out.

Tuberculosis

Oral tuberculosis is rare. It is a complication of advanced 'open' pulmonary disease with infected sputum. Men of middle age or over are affected;

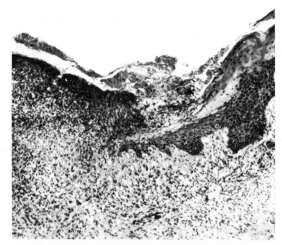

Fig. 15.47 Traumatic ulcer. Section shows destruction of the epithelium and dense inflammatory cellular infiltration of the corium extending up to the raw surface (× 45).

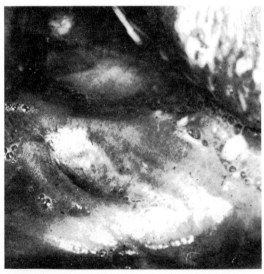

Fig. 15.46 Traumatic ulcer. An enlarged picture of an ulcer forming under the lingual flange of a denture. The ulcer was large and secondarily infected but quickly healed when the denture was removed.

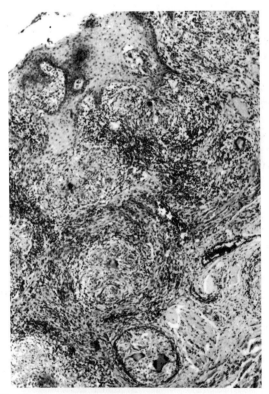

Fig. 15.48 Tuberculous ulcer of the tongue. Part of a biopsy from a man of 50 with chronic pulmonary tuberculosis, showing the typical rounded follicles of pale-staining reticulo-endothelial cells, and some giant cells. The follicles are surrounded by chronic inflammatory cells and early, poliferating connective tissue (× 45.)

the typically lesion is ulceration of the tongue but other parts of the mouth may occasionally be affected. The ulcer is characteristically stellate in shape with overhanging edges and pale, watery granulations in the floor, but the appearance is variable. The lesion may occasionally be indurated, resembling a malignant ulcer, or granulomatous. Severe pain is characteristic of the later stages. The regional lymph nodes are usually unaffected.

Biopsy should always be carried out, and the diagnosis is rarely suspected until after a biopsy has shown tubercle follicles. *M. tuberculosis* can be demonstrated by Ziehl–Neelsen's stain in the sputum, and chest X-rays show advanced infection.

No local treatment is needed; oral lesions clear up rapidly when adequate systemic chemotherapy is given for the pulmonary infection.

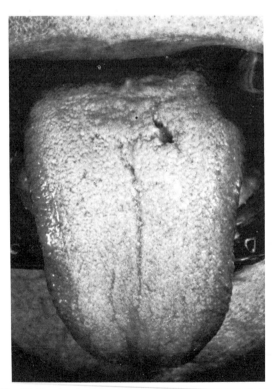

Fig. 15.49 A tuberculous ulcer of the tongue. The rather angular shape and overhanging edges of the ulcer can be seen. The patient was a man of 56 with advanced pulmonary tuberculosis.

Syphilis

On rare occasions the site of the primary infection is the mouth and it causes an isolated lesion (chancre) on the mucous membrane. Syphilis may also cause stomatitis in the secondary stage or a gumma in the tertiary stage. The oral lesions in each stage of syphilis are quite different from each other but are described together here for convenience. Though the incidence of disease has progressively increased in recent years oral syphilis is rarely seen, or perhaps goes unrecognised. It is obviously of great importance to recognise these lesions to prevent further spread of the disease and to ensure early treatment.

Primary syphilis

A chancre appears 3 to 4 weeks after infection. The site may be the lip or tip of the tongue, and the lesion consists of a firm nodule about a quarter of an inch across. The surface breaks down after a few days, leaving a rounded ulcer with raised indurated edges. Sometimes there is a clinical resemblance to a carcinoma. There is no pain or tenderness unless there is secondary infection. The regional lymph nodes are enlarged, rubbery and discrete.

At this stage serological reactions are not usually positive and diagnosis depends on seeing *Treponema pallidum* in material from the chancre. The spirochaete can be seen by dark-ground illumination of a smear but must be distinguished from other spirochaetes found in the mouth. The rarity of oral chancres makes their recognition difficult, but it is important that they should not be missed; they are highly infective, and treatment is most effective at this early stage.

After 8 or 9 weeks the chancre heals, often without scarring.

Secondary syphilis

The secondary stage develops 1 to 4 months after infection, and gives rise to generalised effects. There is usually a mild, febrile illness with malaise, headache, a sore throat and generalised enlargement of the lymph nodes. A rash and stomatitis soon follow.

The rash may be of almost any form, but often consists first of pinkish macules, usually generalised, symmetrically distributed and starting on the trunk. The rash is not irritating or painful and may last for only a few hours or for a few weeks. The presence or history of such a rash is a useful aid to diagnosis.

Oral lesions of secondary syphilis are rarely seen without the rash. The tonsils, lateral borders of the tongue and lips are predominantly involved, and the usual appearance is of a flat ulcer covered by greyish membrane. The lesions may be irregularly linear (snail's track ulcers) or may coalesce to form well-defined rounded areas (mucous patches).

The discharge from the ulcers contains large numbers of spirochaetes, and saliva is highly infective. Serological reactions are positive at this stage.

Tertiary syphilis

This late stage of syphilis is usually considered to develop about 3 years after infection, but changes are gradual and their onset impossible to detect. In the intervening latent period the patient may appear well. The characteristic lesion is the gumma, which may involve the oral mucosa, skin, or viscera.

A gumma may vary from one to several inches in diameter and may affect the palate, tongue or tonsils. It begins as a swelling, sometimes with a yellowish centre which undergoes necrosis leaving

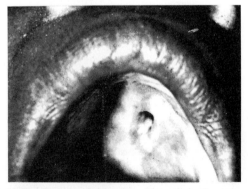

Fig. 15.50 Gumma of the palate. Necrosis in the centre of gumma on the palate has caused perforation of the bone and a typical round punched-out hole.

an indolent deep ulcer. The outline of the ulcer is rounded, with soft, punched-out edges. The floor is depressed and pale, resembling wash-leather in appearance. The lesion is painless and eventually heals with severe scarring. A gumma may, as a result, distort the soft palate or tongue, perforate the hard palate or destroy the uvula.

Leukoplakia of the tongue may also develop during the later stages of syphilis, as discussed later, and other effects of the disease such as aortitis, tabes or general paresis of the insane may be seen.

Congenital syphilis

Mainly as a result of widespread use of serological tests in antenatal clinics, congenital syphilis has now virtually been abolished in Britain. The effects on the fetus depend on the period of gestation when infection is acquired. Live birth is compatible only with infection late in pregnancy, hence congenital syphilis typically affects the permanent teeth.

The early lesions are varied in character but mucous patches are common. Rhagades are infected, painful fissures which form at muco-cutaneous junctions and leave permanent and characteristic radiating scars at the angles of the mouth. The permanent teeth may be hypo-plastic, the incisors being notched and barrel-shaped (Hutchinson's teeth). Rhinitis with a mucopurulent discharge is often present, and other effects are a saddle nose, frontal bossing, interstitial keratitis and sabre shins.

Treatment

Antibiotics are the mainstay of treatment; penicillin is the most commonly used drug but tetracycline and erythromycin are also effective. Treatment must be continued until serological reactions are persistently negative.

TONGUE DISORDERS

The tongue can be involved in generalised stomatitis and show lesions similar to those in other parts of the mouth. The tongue is also the site of lesions or a source of symptoms peculiar to itself and, for quite unknown reasons, can produce the earliest symptoms of latent defects of haemopoiesis.

Sore tongue and glossitis

Glossitis is used to describe the red, smooth and sore tongue particularly characteristic of anaemia. It is important to appreciate that these characteristic features are a combination of *signs* (redness and smoothness) and a *symptom* (soreness) and these are by no means consistently associated. Tongues can be sore in the absence of visible changes or smooth but asymptomatic. Sore tongue is a not uncommon complaint and there are four clinical variants:

1. Ulceration of the tongue
2. Glossitis
3. The sore, physically normal tongue
4. Geographical tongue (erythema migrans linguae).

Ulceration of the tongue

The tongue may be involved in, or even the predominantly affected site of, various types of stomatitis such as herpes simplex or, more often, lichen planus (see Fig. 15.32). The tongue may also be the site of solitary ulcers, particularly carcinoma, which when far back may be difficult to see.

In general, when there are definable lesions of these kinds diagnosis is straightforward and depends on clinical recognition of the type of lesion or biopsy.

Glossitis

The tongue is red (inflamed), smooth (atrophy of the papillae) and sore. The main causes are as follows.

a. *Anaemia.* Iron deficiency and pernicious anaemia are the main causes. Women are more frequently affected than men. Detailed haematological examination is essential. These investigations are important, as a fall in haemoglobin level may lag behind other changes. Thus there

may be glossitis, haematological signs of a deficiency state, but a haemoglobin level within normal limits.

b. *Candidosis.* The tongue can be red, sore and oedematous due to candidal infection. This is characteristic of acute antibiotic stomatitis and is often then associated with angular stomatitis and other features of candidosis. This condition is rarely seen now that antibiotics are used somewhat less wildly than in their early days and topical oral antibiotics have now been discredited for the treatment of oral infections.

c. *Vitamin B group deficiencies.* These are exceedingly rarely seen but glossitis with angular stomatitis is characteristic of riboflavin and to some extent of nicotinic acid deficiency. The diagnosis of vitamin deficiency should not be made on oral signs alone in an otherwise healthy patient. The giving of B group vitamins is nevertheless a common gesture in an attempt to deal with the complaint. The measure is virtually invariably ineffective, but the ineffectiveness itself can be said to serve some purpose, in that it makes it clear that deficiency of these vitamins is not a cause.

d. *Lichen planus.* This can produce a smooth tongue due to atrophy of the papillae (particularly in the late stage of long-standing disease) but

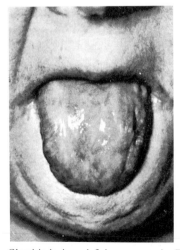

Fig. 15.51 Glossitis in iron-deficiency anaemia. The tongue is smooth due to atrophy of the papillae, and is red and sore. Anaemia is the commonest diagnosable cause of glossitis and must always be looked for by haematological examination.

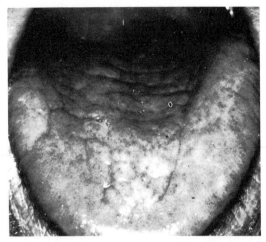

Fig. 15.52 Glossitis in antibiotic stomatitis. The tongue is red, smooth and sore as in anaemic glossitis but the appearance of the tongue is partly due to inflammatory oedema, similar changes affect the rest of the mucosa, and other features of candidosis, such as thrush, are often present.

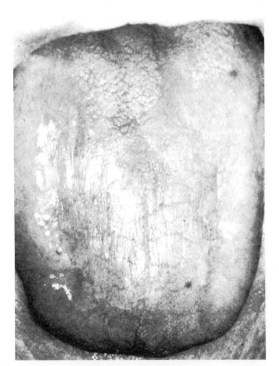

Fig. 15.53 Smooth tongue due to lichen planus. This is a late change due to long standing disease. The tongue is smooth due to atrophy of papillae but has a faint silvery sheen. There are usually no symptoms at this stage.

there is then no soreness. The condition can usually be readily recognised. There is often a bluish-white sheen to the surface of the tongue, and other signs of lichen planus are likely to be seen in other parts of the mouth.

The sore, physically normal tongue

This is perhaps the most common type and presents the most difficult problems. In the absence of visible signs the tendency is often of course to label the complaint as 'neurotic' but, though the symptoms can be psychogenic, it is essential first to exclude organic disease. The main conditions that must therefore be considered are as follows.

Haematological deficiency states. Soreness can precede visible, physical changes. The haemoglobin is usually within normal limits but abnormalities of the red cells may be seen in a stained film, and serum levels of iron, B12 or folate (as the case may be) are depressed. When abnormalities such as these are found, specific treatment quickly relieves the symptoms.

Psychogenic disorders. Sore tongue seems in some patients to be of psychogenic origin and in this respect comparable to atypical facial pain. Depression is sometimes the underlying disorder, but is often effectively disguised or replaced by what seems to be a physical symptom. Recog-

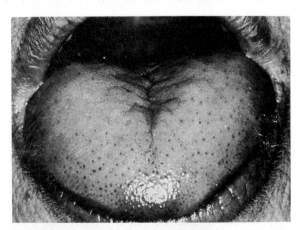

Fig. 15.54 A normal-looking but persistently sore tongue in a doctor's wife who had repeated but inadequate haematological investigations which failed to detect early pernicious anaemia.

nition of psychogenic symptoms such as these can be difficult, and the general problem is discussed in more detail in Chapter 18. Once the basis of the symptoms is recognised, adequate treatment with an antidepressant agent such as amitriptyline can sometimes abolish the soreness of the tongue and bring about great improvement in the patient's general sense of well-being in many cases.

In a few patients the underlying problem seems to be an anxiety state. This can occasionally be dealt with by reassurance, especially if there is an unfounded fear, particularly of cancer of the mouth. In other cases the basis for the anxiety state seems to be less specific. A short course of diazepam may sometimes be helpful.

As with atypical facial pain, there seems also to be a hard core of patients who complain bitterly and persistently of sore tongue, in whom no organic disease can be found and who show no response to psychoactive drugs or any other form of treatment.

Geographical tongue (erythema migrans linguae)

This common condition is characterised by the recurrent appearance and disappearance of red areas on the tongue.

The cause is unknown but, in some at least, the condition is familial and has been described in several succeeding generations of a family. The abnormality can therefore be seen at a very early age, though it is probably not often noticed. Most cases are seen in middle-aged patients. It seems improbable (but not impossible) that the condition has remained unnoticed for so long.

Apart from the fact that in many patients geographical tongue seems to be a developmental anomaly, the cause is unknown.

Histologically there is thinning of the epithelium in the centre of the lesion and there may be mild hyperplasia and hyperkeratosis at the periphery; there are chronic inflammatory cells in the underlying connective tissue.

Clinically the condition may be seen at any stage. An irregular, smooth, red area appears, usually with a sharply defined edge, where the filiform papillae stop short; it extends for a few days, then heals, only to appear again in another area. Sometimes the lesion is annular with a slightly raised pale margin, and several of these areas may coalesce to form a scalloped pattern.

Most patients have no symptoms but some adults complain of soreness. One possible reason may be that the patient has become anxious that the lesion may be due to cancer. Reassurance is

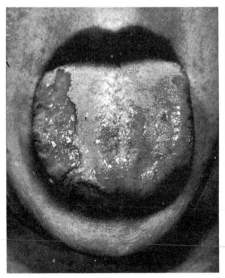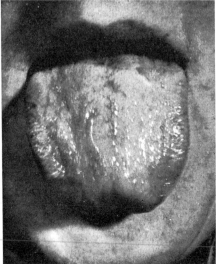

Fig. 15.55 Geographical tongue. The irregular, sharply defined red area with loss of papillae, is characteristic. Ten days later the lesion had disappeared (as shown on the right) but reappeared again later on another part of the tongue.

then necessary and may be effective. In others soreness may be due to an underlying haematological deficiency state, and the lesion is coincidental.

It is noticeable, however, that even some children with geographical tongue complain that it is sufficiently hypersensitive to prevent them eating certain foods. The areas of thinning of the epithelium, together with the inflammatory changes, may therefore cause symptoms, but this does not explain their frequent absence.

Soreness in association with geographical tongue may also be psychogenic, and may then respond to appropriate treatment. Some evidence has been produced to show an apparently significant association between geographical tongue and emotional disturbance. However, there remains a group where no cause for the soreness can be found and no treatment seems to be effective.

Hairy tongue

The filiform papillae can become elongated and hair-like, forming a thick fur on the dorsum of the tongue. The filaments may be up to half a centimetre long and pale brown to black in colour. Adults are affected but the cause is unknown. Heavy smoking, excessive use of antiseptic mouthwashes, and defective diet have been blamed, but their effect is questionable. The discolouration is

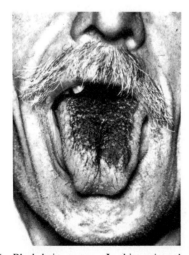

Fig. 15.56 Black hairy tongue. In this patient there is only slight overgrowth of the papillae but dense black staining. In other cases the filiform papillae may be much more elongated and hair-like. The posterior part of the tongue is the characteristic site.

probably caused by pigment-producing bacteria and fungi but not *Candida albicans*.

Treatment is far from satisfactory. Generally the measure most likely to succeed is probably that of persuading the patient to scrape off the hyperplastic papillae and vigorously cleanse the dorsum of the tongue using a firm toothbrush. This has the effect of removing large numbers of microorganisms mechanically and also, by removing the overgrown papillae, making conditions less suitable for their continued proliferation.

Black tongue

The dorsum of the tongue may sometimes become black without overgrowth of the papillae. This may simply be staining due to drugs such as iron compounds used for the treatment of anaemia, but is then transient. Occasionally the sucking of antibiotic lozenges causes the tongue to become black, and this may be due to pigment-producing organisms, particularly aspergillus strains.

Furred tongue

This condition, in which the tongue becomes coated with desquamating cells and debris, is seen in those who smoke heavily, and in many systemic upsets, especially of the gastrointestinal tract, and infections in which the mouth becomes dry and little food is taken. A furred tongue is often seen in the childhood fevers, especially scarlet fever.

Median rhomboid glossitis

Median rhomboid glossitis is a lesion of the midline of the dorsum of the tongue at the junction of the anterior two thirds with the posterior third.

The appearance (from which the name derives) is a red or pink rhomboid (lozenge-shaped) area of depapillation. Nevertheless the appearance is variable and the area may be white or pink and lobulated.

The nature of this lesion is controversial. The site suggests that it is developmental but few now believe the theory that it is the result of persistence of the tuberculum impar.

Histologically the appearances are also variable and include irregular (pseudoepitheliomatous) hyperplasia with an inflammatory infiltrate, granu-

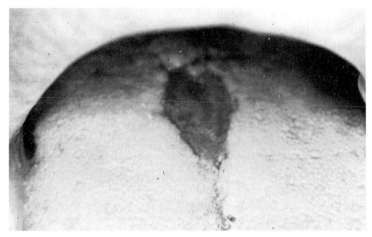

Fig. 15.57 Median rhomboid glossitis. There is the typical lozenge-shaped area of depapillation in the midline of the tongue.

lar cell tumour (Ch. 16), or candidosis (the white variant).

Clinically, median rhomboid glossitis is seen in adults and is typically symptomless. Its chief importance is that the histological features have been mistaken for a carcinoma and treated accordingly. Quite apart from the need for proper histological assessment, carcinoma hardly ever develops in this site.

SUGGESTED FURTHER READING

Allen C M, Beck F M 1987 Differences in mucosal reaction related to *Candida albicans* isolates. J Oral Pathol 16: 89–93

Arbesfeld S J, Kurban A K 1988 Behcet's disease. New perspectives on an enigmatic syndrome. J Am Acad Dermatol 19: 767–779

Bagg J, Williams B D, Amos N et al 1987 Absence of circulating IgG immune complexes in minor recurrent apththous ulceration. J Oral Pathol 16: 53–56

Barrett A P 1987 Clinical characteristics and mechanisms involved in chemotherapy-induced oral ulceration. Oral Surg, Oral Med, Oral Pathol 63: 424–428

Bolewska J, Holmstrup P, Moller-Madsen B, Kenrad B 1990 Amalgam-associated mercury accumulations in normal oral mucosa, oral lesions of lichen planus and contact lesions associated with amalgam. J Oral Pathol Med 19: 39–42

Burge S M, Frith P A, Millard P R, Wojnarowska F 1989 The Lupus band test in oral mucosa, conjunctiva and skin. Br J Dermatol 121: 743–752

Cannell H 1988 The development of oral and facial signs in B-thalassaemia major. Br Dent J 164: 50–53

Cawson R A 1987 Oral pathology—colour aids in dentistry. Churchill Livingstone, Edinburgh

Cawson R A, Eveson J W 1987 Oral pathology and diagnosis. William Heinemann Medical Books, London and Gower Medical Publishing, London

Chan H-L, Stern R S, Arndt K A et al 1990 The incidence of erythema multiforme, Stevens-Johnson syndrome and toxic epidermal necrolysis. Arch Dermatol 126: 43–47

Dreizen S, McCredie K B, Bodey G P, Keating M J 1986 Quantitative analysis of the oral complications of antileukemia chemotherapy. Oral Surg, Oral Med, Oral Pathol 62: 650–653

Eisenbud L, Horowitz I, Kay B 1987 Recurrent aphthous stomatitis of the Behcet's type: successful treatment with thalidomide. Oral Surg, Oral Med, Oral Pathol 64: 289–292

Farthing P M, Matear P, Cruchley A T 1990 The activation of Langerhans' cells in oral lichen planus. J Oral Pathol Med 19: 81–85

Firth N A, Reade P C 1989 Angiotensin-converting enzyme inhibitors implicated in oral mucosal lichenoid reactions. Oral Surg, Oral Med, Oral Pathol 67: 41–44

Fleming M G, Valenzuela R, Bergfeld W F, Tuthill R J 1988 Mucous gland basement membrane immunofluorescence in cicatricial pemphigoid. Arch Dermatol 124: 1407–1410

Gilhar A, Pillar T, Winterstein G, Etzioni A 1989 The pathogenesis of lichen planus. Br J Derm 120: 541–544

Grinspan D, Blanco G F, Aguero S 1989 Treatment of aphthae with thalidomide. J Am Acad Dermatol 20: 1060–1063

Hay K D 1988 Candidosis of the oral cavity. Drugs 36: 633–642

Herrod H G 1990 Chronic mucocutaneous candidiasis in childhood and complications of non-*Candida* infection. J Pediatr 116: 377–382

Hietanen J, Pihlman K A, Forstrom L et al 1987 No evidence of hypersensitivity to dental restorative materials in oral lichen planus. Scand J Dent Res 95: 320–327

Hill L V H, Tan M H, Pereira L H, Embil J A 1989 Association of oral candidiasis with diabetic control. J Clin Pathol 42: 502–505

Ho C, Gupta A K, Ellis C N et al 1990 Treatment of severe lichen planus with cyclosporine. J Am Acad Dermatol 22: 64–68

Holmstrup P, Thorn J J, Rindum J, Pindborg J J 1988 Malignant development of lichen planus-affected oral mucosa. J Oral Pathol 17: 219–225

Huff J C, Weston W L 1989 Recurrent erythema multiforme. Medicine 68: 133–141

Hughes A M, Hunter S, Still D, Lamey P J 1989 Psychiatric disorders in a dental clinic. Br Dent J 166: 16–18

Hunter L, Addy M 1987 Chlorhexidine gluconate mouthwash in the management of minor aphthous ulceration. Br Dent J 162: 106–109

International Study Group for Behcet's Disease 1990 Criteria for the study of Behcet's disease. Lancet 335: 1078–1080

James J, Ferguson M M, Forsyth A et al 1987 Oral lichenoid reactions related to mercury sensitivity. Br J Oral Maxillofac Surg 25: 474–480

Korman N 1988 Pemphigus. J Am Acad Dermatol 18: 1219–1238

Krusinski P A 1988 Treatment of mucocutaneous herpes simplex infections with acyclovir. J Am Acad Dermatol 18: 179–181

Lamey P J, Lewis M A O, Rees T D et al 1990 Sensitivity reaction to the cinnamonaldehyde component of toothpaste. Br Dent J 168: 115–118

Lamey P J, Lamb A B 1988 Prospective study of aetiological factors in burning mouth syndrome. Br Med J 296: 1243–1246

Lamey P J, Lewis M A O 1989 Oral medicine in practice: Oral ulceration. Br Dent J 167: 127–132

Lamey P J, Lewis M A O 1989 Oral medicine in practice: viral infection. Br Dent J 167: 269–274

Lamey P J, Taylor J A, Devine J 1988 Giant cell arteritis. A forgotten diagnosis. Br Dent J 164: 48–50

Leading article 1989 Behcet's disease. Lancet 354: 761–762

Lemak M A, Duvic M, Bean S F 1986 Oral acyclovir for the prevention of herpes-associated erythema multiforme. J Am Acad Dermatol 10: 50–54

Lewis M A O, Lamey P-J, Forsyth A, Gall J 1989 Recurrent erythema multiforme: a possible role of foodstuffs. Br Dent J 166: 371–373

Lind P O 1988 Oral lichenoid lesions related to composite restorations. Acta Odontol Scand 46: 63–65

Littner M M, Dayan D, Gorsky M et al 1987 Migratory stomatitis. Oral Surg, Oral Med, Oral Pathol 63: 555–559

Lovas J G L, Harsani B B, El Geneidy A K 1989 Oral lichenoid dysplasia: A clinicopathologic analysis. Oral Surg, Oral Med, Oral Pathol 68: 57–63

Lozada-Nur F, Gorsky M, Silverman S 1989 Oral erythema multiforme: clinical observations and treatment of 95 patients. Oral Surg, Oral Med, Oral Pathol 67: 36–40

Main D M G 1989 Acute herpetic stomatitis: referrals to Leeds Dental Hospital 1978–1987. Brit Dent J 166: 14–16

Malmstrom M, Konttinen Y T, Jungell P et al 1988 Lymphocyte activation in oral lichen planus in situ. Am J Clin Pathol 89: 329–334

Masuda K, Urayama A, Kogure M et al 1989 Double-masked trial of cyclosporin versus colchicine and long-term open study of cyclosporin in Behcet's disease. Lancet 1: 1093–1096

Murti P R, Daftary D K, Bhonsle R B et al 1986 Malignant potential of oral lichen planus; observations in 722 patients from India. J Oral Pathol 15: 71–77

Nowak A J 1988 Oropharyngeal lesions and their management in epidermolysis bullosa. Arch Dermatol 124: 742–745

O'Duffy 1990 Behcet's syndrome. New Engl J Med 322: 326–327

Yazici H, Pazarli H, Barnes C G et al 1990 A controlled trial of azathioprine in Behcet's syndrome. New Engl J Med 322: 281–285

Pedersen A 1989 Psychologic stress and recurrent aphthous ulceration. J Oral Pathol Med 18: 119–122

Phenal J A, Levin S M 1986 A prevalence study of denture stomatitis in subjects with diabetes mellitus or elevated plasma glucose levels. Oral Surg, Oral Med, Oral Pathol 62: 303–305

Porter S R, Scully C, Flint S 1988 Hematologic status in recurrent aphthous stomatitis compared with other oral disease. Oral Surg, Oral Med, Oral Pathol 66: 41–44

Potts A J C, Hamburger J, Scully C 1987 The medication of patients with oral lichen planus and the association of nonsteroidal anti-inflammatory drugs with erosive lesions. Oral Surg, Oral Med, Oral Pathol 64: 541–543

Pye M 1988 Lingual and scalp infarction as a manifestation of giant cell arteritis: delay in diagnosis leading to blindness. J Rheumatol 15: 1597–1598

Rush C B, Stram J R, Chasin W D 1988 Treatment of severe recurrent aphthous stomatitis with colchicine. Arch Otolaryngol Head Neck Surg 114: 671–675

Samaranayake L P 1990 Oral candidosis: and old disease in new guises. Dental Update 15: 36–49

Samaranayake L P, Holmstrup P 1989 Oral candidiasis and human immunodeficiency virus infection. J Oral Pathol Med 18: 554–564

Scully C, Cawson R A 1988 Oral medicine—colour aids in dentistry. Churchill Livingstone, Edinburgh

Scully C, Porter S R 1989 Recurrent aphthous stomatitis: current concepts of etiology, pathogenesis and management. J Oral Pathol Med 18: 21–27

Sedano H O, Gorlin R J 1989 Epidermolysis bullosa. Oral Surg, Oral Med, Oral Pathol 67: 555–563

Stephenson P, Lamey P-J, Scully C, Prime S S 1987 Angina bullosa haemorrhagica: clinical and laboratory features in 30 patients. Oral Surg, Oral Med, Oral Pathol 63: 560–563

Straus S S (Moderator) 1988 Varicella-zoster infections. Biology, natural history, treatment and prevention. Ann Intern Med 108: 221–237

Thorn J J, Holmstrup P, Rindum J, Pindborg J J 1988 Course of various forms of oral lichen planus. A prospective follow-up study of 611 patients. J Oral Pathol 17: 213–218

Wassilew S W, Reimlinger S, Nasemann T, Jones D 1987 Oral acyclovir for herpes zoster: a double blind controlled trial in normal subjects. Br J Dermatol 117: 495–501

Wheeler C E 1988 The herpes simplex problem. J Am Acad Dermatol 18: 163–168

Williams D M 1989 Vesiculobullous mucocutaneous disease: pemphigus vulgaris. J Oral Pathol Med 18: 544–553

Williams D M 1990 Vesiculo-bullous mucocutaneous disease: benign mucous membrane and bullous pemphigoid. J Oral Pathol Med 19: 16–23

16. Oral white lesions, pre-cancer, cancer and other soft-tissue tumours

Because of their importance, white and precancerous lesions and cancer of the mouth are considered first here.

WHITE LESIONS (KERATOSES) AND LEUKOPLAKIAS

Terminology

The World Health Organization definition of leukoplakia is that of a white patch or plaque that cannot be characterised clinically or pathologically as any other condition (or, in other words, a white plaque is a white plaque). This definition does not and should not be used to imply any specific histological changes. However, the term 'syphilitic leukoplakia' persists. Unfortunately also, many doctors are unshakably convinced that all persistent white lesions of the mouth are 'leukoplakias' and that *all* are premalignant. In the writer's experience for example, a patient was refused life insurance because he had 'oral leukoplakia', even though it was merely lichen planus.

Histologically, oral white plaques show three main features:

1. Abnormal keratinisation
2. Variable hyper- or hypoplasia of the epithelium
3. Variable degrees of disordered maturation of the epithelium (atypia).

Abnormal keratinisation. Keratinisation produces the white appearance of these plaques and can be of two types. Hyperorthokeratosis (usually abbreviated to hyperkeratosis) is the overproduction of mature keratin. A deeply staining layer of granular cells containing pre-keratin (eleidin) granules underlies the keratin layer.

Parakeratosis (hyperparakeratosis) denotes the persistence of degenerating nuclei in the superficial cells, and there is therefore no sharp dividing line between the prickle cell layer and the parakeratotic cells, since the nuclei mature and become progressively more effete as they approach the surface. There is no granular cell layer.

A plaque may show both hyperortho- and parakeratosis in different parts or they may alternate along the length of the specimen.

Epithelial hyperplasia and hypoplasia. The prickle cell layer may be hyperplastic—a change known as acanthosis (Acanthus—a prickly, thistle-like plant, hence 'acanthosis' for overgrowth of the prickle cells). In many cases, however, the epithelium is hypoplastic (thinner than normal), when it is often termed 'atrophic'.

The thickness of the prickle cell layer bears no regular relationship to the degree of keratinisation, and gross hyperkeratosis can be associated with hypoplasia of the underlying epithelium. There is also no constant relationship between the degree of hyperplasia and premalignancy, and the idea that cancer is the end-stage of progressive hyperplasia is antiquated and grossly misleading. Frequently the opposite is true and premalignant lesions are often atrophic with an epithelium only a few cells thick.

Disordered maturation of the epithelium. The epithelial cells normally undergo orderly, progressive development from the basal cell layer, through the prickle cell layer to the surface, where effete cells are shed. This sequence can be normal in hyperkeratotic lesions or disordered to any degree (*atypia, dysplasia*), as discussed later. Dysplasia is not recognisable clinically but is the main feature that must be looked for histologically as the only significant guide to the possibility of malignant change.

The best—but by no means wholly reliable—guide to the potentialities of leukoplakias is the histology. As a consequence all leukoplakias should be biopsied.

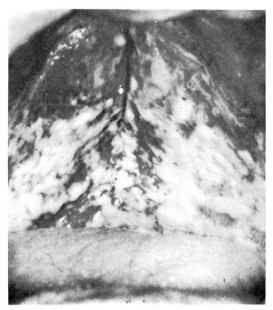

Fig. 16.1 White plaque of thrush. Patches of thrush have become confluent, forming extensive plaque on each side of the palate. The soft, easily detached character of the plaque and the presence of hyphae in a direct smear make the diagnosis clear.

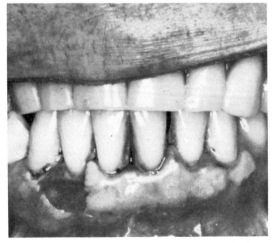

Fig. 16.2 Chemical burn. Over-use of chromic acid for an attack of ulcerative gingivitis has resulted in a burn of the attached gingiva. To the left of the picture part of this necrotic epithelium has separated.

Types of white lesion

1. *Transient white plaques*
   a. Thrush (Ch. 15)
   b. Chemical burns (Ch. 15)

2. *Persistent white plaques*
   a. Developmental; white sponge naevus
   b. Frictional keratosis

c. Smoker's keratosis
d. Syphilitic leukoplakia
e. Chronic candidosis
f. Hairy leukoplakia
g. Lichen planus
h. Leukoplakia of unknown cause
i. Dysplastic leukoplakia
j. Early carcinoma
k. Skin grafts.

White sponge naevus

This uncommon condition is inherited as a simple dominant and characterised by widespread, soft, uneven thickening of the superficial layers of the epithelium. Almost the whole of the oral cavity may be involved, with the characteristic changes extending even into the sulcuses, the inner aspect of the lips and sometimes the dorsum of the tongue. The uneven surface is due to fragments being shed or chewed off, and this roughness is usually the only symptom. The lesion has no definable boundary and fades away into normal mucosa at its margins. Other mucous membranes may also be affected.

Histopathology. The epithelium is hyperplastic with a greatly thickened superficial layer. This shows such gross intracellular oedema that only

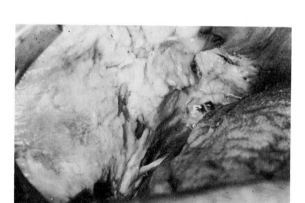

Fig. 16.3 White sponge naevus. The typical features are the widespread distribution of the plaque, its great variation in thickness and irregular surface.

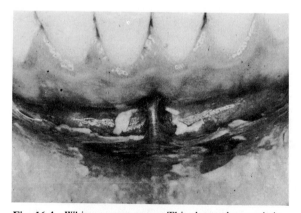

Fig. 16.4 White sponge naevus. This shows characteristic spread of the defect along the sulcus and inside the lower lip across the midline. The irregular thickness, partial shedding and thinner areas produced as a consequence can be seen.

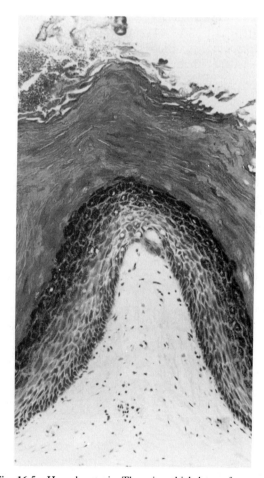

Fig. 16.5 Hyperkeratosis. There is a thick layer of eosinophilic keratin, beneath which is a prominent basophilic granular cell layer. In spite of the excessive keratinisation, the epithelium is not hyperplastic, and inflammatory changes are absent.

the cell margins are visible, giving a so-called basket-weave appearance. There are no inflammatory changes.

Management. Patients need only to be reassured that the condition, though untreatable, is benign.

Frictional keratosis

This is caused by continued abrasion of the mucous membrane by such irritants as a sharp tooth, cheek biting or, in elderly patients, prolonged denture wearing.

In their early stages these patches are pale and translucent rather than white, but later become dense and white, sometimes with a rough surface. Cheek biting, a nervous habit, causes a lesion with a more uneven surface, patchily red and white in colour.

Histopathology. Biopsy shows a moderately hyperplastic epithelium with a prominent granular cell layer and thick keratin on the surface. There is often a scattered infiltrate of chronic inflammatory cells in the corium.

Management. Removal of the irritant by smoothing off or extracting a sharp tooth, or remaking a faulty denture, as appropriate, causes the patch quickly to disappear. If this fails the diagnosis must be reconsidered and a biopsy may then be necessary. True frictional keratosis is completely benign, and there is no evidence that continued minor trauma of this sort alone has any carcinogenic action.

Smoker's keratosis

The most characteristic type of lesion is seen on the palate of men who are heavy pipe smokers. The lesions are probably the result of irritation by heat (low-grade burns) but the chemical components of the smoke presumably also contribute.

Histopathology. Unlike other keratotic lesions there are two components: (1) hyperkeratosis and (2) inflammation and swelling of minor palatal salivary glands. The latter is said to be caused by blockage of the ducts by the overproduction of keratin, with consequent inflammation and swelling.

Apart from the effects on mucous glands the changes are essentially similar to those of frictional keratosis. There are varying degrees of keratosis or parakeratosis, and acanthosis. In the corium

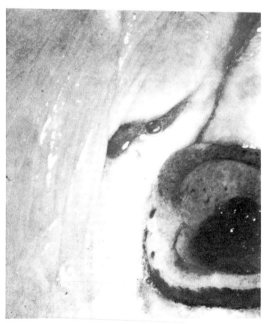

Fig. 16.6 Frictional keratosis and ulceration. Chronic abrasion of the cheek has provoked hyperkeratosis of the mucosa; the sharp enamel edge has also cut into the tissue, causing a traumatic ulcer.

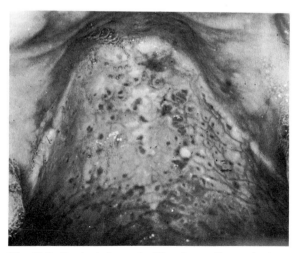

Fig. 16.7 Smoker's keratosis. The plaque affects only the unprotected area of the palate behind the upper denture; it shows a tessellated pattern and is studded with many papular swellings, each with an umbilicated red centre. These are inflamed mucous glands.

there is usually infiltration by chronic inflammatory cells.

Clinically, smoker's keratosis is readily recognisable by the white thickening of the palate and the multiple small glandular swellings. The soft palate is typically most severely affected, but the keratosis can also involve almost the whole of the hard palate. If a denture is worn, the latter is protected and the anterior margin of the white area is sharply demarcated from the normal mucosa of the denture-bearing area.

The white component of the lesion is variable; it may be thin and translucent or thick and white with a rough surface, often with a paving stone (tessellated) pattern.

The mucous glands form swellings, usually from 2 to 4 mm in diameter, which are umbilicated and have a red centre. These swellings may be few and large or many and small.

Prognosis. Circumstantial evidence suggests that continued heavy pipe smoking may be a factor in the production of mouth cancer. These palatal changes may perhaps serve as a warning to the patient and are reversible if smoking is stopped.

However, when cancer does develop in a pipe smoker's mouth it is in the retromolar or faucial region and *not* in the area of keratosis. Different factors may therefore be acting to produce the keratosis from those which contribute to the malignant change.

Cigarette smokers do not show any very characteristic changes. White plaques may rarely form on the lips where a cigarette end is habitually allowed to burn down too far.

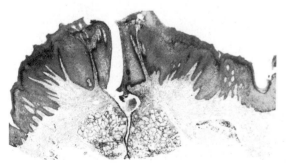

Fig. 16.8 Mucous gland in smoker's keratosis. The epithelium is hyperplastic and hyperkeratotic, especially around the orifice of the duct where there is a concentration of inflammatory cells (× 15).

White patches on the anterior floor of the mouth sometimes seem to be the result of excessive cigarette or cheroot smoking. These are irregular in shape, soft, white or grey, have a slightly wrinkled surface, and there is often some erythema at the margin.

Management. The main aim should be to stop the patient from smoking, to protect the mouth (pipe smoking) or the bronchi (cigarette smoking).

Even severe smoker's keratosis will clear up if smoking is stopped, and this confirms the diagnosis more convincingly than a biopsy.

White lesions due to 'smokeless' tobacco

Tobacco chewing is a habit that had virtually disappeared from Britain. In the USA by contrast the habit has persisted, and, in southern states particularly, the habit of 'snuff dipping' is prevalent and is increasing among young people in other areas also. This term is given to holding a quid of tobacco in the lower buccal sulcus for long periods. More recently an attempt has been made to promote a preparation (Skoal Bandits) for this purpose into Britain. Its production and sale was banned in 1990 but the ban was later overturned.

Use of smokeless tobacco causes extensive leukoplakia-like lesions in the area of mucosa in contact with it. Microscopically there are no specific features but, typically, hyperkeratosis with stromal inflammation and in some cases, dysplasia.

In the earlier stages the changes are reversible if the habit is stopped. However, there is a significant risk of malignant change if the habit is maintained, but usually only after several decades. Most such carcinomas are low grade or verrucous in character.

Syphilitic leukoplakia

Leukoplakia of the dorsum of the tongue is one of the characteristic effects of tertiary syphilis. It is exceedingly rare now.

Histopathology. In addition to the hyperkeratosis and acanthosis with or without dysplasia, typical changes of the late syphilitic granuloma may be seen in the connective tissue with a chronic inflammatory cellular infiltrate, mainly of plasma cells. Giant cells may also be present, and, rarely,

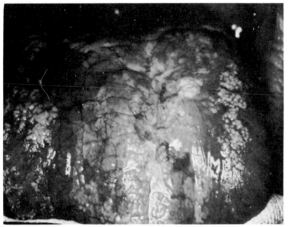

Fig. 16.9 Syphilitic leukoplakia and carcinoma. The plaque has ill-defined margins but there is widespread atrophy of the papillae. In the thickest part of the plaque just to the left of the midline are small erosions which proved to be squamous cell carcinoma on biopsy.

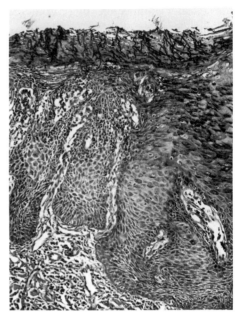

Fig. 16.10a Candidal leukoplakia. The gross acanthosis and infiltration of superficial plaque by candidal hyphae can be seen.

granulomas may be seen. Endarteritis of small arteries is particularly characteristic. One or more foci of malignant change may be found in the epithelium.

Clinically the features of syphilitic leukoplakia are variable apart from its site on the anterior two-thirds of the dorsum of the tongue. The plaque may be thick and widespread or extend over a limited area. Typically it is of irregular thickness with ill-defined margins and may show small red erosions which may indicate foci of malignant change.

Management. After biopsy, the diagnosis must be confirmed by serology. If the disease is still active and unsuspected the patient should be referred for treatment and examination, as syphilitic aortitis or CNS disease may also be present or develop later.

Antibiotic treatment does not cure the leukoplakia, which persists and may undergo malignant change in spite of normal serology. The risk of malignant change is high.

Chronic hyperplastic candidosis (Candidal leukoplakia)

Candida albicans can cause chronic lesions of the oral mucosa, forming persistent tough white

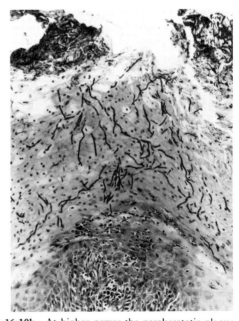

Fig. 16.10b At higher power the parakeratotic plaque, invading hyphae and inflammatory infiltrate at the base of the plaque can be seen.

plaques which are indistinguishable clinically from leukoplakia due to other causes. The diagnosis can only be made with certainty by biopsy, but other features of candidal infection such as angular stomatitis may also be associated.

Pathology

The same essential features are seen in chronic hyperplastic candidosis as in thrush. The differences are merely those of the intensity of the changes related to the chronicity of the infection.

The plaque consists of a thick layer of parakeratotic epithelium invaded by hyphae of candida. These grow into the epithelium approximately at right angles to the surface. There is an inflammatory infiltrate in the plaque consisting of fluid exudate, seen as beads of oedema separating the epithelial cells, and leucocytes both within the plaque but particularly concentrated at its base. The underlying epithelium is hyperplastic, often grossly so, and there are chronic inflammatory changes in the underlying connective tissue.

Some believe that these plaques are merely candidal infection 'superimposed' on another lesion. Nevertheless, no evidence has ever been produced to show the presence of any pre-existing lesion which has become infected. Experimentally it has also been shown that invasion of an epithelium by *Candida albicans* induces epithelial hyperplasia.

Clinical features

Chronic hyperplastic candidosis is typically seen in middle-age but very occasionally one of the rare mucocutaneous candidosis syndromes may pass unrecognised until middle-age is reached. The plaques of candidal leukoplakia are firm, whitish and speckled or of irregular thickness and outline. Underlying and peripheral inflammation of the mucous membrane is usually also seen. Unlike the plaques of thrush, these lesions (as the histology suggests) are tough and adherent and cannot be wiped off.

Common sites are the buccal mucosa, particularly just inside the angle of the mouth, and the dorsum of the tongue; occasionally the palate and other sites may be affected. Chronic angular stomatitis may be associated and help to identify the candidal nature of the lesions.

Rare mucocutaneous candidosis syndromes

Rare types of candidosis involve the mouth and, to a lesser extent, the skin and are known as chronic mucocutaneous candidosis. Several of these uncommon syndromes appear to be genetically determined and inherited as an autosomal recessive trait. One well-known but also uncommon type is associated with endocrine disturbances such as hypoparathyroidism or Addison's disease or both (endocrine-candidosis syndrome). Another type is very severe and is characterised by the appearance of gross proliferative lesions of the skin (candida 'granuloma') as well as oral changes. In these rare disorders the infection starts in early childhood as infantile thrush. Then as the disease persists the lesions progressively change to a leukoplakic character. Chronic mucocutaneous candidosis is one of the very few causes of leukoplakia-like lesions in children.

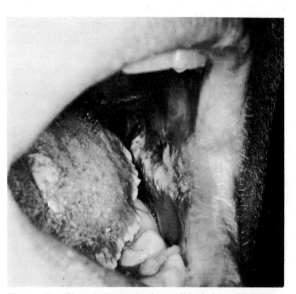

Fig. 16.11 Chronic hyperplastic candidosis in a child. The tough leukoplakia-like lesions affected the buccal mucosa and the tongue on both sides. This was one of several affected siblings. (Reproduced from *Scientific foundations of dentistry* 1976 by courtesy of William Heinemann Medical Books, London)

These diseases, particularly the more severe variants, may sometimes be associated with limited defects of cell-mediated immunity. Iron deficiency is often associated.

Diagnosis

The diagnosis of chronic candidosis cannot be made on clinical grounds alone but may be suspected in the presence of other signs of candidal infection, especially angular stomatitis. A speckled plaque is also suggestive, as there is evidence that these more frequently show candidal infection than do homogeneous plaques.

A scraping from the lesion shows gram-positive hyphae embedded in clumps of epithelial cells. Biopsy shows hyphae invading a parakeratotic plaque which is infiltrated with inflammatory cells and exudate. Deeply there is acanthosis and chronic inflammatory changes in the dermis.

Management

Treatment is difficult, as the response of these long-established infections to topical antifungal drugs is poor and systemic administration can have severe toxic effects. Imidazoles such as miconazole or ketoconazole appear, however, to be more effective than earlier anti-fungal drugs.

Iron deficiency, when present, needs to be treated vigorously.

Hairy (AIDS-associated) leukoplakia

Patients with HIV infection may develop a distinctive type of leukoplakia. The plaque usually affects the lateral margins of the tongue and is soft, white and typically asymptomatic. The surface is corrugated or can have white filamentous projections.

Microscopically there is hyperkeratosis and acanthosis. The surface is frequently corrugated rather than 'hairy' (fine keratin projections). More deeply there are vacuolated and ballooned prickle cells with pyknotic nuclei surrounded by clear halo (*koilocytes*). There is little or no inflammatory infiltrate in the corium. *Candida albicans* infection of the epithelium may be associated.

Replication of EB virus within the epithelial cells and response to acyclovir, with recurrence after cessation of treatment, have been reported.

Diagnosis and management. Patients with 'hairy' leukoplakia are usually HIV positive, and over 60% of these are likely to develop AIDS. Hairy leukoplakia therefore appears to be a sign of a poor prognosis (see Fig. 8.15).

Treatment of asymptomatic cases of hairy leukoplakia may not be necessary. It does not appear to be precancerous, but acyclovir can be given.

Lichen planus

Lichen planus is the most common cause of persistent white lesions in the mouth but these are usually in the form of striae, often forming well-defined patterns as described earlier.

Lichen planus occasionally causes plaque-like lesions, particularly on the dorsum of the tongue.

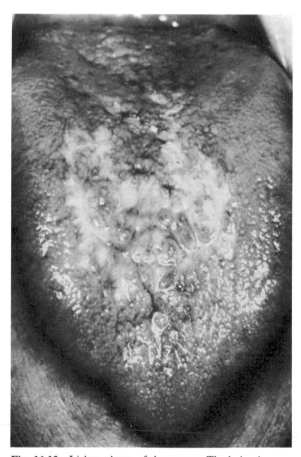

Fig. 16.12 Lichen planus of the tongue. The lesion is plaque-like in this case and simulates the hyperkeratosis seen in other types of leukoplakia.

This plaque may be thick, is characteristically snowy white and may have ill-defined margins having a fluffy or cotton wool-like appearance. Long-standing lichen planus of the buccal mucosa can also become plaque-like. Lichen planus, as mentioned earlier, has some premalignant potential, and up to 1% may undergo malignant change over a 10-year period. However, it is suggested that this is more likely in atrophic rather than plaque-like lesions.

Sublingual keratosis

The typical appearance is an irregular, but frequently symmetrical, white soft plaque with a wrinkled surface and an irregular but well-defined margin. The plaque typically extends from the anterior floor of the mouth to the undersurface of the tongue and may have a roughly butterfly shape. There is usually no associated inflammation.

Histologically, sublingual keratosis is not distinctive, but the frequency of dysplasia or malignant change has been reported to be exceptionally high and may be as great as 15%.

Sublingual keratosis was at one time thought to be a naevus (developmental). This is not the case, and the appearance alone readily enables sublingual keratosis to be distinguished from true white sponge naevus.

Idiopathic leukoplakia

These form the majority of persistent white plaques. From the present (inadequate) basis of knowledge, no aetiological factor can be identified. The histopathology is also highly variable, ranging from 'simple' hyperkeratosis and hyperplasia to severe dysplasia.

The most extensive study on leukoplakia so far carried out suggests that this group has a higher risk of developing cancer than the other types described. In most lesions of definable cause the risk of malignant change is very low, especially now that late-stage syphilis forms a negligibly small group.

Management. Biopsy is essential. If then there is no sign of dysplasia microscopically, the lesion can be kept under observation and biopsies repeated if, for example, the lesion enlarges or develops red

areas. Alternatively, small lesions can be excised entire.

If biopsy shows dysplasia then the risk of malignant change is high and the management becomes more difficult, as discussed below.

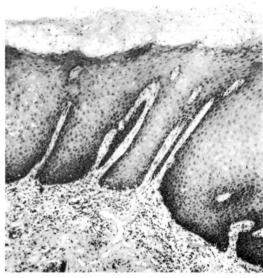

Fig. 16.13 Leukoplakia. There is parakeratosis (i.e. nuclei can be seen in the superficial plaque), gross irregular hyperplasia of the epithelium (acanthosis) and inflammatory changes in the corium indicated by the infiltrate of chronic inflammatory cells.

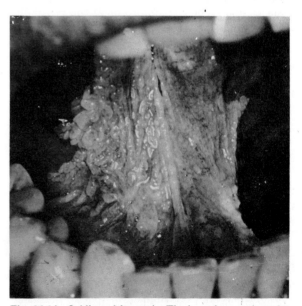

Fig. 16.14 Sublingual keratosis. The irregular margin and wrinkled surface are typical. This patient developed a carcinoma at the edge of this plaque.

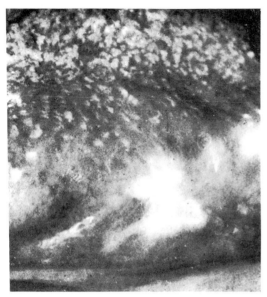

Fig. 16.15 Carcinoma mimicking leukoplakia. This early carcinoma has itself produced a layer of keratin on its surface; it appears clinically as a small patch of leukoplakia but did not develop in a pre-existing white lesion.

Histologically, dysplastic lesions (apart from syphilitic lesions) are mostly a subgroup of leukoplakias of unknown cause. They form only a minority of chronic white lesions but are particularly important because of the risk of malignant change. The only indicator of the possibility of this change is the histological features of dysplasia, as discussed below.

Skin grafts

Grafts form a smooth white area usually flush with the surrounding surface and with a well-defined regular margin. One or two hairs may persist in the area and make the diagnosis obvious, even if it has not already been revealed by the patient's history.

PREMALIGNANT LESIONS OF THE MOUTH

Though a minority of white lesions undergo malignant change, it should not be assumed that all leukoplakias are premalignant or that all premalignant lesions are white. Only a minority of cancers develop in detectable premalignant lesions.

The term 'premalignant' is itself misleading in that it indicates some identifiable change which ultimately progresses to cancer. There is however no completely reliable way of predicting the progress of such a lesion. Some with suspect features later regress. As a consequence it is only justifiable to use the term premalignant *after* malignant change has supervened. The term should be used only retrospectively—that is, from a knowledge of its behaviour one can say that a lesion *was* premalignant.

There is no doubt about the potentialities of some leukoplakias to undergo malignant change but the level of risk cannot be accurately assessed. Most figures have been based on small series and have often been highly selective. The largest single study, carried out in Sweden, was based on no fewer than 782 cases of unspecified white lesions followed for an average of 12 years. Of these only 2.4% underwent malignant change in 10 years and almost twice as many after 20 years. Even this low rate represents a risk of malignant change 50 to 100 times that in the normal mouth. Other (smaller) series have suggested transformation rates of 10% to 30% or more, though in many cases no time scale has been indicated.

Other lesions, particularly red ones (*erythroplasia*), have been shown to have greater precancerous potentialities; many erythroplasias are histologically carcinoma-in-situ when first seen. Others show a mixed picture of white and red change and have been called 'speckled leukoplakias'.

The only guide as to the potentialities of these lesions is provided by the histology and, in particular, by the presence of dysplasia. Unfortunately the assessment of the severity of dysplasia under the microscope cannot be completely objective, and the presence of this change does not allow reliable predictions to be made as to what may ultimately happen.

Overall, genuinely premalignant lesions of the mouth are rare and much less common than frank carcinoma.

Dysplasia (dyskeratosis)

Dysplasia is a histological term. It is not characterised by a specific clinical appearance. Small and innocent-looking white patches are just as likely to

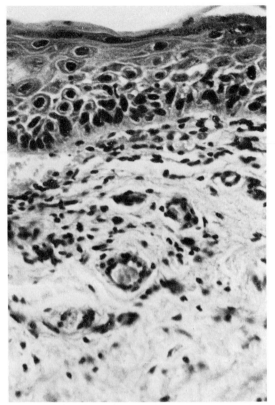

Fig. 16.16 Dysplasia. The epithelium shows greatly disordered maturation. The basal cells lie haphazardly and the nuclei are irregular in size and hyperchromatic. Disorder of the prickle cell layer is also obvious but the epithelium (as is often the case) is not hyperplastic. This patient subsequently developed several carcinomas of the mouth.

show dyskeratosis as large ones. Red, atrophic areas in combination with white, giving a speckled appearance, are suggestive of dysplasia, but dysplastic lesions do not always have this appearance.

Dysplasia, dyskeratosis and atypia are terms which denote disordered proliferation, maturation and organisation of the epithelium. Dysplastic lesions progress to cancer in many but not all cases, but, as mentioned earlier, those which are not going to progress cannot be identified histologically.

Histological features

The epithelium may or may not be hyperplastic and is often thinner than normal (atrophic). The surface usually shows keratosis (though this may be slight) but usually keratinisation is incomplete and the effete cells contain degenerate nuclei (parakeratosis).

The epithelium itself is characterised by some or all of the following changes.

1. *Nuclear hyperchromatism.* The nuclei stain more densely due to increased nucleic acid content.
2. *Nuclear pleomorphism* and altered nuclear/cytoplasmic ratio. The nuclei are variable in size out of proportion to the size of the cell; there may then be little cytoplasm surrounding the nucleus.
3. *Mitoses.* Mitoses may be seen, sometimes at superficial levels.
4. *Loss of polarity.* The basal cells in particular may lie higgledy-piggledy at angles to one another.
5. *Deep cell keratinisation.* Individual cells may start to degenerate long before the surface is reached and show the characteristic eosinophilic change deeply within the epithelium. Strictly speaking, the term 'dyskeratosis' applies only to this particular cellular change.
6. *Differentiation.* The organisation of the individual cell layers becomes lost and no clearly differentiated basal and spinous cell layers can be identified.
7. *Loss of intercellular adherence.* The boundaries of the cells may become separated.

These changes are by no means always seen together and there is no objective way of assessing their severity. It is usually possible to distinguish 'mild' atypia (where the overall differentiation and organisation of the epithelium is not significantly disturbed and few abnormal cells are present) from severe dysplasia. In severe dysplasia the epithelium is conspicuously disorganised and has an irregularly dark and smudgy appearance due to enlarged, hyperchromatic and irregularly shaped nuclei scattered throughout the thickness of the epithelium.

It must be emphasised therefore that the assessment of dyskeratosis is essentially subjective and it is not possible to prognosticate on the basis of the histological changes.

The reason for this unsatisfactory situation is that these changes are so uncommon that it has never been possible to plot the successive changes

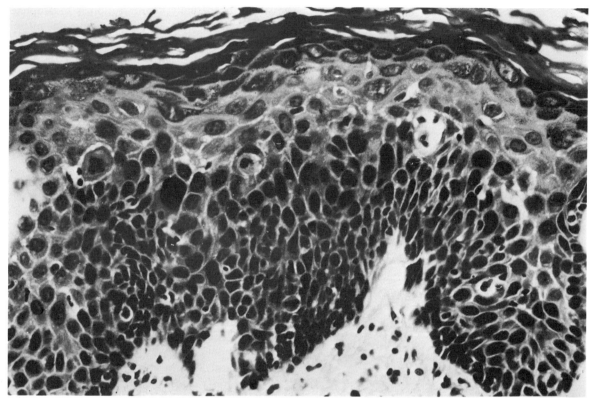

Fig. 16.17 Dysplasia. Many of the epithelial cells are hyperchromatic, irregular in shape and size, have scanty cytoplasm and lack orderly arrangement. Some nuclei are excessively large and mitotic figures can be seen. Malignant change followed within a year (× 300).

in sequential biopsies on an adequate scale. Further, in view of the multiplicity of these changes, it is not possible to quantify them in any reliable way. There is also no satisfactory way of sampling such lesions. If part is taken for biopsy purposes there is no certainty that it is representative of the whole lesion.

Carcinoma-in-situ is a term sometimes used for severe dysplasia where the abnormalities extend throughout the thickness of the epithelium: a state sometimes graphically called 'top-to-bottom change'. All the cellular abnormalities characteristic of malignancy may be present; only invasion of the underlying connective tissue is absent.

This degree of dysplasia is rarely seen in the mouth, and there is no characteristic clinical appearance.

Erythroplasia

Erythroplasias are red and their surface is usually velvety in texture. The term 'erythroplakia' (literally 'red plaque') is frequently used to mean erythroplasia in spite of the fact that these lesions typically do not form raised plaques and their surface is often depressed below the level of the surrounding mucosa. Erythroplasia is also the established term for exactly comparable lesions of the skin. The margin may be sharply defined and there is an obvious difference in surface texture from the surrounding epithelium apart from the difference in colour.

Erythroplasia is rarely seen in the mouth but with few exceptions these lesions prove to be carcinoma-in-situ or invasive carcinoma and must be biopsied.

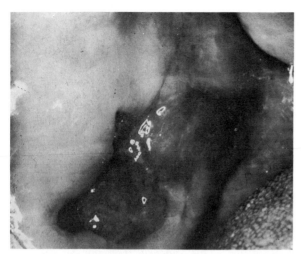

Fig. 16.18 Erythroplasia. This buccal plaque was red and velvety with an irregular shape but sharply defined outline. Histologically this showed carcinoma-in-situ but early invasive carcinoma can also have this appearance.

Speckled leukoplakia

This term denotes a lesion consisting of white flecks or nodules on an atrophic erythematous base. It can be regarded as a combination of leukoplakia and erythroplasia and it has been shown that speckled leukoplakia more frequently shows dysplasia than the more homogeneous looking lesions.

Many cases of chronic candidosis have this appearance.

Management of dysplastic lesions

There is no completely satisfactory method of managing dysplastic epithelial lesions. Total excision (with skin grafting if necessary) is the most obvious approach. Nevertheless, excision does not necessarily prevent the development of cancer later, and one very large survey found that malignant change was more frequent in those which had been treated by surgery. Other evidence suggests that those with dysplastic lesions have a high risk of developing multiple carcinomas. By contrast, it is also known that even severely dysplastic lesions can remain static or regress spontaneously. This cannot be predicted but it does suggest that a more

conservative approach may also be justified. If, therefore, the lesion, after biopsy, is kept under observation, close and frequent follow-up is necessary to enable immediate treatment to be given if carcinomatous change is detected in a later biopsy or shown by the clinical behaviour.

An alternative approach that has been advocated is cryotherapy ablation. However, there have been reports of invasive carcinomas developing in areas treated in this way, and some experimental evidence has been produced to suggest that cryotherapy may increase the risk of malignant change.

CARCINOMA OF THE MOUTH

Carcinoma is the most common malignant tumour of the mouth, but is uncommon compared with other sites such as the bronchus, breast and gastrointestinal tract. Cancer of the mouth accounts for only about 2% of all malignant tumours in such countries as the United Kingdom and the United States. In most countries where data are available, the incidence of cancer of the mouth, though variable, is low. India and Sri Lanka are, however, exceptional, and cancer of the mouth accounts for approximately 40% or more of all cancer there, though the incidence varies widely in different parts of this sub-continent.

Over 90% of these tumours are squamous cell carcinomas. Most of the remainder are adenocarcinomas of minor salivary glands, and a few are undifferentiated.

In round figures approximately 1300 cases of intraoral cancer and just over 250 cases of cancer of the lip are registered in England and Wales each year.

Sites of oral cancer

The lower lip is the most frequent site of oral cancer overall, while the tongue is the most frequently affected site *within* the mouth. The palate is rarely affected and, within the oral cavity, the majority of cancers are concentrated in the lower part of the mouth, particularly the lateral borders of the tongue, the adjacent floor of the mouth and lingual aspect of the alveolar margin, forming a U-shaped area extending back towards the mesopharynx. This accounts for only about 20% of the whole area of the interior of the oral cavity, but 70% of oral cancers are concentrated there.

Age and sex incidence

Oral cancer is an age-related disease, and 98% of patients are over the age of 40. While the overall incidence in the population is only about 1 in 20 000, this increases to 1 in 1100 in males of 75 and over. There is a sharp and virtually linear increase of incidence of mouth cancer with age, as there is with carcinoma in many other sites.

Cancer of the mouth is more common in men than women in most countries, and carcinoma of the lip is at least 8 times as common in men as in women in Britain. Intraoral cancer used to be several times more frequent in men than women, but the male to female ratio is overall about 3 to 2, and in south-east England recent figures show little difference in incidence between the sexes. The change is the result of the gradual decline in oral cancer in men associated with a low but static rate in women.

Aetiology

In considering the aetiology of cancer of the mouth, it is important to take into account the quality of the statistics and in particular the fact that assertions are made about the incidence of the disease (in relation, for example, to tobacco consumption) even when there is no unbiased, national source of data on which to base them. Further, any causative factor has to operate over a long period or the process of malignant change is so slow that there is a prolonged lag period before it becomes evident. This has been shown strikingly in Japan, where cancers are still developing half a century after the gross but instantaneous radiation exposure from the atomic bombs.

Significant or speculative risk factors for oral squamous cell carcinoma include the following:

1. Increasing age
2. Tobacco use
3. Alcohol
4. Infectious agents
   a. Viruses
   b. Syphilis
   c. Chronic candidosis
5. Malnutrition
6. Oral sepsis
7. 'Betel' chewing
8. Sunlight (lip cancer)
9. Genetic factors and oncogenes
10. Precancerous lesions.

Age

As with other carcinomas, oral cancer is rare in the young and rises steeply in incidence with increasing age. This suggests that any carcinogens have to act over a long period.

Tobacco use

The effects of tobacco on the mouth depend on the way it is used, and this varies in different countries. In Westernised countries, cigarette smoking predominates and pipe smoking has declined. In some countries, notably in India and the southern states of the USA, tobacco chewing (more precisely, held unsmoked in the mouth for prolonged periods) is a habit. In addition the methods of processing tobacco before use vary widely, so that its products released into the mouth differ considerably. This is particularly noticeable in India where, in some areas, the use of a particular type of tobacco appears to be associated with a very high incidence of the disease.

Cigarette smoking. This habit which, though declining now in health-conscious countries, is held in the USA to be a major etiological factor, particularly in association with alcohol, and some epidemiological evidence has been produced to support this idea. In Britain, unlike the USA, there is a National Cancer Registry and more accurate information exists as to the incidence of the disease, and it is noteworthy that mouth cancer in males has steadily *declined* over a period of more than three-quarters of a century while cigarette smoking became more and more widespread. During this same period, mouth cancer did not increase in women despite their increasing adoption of cigarette smoking.

In addition, surveys of dysplastic, premalignant leukoplakias have found that the majority developed in non-smokers.

As discussed later, there is rarely any oral lesion that is consistently related to prolonged heavy cigarette smoking. Patients can be seen with apparently healthy oral mucosa despite having smoked heavily for many decades.

In the Indian subcontinent, where the mouth is one of the most common sites of cancer and the prevalence of the disease is probably the highest in the world, tobacco is processed in a variety of ways. It is also smoked in a variety of ways and also chewed as a component of pan ('betel'). Several studies have linked tobacco use there with mouth cancer.

Pipe smoking. This habit has steadily declined in most Westernised countries, and, in Britain in particular, mouth cancer in males has also decreased virtually at the same rate. In women by contrast, pipe smoking has not been a habit and the mouth cancer rate has remained little changed over many decades. In other countries also, epidemiological evidence has associated mouth cancer with pipe smoking.

In general, pipe smoke and other tobacco products tend to be held in the mouth and are thus more likely to have a local effect. Cigarette smoke, by contrast, is inhaled and has well-recognised effects on the lungs.

Tobacco chewing (smokeless tobacco). In the southern USA there has long been the habit of 'snuff dipping' in which a quid of tobacco with various other ingredients is held in the lower buccal sulcus for a prolonged period. This results in an extensive hyperkeratotic plaque and later, in many cases, the development of a low-grade carcinoma. There appears therefore to be little doubt that tobacco applied locally over a long period is carcinogenic.

Recently, smokeless tobacco in a preparation resembling a tea bag (Skoal Bandits) has been promoted in the USA, Britain and elsewhere, as mentioned earlier. Its use has lead to similar keratoses. However, this particular preparation has not been available long enough to have any significant effect on mouth cancer incidence, and its production in Britain has been banned. Tobacco is frequently included in the quid in betel leaf chewers and may account in part for the high incidence of oral cancer in them.

Alcohol

Alcohol consumption has steadily increased in Britain particularly in the past half century. However, as with cigarette-smoking, this increased consumption has been associated with a decline in oral cancer.

In the USA it is generally believed that the combination of smoking and drinking are the most important factors contributing to mouth cancer. Among other considerations, the low incidence of mouth cancer among Mormons, who neither drink nor smoke, is quoted in support of this idea. However, health-conscious groups such as these, like many in south-east England also have a low oral cancer incidence, and it is not clear what protective factors are operating.

In Denmark an increase in oral cancer has been reported and this has been related to increasing alcohol consumption.

Alcoholic drinks are not usually allowed to reside in the mouth for long periods, and there is no consistently found local alcohol-related oral lesion. However, some of the epidemiological evidence from the USA suggests a systemic effect via liver damage, and some studies there have found a stronger correlation between mouth cancer and cirrhosis of the liver than with calculated alcohol consumption. It is suggested therefore that depressed metabolism of potential carcinogens is the operative factor. However, in Britain and probably in other countries, alcohol is not the main cause of hepatic cirrhosis. A high proportion are of unknown cause or due to the several hepatitis viruses.

Infectious agents

Viruses. Earlier attempts have been made to link herpes simplex virus with mouth cancer but the evidence is slender. More recently, human papilloma viruses, particularly type 16, have been found to be associated with mouth cancer. However, they are also associated with papillomas, which have no malignant potential, and with normal mucosa, so that their role is questionable.

Syphilis. Syphilitic leukoplakia, developing in late-stage disease, has a high malignant potential but is no longer a significant risk factor.

Chronic candidosis. As discussed earlier, chronic candidosis can lead to the formation of hyperkeratotic plaques or speckled leukoplakias in which the epithelium is dysplastic. There have been isolated reports of malignant change in such lesions, but, overall, this accounts for a very small proportion of cases.

Malnutrition

There is a high incidence of mouth as well as oesophageal cancer in Paterson–Kelly syndrome (Ch. 20), in which iron deficiency is usually a feature. However, this disease has declined in frequency to such a degree that it is no longer a significant risk factor.

A low intake of vitamin A has been reported in some mouth cancer patients but the significance and validity of this finding are unclear.

In India malnutrition may contribute to the high incidence of mouth cancer. However, there appears to be no comparably high frequency of mouth cancer in other areas, such as many parts of Africa, where malnutrition is at least as severe.

Oral sepsis

Oral sepsis has traditionally been regarded as contributing to mouth cancer but any association has never been quantified. However, oral cancer is most common in low socioeconomic groups, which tend to have the most neglected mouths, and it has also progressively decreased in frequency in Britain, where a slow but steady improvement in oral health (Ch. 26) is well documented. Much of the oral cancer in the Indian subcontinent also appears to be associated with oral neglect.

Despite such considerations the aetiological role of oral sepsis in mouth cancer must be regarded as unproven.

Betel chewing

A widespread habit in the Indian subcontinent is the chewing of a quid of a variety of substances wrapped in betel leaf. The components vary but frequently include areca nut, tobacco and lime. Areca nut releases arecolin which, experimentally, is carcinogenic, while tobacco used in this way is associated with oral cancer in humans as discussed earlier. Oral submucous fibrosis (Ch. 20) is also thought to be a result of exposure to areca nut and to have a potential for malignant change. Nevertheless, these considerations do not apply to oral cancer in other countries.

Sunlight

Exposure to the ultraviolet component of sunlight is a risk factor, with the result that lip cancer is predominantly a disease of outdoor workers, particularly farmers and fishermen. As with other skin cancers, fair-skinned persons are at most risk.

The relationship between exposure to sunlight and lip cancer has been clearly shown in hot countries such as Australia and the USA with large immigrant, fair-skinned populations of European origin. In the USA for example the risk of lip cancer approximately doubles for every 250 miles nearer the equator the site of residence is.

Genetic factors and oncogenes

There are a few genetic disorders, notably dyskeratosis congenita, of which oral cancer is a frequent feature, but these disorders are all rare. Mice with a high susceptibility to oral cancer have also been bred. However, there is no convincing evidence of any genetic trait predisposing to oral cancer in humans apart from rare genetic disorders mentioned earlier.

The c-myc oncogene product and epidermal growth factor receptor protein have been identified in some oral cancers but their role is as yet unclear.

Precancerous lesions

It seems reasonable to suppose that the aetiological factors for precancerous lesions are the same as those for cancer itself. However, there are often no discernable aetiological agents leading either to dysplastic keratotic lesions or to cancer itself. As mentioned earlier, surveys have shown that the majority of dysplastic, potentially premalignant leukoplakias are of unknown cause.

In addition, cancers can also arise in long-standing lesions of lichen planus. However, these and idiopathic dysplastic lesions precede only a relatively few oral carcinomas. In India, an unknown proportion of cancers arise in lesions of oral submucous fibrosis; some of these lesions are associated with betel chewing but many appear to be of unknown cause.

Summary

It is a tenaciously held, traditional belief that cigarette smoking and alcohol consumption are major risk factors for oral cancer, but the epidemiological evidence is conflicting. More certain risk factors such as tobacco chewing or chronic syphilis apply to only a small proportion of carcinomas overall, and in very many patients no risk factor may be identifiable. In the Indian subcontinent, a variety of factors, including tobacco use, betel chewing (often including tobacco), malnutrition and diseases such as oral submucous fibrosis are suspected of being major contributory factors. However, even in this area of the world, where the mouth is one of the most common sites of cancer, the risk factors have not all been identified with certainty.

Survival rates for oral cancer

Duration of survival after treatment depends on a variety of factors, such as the site of the tumour and the stage when treatment started. Other factors are the age and sex of the patient. In all cases the crude survival rates have to be corrected for general mortality from a wide variety of causes, especially in the older age-groups. When sample sizes are sufficiently large and several of these groups can be combined, the survival curves show that the highest mortality is in the first 2 years, the disease then continues to claim victims but at a slower rate, and those few that survive for 10 years have a reasonable chance of having been cured.

The stage of disease at the start of treatment makes it one of the main factors affecting the duration of survival.

As a rough guide it can be said that of males with early-stage disease, nearly 90% survive the first year, about 65% survive for up to 5 years, while just under 55% survive for 10 years.

Of males with late-stage disease, by contrast, well under 45% survive the first year, about 16% survive for 5 years, and 12% survive for 10 years.

The site of the growth has a strong effect on survival. The extremes are seen in cancer of the lip, where the 5-year survival rate for males is over 77%, while for cancer of the tongue it is 26%, and for the mesopharynx it is only 17.6%, and in general the further back the tumour is, the poorer the survival rate. As might be expected, the older the patient, the shorter the duration of survival, partly because older people are less able to withstand radiotherapy or surgery.

Pathology

Carcinoma of the oral cavity is, in over 90% of cases, squamous cell in type and usually well differentiated.

The characteristic microscopic features are invasion of the deeper tissues together with cellular abnormalities. These include pleomorphism and intense nuclear staining.

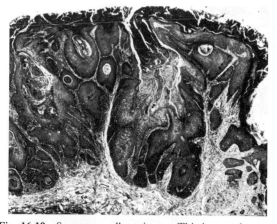

Fig. 16.19 Squamous cell carcinoma. This is an early lesion which formed a small nodule on the side of the tongue. The darkly-staining carcinoma cells are actively invading the underlying tissues and are surrounded by a well-marked inflammatory reaction. The tumour is well differentiated and there are cell-nests within the epithelial processes (× 12).

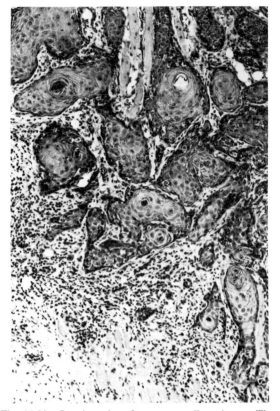

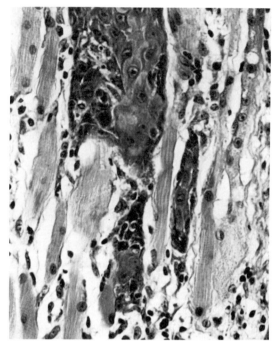

Fig. 16.21 At higher power a group of tumour cells shows typical cytological irregularity. Surrounding and beneath the tumour, muscle fibres are in process of destruction.

Fig. 16.20 Growing edge of squamous cell carcinoma. The invading processes of tumour cells retain the arrangement of squamous epithelium but there are several cell nests formed by premature keratinisation deep within the tissues. Muscle fibres have been surrounded in the upper part of the picture and are in process of destruction. There is lymphocytic infiltrate surrounding the tumour margins.

The invading carcinoma cells grow into the tissues, forming irregular branching processes, the tips of which are often cut off in a section to give the appearance of separate islands of cells beyond the main growth. Tumour cells invade deeper tissues regardless of their nature; muscle, glands, nerves and eventually bone are infiltrated and destroyed.

The nuclei of the cancer cells are enlarged and darkly staining and, especially along the growing edges of the tumour, have little cytoplasm. In the central parts of the better differentiated tumours, the cells have more cytoplasm which stains palely with eosin or may form concentric layers of keratin

(cell-nests). In poorly differentiated tumours the cells tend to more irregular and darkly staining, and little evidence of a squamous pattern may be discernible. Mitoses are more frequent and tend to be abnormal in character. Invading cancer cells excite an inflammatory reaction and become surrounded by lymphocytes and plasma cells. Spread is by infiltration of the surrounding tissues and by lymphatics to the regional lymph-nodes. Bloodstream spread is a late feature of the disease and is rarely seen.

Carcinoma of the lip

Cancer of the lip is the most common single site of oral cancer but is rarely seen by the dentist.

This disease is often recognised at a very early stage and so has a better prognosis than cancer within the mouth.

Clinically the usual site is the vermilion border of the lower lip to one side of the midline. Men of middle age or over are predominantly affected.

An area of thickening, induration, crusting or shallow ulceration of the lip, less than a quarter of an inch in diameter, is often an early carcinoma and should be so regarded until shown to be innocent by histological examination. Later these lesions, if neglected, grow and develop the obvious features of a cancer: either a hard, prominent mass or spreading ulceration. Spread to the lymph nodes tends to be slow; the submental nodes are usually the first to be affected.

Diagnosis of an early carcinoma of the lip depends on histological examination. Some surgeons prefer to excise such lesions widely without taking a preliminary fragment for biopsy; this can be done without danger to the patient or disfigurement and is a justifiable procedure which in many cases brings about a cure. Radiation of the lip is also effective but, whatever the method of treatment, the more advanced the lesion the poorer the prognosis.

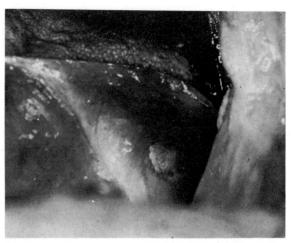

Fig. 16.22 Early squamous cell carcinoma in a heavy pipe smoker. A mirror overlies the dorsum of the tongue. The edge of the minute warty lesion on the lingual aspect of the retromolar area can be seen near the right of the picture and its surface in the mirror below and slightly to the left. There was also typical smoker's keratosis of the palate.

Carcinoma of the tongue

The anterior part of the tongue, particularly the lateral border, is most frequently involved. It is important to note that in its early stages a carcinoma is painless. By the time the patient is first seen there is often, however, either an ulcer, or a swelling and pain may have developed.

In the *early* stages the lesion can be detected when only about 5 mm in diameter. At this stage all that usually can be seen is a small white or red patch, an erosion or a small nodule. More often the lesion is up to 2 cm across. Pain, if present, is not severe or continuous. The growth may, however, be ulcerated and there may be soreness, or stinging pain when sharply flavoured food is eaten. The ulcer is firm with raised edges and has an inflamed, granulating floor which bleeds easily; the base is indurated. The lymph nodes are not usually clinically involved at this stage.

Approximately two out of three patients having localised lesions less than 2 cm in diameter survive for 5 or more years after treatment.

In more advanced disease the usual picture is of a typical malignant ulcer several centimetres in diameter, hard in consistency, with rolled or irregular raised edges, a rough infected floor,

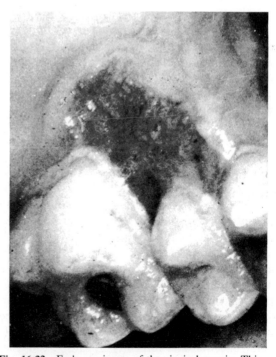

Fig. 16.23 Early carcinoma of the gingival margin. This early lesion in a young woman shows the typical raised, rounded edge and granulating floor.

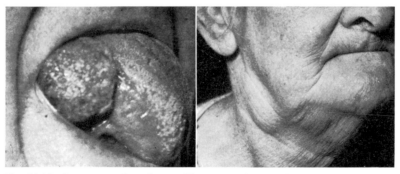

Fig. 16.24 Squamous cell carcinoma. The tumour forms a rounded nodule on the side of the tongue and has not yet ulcerated. The regional lymph nodes are already involved and form a clearly visible swelling in the neck.

which bleeds easily, and an indurated base due to infiltration of surrounding tissues by tumour and inflammatory cells. The growth is fixed to the surrounding tissues and infiltrates the tongue, which becomes progressively stiffer and more painful; eating, swallowing and talking become difficult. By this time pain is usually the main symptom and severe stabbing pain may radiate widely. The lymph nodes also become involved.

Lymphatic drainage from the tip of the tongue is to the submental nodes and then to the juguloomohyoid group, low down in the neck; from the dorsum and sides of the tongue, drainage is to the submaxillary nodes and then to the jugulodigastric group. Spread of cancer may be by an abnormal route, and all the lymph nodes of both sides of the neck must be examined. Affected lymph nodes are enlarged and hard, the surface becomes irregular and the mass becomes fixed to deeper tissues and to the skin. The growth has spread beyond the tongue when the majority of patients are first seen; in these circumstances the prognosis is poor. Only one patient in six survives for 5 years or longer.

In the *late* stages, local spread of the growth causes gross destruction of adjacent parts with widespread sloughing. The tongue becomes fixed; pain is severe and persistent; swallowing and speech are difficult. Affected lymph nodes may ulcerate through the skin. The combination of pain, infection and difficulty in eating, cause loss of weight, anaemia and deterioration of general health; this state, known as malignant cachexia, is ultimately fatal. In other patients aspiration of

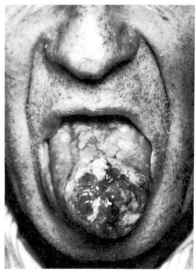

Fig. 16.25 Squamous cell carcinoma. Cancer has developed in a patch of leukoplakia on the tongue of a patient who had had syphilis for many years.

septic material from the mouth causes bronchopneumonia, and, in a few, haemorrhage from the growth is the cause of death.

A small, but possibly increasing, proportion of patients survive treatment of the primary growth but die later from distant metastases.

One factor explaining the high mortality from cancer of the tongue is the fact that lesions affecting the posterior third are less readily detectable and cannot be seen directly. Detection is aided by use of a laryngeal mirror, determined palpation with the finger tip and the use of

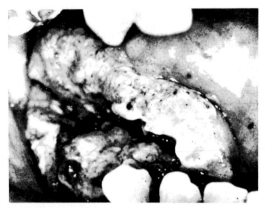

Fig. 16.26 Squamous cell carcinoma. An advanced lesion showing gross destruction and heaped-up, proliferating edges of the ulcer spreading from the floor of the mouth upwards into the side of the tongue, laterally over the alveolar ridge and backwards towards the pharynx.

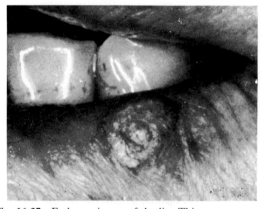

Fig. 16.27 Early carcinoma of the lip. This innocent-looking crusted nodule on the lip of a man of 47 is an invasive, squamous cell carcinoma. Such a tumour should be completely excised with a wedge-shaped piece of the lip.

special radiographic techniques. Nevertheless the diagnosis is often not made until the disease is well advanced.

Carcinoma of the floor of the mouth, alveolar ridge, cheek and palate

These show essentially the same features as carcinoma of the tongue and form indurated masses which usually ulcerate early. Treatment of these tumours, especially when they are close to bone,

is difficult and the prognosis of cancer in any of these sites is also poor.

Management

The nature of a chronic ulcer, white or red lesion, or swelling of the mucous membrane must be confirmed by biopsy. It is only when treatment is started as early as possible that there is a reasonable chance of success.

Biopsy examination of any chronic lesion in the mouth, especially in patients of middle age or older, is therefore essential.

Indecision about taking a biopsy or an attempt to try the effect of local measures or antibiotics usually proves fatal to the patient.

Sepsis in the mouth must be dealt with before beginning treatment, particularly if this is to be by irradiation. In many cases, the teeth should be extracted before radiotherapy, especially if the teeth are in poor condition and clearance is doubly important. The sockets should be healed, as nearly as possible, before treatment is begun. If the teeth are not cleared in this way, irradiation necrosis of the jaws is likely to follow extractions or dental infection later on.

Treatment is frequently by irradiation, and is usually more acceptable to the patient, but surgery is used in such cases as indicated below. Radiotherapy is carried out by implantation of radioactive material into the neoplasm, by means of ultra-high-voltage apparatus or by radioactive isotopes such as cobalt. The affected area can be accurately irradiated and the dose controlled to give the minimum possible damage to surrounding tissues, and reduce the danger of bone necrosis. Surgery is mainly indicated for the following types of case:

1. Very small lesions (about half a centimetre across) should be treated by excision biopsy and removed with the cone of tissue forming the base.
2. Where cancer has invaded bone, the mandible of that side may have to be excised.
3. Where there has been a poor response to irradiation, or the growth has recurred soon after, wide excision may be carried out, but the prognosis is poor.

4. Regional lymph nodes may be removed by block dissection.

The value of chemotherapy is not yet established and is mainly used when all else has failed.

Verrucous carcinoma

This variant of squamous cell carcinoma is of low-grade malignancy. It is more frequent in the elderly, particularly males, and has a characteristic white, warty appearance, forming a well-circumscribed mass raised above the level of the surrounding mucosa.

Microscopically, verrucous carcinoma consists of close-packed papillary masses of well-differentiated squamous epithelium which is heavily keratinised. The lower border of the lesion is well defined and formed by blunt rete processes which 'push down' but do not invade the underlying tissues. There is typically a chronic inflammation in the stroma.

Verrucous carcinoma is slow growing and usually responds well to excision. Metastases are very rare.

BENIGN EPITHELIAL TUMOURS

Squamous cell papilloma

Papillomas mainly affect adults and have a distinctive and clinically recognisable, cauliflower-like or branched structure of finger-like processes. The papillae consist of stratified squamous epithelium supported by a vascular connective tissue core. They are frequently keratinised and cause the lesion to be white (Fig. 16.33).

Human papilloma virus (HPV) of various subtypes are associated. They are not known to be causative, and no inclusion bodies or other indications of a viral origin are histologically evident.

Oral papillomas appear to have no potential for malignant change and respond to local excision.

Infective warts (verruca vulgaris)

These are uncommon but seen particularly in children and frequently appear to have resulted from autoinoculation from warts on the hands.

Histologically the structure is generally similar to that of papillomas but there are typically large clear cells (koilocytes) with pyknotic nuclei and prominent keratohyaline granules in the superficial layers of the prickle cells. There is also positive staining of the nuclei with peroxidase-labelled antiserum to HPV.

Adenoma

Intraoral adenomas arise from minor salivary glands. They typically form smooth, round or lobulated, painless firm swellings and are most frequently found on the palate. Salivary gland adenomas and other tumours are discussed in Chapter 17.

CONNECTIVE-TISSUE TUMOURS AND TUMOUR-LIKE NODULES

Fibrous polyps, epulides and denture-induced granulomas

Fibrous nodules are the most common soft-tissue swellings of the mouth. They are not neoplasms but hyperplastic lesions that develop in sites subject to chronic minor injury and/or low-grade infection. The term *epulis* (literally 'upon the gum') refers only to the site of origin, and, though the great majority of epulides are fibrous, it has no implication as to the histological structure. Less common types of epulis, as described later, are the giant-cell epulis and pyogenic granuloma, and, very rarely, other tumours can appear clinically as an epulis.

Irritation of the gingival margin by the sharp edge of a carious cavity or by calculus may lead to the formation of a fibrous epulis; irritation of alveolar or palatal mucosa by a rough area on a denture may provoke development of a denture granuloma. Though different names are given to these lesions they are similar in origin and structure.

The events leading to the formation of these hyperplastic nodules are probably persistent minor injury, and infection by oral bacteria, causing chronic inflammation and proliferation of granulation tissue. Epithelium covers the nodule, and inflammation gradually subsides; the granulation

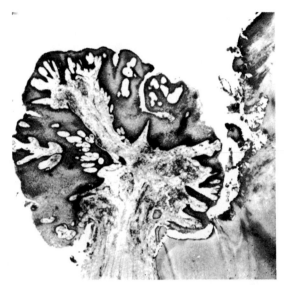

Fig. 16.28 Polyp of the gum. Irritation of gingival tissues by the sharp edge of a carious cavity has caused chronic inflammation and proliferation of connective tissue. The nodule has acquired a covering of epithelium. The similarity of structure of a polyp of the gum and of the pulp (Fig. 4.14) can be seen (× 15).

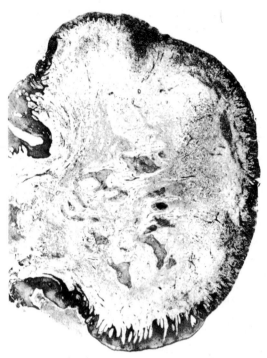

Fig. 16.29 Fibrous epulis. The nodule consists of hyperplastic connective tissue covered by stratified squamous epithelium. Where the surface has been abraded the epithelium is thin and the tissues are infiltrated by inflammatory cells. In the centre of the mass there is irregular bone formation (× 10).

tissue becomes replaced by collagenous fibrous tissue in which inflammatory cells may still be seen.

Bone formation is sometimes seen in a fibrous epulis, and in American texts a fibrous epulis is termed (in an apparent desire to cause confusion) a 'peripheral ossifying fibroma' even though it is not thought to have any relation to the ossifying fibroma of bone nor to be a fibroma.

Clinical features

A fibrous epulis is most common near the front of the mouth between two teeth on the buccal or labial aspect of the gingival margin. A denture granuloma denture-induced hyperplasia often forms in relation to the edge of a denture. These swellings are pale and firm but may be abraded and ulcerated. Obvious inflammation then becomes superimposed.

Fibrous nodules should be excised together with the small base of normal tissue from which they arise. In the case of the fibrous epulis the underlying bone should be curetted. There should be no recurrence if this is done thoroughly and the

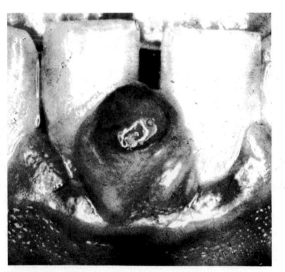

Fig. 16.30 Fibrous epulis. An enlarged photograph showing an epulis arising from the gingival margin between the lower central incisors. The upper part of the surface is ulcerated as a result of injury.

source of irritation is removed. The clinically similar type of epulis which may develop during pregnancy is described below.

On very rare occasions a malignant tumour, particularly a metastasis from elsewhere in the body, may develop on the gingival margin and simulate a simple epulis; this emphasises the need for histological examination of these nodules.

'*Leaf fibroma*'. A leaf fibroma is another fibrous overgrowth which forms under a denture and is flattened against the palate. Often, therefore, it is difficult to see until it is lifted away from its bed. It should be excised.

Pyogenic granuloma and pregnancy epulis

Pyogenic granuloma is a relatively uncommon type of epulis. Clinically it is usually red and relatively soft. Microsopically it consists of many dilated blood vessels in a loose oedematous connective tissue stroma. There is typically a dense acute inflammatory infiltrate but this is sometimes scant or absent.

A pregnancy epulis has the same histological appearances and can only be distinguished by the nature of the patient and usually an associated pregnancy gingivitis (Ch. 6).

Giant-cell epulis

The giant-cell epulis is less common but, like the fibrous epulis, is probably hyperplastic. Just as the fibrous epulis may show osteoblastic activity, the giant-cell epulis shows osteoclasts in proliferating granulation tissue.

Histologically a giant-cell epulis consists of multinucleate cells in a vascular stroma of plump spindle-shaped cells. The appearance is similar to that of a giant-cell granuloma of the jaw but for the fact that the epulis has a covering of stratified squamous epithelium. All gradations are seen between this highly cellular and vascular lesion and a fibrotic nodule containing a few scattered multinucleate cells in the centre. This presumably represents a late stage and an attempt at healing.

Clinically a giant cell epulis is usually found growing from the gingival margin between teeth anterior to the permanent molars. Its development may therefore be related to the resorption of the

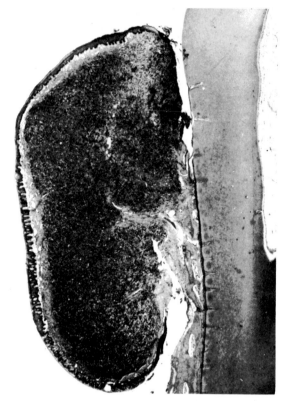

Fig. 16.31 Giant-cell epulis. This has arisen from the periodontal tissues to which it is still attached. The central area of multinucleate and stromal cells is separated from the epithelial covering by a clearly defined zone of connective tissue (× 12).

deciduous teeth. The swelling is rounded, soft, and maroon or purplish in colour; it may grow rapidly in its early stages and bleeds easily.

The treatment is excision of the nodule together with the base of gum from which it arises and curettage of the underlying bone. Adjacent teeth need not be extracted if they are healthy, and if treatment is thorough there should be no recurrence.

Rarely a giant-cell granuloma of the jaw may erode through the bone and appear on the surface as a broad-based, flattened or rounded nodule of purplish colour. The appearance is different from that of a giant-cell epulis, which is pedunculated or forms a prominent polypoid swelling, clearly arising from the gingival margin. A radiograph will confirm the presence of a giant-cell granuloma of the jaw by showing widespread bone destruction

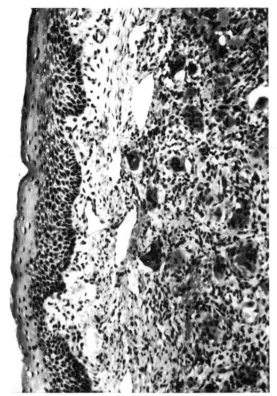

Fig. 16.32 Giant-cell epulis. Part of the same specimen as Fig. 16.31 at higher magnification shows the large multinucleate cells and the plump stromal cells beneath the epithelial covering (× 145).

within the jaw. A giant-cell epulis may cause no bone changes or, at most, superficial resorption.

Fibromas and neurofibromas

Fibroma. The true fibroma is rare in the mouth. Simple connective-tissue overgrowths described earlier are of similar appearance and much more common. However, some authorities regard the latter as fibromas. In any case fibromas cannot be distinguished histologically from hyperplastic nodules with certainty.

Giant-cell fibroma. Despite the rarity of true fibromas this variant is relatively common. It is distinguished microscopically by the presence of large, stellate, darkly-staining cells (quite unlike the multinucleate cells of a giant-cell granuloma) scattered between short, coarse fibrous tissue bundles. Clinically, giant-cell fibromas are typically pedunculated and usually arise from the gingivae. The surface is frequently verrucous.

Neurofibromas. These are uncommon tumours arising from nerve sheaths. They form smooth lumps in the mouth, and microscopically they are cellular with plump nuclei separated by fine, sinuous collagen fibres among which mast cells can usually be found. In many cases they are a feature of neurofibromatosis.

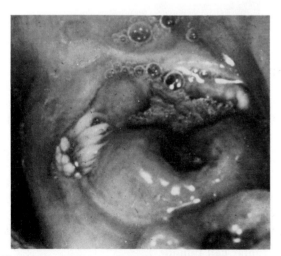

Fig. 16.33 Squamous cell papilloma. The papilloma growing on the gingival margin shows the typical pointed processes of epithelium which are extending up the lingual aspect of the molar. The white appearance is caused by keratinisation.

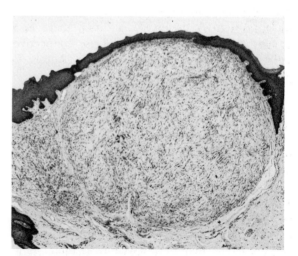

Fig. 16.34 Submucosal neurofibroma. The highly cellular structure with little formation of collagenous fibrous tissue and sharp demarcation from the surrounding connective tissue are characteristic.

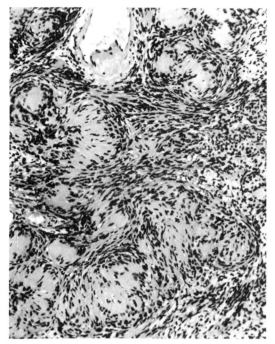

Fig. 16.35 Neurilemmoma. The compact bundles of fibroblast-like cells with grouped nuclei (palisading) (Antoni A tissue) is characteristic (× 135).

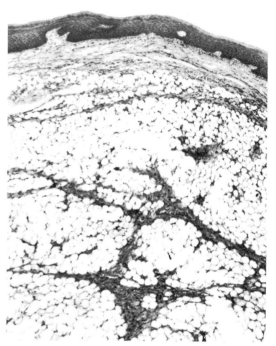

Fig. 16.36 Lipoma. The fat globules (dissolved out during preparation) are held together by areolar tissue and surrounded by a thin fibrous layer (× 45).

Neurilemmomas. These arise from axon sheaths and are also uncommon. They form painless smooth swellings. Microscopically the appearance is distinctive with multiple rounded masses of elongated spindle cells with palisaded nuclei (Antoni A tissue). In addition there is a variable amount of unorganised loose connective tissue with scanty pleomorphic nuclei (Antoni B tissue). Excision is curative.

Lipoma and fibrolipoma

The lipoma is common in subcutaneous tissues, but rare in the mouth. It consists of normal fatty tissue; that is, globules of fat supported by areolar tissue. In some specimens fibrous tissue forms a large part of the tumour, which is then known as a fibrolipoma.

The tumour appears as a soft, rounded, pale swelling which may have a yellowish tinge. It is painless and may be pedunculated. Growth is slow and there are usually no symptoms until the swelling is bitten, or becomes conspicuous because of its size. It should be excised.

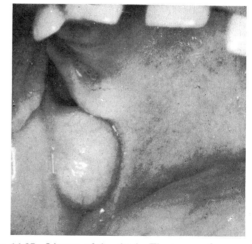

Fig. 16.37 Lipoma of the cheek. The tumour forms a pale, very soft yellowish swelling.

Granular cell tumour

This peculiar entity is rare but the tongue is said to be the most common site.

Histopathology. The two main features are large granular cells (which form the bulk of the lesion)

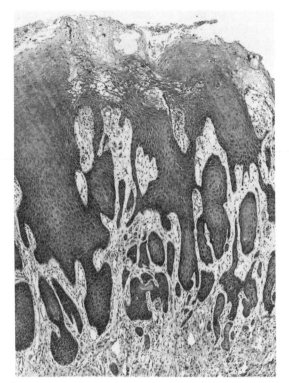

Fig. 16.38 Granular cell tumour. The irregular proliferation of the epithelium (pseudoepitheliomatous hyperplasia) mimics a squamous cell carcinoma strikingly closely.

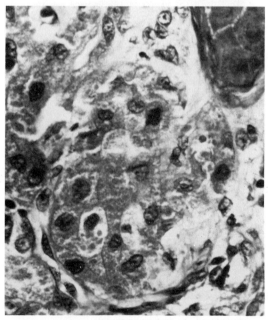

Fig. 16.39 Granular cell tumour. At higher power the granular cells in the connective tissue are apparent and would be diagnostic.

and pseudoepitheliomatous hyperplasia of the overlying epithelium. The granular cells by electron microscopy appear to originate from Schwann cells. However, the striking histological feature is that all stages of apparent transition of striped muscle cells into granular cells may be seen. The granular cells are large, with clearly defined cells membranes and filled with pale granular material which takes up stains for mucopolysaccharides.

The pseudoepitheliomatous hyperplasia can be mistaken for carcinoma, especially when granular cells are not prominent.

Clinically, granular cell myoblastoma typically forms a painless smooth swelling sometimes on the dorsum of the tongue. In this site the lesion has been mistaken for a carcinoma and patients have suffered the unpleasantness and hazards of unnecessary surgery or radiotherapy. Simple excision should, however, be curative.

The *congenital epulis* shows similar cellular appearances to granular cell tumours but lacks pseudoepitheliomatous hyperplasia of the epithelium.

MALIGNANT CONNECTIVE-TISSUE TUMOURS

Sarcomas

Sarcomas of virtually any type can affect the oral soft tissues. All are rare apart from Kaposi's sarcoma in some areas, but among HIV-negative persons, rhabdomyosarcoma is the most common; fibrosarcomas are very rare. These neoplasms tend to affect a considerably younger age group than carcinomas, and rhabdomyosarcomas in particular may be seen in children. Sarcomas grow rapidly, are invasive and destructive of surrounding tissues, and are usually spread by the bloodstream. Many of the sarcomas are clinically indistinguishable from one another, but others such as Kaposi's sarcoma and malignant melanoma are pigmented and must be differentiated from benign pigmented lesions. Pigmented tumours and benign pigmented lesions are therefore discussed together.

Rhabdomyosarcoma. This can affect children or young adults and forms a rapidly growing soft swelling. Microscopically, several types are recognised. The embryonal type, which more frequently affects children, consists of cells of variable shape and size. Some are strap or tadpole-shaped, while cells with cross striations may be difficult to find. The alveolar type consists of slit-like spaces into which hang tear-shaped, darkly-staining cells attached to the walls. These alveoli are separated by a fibrous stroma.

Treatment is by excision and combination chemotherapy but the prognosis is poor.

Fibrosarcomas. There consist of broad interlacing bands of fibroblasts with a streaming or herring bone pattern. They vary from those which produce abundant collagen to those which are highly cellular with closely packed nuclei among which there are often mitoses.

Treatment is by radical excision. Local recurrence and spread is common but metastasis is rare.

Other sarcomas of oral soft tissues. Neurofibrosarcomas, liposarcomas, leiomyosarcomas and even soft-tissue osteosarcomas and chondrosarcomas may be seen, but all are rare.

Lymphomas

Lymphomas can arise from any type of lymphocyte, but most frequently from B cells; they are all malignant. They comprise Hodgkin's disease and the more common non-Hodgkin lymphoma.

Lymphomas relatively frequently involve the cervical lymph nodes but are rare in the mouth. However, in AIDS, lymphomas may account for 2% of oral neoplasms.

Non-Hodgkin lymphomas

Clinically adults are predominantly affected, and, within the mouth, lymphomas form nondescript, usually soft, painless swellings, which may become ulcerated by trauma.

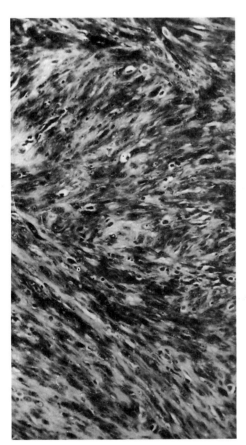

Fig. 16.40 Fibrosarcoma of the tongue. There are streams of neoplastic fibroblasts, but the striking feature is the dense masses of spindle-shaped, darkly-staining nuclei and their variation in size (× 125).

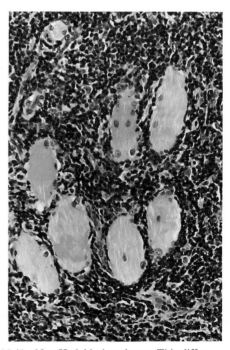

Fig. 16.41 Non-Hodgkin lymphoma. This diffuse lymphoma consists of small neoplastic lymphocytes which have invaded and are destroying muscle.

Nasopharyngeal (T cell) lymphoma is a rare cause of midline granuloma syndrome (Ch. 20) and can cause swelling and ulceration of the palate as a presenting feature.

Microscopically lymphomas frequently present difficulties of precise diagnosis. Non-Hodgkin lymphomas may be *diffuse* and appear as solid sheets of lymphocytes which may be predominantly small or large. Alternatively they may have a *follicular* pattern. Most follicular lymphomas are low grade and have a better prognosis. Invasion of adjacent tissues may be seen and helps to confirm the malignant nature of these tumours.

If traumatised, inflammatory cells can obscure the lymphomatous nature of the tumour. However, lymphoma cells are monoclonal and this can be recognised by immunocytochemistry by the production particularly of kappa light chains only.

Management. In addition to biopsy, staging is necessary to determine the extent of spread of the tumour. In general, localised disease is treated by irradiation while those (the majority of patients) with disseminated disease are treated by combination chemotherapy. Oral complications of such treatment, such as ulceration and infection, are common.

Burkitt's lymphoma. This is unusual in that its onset is in childhood, is endemic in East Africa and has an association with the Epstein Barr virus (EBV).

Clinically it is also unusual in its predominantly extranodal distribution. The jaw is the single most common initial site, and spread to the parotid glands is common. Over 95% of cases respond completely to single-dose chemotherapy.

Microscopically Burkitt's lymphoma is a small-cell lymphoma containing scattered pale histiocytes which give the otherwise dark sheets of cells a so-called 'starry sky' appearance.

Lymphoma resembling Burkitt's lymphoma microscopically, can also be a complication of immunosuppressive treatment and of AIDS but does not behave like African Burkitt's lymphoma.

Hodgkin's disease

The cervical lymph nodes are frequently affected and are typically firm and rubbery but not tender. Lesions are exceptionally rare in the mouth and are not clinically distinguishable from non-Hodgkin lymphoma. Microscopically, the characteristic features are the mixed cellular picture and occasional Reed–Sternberg giant cells with paired (mirror-image) nuclei.

Permanent cure of some types of Hodgkin's disease is possible as a result of irradiation of localised disease or combined chemotherapy, and the overall 5-year survival rate may be up to 80%.

Melanoma and other pigmented lesions

Some uncommon but malignant oral tumours, notably melanomas and Kaposi's sarcoma, can appear as pigmented patches and must therefore be distinguished from the many benign causes of pigmentation.

Oral melanotic naevi

Pigmented naevi are benign lesions of melanocytes which form circumscribed brown to black patches about 5 or 6 mm across, usually on the hard palate. They are asymptomatic but should be excised and sent for microscopy as they cannot be distinguished clinically from early malignant melanomas.

Microscopically the main features are modest numbers of pigmented melanocytes in the basal cell layer but many clumps of melanocytes in the corium. Rarely, intraepithelial foci of proliferating melanocytes project into the corium and appear to be dropping off the basal layer (junctional activity). Equally rarely, junctional activity is associated with circumscribed nests of melanocytes in a limited area of the upper corium (compound naevus).

In the *blue naevus*, the epithelium is normal, but beneath and separate from it is a focus of spindle-shaped pigmented melanocytes.

All these variants should be excised.

Malignant melanoma

Intraoral melanomas are rare. They are usually dark brown or black or, if non-pigmented, red. They are macular or nodular and may ulcerate.

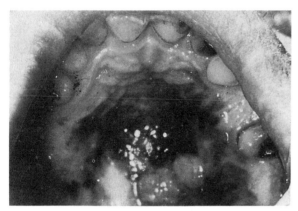

Fig. 16.42 Malignant melanoma. As can be seen the tumour was already extensive when first seen, and survival was short.

The palate is most frequently affected. Melanomas may be noticed by chance but more frequently cause soreness, bleeding, or a neck mass. The peak age incidence is between 40 and 60.

Early diagnosis, by biopsy of all pigmented patches, is essential, though most will be found to be amalgam tattoos or, less frequently, melanotic naevi.

Microscopically melanomas consist of neoplastic melanocytes often surrounded by clear halos, both within the epithelium and invading deeper tissues. These cells are round to spindle shape and typically speckled or intensely pigmented with melanin. However, in amelanotic melanomas, the absence of pigment makes these cells more difficult to recognise.

Melanomas of the superficial spreading type are rare in the mouth and they are usually invasive unless recognised unusually early. The prognosis is consequently poor as there is early involvement of lymph nodes. Distant spread is to the lungs, liver, bones and other organs.

Treatment is by radical excision and usually chemotherapy or radiotherapy or both. In a recent series the median survival for mucosal melanomas was less than 2 years.

Amalgam tattoo

Fragments of amalgam frequently become embedded in the oral mucosa and form the most common pigmented patches which may simulate melanomas clinically. They are usually close to the dental arch, tend to be bluish rather than brown and may be 5 mm or more across. Dense tattoos may be radiopaque.

Microscopically amalgam is seen as brown or black granules deposited particularly along collagen bundles and round small blood vessels. There may be no inflammatory reaction or there may be a foreign body reaction with amalgam granules in the macrophages or giant cells.

Excision is necessary only to exclude the possibility of a melanoma.

Melanotic neuroectodermal tumour of infancy

One of these tumours (Ch. 11) may very rarely show through the mucosa as an ill-defined pigmented area in the palate.

Other mucosal pigmentations

These include multiple pigmented macules in Peutz Jeghers syndrome, diffuse pigmentation due to Addison's disease or drugs, racial pigmentation (mainly gingival), and pigmentation occasionally associated with chronic lichen planus or AIDS.

Red or purple lesions

Red or purple lesions are frequently tumours or other lesions of blood vessels. However, amelanotic melanomas are also red.

Erythroplasia

As described earlier, these red and often velvety circumscribed areas are frequently dysplastic with a high risk of carcinomatous change, or are early carcinomas.

Other causes of red mucosal areas

These are usually diffuse and readily distinguished clinically from erythroplasia, but occasionally the latter needs to be excluded by biopsy. They include:

— Candidosis (particularly denture stomatitis)
— Pernicious and other anaemias
— Median rhomboid glossitis.

Exceptionally rarely, pernicious anaemia can cause red areas simulating erythroplasia, but these are transient, only to reappear in another site. More characteristic are patterns of red streaks on, or generalised redness of, the dorsum of the tongue, as may be the case in any type of anaemia.

Haemangiomas

Haemangiomas are mostly hamartomas of blood vessels; vascular neoplasms (apart from Kaposi's sarcoma) are rare.

Haemangiomas may be localised but are occasionally diffuse and associated with similarly affected areas of the face and rarely also of the meninges (Sturge Weber syndrome) when epilepsy and mental defect are associated.

Isolated haemangiomas form purple, flat or nodular lesions which blanch on pressure. *Micros-*

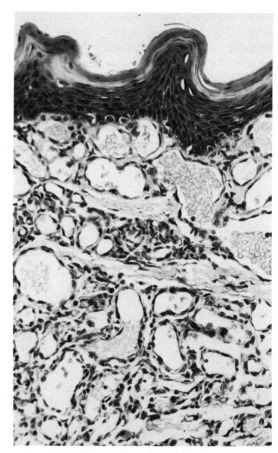

Fig. 16.44 Capillary haemangioma. At higher power the multitude of small vessels is more obvious.

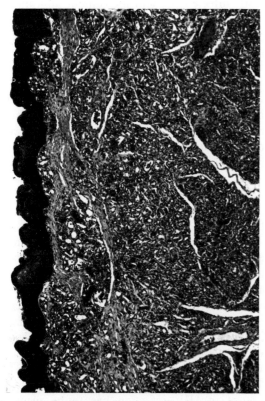

Fig. 16.43 Capillary haemangioma. The innumerable small blood vessels extending immediately under the epithelium give it the characteristic red colour. A vascular naevus of the face was associated (× 48).

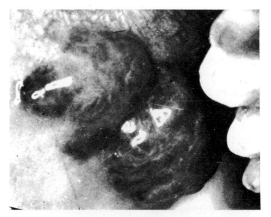

Fig. 16.45 Cavernous haemangioma of the cheek. The colour is deep purple and the structure, i.e. a mass of thin-walled blood sinuses, is apparent from the clinical appearance. A mass engorged with blood and as prominent as this, is liable to be bitten and bleed severely.

copically they are either capillary or cavernous or mixed. The capillary type consists of innumerable minute blood vessels and vasoformative tissue—mere rosettes of endothelial cells. The cavernous type consists of large blood-filled sinusoids.

Excision of mucosal haemangiomas should be avoided unless they cause repeated episodes of bleeding due to trauma. However, excision can sometimes be achieved without severe bleeding, especially if cryosurgery is used.

Lymphangioma

These uncommon tumours have an essentially similar structure to haemangiomas but normally

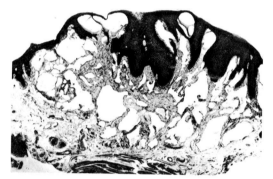

Fig. 16.46 Lymphangioma. There is a localised aggregation of dilated lymph vessels which formed a pale superficial swelling. Bleeding into these lesions causes them suddenly to become purple or almost black (× 14).

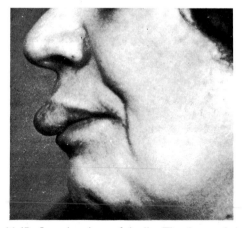

Fig. 16.47 Lymphangioma of the lip. The characteristic swelling of the lip (macrocheilia) sometimes produced by these tumours is shown here.

form pale, translucent, smooth or nodular elevations of the mucosa. However, they may be noticed because they suddenly swell and become dark purple due to bleeding into the lymphatic spaces. Rarely lymphangiomas are diffuse and extensive, and cause generalised enlargement of the tongue (macroglossia) or of a lip (macrocheilia).

Localised lymphangiomas can be excised but this is more difficult in the diffuse type where the operation may have to be done in stages.

Kaposi's sarcoma

Since the outbreak of AIDS, Kaposi's sarcoma has become the most common type of intraoral sarcoma. It mainly affects male homosexuals with AIDS, but has occasionally been seen in immunosuppressed patients such as those who have had organ transplants.

Within the mouth, the palate is the most frequently affected site and the tumour appears as a purplish area or nodule which bleeds readily. In any male below the age of about 50, with such a lesion, Kaposi's sarcoma must be excluded since (in the absence of immunosuppressive treatment) it is pathognomonic of AIDS.

Microscopically Kaposi's sarcoma is a vascular tumour in which the factor VIII antigen (a marker for endothelial cells) can be identified. The early 'pre-sarcomatous' lesion consists of a mass of capillary-size blood vessels, sometimes with mononuclear cell cuffing. It resembles granulation tissue, particularly in the mouth where superficial lesions can be traumatised and become secondarily inflamed.

Later, there is increasingly widespread angiomatous proliferation, and in some areas the vessels may be slit-shaped when obliquely sectioned. There is also proliferation of angular or spindle-shaped interstitial cells. Ultimately, the latter predominate and show increasing numbers of mitoses. Central necrosis may develop and extravasation of red cells can leave deposits of haemosiderin.

Biopsy will confirm the diagnosis but the presence of HIV infection has to be made by other means, particularly other clinical manifestations (such as opportunistic infections), the blood

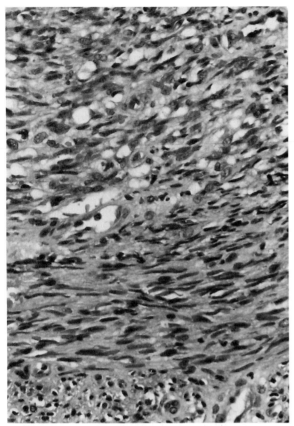

Fig. 16.48 Kaposi's sarcoma. Spindle-shaped cells predominate in this well-advanced lesion but there are minute vascular spaces in the upper part of the picture.

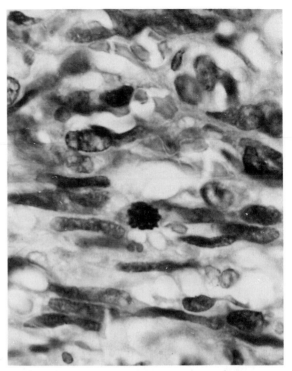

Fig. 16.49 Kaposi's sarcoma. At high power a single mitosis can be seen in this field among the spindle cells.

picture, showing lymphopenia, and, if possible, an HIV antibody test.

Kaposi's sarcoma must be distinguished from AIDS-associated thrombocytopenic purpura, which may appear similar clinically. However, the latter may be seen earlier and is distinguishable by haematological testing.

Other red or purple tumour-like nodules

These include:

—Pyogenic granuloma
—Pregnancy epulis
—Giant-cell epulis
—Purpura and other blood blisters
—Telangiectases
—Lingual varices.

Purpura and blood blisters.

Purpura, as mentioned above, may have to be distinguished from Kaposi's sarcoma in some patients. It is described in more detail in Chapter 20.

Blood blisters. These may be a manifestation of purpura or the result of bleeding into a bulla, in for example, mucous membrane pemphigoid.

Telangiectases. These may result from hereditary haemorrhagic telangiectasia (HHT) where there are multiple pinhead size, purplish lesions scattered about the oral mucosa and skin. Significant oral bleeding from this cause is rare.

Post-irradiation telangiectasia is recognisable from the history and by the ischaemic pallor of the surrounding mucosa.

Lingual varices form symmetrically on the underside of the tongue in the elderly. If they are noticed and alarm the patient, reassurance should be given.

Localised oral purpura is characterised by blood blisters forming in the oral mucosa as a result of minor or unnoticed trauma, but there is no abnor-

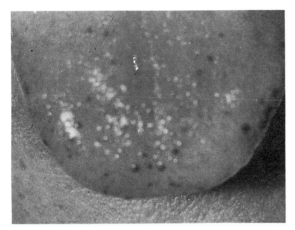

Fig. 16.50 Hereditary haemorrhagic telangiectasia. Multiple 1–2 mm telangiectasia were scattered in the mucosa of the tongue and the rest of the mouth but had not bled significantly.

mality of haemostasis. Occasionally such blisters form in the throat and cause a choking sensation ('angina bullosa haemorrhagica'). Systemic purpura can be firmly excluded by haematological examination and the patient can thus be reassured.

Metastatic tumours

Exceedingly rarely, metastatic deposits form in the oral soft tissues and may, for example, clinically mimic a non-neoplastic epulis. The appearance of soft-tissue metastases is variable. The diagnosis can only be made by microscopy, and this emphasises the need to biopsy all soft-tissue swellings.

SUGGESTED FURTHER READING

Abdel-Salam M et al 1990 Which oral white lesions will become malignant? An image cytometric study. Oral Surg, Oral Med, Oral Pathol 199: 345–350

Archibald D, Lockhart P B, Sonis S T et al 1986 Oral complications of multimodality therapy for advanced squamous cell carcinoma of the head and neck. Oral Surg, Oral Med, Oral Pathol 61: 139–141

Blatchford S J, Koopman C F, Coulthard S W 1986 Mucosal melanoma of the head and neck. Laryngoscope 96: 929–934

Bouquot J E, Weiland L E, Kurland L T 1988 Leukoplakia and carcinoma in situ synchronously associated with invasive oral/oropharyngeal carcinoma in Rochester Minn., 1935–1984. Oral Surg, Oral Med, Oral Pathol 65: 199–207

Brahim J S, Katz R W, Roberts M W 1988 Non-Hodgkin's lymphoma of the hard palate mucosa and buccal gingiva associated with AIDS. J Oral Maxillofac Surg 46: 328–330

Bryne M, Koppang H S, Lilleng R et al 1989 New malignancy grading is a better prognostic indicator than Broders' grading in oral squamous cell carcinomas. J Oral Pathol Med 18: 432–437

Buchner A, Hansen L S 1987 Pigmented nevi of the oral mucosa: A clinicopathological study of 36 new cases and review of 155 cases from the literature. Oral Surg, Oral Med, Oral Pathol 63: 566–572

Buley I D, Gatter K C, Kelly P M A et al 1988 Granular cell tumours revisited. An immunohistochemical and ultrastructural study. Histopathology 12: 263–274

Burton G V et al 1990 Extranodal head and neck lymphoma. Arch Otolaryngol Head Neck Surg 116: 69–73

Corey J P, Calderelli D D, Hutchinson J C et al 1986 Surgical complications in patients with head and neck cancer receiving chemotherapy. Arch Otolaryngol Head Neck Surg 112: 437–439

Eveson J W 1981 Animal models of intraoral chemical carcinogenesis: A review. J Oral Pathol 10: 129–146

Eveson J W 1983 Oral premalignancy. Cancer Surveys 2: 403–424

Forastiere A A 1986 Review: Management of advanced stage squamous cell carcinoma of the head and neck. Am J Med Sci 291: 405–415

Freedman A M, Reiman H M, Woods J E Soft tissue sarcomas of the head and neck. Am J Surg 158: 367–372

Hogewand W F C et al 1989 The association of white lesions with oral squamous cell carcinoma. Int J Oral Maxillofac Surg 18: 163–164

Howell R E, Handlers J P, Abrams A M et al 1987 Extranodal oral lymphoma. Part II: Relationship between clinical features and the Lukes–Collins classification of 34 cases. Oral Surg, Oral Med, Oral Pathol 64: 597–602

Hoyt D J, Jordan T, Fisher S R 1989 Mucosal melanoma of the head and neck. Arch Otolaryngol Head Neck Surg 115: 1096–1099

Jones G M, Sheperd J P, Scully C 1987 A case of squamous cell carcinoma arising in an area treated with a carbon dioxide laser. Br J Oral Maxillofac Surg 25: 57–60

Kashima H K et al 1990 Human papilloma virus in squamous cell carcinoma, leukoplakia, lichen planus, and clinically normal epithelium of the oral cavity. Ann Otol Laryngol 99: 55–61

Katsikeris N, Kakarantza-Angelopolou E, Angelopoulos A P 1988 Peripheral giant cell granuloma. Clinicopathological study of 224 new cases and review of 956 reported cases. Int J Oral Maxillofac Surg 17: 94–99

Kaugars G E, Burns J C, Gunsollwy J C 1988 Epithelial dysplasia of the oral cavity and lips. Cancer 62: 2166–2170

Leading article 1989 Oral cancer. Lancet 335: 311–312

Lind P O 1987 Malignant transformation in oral leukoplakia. Scand J Dent Res 95: 449–455

McAndrew P G 1990 Oral cancer and precancer: treatment. Br Dent J 168: 191–198

MacDonald D G, Critchlow H A 1987 Effects of 2 episodes of cryosurgery on carcinogen-treated hamster cheek pouch. Int J Oral Maxillofac Surg. 16: 90–94

Mashberg A, Feldman L J 1988 Clinical criteria for identifying early oral and oropharyngeal carcinoma: erythroplasia revisited. Am J Surg 156: 273–275

Moller H 1989 Changing incidence of cancer of the tongue, oral cavity and pharynx in Denmark. J Oral Pathol Med 18: 224–229

Murti P R, Daftary D K, Bhonsle R B et al 1986 Malignant potential of oral lichen planus; observations in 722 patients from India. J Oral Pathol 15: 71–77

Murti P R et al 1990 Effect on the incidence of oral submucous fibrosis of intervention in the areca nut chewing habit. J Oral Path Med 19: 99–100

Palmer R M 1987 Tobacco smoking and oral health. Health Education Authority

Palmer R M 1988 Tobacco smoking and oral health. Br Dent J 166: 258–260

Patton L L, McMillan C W, Webster W P 1990 American Burkitt's lymphoma: a 10-year review and case study. Oral Surg, Oral Med, Oral Pathol 69: 307–316

Peters E, Cohen M, Altini M, Murray J 1989 Rhabdomyosarcoma of the oral and paraoral region. Cancer 63: 963–966

Pospisil O A, MacDonald D G 1981 The tumour potentiating effect of cryosurgery on carcinogen treated hamster cheek pouch. Br J Oral Surg 19: 96–104

Rao B N, Santana V M, Fleming I D et al 1989 Management and prognosis of head and neck sarcomas. Am J Surg 158: 373–377

Scully C 1988 Viruses in the aetiology of cancer. Br Dent J 166: 362–364

Scully C et al 1988 Papillomaviruses: The current status in relation to oral disease. Oral Surg, Oral Med, Oral Pathol 65: 526–532

Shibuya H et al 1986 Leukoplakia-associated multiple carcinomas in patients with tongue carcinoma. Cancer 57: 843–846

Stewart C M, Watson R E, Eversole L R et al 1988 Oral granular cell tumors: a clinicopathological and immunocytochemical study. Oral Surg, Oral Med, Oral Pathol 65: 427–435

Wey P D, Lotz M J, Triedman L J 1987 Oral cancer in women nonusers of tobacco and alcohol. Cancer 60: 1644–1650

Williams J L L 1990 Oral cancer and precancer: clinical features. Br Dent J 168: 13–17

Woods J E 1989 Management of malignant melanoma of the head and neck. May Clin Proc 64: 861–863

17. Diseases of the salivary glands

Normal function and health of the mouth depend on normal secretion of saliva by the major and minor glands. Failure of salivary secretion causes a dry mouth which, apart from being distressing, encourages oral infection.

OBSTRUCTION

Salivary calculi

A stone occasionally forms in a salivary gland or duct, usually by deposition of calcium salts around a nidus of organic material, and has a layered microscopic structure.

At least 80% of calculi form in the submandibular gland, about 6% in the parotid and about 2% in the sublingual and minor salivary glands.

Clinical features

Adults are mainly affected—males twice as often as females. Salivary calculi are usually unilateral and the classical symptom is pain related to eating, when the smell or taste of food stimulates salivary secretion. Alternatively obstruction of the duct leads to infection, pain and swelling of the gland.

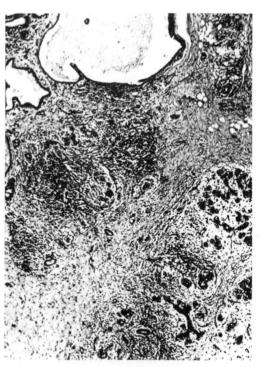

Fig. 17.1 Salivary obstruction. A grossly dilated duct is seen at the top of the picture. Below, the secretory tissue has atrophied and is extensively infiltrated with chronic inflammatory cells (× 40).

Occasionally there may be no symptoms until the stone passes forward along the duct and is felt within the mouth. Alternatively the stone may be noticed on a routine radiograph.

The diagnosis can be confirmed if the calculus can be palpated in the duct or seen at the duct orifice. If further back the calcified material can frequently be visualised in a radiograph. About 40% of parotid and 20% of submandibular stones are not radiopaque, and sialography may be needed to locate them.

Calculi are *not* a cause of dry mouth.

Management

If sufficiently far forward in the duct a stone may sometimes be milked forward and manipulated out of the duct orifice. Otherwise the duct has to be opened to gain access. This may be done by an incision under local anaesthesia along the line of the duct just long enough to release the mass. A temporary suture should be put through the duct behind the calculus to prevent it from slipping backwards. The papilla should be left unsutured or the margins of the opening sutured to the mucosa on either side to prevent subsequent scarring and fibrous obstruction.

If the gland has become damaged by recurrent infection and fibrosis or calculi have formed within the gland itself, it may have to be excised.

Duct obstruction

The usual cause of obstruction of the papilla is chronic trauma (from such causes as projecting clasps, faulty restorations or sharp edges of broken teeth) leading to fibrosis. Fibrosis makes the duct papilla difficult to find and may prevent insertion of a probe.

Fibrosis and stenosis of a duct may be caused by ulceration round a calculus or result from incompetent surgery.

Sialography should show the degree of narrowing of the duct or papilla and dilatation behind. Once the cause has been removed treatment depends on the site of the obstruction. The papilla may have to be excised and the duct lining sutured to the oral mucosa on either side. Alternatively the duct may be dilated with bougies.

Salivary fistula

Salivary fistula, a communication between the duct system or gland with the skin or mucous membrane, is uncommon. Internal fistulae drain into the oral cavity and cause no symptoms. A fistula on the skin, however, is troublesome and often persistent. It may be the result of an injury to the cheek or a complication of surgery. Infection often becomes superimposed and the persistent leakage of saliva prevents healing. The treatment is primarily by surgical repair but is difficult. The problem is such that external incisions into the parotids should be avoided at all costs as there is also the possibility of damage to branches of the facial nerve.

Mucoceles—cysts

The most common type of salivary and soft-tissue cyst is the mucous extravasation cyst (mucocele) but retention cysts occasionally also form.

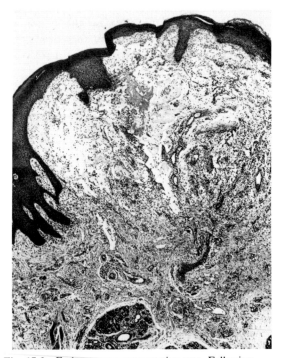

Fig. 17.2 Early mucous extravasation cyst. Following damage to the duct, secretion is escaping into the tissues, forming irregular pools of fluid just beneath the surface and provoking an acute inflammatory response ($\times$ 18).

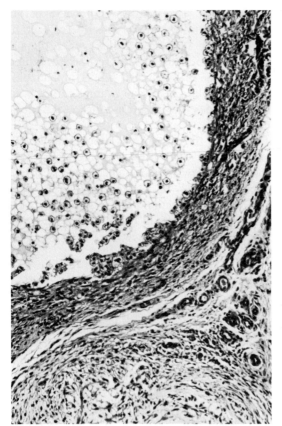

Fig. 17.3 Mucous extravasation cyst. A completely enucleated cyst shows a wall of compressed connective tissue and granular contents containing disintegrating cells. Against the wall, lower right, there is some compressed glandular tissue ($\times$ 12).

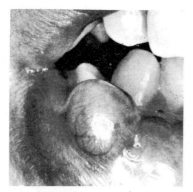

Fig. 17.4 Mucous cyst. This is the commonest site. The rounded, bluish, translucent appearance is characteristic.

Mucoceles mainly affect the minor salivary glands, particularly of the lip.

Aetiology and pathology

The cause is usually damage to the duct of a mucous gland. This may be caused by a blow on the lip, as might happen to a football referee holding a whistle in his mouth.

Microscopically saliva that has leaked into the superficial surrounding tissues excites an inflammatory reaction. The pools of saliva gradually coalesce to form a rounded cyst usually surrounded by compressed connective tissue without an epithelial lining. Occasionally the duct may become obstructed but less severely damaged so that saliva does not escape into the surrounding tissues. A retention cyst thus forms with a lining of compressed duct epithelium.

Clinical features

Mucoceles most often form in the lower lip and occasionally on the buccal mucosa or floor of the mouth (ranula).

They are usually superficial and rarely larger than 1 cm in diameter. In the early stages they appear as rounded fleshy swellings. When fully developed they are obviously cystic, hemispherical, fluctuant and bluish due to the thin wall.

It is not possible to distinguish a mucous extravasation cyst from a retention cyst clinically, but this is of little practical importance.

Treatment

A small superficial mucocele is treated by excision with the underlying glandular tissue. No deep dissection is necessary and the small gland is usually found to have been removed with the cyst.

Ranula

This term is often used loosely for any cyst of the floor of the mouth, but is more properly applied to mucoceles arising from the sublingual or submandibular salivary glands. They are uncommon.

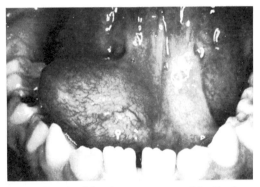

Fig. 17.5 Ranula. Like the mucous cyst of the lip the ranula forms a bluish, translucent swelling in the floor of the mouth.

The structure is essentially the same as other mucoceles, though there is usually an epithelial lining.

Ranulae are usually unilateral and 2 or 3 cm in diameter. Occasionally they extend across the whole of the floor of the mouth. They are soft, fluctuant and bluish in colour. A ranula is typically painless but may interfere with speech or mastication.

Treatment is preferably by marsupialisation with removal of the related gland. A simple incision leads to recurrence, and enucleation is difficult because of the very thin wall.

SIALADENITIS

Mumps

Mumps is an acute infection by a paramyxovirus (the mumps virus) causing painful swelling of the parotids and sometimes other glands. It is highly infectious and is the most common cause of acute parotid swelling.

Clinical features. Children are mainly affected. An incubation period of about 21 days is followed by headache, malaise, fever and tense, painful and tender swelling of the parotids.

Adults who contract mumps often have more serious effects such as orchitis or oophoritis. The malaise may also be more severe and prolonged. Meningitis or permanent nerve deafness are possible complications.

After an attack immunity is long lasting.

The diagnosis is usually obvious from the history and clinical features, and mumps is rarely a dental problem. Unilateral swelling of a parotid may be mistaken for a dental infection or bacterial sialadenitis. On the rare occasions when the submaxillary or sublingual glands are affected, mumps may have to be differentiated from lymphadenitis. In cases of doubt a history of mumps earlier in life usually excludes this diagnosis since recurrence is so rare.

If necessary the diagnosis of mumps can be confirmed by a rise in titre of complement-fixing antibodies. Afterwards antibodies to the S antigen disappear relatively quickly, and their presence indicates recent infection. The V antibody is persistent and its presence in the serum only indicates an infection at some time in the past.

Suppurative parotitis

Suppurative parotitis traditionally affected debilitated patients, particularly postoperatively, as a result of xerostomia secondary to restricted fluid intake.

Currently, suppurative parotitis can still be a complication of debilitating conditions or septicaemia but is probably more commonly seen in ambulant patients with severe xerostomia, particularly Sjögren's syndrome, and has even been reported as a complication of tricyclic antidepressant treatment.

Important bacterial causes include *Staphylococcus aureus*, streptococci and anaerobes.

Typical clinical features are pain in one or both parotids with swelling, redness and tenderness and often increasing malaise. The regional lymph nodes are enlarged and tender, and pus exudes or can be expressed from the parotid duct. The progress of the infection depends largely on the patient's underlying physical state.

Management. Pus must be obtained for culture and sensitivity testing. In the interim, treatment can be started with a penicillin but changed if necessary according to the bacteriological findings. Frequently drainage is necessary.

Chronic sialadenitis

This is usually a complication of chronic duct obstruction. It is usually unilateral and asymptomatic or with intermittently painful swelling of the gland. Sialography may show dilatation of ducts behind the obstruction.

Microscopically there are varying degrees of destruction of acini, duct dilatation and a scattered chronic inflammatory cellular infiltrate, usually predominantly lymphocytic. Extensive interstitial fibrosis, and sometimes squamous metaplasia in the duct epithelium, follow. Calculus formation may be seen in the dilated ducts.

The treatment is to remove the obstruction if possible, but more often the gland has to be excised and the mass examined histologically to make sure that it was not a tumour.

ACINAR DESTRUCTION

Destruction of salivary tissue can result from Sjögren's syndrome or severe radiation damage and leads to complete, or almost complete, failure of salivary secretion. This is persistent, distressing and leads to secondary changes in the mouth and teeth. Once salivary acini have been destroyed they cannot be replaced and the changes are irreversible. Treatment is therefore essentially symptomatic, but is nevertheless important.

Sjögren's syndrome

In 1933 Sjögren noticed the association of dryness of the mouth and dryness of the eyes. Later he found that this disorder had a significant association with rheumatoid arthritis. However, there are two closely related but distinct diseases which can be defined as follows:

1. *Sjögren's syndrome* comprises dry mouth, dry eyes associated with rheumatoid arthritis or other connective tissue disease (secondary Sjögren's syndrome).

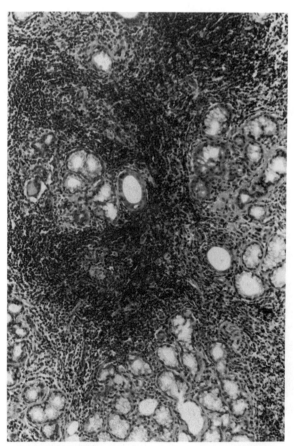

Fig. 17.6a Sjögren's syndrome. There is a widespread lymphocytic infiltrate and destruction of salivary gland acini.

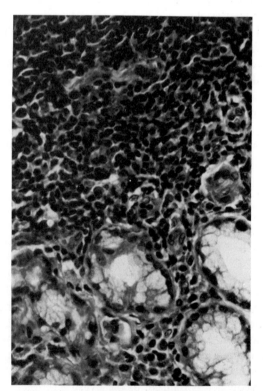

Fig. 17.6b Sjögren's syndrome. The acini above have been destroyed and the remaining acini (below) are surrounded by lymphocytes.

2. *Sicca (dry) syndrome* comprises dry mouth and dry eyes unassociated with connective tissue disease (primary Sjögren's syndrome).

There is an increased risk of lymphoma, particularly in sicca syndrome which tends to be more severe.

Aetiology and pathology

Sjögren's and sicca syndrome are characterised by a variety of immunological abnormalities. These help to establish the diagnosis (and to distinguish one from the other) and have much in common with those in other connective-tissue diseases. Rheumatoid factor, antinuclear and antisalivary duct and antithyroid autoantibodies can be detected with variable frequencies and, more specifically, the SS-antibodies. However, the pathogenesis of the destruction of glandular tissue is obscure.

Histologically, these syndromes are characterised by infiltration and replacement of the salivary and lacrimal glands by lymphocytes and plasma cells, at first in the periductal areas but gradually spreading throughout the glandular tissue. The secretory acini are progressively destroyed but duct tissue tends to survive and proliferate. The final result is replacement of the whole gland tissue by a dense lymphocytic infiltrate in which islands of proliferated duct epithelium stand out. The lymphocytes, however, remain confined within the gland capsule and do not cross the intraglandular septa.

Clinical features

These syndromes predominantly affect women of middle age or older, nearly 10 times as frequently as men. Sjögren's syndrome affects 10% to 15% of patients with rheumatoid arthritis, possibly 30% of patients with lupus erythematosus and a variable proportion of patients with other connective-tissue diseases. Sjögren's and sicca syndromes are therefore relatively common. They are the main cause of dry mouth unrelated to drug treatment or radiotherapy, but their most serious consequence is damage to the eyes.

Sicca syndrome tends to cause more severe oral and ocular changes than Sjögren's syndrome.

The mouth

In addition to discomfort, xerostomia can cause difficulties with eating or swallowing, disturbances of taste sensation, can affect the quality of speech and predispose to infection.

In the early stages, there may be little visible clinical change though objective testing shows diminished parotid secretion.

In established cases the oral mucous membranes are obviously dry, often red, shiny and parchment-like. The tongue is typically red, the papillae characteristically atrophy and the dorsum of the tongue becomes lobulated with a cobblestone appearance.

With the reduction in salivary secretion the oral flora changes and candidal infections are common. The latter are the main cause of soreness of the mouth in Sjögren's syndrome and are characterised by generalised erythema of the mucosa, often with angular stomatitis.

Other effects are rapidly progressive dental caries and periodontal disease in the dentate patient. In the edentulous patient there may be difficulty with retention of dentures, but this is surprisingly uncommon.

The most severe infective complication is suppurative parotitis.

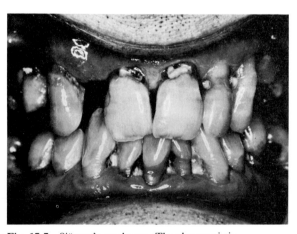

Fig. 17.7 Sjögren's syndrome. The characteristic accumulations of plaque and deterioration of periodontal state result from the much-impaired oral clearance.

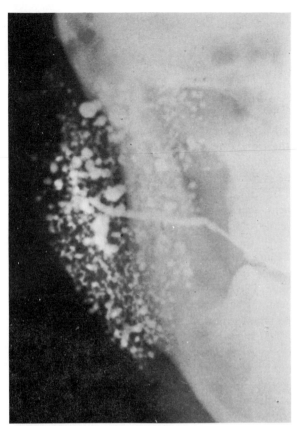

Fig. 17.8 Sjögren's syndrome. The sialogram shows the typical snowstorm appearance of blobs of contrast medium that has leaked from the duct system. Emptying and clearance are also much delayed.

Swelling of the parotids is not commonly seen, but a history of swelling at some time may be obtained in about 30% of patients. Swelling due to the syndrome itself shows no inflammation and is rarely painful.

Later, in advanced disease, ascending parotitis can produce a hot, tender parotid swelling with red, shiny overlying skin. Malaise and fever are often associated.

Parotid swelling appearing years after the onset is strongly suggestive of the development of a lymphoma.

The eyes

Failure of tear secretion prevents the clearance of foreign particles from the cornea and conjunctiva with resulting inflammation (keratoconjunctivitis sicca), a gritty sensation in the eyes and obvious redness due to conjunctivitis. Even in mild cases there are often soft crusts formed at the canthus.

Keratoconjunctivitis is one of the most important complications of Sjögren's syndrome, in that it can damage sight or ultimately cause blindness.

Diagnosis

The findings in Sjögren's syndrome are highly variable and no single test will reliably confirm the diagnosis. A wide variety of tests may therefore have to be carried out.

Parotid flow rate is a sensitive test of salivary function. Normal parotid flow is between 1 and 2 ml per minute but may be reduced to 0.5 ml/min or less. Parotid flow rate is measured by cupping the papilla and stimulating salivary flow with dilute citric acid.

Sialography is carried out by instilling a water-soluble contrast medium into the salivary duct system. The characteristic finding is so-called sialectasis. The appearances are of dots or blobs of radiopaque material scattered within the gland area and often have a snowstorm appearance.

Labial gland biopsy is often informative as the changes in these minor salivary glands in the lower lip show a close correlation with those in the parotid. Biopsy of the labial glands is much safer and simpler than biopsying the parotid, where damage to the facial nerve or a parotid fistula are serious risks.

Immunological findings. In Sjögren's syndrome rheumatoid factor is found in about 90% of patients, while antinuclear factors and antisalivary duct antibodies are present in over 50%. In sicca syndrome, by contrast, rheumatoid factor is found in only about 50%, antinuclear factors in about 50% and antisalivary duct antibody in only 10%. In addition, the autoantibody anti SS-B is more prevalent in sicca syndrome. Other autoantibodies such as antithyroid antibodies are often also detectable. The ESR is typically raised.

Additional investigations. Haematological investigation is needed as anaemia is commonly associated, particularly when there is rheumatoid arthritis. The presence of rheumatoid arthritis or other connective-tissue disease may need to be confirmed but is typically of long standing before Sjögren's syndrome develops.

Most important of all is *ophthalmological examination* to exclude keratoconjunctivitis sicca which, in its early stages, is symptomless.

Management

The damage to the salivary glands is progressive and irreversible. Treatment of the oral changes is therefore essentially symptomatic.

Dryness of the mouth can be relieved partially by providing artificial saliva. Dryness of the eyes is treated with artificial tears of methyl cellulose solution.

If the patient is dentate then sweet-eating should be prohibited, a high standard of oral hygiene maintained and frequent dental checks are necessary. Topical fluorides should be applied regularly. In addition 0.2% chlorhexidine mouth rinses may help to reduce plaque formation.

Soreness of the mouth is usually due to infection by *Candida albicans*. This can be treated, with nystatin or amphotericin mixture, *not* tablets.

Ascending parotid infection indicated by pain, increase in size of the swelling and inflammation of the overlying skin must be treated with antibiotics such as flucloxacillin, with metronidazole if necessary.

Medical management of other features such as rheumatoid arthritis in Sjögren's syndrome is along conventional lines.

Other complications

A recognised complication of Sjögren's syndrome is the development of malignant lymphoma. For this reason immunosuppressive treatment with drugs such as corticosteroids, or irradiation, to reduce the size of the swollen glands is contraindicated. In any case, neither of these measures has any lasting benefit in Sjögren's syndrome.

Sjögren-like syndrome in graft-versus-host disease

A disease in virtually all respects similar to primary Sjögren's syndrome develops in about a third of all cases of graft-versus-host disease (Ch. 20), particularly when severe. The histological

changes in lip biopsies are the same as in Sjögren's syndrome and serve to distinguish GVHD from salivary gland damage secondary to irradiation used for immunosuppression.

Irradiation

Salivary tissue is highly sensitive to ionising radiation, and some damage to the salivary glands is an almost inevitable consequence of irradiation in the region of the mouth.

In most cases, with properly regulated treatment, salivation should recover after a period of weeks or months. Irradiation leads to irreversible destruction of acini and fibrous replacement.

Rampant dental caries is a well known consequence of therapeutic radiation of the head and neck. The precise mechanism is not clear but it is apparent that the flow is not merely reduced but the composition of the saliva also changes.

The management of dry mouth is as described for Sjögren's syndrome. However, it is even more important to control dental caries and its sequelae because of the danger of irradiation-associated osteomyelitis (Ch. 8) secondary to periapical infection or extractions.

DRY MOUTH

This is an unpleasant symptom and, if severe and persistent, as when the salivary glands are damaged, can be only partially relieved. The main causes are as follows:

1. Transient conditions
   —Emotional disturbances, acute anxiety, etc.
2. Chronic conditions
   a. Functional
      (i) Local causes—mouth breathing
      (ii) Systemic causes (factors affecting function of the glands):
      — neuroses, particularly chronic anxiety states
      — organic disease, tumours, infections, or injuries of the brain or affecting the autonomic outflow
      — drugs
      — dehydration—excessive sweating, vomiting, polyuria, haemorrhage, fluid restriction

b. Disease of the salivary glands
— Sjögren's syndrome
— Irradiation damage
— HIV infection.

Many patients with severe xerostomia make no complaint of dry mouth, though they may, for instance, admit that they have difficulty in eating dry food. Some who make this complaint, often also complain of an unpleasant taste in the mouth but have no detectable disturbance of salivary flow and the problem is neurotic in nature. Objective tests (salivary flow studies) are therefore desirable when patients complain of dry mouth.

Local causes—mouth breathing

The front of the mouth is mainly affected, causing chronic gingivitis. Some patients complain of dryness of the mouth in the morning because the mouth falls open during sleep. In some cases, particularly where there is faulty lip seal, the periodontal state may be helped by use of a mouth guard.

Systemic causes

A dry mouth is a common feature of anxiety. Many drugs used in the treatment of depression also cause a dry mouth. If no drugs are being taken, organic causes should be excluded. Reassurance or a lubricant mouth rinse may be helpful. Occasionally referral to a psychiatrist may be necessary.

Dehydration

Salivary secretion is diminished whenever there is severe fluid loss from such causes as those enumerated above. Thirst is severe but the problem is not a dental one. Treatment is that of the underlying condition by restoration of fluid and electrolyte loss.

Drugs

The main types of drugs liable to cause a dry mouth include the following:

1. Sympathomimetic agents. Amphetamine and related drugs are mainly used as appetite suppressants or drugs of abuse. Others are used in the control of asthma and other allergies.
2. Atropine and related drugs (anticholinergic agents) are mainly used for the control of asthma (ipratropium), Parkinson's disease and to a lesser extent for peptic ulcer.
3. Antihistamines. These also have atropinic effects.
4. Phenothiazine neuroleptics ('major tranquillizers').
5. Tricyclic and some other antidepressants.
6. Hypotensive agents, especially ganglion blockers (largely obsolete).

Among drugs in common use the most potent cause of dry mouth are the tricyclic antidepressants. If their continued use is essential for the patient's health, a dry mouth must be accepted as an inevitable consequence but a lubricant mouth rinse such as methyl cellulose solution may be helpful.

Disease of the salivary glands

The main causes, particularly Sjögren's syndrome, have been discussed earlier.

Other organic causes have been described, such as aplasia, obstruction, infection or excision, but these are not a practical problem, in that aplasia is exceedingly rare and other causes do not affect a sufficient number of glands to have a serious effect on salivary secretion. Salivary calculi do *not* cause dryness of the mouth.

SALIVARY GLAND NEOPLASMS

Salivary gland tumours comprise a significant proportion of oral tumours, and carcinomas arising from these glands are the next most common neoplasms of the mouth after squamous cell carcinoma. However, tumours of the minor intraoral salivary glands are less common than in the parotids. The histopathology of salivary gland tumours is notoriously difficult, and it is not always possible to be certain that a particular tumour is malignant from the histological features alone.

The incidence of salivary gland cancers in Europe is estimated to be about 1.2 per 100 000 and in England and Wales about 600 salivary gland cancers are registered each year. However, over 75% of salivary gland tumours are benign, so that the total number seen in a year in Britain may be approximately 2400.

Unlike other cancers women are slightly more frequently affected.

About 70% of salivary gland tumours develop in the parotid and a few affect the submandibular glands. Tumours in the sublingual glands are a rarity but usually malignant.

Aetiology

Little is known of the aetiology of salivary gland tumours except that they can result from irradiation to the head area. In survivors of the atomic blasts at Hiroshima and Nagasaki there has been an excess of salivary gland tumours. Similarly these tumours can follow therapeutic irradiation of, for example, the thyroid and, it is suggested, multiple dental diagnostic radiographs.

Classification

The World Health Organization 1972 classification of salivary gland tumours is as follows:

1. EPITHELIAL TUMOURS
   a. Adenomas
      (i) Pleomorphic adenoma ('mixed tumour')
      (ii) Monomorphic adenomas
         — Adenolymphoma
         — Oxyphilic adenoma
         — Other types
   b. Mucoepidermoid tumour
   c. Acinic cell tumour
   d. Carcinomas
      (i) Adenoid cystic carcinoma
      (ii) Adenocarcinoma
      (iii) Epidermoid carcinoma
      (iv) Undifferentiated carcinoma
      (v) Carcinoma in pleomorphic adenoma (malignant mixed tumour)
2. NON-EPITHELIAL TUMOURS
3. UNCLASSIFIED TUMOURS
4. ALLIED CONDITIONS
   a. Benign lymphoepithelial lesion
   b. Sialosis
   c. Oncocytosis.

Pleomorphic adenoma

The pleomorphic adenoma (mixed tumour) accounts for about 75% of parotid tumours but a slightly lower proportion of intraoral salivary gland tumours. It probably arises mainly from duct epithelium (duct-like structures are a common feature) and myoepithelial cells. It is usual to see a wide variety of epithelial structures, ranging from ducts, sheets of epithelial cells and areas of squamous metaplasia often with keratinisation.

In addition to the obviously epithelial element there are usually extensive areas of connective-tissue products, either fibrous, myxoid, or cartilaginous. These mesenchymal elements are due to the pluripotential properties of myoepithelial cells. Many tumours are predominantly myxoid and can burst at operation if not gently handled, and then recur.

Myoepithelial cells cannot be identified by light microscopy and can appear dark and angular, spindle-shaped or resemble plasma cells. However, immunocytochemistry shows their typical double staining with epithelial (cytokeratin) markers and mesenchymal markers, particularly S-100 protein, vimentin and myosin.

Clinical features

Adults are predominantly affected: the usual intraoral site is the palate, often at the junction of the hard and soft palate, or occasionally the cheek or lip. Growth is usually slow and it sometimes takes several years for the tumour to reach an inch in diameter.

Pleomorphic adenomas form rubbery, often slightly lobulated swellings. When close under the mucosa the tumour may have a bluish colour. The swelling is usually attached to the overlying mucous membrane but freely mobile on the deeper tissues. If neglected, salivary adenomas grow to a great size and occasionally undergo malignant change.

Treatment is wide excision of the tumour; recurrence is inevitable if excision is inadequate.

The reputation of the pleomorphic adenoma for recurrence is, however, due to the very considerable surgical difficulties of complete removal of tumours from the parotid (the common site) where the facial nerve, in particular, makes dissection hazardous. In addition, pleomorphic adenomas have an unusually strong tendency to seed and recur in the incision scar if opened at operation or if incompletely excised. In the case of parotid tumours, therefore, recurrences are prevented only by removing the gland with the tumour intact. Recurrences are typically multifocal and difficult to deal with. Even so, the recurrence rate is low in skilled hands.

Other adenomas

Monomorphic adenomas

As their name implies, these tumours have a uniform cellular structure often with a tubular or trabecular pattern and lack the connective-tissue components of the pleomorphic adenoma.

The canalicular monomorphic adenoma affects the lower lip and consists of small darkly-staining cells in a tubular or trabecular pattern but sometimes resembling an adenoid cystic carcinoma.

Adenolymphoma (Warthin's tumour, cystadenoma lymphomatosum)

Adenolymphoma is probably the worst choice of name for this tumour since it misleadingly implies that it is a variant of malignant lymphoma. The term Warthin's tumour is more satisfactory (Fig. 17.11).

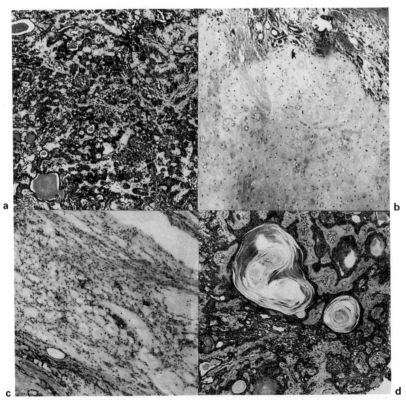

Fig. 17.9 Pleomorphic salivary adenoma. Four areas from the same tumour show the variety of appearances. The first (a) is highly cellular and shows many duct-like spaces among the darkly-staining cells. The second (b) shows pale-staining material resembling cartilage and containing scattered nuclei in well-defined lacunae; there are a few glandular elements at the upper margin. The third (c) shows the darkly-staining cells spread apart by what appears to be glandular secretion. The last area (d) shows glandular elements but, in addition, there is squamous metaplasia and keratinisation forming cell nests (× 42).

Warthin's tumour is seen only in the parotids and accounts for about 9% of tumours there. It has a highly characteristic appearance and consists of tall, eosinophilic columnar cells which form a much-folded covering to aggregations of lymphoid tissue (including many germinal follicles) and line cystic spaces.

Warthin's tumour is benign but sometimes multiple.

Oxyphilic adenoma

Oxyphilic adenoma is a rare benign tumour that virtually only affects the parotid, particularly in the elderly. It consists of large strongly eosinophilic cells with small compact nuclei ('oncocytes') which are typically arranged in solid cords.

Oncocytosis is the term given to replacement or transformation of acinar cells of the parotid (or rarely other glands) by cells having the same appearance as those of the oxyphilic adenoma but without loss of the normal lobular architecture. Oncocytosis is usually an age-related change and when widespread the gland becomes swollen and soft.

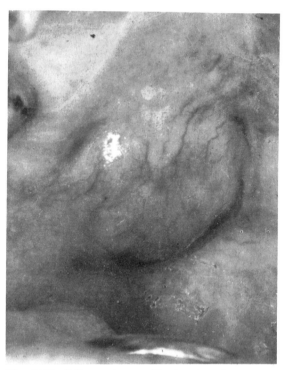

Fig. 17.10 Salivary adenoma. The junction of hard and soft palates is a common site; the tumour usually feels rubbery and lobulated on palpatation.

Mucoepidermoid tumour/carcinoma

These, which account for between 3% and 9% of salivary gland neoplasms, are termed mucoepidermoid carcinoma in the USA and increasingly elsewhere, because of their unpredictable behaviour.

This tumour consists of two cell types, namely large, pale mucus-secreting cells which are surrounded by epidermoid (squamous) cells. Either may be predominant. If mainly epidermoid, the tumour is solid, or if mainly mucoid the tumour tends to be cystic. There is no well-defined capsule, but the tumour usually grows slowly.

Mucoepidermoid tumours can be invasive and occasionally metastasise despite a benign histological appearance. Mucoepidermoid tumours which show obviously malignant microscopic features are rarely seen but behave like other carcinomas and are more likely to metastasise.

The clinical features of a mucoepidermoid tumour are essentially similar to those of an adenoma. Treatment is by wide excision, and recurrence is then uncommon.

Acinic cell tumour/carcinoma

Acinic cell tumours are rare and account for about 1% of salivary gland tumours. Their behaviour is also unpredictable. They show an almost uniform pattern of large cells, similar to serous cells, with granular basophilic cytoplasm and more strongly resemble true adenomas than any other salivary gland tumour. A characteristic feature seen in sections is scattered round 'holes', thought to be entrapped secretion. Sometimes these are so numerous as to give the tumour a lace-like appearance. However, despite apparently benign histological appearances, acinic cell tumours can be invasive and occasionally metastasise. More obviously malignant variants with nuclear pleomorphism and hyperchromatism are also occasionally seen microscopically and behave like other carcinomas.

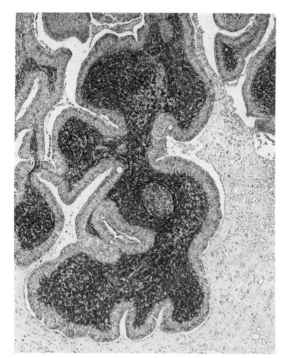

Fig. 17.11a Adenolymphoma. The columnar cells surround dense accumulations of lymphocytes, and the germinal follicle is present in the centre. Around the tumour cells is a cystic space.

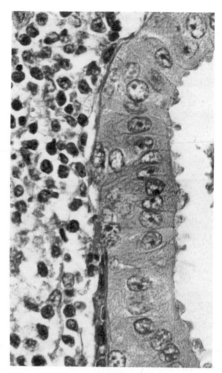

Fig. 17.11b Adenolymphoma. The tall columnar epithelial cells are seen to the right, and beneath them are the lymphocytes.

Malignant salivary gland tumours

The clinical features of malignant salivary tumours are more rapid growth, pain and fixation to surrounding tissues, particularly in the more advanced stages. Malignant change in a pleomorphic adenoma may be unsuspected or may be indicated by a sudden increase in rate of growth or the development of pain or facial palsy in the case of parotid tumours.

Adenoid cystic carcinoma

This tumour usually has a highly characteristic histological pattern consisting of rounded groups of small darkly-staining cells of almost uniform size, surrounding multiple small clear spaces (cribriform or 'Swiss cheese' pattern) (Figs. 17.13 and 17.14).

The adenoid cystic carcinoma usually grows relatively slowly but has a tendency to infiltrate, particularly along nerve sheaths, and may metastasise. The prognosis is poor unless the tumour is vigorously treated. This consists of wide excision at the earliest possible stage often combined with radiotherapy.

Adenocarcinoma and other carcinomas

Adenocarcinomas of the salivary glands show a variety of appearances. Some show attempts at duet formation typical of adenocarcinomas, while others have a papillary cystic pattern.

Some are so poorly differentiated that their glandular origin is difficult to discern.

These adenocarcinomas tend to show more rapid progress and more malignant behaviour than adenoid cystic carcinoma.

Squamous cell carcinoma can also affect salivary glands by metaplasia of glandular cells, as seen in pleomorphic adenoma, but is rare.

Undifferentiated carcinomas usually consist of closely set, small, darkly-staining cells with little

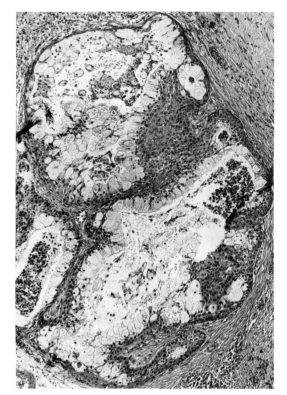

Fig. 17.12a   Mucoepidermoid tumour. The mucous cells surround microcysts. Underlying the mucous cells are the epidermoid (squamous) cells.

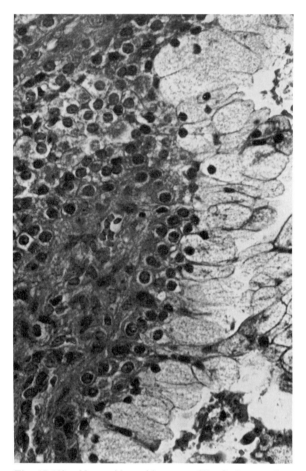

Fig. 17.12b   Mucoepidermoid tumour. The finely granular mucous cells are seen to the right with the underlying epidermoid cells which underly them on the left of the picture.

cytoplasm, and their origin is impossible to discern. Rapid spread and metastasis is typical.

The 5-year survival rate for malignant salivary gland tumours (all variants) is between 70% and 80%.

Malignant change in pleomorphic adenoma (malignant mixed tumour)

Pleomorphic adenoma is one of the few benign tumours that can undergo malignant change. This is suggested by a sudden increase in rate of growth of a tumour that has been growing slowly for a long period. Histologically, malignant change in pleomorphic adenoma is shown by obviously carcinomatous features adjacent to the benign cellular picture of the remainder of the tumour. This is typically a late phenomenon, usually happening only after the tumour has been present for many years or in recurrences after inadequate excision.

Other salivary gland neoplasms and allied conditions

Secondary tumours

Carcinomas and occasionally other tumours can metastasise to the salivary glands, particularly the parotid. Such secondaries can sometimes be difficult to differentiate from primary salivary gland carcinomas, and diagnosis may depend on finding a primary elsewhere. Renal tumours can, for ex-

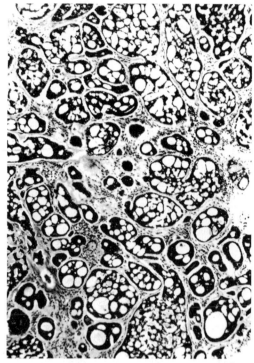

Fig. 17.13 Adenocystic carcinoma. The rounded or irregular 'islands' of darkly-staining cells surrounding multiple small cavities form the highly characteristic 'Swiss cheese' pattern (× 45).

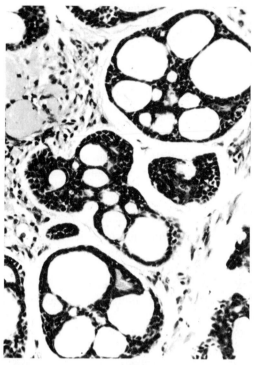

Fig. 17.14 Adenocystic carcinoma. At higher power it can be seen that the darkly-stained tumour cells have little cytoplasm and surround cyst cavities or ducts which usually contain a little pale mucoid material (× 220).

ample, closely resemble clear-cell adenocarcinomas of salivary glands.

Non-epithelial tumours

The most common non-epithelial tumours of salivary glands are lymphomas. Some of these arise as a complication of Sjögren's syndrome, and, occasionally, malignant change in benign lymphoepithelial lesion is seen. In other cases salivary gland lymphoma is the first overt sign of widespread disease. Such a possibility must always be investigated since the prognosis is heavily dependent on the stage the tumour has reached.

Juvenile haemangioma of the parotids

Juvenile haemangioma is a rare tumour of infancy in which the parotid structure is largely replaced by angiomatous tissue among which glandular elements can be seen. This angiomatous proliferation may be so vast as to produce an arteriovenous fistula of such an extent as to precipitate circulatory failure, but this is exceedingly rare.

In most cases juvenile haemangioma responds to excision, but it also appears that some of these tumours regress spontaneously.

Benign lymphoepithelial lesion

This term is given to replacement of glandular tissue by lymphocytes but with persistence of duct tissue which may proliferate to form 'epimyoepithelial' islands. The appearance is indetical to that seen in Sjögren's syndrome but serological changes and other features of that disease may be lacking.

AIDS-related salivary gland diseases

Xerostomia is a recognised manifestation of HIV infection in children. In young adults parotid swellings due to benign lymphoepithelial cysts are reported to be a frequent finding on CT scanning and, in association with cervical lymph-adenopathy, are strongly predictive of HIV seropositivity.

Alternatively, histological changes resembling benign lymphoepithelial lesion may be found but xerostomia may not be associated.

Sialosis

Sialosis is a rare condition in which there is recurrent, non-neoplastic, non-inflammatory, bilateral swelling of the parotids.

Histologically there is hypertrophy of the serous cells, oedema of the interstitial connective tissue and atrophy of striated ducts. The changes may progress to fatty replacement of the glandular tissue.

The cause is unknown but endocrine disturbances and alcoholism are possible factors.

Intraosseous salivary gland tissue

Ectopic salivary gland tissue is occasionally present in the mandible either in a cavity in the bone near the angle (Stafne bone cavity) or entirely enclosed in the bone. Rarely, salivary gland tumours of any type can develop within the jaw (presumably from this ectopic salivary tissue) but are so uncommon as to be little more than pathological curiosities.

Radiographically, benign intraosseous salivary tumours produce cyst-like areas of radiolucency while malignant variants produce less well-defined or ragged areas. The diagnosis can only be made on biopsy.

SUGGESTED FURTHER READING

Atkinson J C, Travis W D, Pillemer S R et al 1990 Major salivary gland function in primary Sjögren's syndrome and its relationship to clinical features. J Rheumatol 17: 318–322

Auclair P L, Langloss J M, Weiss S W, Corio R L 1986 Sarcomas and sarcomatoid neoplasms of the major salivary gland regions. Cancer 58: 1305–1315

Calabrese L H, Wilke W S, Perkins A D, Tubbs R R 1989 Rheumatoid arthritis complicated by infection with the human immunodeficiency virus and the development of Sjögren's syndrome. Arthritis Rheumat 32: 1453–1457

Cawson R A 1987 Oral pathology—colour aids in dentistry. Churchill Livingstone, Edinburgh

Cawson R A, Eveson J W 1987 Oral pathology and diagnosis. William Heinemann Medical Books, London and Gower Medical Publishing, London

Chang E Z, Lee W C 1989 Surgical treatment of salivary gland tumors. J Oral Maxillofac Surg 47: 555–558

Chau M N Y, Radden B G 1989 A clinical-pathological study of 53 intra-oral pleomorphic adenomas. Int J Oral Maxillofac Surg 18: 158–162

De Clerck L S, Couttenye M M, de Broe M E, Stevens W J 1988 Acquired immunodeficiency syndrome mimicking Sjögren's syndrome and systemic lupus erythematosus. Arthritis Rheumat 31: 272–275

Ebbs S R, Webb A J 1986 Adenolymphoma of the parotid: aetiology, diagnosis and treatment. Br J Surg 73: 627–630

Ellis G L, Gnepp D R 1988 Unusual salivary gland tumors. In: Gnepp D R (ed) Pathology of the head and neck. Churchill Livingstone, New York

Ellis G L, Wiscovitch J G 1990 Basal cell adenocarcinomas of the major salivary glands. Oral Surg, Oral Med, Oral Pathol 69: 461–469

Eveson J W, Cawson R A 1985 Tumours of the minor (oropharyngeal) salivary glands: a demographic study of 336 cases. J Oral Pathol 14: 500–509

Eveson J W, Cawson R A 1985 Salivary gland tumours. A review of 2410 cases with particular reference to histological types, site, age and sex distribution. J Pathol 146: 51–58

Eveson J W, Cawson R A 1986 Warthin's Tumor (cystadenolymphoma) of salivary glands. Oral Surg, Oral Med, Oral Pathol 61: 256–262

Finfer M D, Schinella R A, Roithstein S G, Persky M S 1988 Cystic parotid lesions in patients at risk for the acquired immunodeficiency syndrome. Arch Otolaryngol Head Neck Surg 114: 1290–1294

Fox P C, Busch K A, Baum B J 1987 Subjective reports of xerostomia and objective measures of salivary gland performance. JADA 115: 581–584

Fox R I, Robinson C A, Curd J G et al 1986 Sjögren's syndrome. Proposed criteria for classification. Arthritis Rheumat 25: 577–585

Glass R J, Van Dis M L, Langalais R P et al 1984 Xerostomia: diagnosis and treatment planning considerations. Oral Surg 58: 248–252

Gleeson M J, Bennett M H, Cawson R A 1986 Lymphomas of salivary glands. Cancer 58: 699–704

Gnepp D R, Chen J C, Warren C 1988 Polymorphous low grade adenocarcinoma of minor salivary gland. Am J Surg Pathol 12: 461–468

Hamper K, Lazar F, Dietel M et al 1990 Prognostic factors of adenoid cystic carcinoma of the head and neck: a retrospective study of 96 cases. J Oral Pathol Med 19: 101–107

Hickman R E, Cawson R A, Duffy S W 1984 The prognosis of specific types of salivary gland tumors. Cancer 54: 1620–1624

Hui K K, Luna M A, Batsakis J G et al 1990 Undifferentiated carcinomas of the major salivary glands. Oral Surg, Oral Med, Oral Pathol 69: 76–83

Itescuk S, Brancato L J, Wichester R 1989 A sicca syndrome in HIV infection: Association with HLA-DR5 and CD8 lymphocytosis. Lancet 2: 466–468

Janin Mercier A, Devergie A, Arrago J P et al 1987 Systemic evaluation of Sjögren-like syndrome after bone marrow transplantation in man. Transplantation 43: 677–679

Jensen O J, Poulsen T, Schiodt T 1988 Mucoepidermoid tumors of salivary glands. A long term follow-up study. APMIS 96: 421–427

Katz J, Fisher D, Leviner E et al 1990 Bacterial colonization of the parotid duct in xerostomia. Int J Oral Maxillofac Surg 19: 7–9

Lack E E, Upton M P 1988 Histopathologic review of salivary gland tumors in childhood. Arch Otolaryngol Head Neck Surg 114: 898–906

Lee L A 1988 Anti-Ro (SSA) and anti-La (SSB) antibodies in lupus erythematosus and Sjögren's syndrome. Arch Dermatol 124: 61–62

Lloyd R E, Ho K H 1988 Combined CT scanning and sialography in the management of parotid tumors. Oral Surg, Oral Med, Oral Pathol 65: 142–144

Matlow A, Korentage R, Keystone E, Bphnedn J 1988 Parotitis due to anaerobic bacteria. J Infect Dis 10: 420–423

Maynard J 1988 Management of pleomorphic adenoma of the parotid. Br J Surg 75: 305–308

Neville B W, Damm D G, Weir J C, Fantasia J E 1988 Labial salivary gland tumors. Cancer 61: 2113–2116

Palmer R M 1986 The identification of myoepithelial cells in human salivary glands. A review and comparison of light microscopical methods. J Oral Pathol 15: 221–229

Palmer T J, Gleeson M J, Eveson J W, Cawson R A 1990 Oncocytic adenomas and oncocytic hyperplasias of salivary glands: a clinicopathological study of 26 cases. Histopathology 16: 487–493

Preston-Marin S, Thomas D C, White S C, Cohen D 1988 Prior exposure to medical and dental X-rays related to tumors of the parotid gland. J Natl Cancer Inst 80: 943–949

Scully C 1986 Sjögren's syndrome: clinical and laboratory features, immunopathogenesis and management. Oral Surg, Oral Med, Oral Pathol 62: 510–523

Singh R, Cawson R A 1988 Malignant myoepithelial carcinoma (myoepithelioma) arising in a pleomorphic adenoma of the parotid gland. Oral Surg, Oral Med, Oral Pathol 66: 65–70

Spiro R H 1986 Salivary neoplasms: overview of a 35 year experience with 2,807 patients. Head Neck Surg 8: 177–184

Spiro R H, Armstrong J, Harrison L et al 1989 Carcinoma of major salivary glands. Recent trends. Arch Otolaryngol Head Neck Surg 115: 316–321

Sreebney L M, Valdini A 1988 Xerostomia. Part I: relationship to other oral symptoms and salivary gland hypofunction. Oral Surg, Oral Med, Oral Pathol 66: 451–458

Talal N 1987 Overview of Sjögren's syndrome. J Dent Res 66 (Spec Iss): 672–674

Ulirisch R C, Jaffe E S 1988 Sjögren's syndrome-like illness associated with the acquired immunodeficiency syndrome-related complex. Hum Pathol 18: 1063–1068

Waldron C A, El-Mofty S K, Gnepp D R 1988 Tumors of the intraoral minor salivary glands: a demographic and histologic study of 426 cases. Oral Surg, Oral Med, Oral Pathol 66: 323–333

Wise C M, Agudelo C A, Demble E L et al 1988 Comparison of parotid and minor salivary gland biopsy specimens in the diagnosis of Sjögren's syndrome. Arthritis Rheumat 31: 662–666

Witten J, Hybert F, Hansen H S Treatment of malignant tumors of the parotid glands. Cancer 65: 2515–2520

Wyatt M G, Coleman N, Eveson J W, Webb A J 1989 Management of high grade parotid carcinomas. Br J Surg 76: 1275–1277

18. Pain, anxiety and neurological disorders

Pain is the most common symptom for which patients come for help. Approximately 40% of the population of Britain only visit a dentist for relief of pain. In the lay mind dentistry and pain are inseparable, both because toothache can be so agonising and because of the persistent idea that dental treatment is necessarily painful. This latter fact emphasises the important point that pain has strong emotional associations and these in turn may be determined to a varying degree by patients' preconceptions. Emotional disturbance itself can apparently also produce the symptom of physical pain. These considerations must be borne in mind when seeking the cause of, or trying to control, pain.

By far the most common causes of pain in the region of the jaws and face are pulpitis and periapical periodontitis as sequels of dental caries. Though the source of such pain is usually obvious on examination, there are also very many other sources of pain, some of which can be exceedingly difficult to identify. The main causes of pain have mostly been discussed individually earlier but can be considered under the following categories.

I. The mouth and jaws

● Diseases of the teeth and supporting tissues
1. Pulpitis secondary to:
   a. Deep caries
   b. Large (unlined) or irritant restorations
   c. Thermal damage during cavity preparation
   d. Exposed cervical dentine or cementum
   e. Fracture of crown and cracked tooth syndrome
2. Periapical periodontitis (almost invariably a sequel of pulpitis)
3. Lateral (periodontal) abscess
4. Acute ulcerative gingivitis (when deeply and rapidly destructive)
5. Pericoronitis.

These together account for the vast majority of the causes of pain in this area. Disease of the teeth (usually the result of dental caries) and adjacent tissues must always first be excluded in the investigation of pain.

● Diseases of the oral mucosa
1. Recurrent aphthae

2. Erosive lichen planus
3. Herpes simplex
4. Herpes zoster
5. Tuberculosis
6. Carcinoma and other neoplasms.

Ulcers generally cause soreness rather than pain, but deep ulceration may cause severe aching pain. Carcinoma in particular, though initially painless, characteristically causes severe pain once nerve fibres become involved.

Herpes zoster causes severe aching pain because of involvement of posterior root ganglia.

● Diseases of the jaws
1. Fractures
2. Osteomyelitis
3. Infected cysts (and rarely, infected odontomes)
4. Malignant neoplasms.

Fractures are easily recognised from the history, clinical signs and radiological features. Other lesions of the jaws, by contrast, sometimes have less clear-cut clinical and radiological features, and the differentiation of (say) an infected cyst from a malignant tumour may be difficult.

● Pain in the edentulous patient
1. Trauma from dentures
2. Excessive vertical dimension
3. Diseases of the mucosa (enumerated earlier) affecting the denture-bearing mucosa
4. Diseases of the jaws (enumerated earlier)
5. Teeth or roots erupting under a denture.

These can be regarded as a separate clinical group, first because the immediate cause of pain is a denture pressing on the lesion. Second, other important causes of pain, particularly pulp pain, need not be considered.

● Postoperative pain
1. Alveolar osteitis (dry socket)
2. Fracture of the jaw
3. Osteomyelitis
4. Damage to nerve trunks or involvement of nerves in scar tissue.

This group of complaints is linked by the single precipitating cause. Nevertheless it must also be appreciated that patients may ascribe to a dental operation, pain that is purely coincidental.

● Masticatory pain
1. Diseases of the temporomandibular joint
2. Pain dysfunction syndrome
3. Temporal arteritis
4. Trigeminal neuralgia
5. Diseases of teeth and supporting tissues
6. Salivary calculi.

Calculi, particularly when obstructing the parotid duct, can cause pain when starting to eat. Hence the history of the relationship of the pain to stimulation of salivation, is distinctive.

The most obvious but, in practice, the least common cause of pain during eating is organic disease of the temporomandibular joint itself. Pain during eating comes much more often from the many other structures involved.

II. Extraoral disease

There is a wide and heterogeneous collection of diseases where pain can be felt in the jaws—or even, in the case of herpes zoster, in the teeth—but the cause lies elsewhere. These may be categorised as follows.

● Disease of the maxillary antrum
1. Acute sinusitis
2. Malignant neoplasms, especially carcinoma, particularly when it involves the antral floor.

● Diseases of salivary glands
1. Acute parotitis. Mumps and, rarely, bacterial parotitis
2. Salivary calculi (see above)
3. Severe Sjögren's syndrome
4. Malignant neoplasms.

● Diseases of the ears
Otitis media or neoplasms in this region can cause pre-auricular pain but are rarely mistaken for a dental problem.

● Diseases of the eyes
Glaucoma can very occasionally cause pain in the upper jaw but is rarely mistaken for a dental condition.

● Pain of vascular origin
1. Migrainous neuralgia

2. Temporal arteritis
3. Myocardial infarction (see below).

- Diseases of the nervous system
1. Trigeminal neuralgia
2. Intracranial tumours
3. Post-herpetic neuralgia
4. Multiple sclerosis
5. Bell's palsy
6. Herpes zoster.

- Psychogenic pain
Atypical facial pain and related complaints.

Pain and anxiety

Pain and anxiety are almost inseparably associated. Pain creates anxiety, anxiety increases sensitivity to pain, and occasionally anxiety seems even able to create the symptom of pain.

Pain control can be difficult in the highly nervous patient. Some patients who respond as if they had been physically hurt are merely demonstrating that they are frightened that they are *going* to be hurt. It is essential therefore not to regard the patient as being unreasonable but to realise that this sort of response is the result of failure to allay the patient's anxieties.

In practical terms, therefore, anxiety must be managed in the first place by sympathetic management of the patient and establishing a trusting working relationship. However, if anxiety remains insurmountable, sedation can be given.

Anxiolytic drugs affect the perception of pain and, in effect, may potentiate analgesics. Thus nitrous oxide is particularly valuable for sedation. In addition to being analgesic in itself, its anxiolytic properties are such that it sometimes induces sufficient indifference to pain that local analgesia may not be required.

Clinical aspects and investigation of pain—general considerations

In most cases it is essential first to identify or exclude dental disease. The history is often informative and in most cases patients are clearly aware when pain is dental in origin.

Pulpitis

Pulpitis is usually the cause when pain is precipitated by hot or cold food or drinks. Pulpitis is also the main cause of spasmodic, poorly localised attacks of pain which may be mistaken for a variety of other possible causes.

The pain of acute pulpal inflammation is of a sharp lancinating character peculiar to itself, impossible to describe but unforgettable once experienced. Recurrent attacks of less severe, subacute or chronic pain, often apparently spontaneous, are suggestive of a diseased and dying pulp.

Examination. The investigation of pulpitis has been discussed earlier (Ch. 4).

The only non-dental condition that is indistinguishable from pulp pain by the patient is the pain of *herpes zoster*. If, therefore, after the most careful search, no local cause can be found, it is important to look for early signs of the characteristic rash. Herpes zoster is a rare cause of toothache, but countless teeth have been extracted in patients with early pain from zoster under the mistaken impression that the pain was dental in origin.

Acute periodontitis

Pain from acute periapical periodontitis is very much easier to identify as it is precisely localised. The characteristic feature is tenderness of the tooth in its socket (Ch. 5).

Radiographs are of little value in the early stages but useful after there has been sufficient destruction to show as loss of definition of the periapical lamina dura. In other cases acute inflammation may supervene on chronic, and a well-defined rounded area of radiolucency is seen.

Acute maxillary sinusitis occasionally causes tenderness of a group of teeth, particularly upper molars, as discussed later.

Lateral, periodontal abscess

This also causes tenderness of the tooth in its socket, but the tooth is usually vital and there is deep localised pocketing (Ch. 6).

Occasionally both a periodontal and periapical abscess may form together on a non-vital tooth with severe periodontal disease, or a periodontal abscess may be precipitated by endodontic treatment when a reamer perforates the wall of the root canal.

Acute ulcerative gingivitis

This usually causes soreness, as do other types of oral ulceration, but when it extends deeply and rapidly, destroying the underlying bone, there may be severe aching pain. In such cases the diagnosis is usually obvious (Ch. 6).

Acute pericoronitis

Pericoronitis usually produces a characteristic clinical picture as described in Chapter 9.

Diseases of the oral mucosa

The common types of oral ulceration, that is to say herpes simplex, recurrent aphthae and erosive lichen planus, usually cause *soreness* but not, in a strict sense, pain. Herpes zoster, by contrast, can cause deep-seated aching pain sometimes indistinguishable from toothache (Ch. 15) because of involvement of the posterior root ganglia.

It is important to emphasise again that early carcinoma is *painless*; pain is a late symptom. By the time that pain becomes troublesome the tumour is usually easily seen unless it is far back in the mouth. Special radiographic techniques can also be used to visualise some neoplasms of the posterior third of the tongue.

Disease of the jaws

The salient feature is that, having taken into account the history and clinical presentation, the provisional diagnosis depends on the radiographic findings. With the exception of fractures and osteomyelitis, diagnosis then depends on biopsy and histological examination (Ch. 13 and 18).

The edentulous patient

In the edentulous patient the range of diseases causing pain is narrowed. Common causes such as pulpitis, periodontitis and gingivitis do not need

to be considered. The chief problem is to decide whether the pain is due to (a) the dentures themselves, or (b) some condition of the mucosa or jaws underlying the dentures.

The most obvious kind of denture-induced pain is traumatic. *Traumatic ulcers*, usually the consequence of over-extension, often cause trouble shortly after the denture has been first fitted. These ulcers heal within 24 to 48 hours when the denture has been relieved. Persistence of ulceration after adequate relief of the denture is likely to be due to some more serious cause, particularly a neoplasm. Biopsy must therefore be carried out.

Later, dentures cause traumatic pain when the bone has become severely resorbed, allowing the denture to bear on the mylohyoid ridge or genial tubercles. These result from the patient's having worn the denture too long, and a new denture, properly designed to overcome these problems, is necessary.

Lack of freeway space due to excessive vertical dimension of the dentures prevents the mandible and masticatory muscles from reaching their natural rest position. This causes the teeth to be held permanently in contact. Aching pain may be felt in the fatigued masticatory muscles, while in some patients the excessive stress imposed on the denture-bearing area causes pain in this region.

Very occasionally patients seem unable to tolerate dentures, however carefully they are constructed, and complain of such symptoms as gripping, burning, or 'drawing' pain, particularly under the upper denture. These symptoms are not associated with any physical changes and are psychogenic.

It is usually straightforward to decide whether pain is caused by the dentures themselves or by some lesion under the dentures. Surprisingly few mucosal diseases affect the denture-bearing area itself, but lichen planus can extend to the sulcus and impinge on the margin of the denture-bearing area.

The most important condition to be excluded is *carcinoma*, either affecting the alveolar margin or in the labial or buccal sulcus or floor of the mouth. Persistent lesions, whether ulcerated or not, developing beneath or at the margins of dentures, must be biopsied without hesitation, as it is in the edentulous age-group that the incidence of carcinoma is highest. A carcinoma can persist for a long time with minimal symptoms, and the patient may notice no more than the fact that the fit of the denture has deteriorated.

Intraosseous lesions causing pain in the edentulous patient may be associated with a swelling or an area of radiolucency. A painful swelling of the jaw in the edentulous patient is probably most often due to an infected residual cyst. Malignant tumours are very much less common but must be considered, as they cannot be distinguished from cysts and other benign conditions with certainty on radiographs alone. Histological examination is therefore essential.

Osteomyelitis of the jaws must be considered virtually only in the edentulous patient who has had radiotherapy to the region of the mouth. In these patients denture ulceration can allow infection to penetrate and set up persistent painful chronic osteomyelitis of the ischaemic bone.

Retained roots or, rarely, late eruption of a buried tooth beneath a denture become painful as they reach the surface, when the mucosa is pinched between the denture and erupting root or tooth. This trouble will be obvious on clinical or radiographic examination, as are the late effects of a healed malaligned fracture.

Postoperative pain

By far the most common cause of pain following dental extractions is *alveolar osteitis (dry socket)*, which can usually be readily recognised on clinical examination (Ch. 9).

Osteomyelitis or fracture of the jaw following operative treatment is rare but can also be recognised from the history, and by clinical and radiographic examination.

Persistent postoperative pain is sometimes ascribed to damage to nerve fibres either as a result of operative trauma or by involvement in scar tissue. However, if there is no associated objective evidence of disturbed sensation there is little or nothing abnormal to be found. Operative intervention in the attempt to relieve such pain is often also ineffective. In some such cases there is complaint of persistent pain unresponsive to treatment but it is unlikely that there is an organic cause. However, damaged nerve tissue may *rarely*

proliferate to form a traumatic neuroma, which is tender to pressure; its excision should lead to relief of the pain.

Forcible opening of the mouth under general anaesthesia particularly for removing wisdom teeth can damage the temporomandibular joint and lead to persistent pain on opening or during mastication.

Solitary bone islands

A postoperative radiograph occasionally shows an area of bone sclerosis which may be thought to result from low-grade chronic infection. However, these bone islands are a natural variation and seen as chance findings in other, asymptomatic patients. Operative intervention is likely to do more harm than good.

Masticatory pain

The common dental cause for pain on mastication is apical periodontitis, but any condition which causes the tooth to be tender in its socket, whether it be a lateral periodontal abscess or, occasionally, maxillary sinusitis, can produce this symptom.

Disorders of the temporomandibular joint

Fractures and dislocations are usually obvious from the history, their effects on the occlusion and the radiographic changes (Ch. 13).

True arthritis of the temporomandibular joint is rare. Rheumatoid arthritis frequently affects the temporomandibular joint, but pain is rarely prominent.

Osteoarthritis of the temporomandibular joint is not a significant cause of symptoms. It is mainly an autopsy finding or occasionally a chance radiographic finding.

Conditions affecting the masticatory muscles

Pain dysfunction syndrome has been discussed in Chapter 14. The pain is usually dull and aching in character, and often associated with clicking sounds from the joint, episodes of locking and some limitation of opening, in varying combinations.

Young women are predominantly affected and there is typically a strong neurotic element.

Temporal arteritis

Temporal (giant-cell) arteritis is a rare cause of masticatory pain, but should be considered particularly in patients over middle age with pain on mastication. The pain is due to ischaemia of the masticatory muscles, caused by the arteritis. It is comparable to intermittent claudication.

The typical manifestation of temporal arteritis is headache. The superficial temporal artery is usually tortuous and thickened, while biopsy shows inflammatory thickening of the wall associated with the characteristic giant cells.

Recognition of this disease is important, as there is a high risk of blindness caused by optic ischaemia. Corticosteroids are effective in arresting the progress of the disease and relieving symptoms.

Trigeminal neuralgia

The characteristic pain of trigeminal neuralgia is occasionally triggered by mastication. Trigeminal neuralgia may then be misdiagnosed as pain dysfunction syndrome. However, the characteristics of the two types of pain are quite different, as discussed later.

EXTRAORAL DISEASE

Diseases of the maxillary antrum

Acute sinusitis is by far the most common disease of the paranasal sinuses which causes facial pain.

Pain is felt over the involved antrum but may be referred to teeth whose roots are in close proximity to the floor of the sinus. Several adjacent molars may therefore be tender, and there should be little difficulty in distinguishing sinusitis from periodontitis. There is usually a history of an upper respiratory infection, nasal congestion, purulent nasal discharge, some fever and malaise. Radiographs show antral opacity.

Tumours of the maxillary antrum

Carcinoma of the antrum is rare. As with cancer of the mouth, pain is not an early symptom. Later, anaesthesia of the distribution of any sensory nerves involved is almost as common as pain.

Oral and dental symptoms from a tumour of the antrum result from involvement of its floor. This may be felt as pain in the teeth or pain under a denture as the fit deteriorates. As the disease advances, teeth may become loose and a palatal swelling becomes obvious.

Radiographs must be taken for signs of destruction of the bony antral walls. It is a general rule that an opaque maxillary antrum in a person over 40 years of age without obvious underlying dental or nasal disease should have the antrum explored. If a mass is found biopsy must be carried out.

Diseases of salivary glands

Acute parotitis

Mumps is a common cause of pain from the parotids, associated with swelling. In children the diagnosis is usually made on clinical grounds very quickly. In adults the diagnosis may not be immediately suspected and, occasionally, these patients think they have dental pain.

Suppurative parotitis

Suppurative parotitis is uncommon and is virtually only seen as a complication of dry mouth. Acute parotitis may therefore be seen as a complication of Sjögren's syndrome or irradiation damage to the glands.

Sjögren's syndrome

When severe, this can cause parotid pain, though it is *rare* for it to do so. Pain is usually associated with swelling of the glands and is difficult to treat.

Malignant tumours of salivary glands

Pain is rarely an early symptom. Swelling is usually the first feature and in the case of malignant change in pleomorphic adenoma, a swelling may have been present for years before pain starts. A painful firm swelling of a salivary gland is strongly suggestive of a malignant tumour. Later there may be nerve palsies and, finally, ulceration and fungation.

DISEASES OF THE NERVOUS SYSTEM

Trigeminal neuralgia

The classical features are as follows.

1. *Trigeminal distribution.* Pain is confined to the areas supplied by the trigeminal nerve.
2. *Paroxysmal character.* The pain is severe, sharp and stabbing in character but lasts only seconds or minutes. In severe cases there may be frequently repeated attacks of pain.
3. *Trigger zones.* Stimuli applied to an area within the distribution of the trigeminal nerve can provoke an attack of pain. Common stimuli are touching, draughts of cold air, or toothbrushing. Occasionally, masticatory effort induces the pain.
4. *Absence of objective sensory loss.* Elderly patients are affected, and though the pain is excruciatingly severe, there is complete (or almost complete) relief of pain between spasms. During an attack the patient's face is often distorted with anguish, while between attacks the general expression is one of apprehension at the thought of recurrence of the pain. The pain may also make the patient depressed.

There are no objective signs and, though diseased teeth may be found (as in any other patients), their treatment has no effect on the pain.

Either the second or third division of the trigeminal nerve is usually first affected, but the pain soon involves both. The first division is rarely affected and the pain does not spread to the opposite side.

Less typical features of trigeminal neuralgia which make diagnosis difficult are more continuous, long-lasting, burning or aching pain, absence of trigger zones, and extension of the pain beyond the margins of the trigeminal area, though not to the opposite side.

Characteristically the disease undergoes spontaneous remissions, leaving the patient free from pain for weeks or months. These remissions may make it difficult to decide whether treatment has been effective.

Diagnosis

In typical cases, the diagnosis should be readily made from the features described.

A careful search should be made for diseased teeth, though paroxysms of pain of this severity are unlikely to be due to dental disease. An inflamed pulp can cause stabs of severe pain in its early stages, but the pain changes in character and soon becomes more prolonged. Pulpitis can usually also be identified as toothache by most patients and is felt to be different in character from pain in the face due to neuralgia. Any diseased teeth should of course be treated, though this does not affect the neuralgia.

In the absence of disease, the teeth should not be arbitrarily extracted, as this only adds to the patient's misfortunes. Pulp stones in particular, seen on a radiograph, are not a reason for extracting teeth.

Treatment

The most effective drugs are anticonvulsants, particularly carbamazepine (Tegretol) and to a lesser extent phenytoin (Epanutin). Carbamazepine, with or without phenytoin in addition, will usually relieve the pain of trigeminal neuralgia, at least for a time. The action seems specific and other types of pain are not relieved. The abolition of the pain of trigeminal neuralgia by giving an anticonvulsant, such as carbamazepine, also helps to confirm the diagnosis.

Carbamazepine must be given long-term (essentially prophylactically) to reduce the frequency and severity of attacks. It has no effect if used as an analgesic when an attack starts.

If a patient has symptoms suggestive of trigeminal neuralgia but is already taking carbamazepine it will often be found that instructions about continuous use have either not been given or not understood.

Up to 80% of patients are relieved of pain partly or completely by carbamazepine, but minor side-effects are common. Drowsiness, dryness of the mouth, giddiness, diarrhoea, nausea are all to some extent dose related. They may be reduced by giving a small initial dose which is gradually increased; in some patients tolerance to the side-effects may develop. Leucopenia is a rare toxic effect.

Surgical treatment. A few patients are unresponsive to carbamazepine or cannot tolerate the side-effects. If drug treatment fails, the final resort is to surgery. In Britain the preferred operation is thermocoagulation of the Gasserian ganglion or its peripheral branches with alcohol.

This treatment inevitably causes undesired effects, particularly partial or total hemifacial anaesthesia. Patients find this so unpleasant that they must be fully warned about it before surgery is decided on. After operation, outbreaks of herpes simplex in the anaesthetic area are common. Up to 5% of patients develop unpleasant burning or tingling sensations (dysaesthesia) in the face. This condition is persistent and intractable, and a poor substitute for trigeminal neuralgia.

If thermocoagulation fails, section of the sensory root in the posterior fossa may have to be carried out.

Intracranial tumours

Pain resembling that of trigeminal neuralgia can rarely be caused by intracranial tumours. Features suggestive of an intracranial lesion are associated sensory loss or, occasionally, impaired motor function. Frequently also, anatomically related nerves (especially III, IV and VI, causing various disorders of oculomotor function) are affected.

Glossopharyngeal neuralgia

This rare condition is characterised by pain similar to that of trigeminal neuralgia but differently distributed. The pain is sharp, lancinating and transient; it affects the base of the tongue and fauces on one side, but may also radiate deeply into the ear. Pain is often precipitated by swallowing, chewing, or coughing. It may be so severe that the patient is terrified to swallow his own saliva and tries to keep his mouth and tongue in as complete a state of immobility as possible.

Some cases of glossopharyngeal neuralgia respond to carbamazepine but less often than does trigeminal neuralgia. Once an organic cause has been excluded, surgical treatment may be needed.

Post-herpetic neuralgia

Up to 10% of patients who have had trigeminal herpes zoster may develop persistent neuralgia and particularly if elderly. The pain is more variable in character and severity than trigeminal neuralgia. It is typically persistent rather than paroxysmal.

The diagnosis is easy to make when the patient is able to give a history of facial zoster or if scars from the rash can still be seen. Unfortunately, post-herpetic neuralgia is remarkably resistant to treatment. Nerve or root section are ineffective and the response to drugs of any type, including carbamazepine, is poor. When pain is severe, large doses of analgesics can be given, but may not be effective.

An alternative, and sometimes successful, form of treatment is to apply mechanical or electrical stimuli to the affected area by the patient himself. The patient applies the instrument hourly for 5 to 10 minutes every day, and this persistent bombardment of the sensory pathways by the stimulator may prevent perception of pain centrally.

Multiple sclerosis

A minority of patients with multiple sclerosis have pain indistinguishable from trigeminal neuralgia, usually as a late symptom. Large surveys suggest that of patients with 'classical' trigeminal neuralgia, between 2% and 3% may have multiple sclerosis, but younger persons are typically affected. The diagnosis usually therefore depends on the presence of multiple lesions, particularly defects of vision, weakness of the limbs, and sensory defects.

In about a third of these patients, unlike trigeminal neuralgia, pain may be persistent, lack trigger zones, or spread beyond the confines of the trigeminal area.

It is suggested that surgical treatment is the most effective means of relieving the pain. The operations are the same as those for trigeminal neuralgia.

Bell's palsy

As discussed later, facial paralysis is the predominant and most troublesome feature; pain

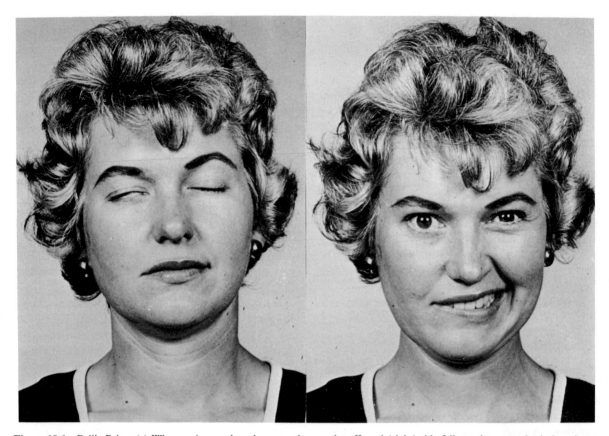

Figure 18.1 Bell's Palsy. (a) When trying to shut the eyes, that on the affected (right) side fails to close completely but the eyeball rolls up normally. (b) When trying to smile the mouth fails to move on the affected side, which remains expressionless having lost all natural skin folds. The difference is made more striking by covering each side of the picture in turn.

This patient, incidentally, complained primarily of facial pain though increasingly aware of the facial disability. The severely disfiguring effect of this disorder and the need for early treatment is obvious. In this case, treatment was completely successful. (Reproduced by kind permission of the patient.)

usually in or near the ear and sometimes spreading down the jaw either precedes or develops at the same time as the facial palsy in about 50% of cases. Rarely a patient with early Bell's palsy seeks a dental opinion for the pain felt in the jaw, since this may precede other symptoms by several days.

Migrainous neuralgia (cluster headache)

Migrainous neuralgia is uncommon and rarely seen in dental practice. Migrainous neuralgia has many features in common with classical migraine (hemicrania) and is probably due to oedema and dilatation of the wall of the internal carotid artery and probably also the external carotid.

Cluster headache mainly affects men, usually young adults but up to the age of 50. Attacks may be precipitated by alcohol or vasodilators or come on spontaneously one to three times a day. In some cases attacks recur at precisely the same time each day. It is also common for sleep to be disturbed by attacks.

The pain is localised to the region of the orbit, temple, or maxilla. The duration is half to two hours. Obvious vascular changes in the affected side of the face typically accompany the pain. The eye may become suffused and water, the nostrils may be blocked, the skin over the cheek may become red and there may be sweating on that side. After one to several months there is usually sudden and spontaneous complete remission of attacks and the patient remains completely free from pain for months, or even years.

A rare variant of cluster headache is a chronic variety with attacks confined to the cheek or lower jaw, known as *lower half headache.*

Unlike migraine there are no visual symptoms and no nausea or vomiting. Cluster headache may respond to simple analgesics or to ergotamine. Ergotamine should be given an hour before the expected attack and is most effective by subcutaneous injection or by suppository. Alternatively ergotamine powder can be inhaled from a spinhaler. Success depends on an accurate idea of the timing of the attacks, and two or three doses a day for the duration of the cluster of attacks may be necessary. Treatment should preferably be stopped for one day each week to see whether there has been spontaneous remission.

In some patients indomethacin is more effective.

Myocardial infarction and angina

Myocardial infarction usually causes constricting or crushing pain substernally, but may radiate down the inside of the left arm or up into the neck or jaw. On rare occasions the pain is felt in the jaw alone. There is even a case on record where a dentist recognised the cardiac cause of jaw pain to the particular dismay of his patient who happened to be a cardiologist. This pain can come on at any time, at rest or during exercise.

The clinical picture is variable, but in typical cases the patient is obviously anxious, pale and sweating with a rapid pulse and low blood pressure.

If an attack comes in the dental chair it must be managed as described in Chapter 21.

PSYCHOGENIC (ATYPICAL) FACIAL PAIN

Pain is not a simple sensation, but has been described as the unpleasant experience felt 'when hurt in body or mind'. The psychological aspects of pain are often of overwhelming importance, and the patient's reaction is affected by such factors as mood, emotional characteristics, personality and cultural background. At one extreme a football player may receive a relatively severe injury in the middle of a game without feeling it. At the other extreme there are patients who complain bitterly and persistently about trivial lesions.

It is also well recognised that pain causes emotional disturbance, and prolonged severe pain, as in rheumatoid arthritis, commonly has so depressing an effect that antidepressant treatment may become necessary. Similarly the patient's perception of pain may be heightened by anxiety, particularly in the dental chair. The successful management of dental patients therefore depends as much on lessening anxiety as on controlling pain effectively.

While it is not difficult to accept that pain can have emotional effects, it is perhaps less easy to accept that emotional disturbances can give rise to pain. Nevertheless, there seems to be a group of patients whose facial pain is psychogenic rather than organic in nature.

It must be emphasised that the diagnosis of psychogenic facial pain is a diagnosis by exclusion, but it is important to try to recognise the condition, however limited the diagnostic methods may be. The symptoms cause real enough suffering to the patient and should if possible be relieved. It is also important not to carry out any unnecessary surgery.

At the risk of oversimplification, three groups of painful conditions can therefore be recognised as follows. (1) The pain is clearly organic and severe; an obvious example is acute pulpitis. Any psychogenic associations are likely to be only a consequence of the severity of the pain. (2) There are both organic and psychogenic components and it is hard to say which is predominant. The best example is pain dysfunction syndrome. (3) There appears to be no organic component to the pain and the patient's predominant problem is psychogenic. The clinical picture is then very much less well defined and diagnosis is often difficult. The following features are suggestive of psychogenic symptoms.

1. *Localisation.* This is not usually precise. Typically pain is not distributed within a recognisable anatomical pattern. Occasionally both sides are involved. A common site is in the maxillary region or in relation to the upper teeth.
2. *Description of the pain.* This may be vague, bizarre ('drawing' or 'gripping') or

exaggerated ('unbearable') but without obvious effect on the patient's health. This is in sharp contrast to conditions such as trigeminal neuralgia where the pain is so agonising in quality that once a patient has been seen while suffering an attack the reaction is not easily forgotten.

3. *Persistence.* The pain is often described as having been continuous, even unremittant, for several years.
4. *Fixity of character.* The pain is often described as being completely unchanging over a very long period, often for several years.
5. *Provocation of pain.* Pain is usually not provoked by any recognisable stimulus such as hot or cold foods or by mastication.
6. *Effects of the pain.* In spite of the fact that the pain may be said to be continuous and unbearable, the patient's sleeping or even eating may be unaffected.
7. *The effect of analgesics.* Analgesics are often said to be completely ineffective but some patients have not even tried analgesics in spite of the stated severity of the pain.
8. *Objective signs.* These are absent. Although teeth have often been extracted and diseased teeth may be present none of these can be related to the pain. As a consequence, treatment of diseased teeth does not relieve the symptoms.
9. *Other signs of psychiatric disturbance.* These are highly variable. Some patients are more or less obviously depressed; some of them mention, in passing, difficulties they have had, for instance, at work with their colleagues. Others may complain how miserable the pain makes them, but it is more likely that the misery is the 'cause' of the pain. Others may complain of bizarre (delusional) symptoms such as 'slime' in the mouth or 'powder' coming out of the jaw.
10. *Response to psychoactive drugs.* In some patients the response to psychoactive drugs, particularly antidepressants, may be dramatic, with relief of pain and striking improvement in the patient's mood.

There have been many reports of pain as a feature of depression. Since mental illness, even now,

carries with it a certain stigma, patients frequently suppress the overt misery of depression. They may also fear (often rightly) that doctors or dentists have contempt for what is regarded as weakness, that is, inability to cope with their life situation. Their pain can therefore be regarded as their cry for help. This is occasionally strikingly evident in a patient who seems otherwise well balanced and emotionally in control but who, when given a chance to describe his complaint at length, suddenly loses control. Acute depression then makes itself obvious as uncontrollable weeping. At the other extreme, there are patients who so strongly reject the idea of mental illness that they insist from the start that the pain is not 'due to their nerves' and typically refuse psychiatric help.

The response of patients with psychogenic pain to sympathetic discussion of the problem therefore tends to fall into fairly well-defined categories. *First*, there is the minority where, having been presented with the opportunity (so to speak), the depression suddenly comes to the surface as uncontrollable crying. *Second*, there are those who welcome the chance to talk, expand upon their problems and welcome the idea of psychiatric help. *Third*, the most difficult group are those who reject—sometimes aggressively—the idea that the pain can be anything other than physical or that 'drugs' might be helpful.

Management

The first essential is to exclude organic disease, and a careful search must be made for all possible sources of pain. If potential sources of pain are found, then they must be dealt with, but there should not be too much optimism as to their effects.

If no organic cause can be found and if the pain and the rest of the clinical picture are suggestive of a psychogenic origin then it is reasonable to refer the patient to a psychiatrist. This can, however, create another problem if the patient is resentful of the idea that he needs such help. Better perhaps is to refer the patient back to the family doctor, explaining why the pain is believed to be of psychogenic origin. The doctor can then refer the patient to a psychiatrist. However, it is important to make an attempt to explain to the patient in simple and sympathetic terms that depression and other emotional disturbances are just as much illnesses and cause just as great suffering as physical diseases, and also that emotional disturbances affect almost everyone to a greater or lesser degree. It is also worthwhile to explain that more common symptoms, particularly headache, are usually also emotional in origin and rarely due to organic disease.

In some patients anxiety may be the predominant feature but this can in turn lead to depression. It is important then to reassure patients that there is no serious disease and that frightening possibilities such as cancer can be confidently excluded. Such reassurance is sometimes remarkably effective.

Sometimes the most effective treatment is to give antidepressants such as amitriptyline. The response of pain to such drugs is itself strongly suggestive of its psychogenic origin.

Unfortunately, there is a hard core of patients who complain of persistent facial pain, have gone the round of specialists (including psychiatrists), have been treated with a wide range of drugs, but still continue to complain of severe pain. This problem may be a reflection of the limited range of treatment available or perhaps such patients 'need' their pain for obscure emotional reasons.

Psychogenic dental pain

This appears to be a variant of the commoner atypical facial pain associated with emotional disturbance. Pain is often exactly referred to one tooth or to a row of teeth which are said either to ache or to be exquisitely sensitive to heat, cold, or pressure. If dental disease is found, treatment has no effect, or if, as a last resort, the tooth is removed the pain moves to an adjacent tooth. Again, if no organic cause can be found and treatment is ineffective, psychiatric assessment is needed.

PARAESTHESIA AND ANAESTHESIA OF THE LIP

Paraesthesia of the lip can be caused by damage to the nerve itself, particularly during the healing phase, or involvement in some lesion of the jaw. Very occasionally it is the result of a neurological disorder. The main causes of most cases of anaesthesia or paraesthesia of the lip are as follows.

1. *Inferior dental blocks.* Persistent anaesthesia or paraesthesia of the lip can occasionally follow inferior dental blocks, possibly as a result of damage of the nerve by the needle or injection into the nerve trunk itself. In most cases, anaesthesia is followed by paraesthesia as recovery takes place.

2. *Trauma.* Paraesthesia of the lip can be a complication of fractures of the mandible where the nerve has become stretched, particularly over the sharp edge of the canal. The effect is temporary but complete recovery may take a few months.

The inferior dental nerve may occasionally be damaged in operations on the mandible and there may be anaesthesia or paraesthesia lasting for many months. It is rare for there to be complete loss of sensation, but if there has been moderately severe damage then recovery may take a year or more.

3. *Acute osteomyelitis.* The inferior dental nerve can be involved in the inflammatory process, but, with effective treatment, recovery is the rule. The condition is now rare.

4. *Malignant tumours of the mandible.* The inferior dental nerve may be compressed by the growing mass or the tumour may infiltrate the nerve sheath. Pain or paraesthesia are strongly suggestive of a malignant tumour, as benign lesions are so slowly growing as to allow the nerve to be pushed gradually aside.

Once a malignant tumour involves the jaw, the prognosis is poor either because it is likely to be secondary carcinoma with widespread metastases or a primary but highly malignant tumour such as osteosarcoma.

5. *Exposed mental foramen.* The mental foramen can become exposed by excessive resorption of mandibular bone in an edentulous patient. The denture can then press upon the nerve as it leaves the foramen. Though these changes are common, paraesthesia of the lip from this cause is surprisingly infrequent.

6. *Herpes zoster.* Herpes zoster affecting the trigeminal nerve can leave residual disturbances of sensation. The most severe and troublesome is post-herpetic neuralgia but in other patients there may be more minor disturbances of sensation, including persistent paraesthesia of the lip.

7. *Multiple sclerosis.* Disturbances of sensation of the face and other regions can be a feature of multiple sclerosis, particularly in its late stages. These disturbances are capriciously distributed according to the sites of lesions in the brain. The lip may be one of the affected sites and the symptoms may range from paraesthesia to extreme and exquisite hypersensitivity whereby the patient will literally jump or scream with pain if the lip is touched. Multiple sclerosis is one of the commoner neurological diseases, nevertheless this is a rare symptom and is virtually only seen in patients with advanced disease and multiple paralyses. There is unlikely to be any doubt about the diagnosis as a consequence.

8. *Tetany.* Tetany is the result of hyopcalcaemic states and characterised by increased neuromuscular excitability together with minor disorders of sensation. One of these is paraesthesia of the lip. Probably the most common cause of tetany is hysterical overbreathing (hyperventilation syndrome).

FACIAL PALSY

Bell's palsy

Bell's palsy is a common cause of facial paralysis possibly resulting from compression of the facial nerve in its canal as a result of inflammation and swelling secondary to a viral infection. Both sexes are equally affected, usually between the ages of 20 and 50. As mentioned earlier pain in the jaw sometimes precedes the paralysis or there may be numbness in the side of the tongue.

Though this disease is uncommonly seen in dental practice, its recognition is important as early treatment may prevent permanent disability and disfigurement.

Function of the facial nerve is tested by asking the patient to perform facial movements. When asked to close the eyes, the lids on the affected side cannot be brought together but the eyeball rolls up normally, since the oculomotor nerves are unaffected. When the patient is asked to smile the corner of the mouth on the affected side is not pulled upwards and the normal lines of expression are absent. The wrinkling round the eyes which accompanies smiling is also not seen on the affected side and the eye remains staring.

The majority of patients recover fully or partially without treatment, but at least 10% of patients with Bell's palsy are unhappy about the final outcome because of permanent disfigurement or other persistent complications.

Persistent facial weakness is itself disfiguring. In some patients the affected part of the face also contracts involuntarily in association with movement of another part. There may, for example, be twitching of the mouth when the patient blinks. More uncommon is unilateral lacrimation when the patient is eating. In the majority of patients with persistent denervation there is contracture of the affected side of the face.

Watering of the eye (epiphora) may remain particularly troublesome. It is due to impaired drainage of tears or occasionally to excessive and erratic lacrimal secretion.

A simple guide to the need for treatment is the severity of the paralysis when the patient is first seen. Full recovery is usual in those patients with an incomplete palsy seen within a week of onset, but more than half of those with a complete lesion fail to recover completely. Electromyography and other electrodiagnostic techniques can be used to assess more precisely the degree of functional impairment as a guide to the need for treatment.

Probably the most effective form of treatment is to give prednisolone, by mouth. A relatively large dose (20 mg four times a day) is given for 5 days and then tailed off over the following 4 days.

Other causes of facial palsy

These include both upper and lower motor neurone lesions:

1. Intracranial causes
   — Strokes
   — Cerebral tumours and other neurological diseases
   — Multiple sclerosis
   — HIV infection
   — Lyme disease
   — Ramsay–Hunt syndrome
   — Trauma to the base of the skull

2. Extracranial causes
   — Malignant parotid neoplasms

—Parotid surgery
—Sarcoidosis (Heerfordt's syndrome)
—Misplaced local anaesthetic.

Strokes. Cerebrovascular accidents (thrombosis or haemorrhage) are a common complication of hypertension in the elderly. Unilateral paralysis (hemiplegia) and often loss of speech (aphasia) are common consequences in those that survive the acute episode.

Unilateral facial palsy is common but differs form Bell's palsy in that the lower part of the face is mainly affected and spontaneous emotional facial reactions may be retained.

As in the case of persistent paralysis in Bell's palsy, an intraoral prosthesis may help to reduce sagging of the affected side of the face in severe cases.

A stroke is occasionally the cause of an emergency in the dental surgery (Ch. 21).

Ramsay–Hunt syndrome is severe facial palsy and pain usually felt in the throat. It is associated with herpes zoster, and vesicles may be seen in the external auditory meatus or throat.

Lyme disease is an infection caused by *Borrelia burgdorferi* which is transmitted by animal ticks. It is increasingly common in the USA but is now seen in many other countries. Arthritis is the chief effect, but in some patients facial palsy or cervical lymphadenopathy may be prominent.

Heerfordt's syndrome is the rare combination of facial palsy, uveitis and parotid swelling, and is caused by sarcoidosis.

Parotid tumours and surgery. Facial palsy is a characteristic manifestation of a malignant parotid tumour. Alternatively a functioning facial nerve may have to be sacrificed during the resection of a malignant tumor, or accidentally damaged during a superficial parotidectomy. The variable course of the facial nerve within the parotid makes it particularly vulnerable to surgical injury and great skill is needed to trace its course during operation.

SUGGESTED FURTHER READING

Dworkin S F, Burgess J A Orofacial pain of psychogenic origin: current concepts and classification. J Am Dent Assoc 115: 565–571

Eversole L R, Stone C E 1987 Vasogenic facial pain (cluster headache). Int J Oral Maxillofac Surg 16: 25–35

Flint S, Scully C 1990 Isolated trigeminal sensory neuropathy: A heterogeneous group of disorders. Oral Surg, Oral Med, Oral Pathol 69: 153–156

Goon W W, Jacobsen P L 1988 Prodromal odontalgia and multiple devitalized teeth caused by herpes zoster of the trigeminal nerve. J Am Dent Assoc 116: 500–504

Hampf G, Vikkula J, Ylipaavalniemi P, Aalberg V 1987 Psychiatric disorders in orofacial dysaesthesia. Int J Oral Maxillofac Surg 16: 402–407

Hillman L, Burns M T, Chander A, Tai Y M A 1989 The management of craniofacial pain in a pain relief unit. Dental Update 16: 431–437

Schielke E, Pfister H E, Einhaupl K M 1989 Peripheral facial nerve palsy associated with HIV infection. Lancet 335: 553–554

Schnetler J, Hopper C 1989 Intracranial tumours presenting with facial pain. Br Dent J 166: 80–83

Scully C, Cawson R A 1991 Medical problems in dentistry, 3rd edn. Wright, Bristol

Sessle B J 1987 The neurobiology of facial and dental pain: Present knowledge, future directions. J Dent Res 66: 962–981

Yontchev E, Hedegard B, Carlsson G E 1987 Outcome of treatment of patients with orofacial discomfort complaints. Int J Oral Maxillofac Surg 16: 312–318

19. Control of pain and anxiety—anaesthesia and sedation in dentistry

Many dental operations such as extractions, major oral surgery and, often, cavity preparation are both painful and prolonged. Pain can usually be abolished by use of local analgesia but, as mentioned in the previous chapter, sedation may also be needed to control anxiety. Pain and anxiety can also be abolished by use of general anaesthetics, but though the use of the latter is declining in dentistry, the use of anaesthesia and sedation are so integral a part of dental practice that some consideration must be given to their special problems.

INFILTRATION AND REGIONAL ANAESTHESIA

Local analgesia can be obtained by injection into the soft tissues immediately around the operation site (infiltration anaesthesia) or by making the injection beside the nerve supplying the area at some distance from the operation site (regional anaesthesia).

Many local anaesthetic agents continue to be produced but none so far seems to have significant advantages over lignocaine.

Local anaesthesia is so safe, simple and effective and, with reasonable care, gives rise to so few complications that general anaesthesia is justified only for special indications.

Advantages of local anaesthesia

These are as follows.

1. No special preparation of the patient is needed.
2. No complicated apparatus or bulky gas cylinders are needed.
3. There is no risk of respiratory obstruction.
4. Anaesthesia lasts for at least an hour and, if the patient is agreeable, can be prolonged as necessary for minor oral surgery or difficult restorative procedures.
5. The patient remains awake and cooperative and needs no after-care.

427

6. Seriously ill patients such as those with heart disease can usually tolerate local anaesthesia without undue risk.
7. An anaesthetist is not required.

Preparation for local anaesthesia

There is no need for any special preparation of the patient before giving a local anaesthetic. The patient should not go without food but if very nervous may be given a sedative such as temazepam 5 mg half an hour before the operation.

Choice of local anaesthetic

Lignocaine and related amide derivatives are safe and effective. Toxic effects and allergy are so rare as to be almost non-existent. Lignocaine, however, is relatively ineffective without a vasoconstrictor. Others such as prilocaine give short-term analgesia without such help. Vasoconstrictors such as adrenaline and noradrenaline, because of their effects on the cardiovascular system, are potentially more toxic than the local anaesthetic itself. Noradrenaline can cause dangerous hypertension, has no advantages and should not be used.

The chief danger of adrenaline is that if it enters the circulation in *significant* amounts, it can cause increased cardiac excitability and arrhythmias. This may be dangerous for patients with unstable cardiac rhythm, such as those who have had a myocardial infarct or severe prolonged hypertension. Nevertheless 2% lignocaine with 1:80 000 or 1:100 000 adrenaline has been used on a vast scale for many years but examples of adverse reactions are hard to find.

Prilocaine (Citanest) 3% can be given alone or with either 1:300 000 adrenaline or felypressin 0.03 i.u. per ml. Felypressin is related to vasopressin (a pituitary extract); its toxicity is very low and it appears effectively to localise the analgesic agent without producing general circulatory effects. These preparations of prilocaine appear to be nearly as effective as the standard preparation of lignocaine and adrenaline, but their advantages appear to be largely theoretical.

Limitations of local anaesthesia

Anxiety and related problems

Some very nervous patients prefer to be unconscious for even the most minor procedures or have a neurotic fear of injections. Children may also be unsuitable for local anaesthesia, particularly if mentally handicapped or uncontrollable for any other reason. Sedation may then be required.

Extensive oral surgery, especially when a bone chisel is used, is particularly unpleasant for the conscious patient.

Local infection

Acute inflammation prohibits the use of a local anaesthetic. Injection into an inflamed area can spread the infection. Moreover, local anaesthetics are frequently ineffective when the pulp or periodontal membrane is inflamed. Where there is no risk of spreading an infection it may be possible to overcome this difficulty by using 5% lignocaine. A regional anaesthetic, injected well away from the area of inflammation, does not have these dangers.

Duration of action

The duration of local anaesthesia using lignocaine 2% with adrenaline 1:80 000 is often much too prolonged. An inferior dental block may be effective for over 2 hours and the face feels stiff and numb long after the operation. This persistence of anaesthesia may allow the patient unknowingly to bite the lip, leaving an extensive ulcer. The duration of local anaesthesia can be controlled to some extent by restraint in the amount injected.

Complications of local anaesthesia

There are many *possible* complications of local anaesthesia. Some of these, such as drug interactions, are theoretical rather than real, and serious complications from local anaesthetics given for dentistry are remarkably rare, provided that a little common sense and restraint are used when these drugs are given.

Palpitations and loss of consciousness (fainting)

These are usually the result of anxiety. In addition, adrenaline increases the heart rate.

Injection into a blood vessel

Experiments suggest that injection needles enter vessels perhaps in as many as 10% of regional blocks. However, it should not be assumed that in such cases anything more than a trace of local anaesthetic enters a blood vessel. If so high a proportion of injections were truly intravascular then inevitably there would be no local anaesthetic effect and 10% of inferior dental blocks would fail. In practice, however, the failure rate of inferior dental blocks is negligible in experienced hands.

It is likely therefore that no more than traces of local anaesthetics may get into the bloodstream and, if so, might cause palpitations or other minor cardiovascular disturbances. The extreme rarity of severe reactions to local anaesthetics indicates that this is not a serious hazard, but anxious practitioners can use an aspirating syringe if they fear possible reactions from intravascular injections.

Cardiovascular reactions

Noradrenaline, when used in high concentration (1:20 000), can, in susceptible subjects, cause severe hypertension and occasionally death. Noradrenaline has no advantages and should not be used.

Adrenaline in a concentration of 1:80 000 or 1:100 000 does not cause trouble clinically but, in overdose can precipitate cardiac arrhythmias by increasing myocardial excitability.

Patients with a history of severe cardiovascular disease, such as prolonged severe hypertension, angina or past myocardial infarcts may be considered to be at risk, but provided that the patient is not anxious and only modest quantities (up to two cartridges) of local anaesthetic solution are given, there is no evidence that the risks are significant. The effectiveness of lignocaine with adrenaline in abolishing pain and hence preventing endogenous catecholamine release probably more than outweighs the suggested dangers of the injection of the small amount of adrenaline. In such cases, some prefer to use prilocaine with felypressin. However, the available statistics provide no support for the idea that it is any safer.

Toxicity of local anaesthetic agents

Lignocaine, prilocaine and related amide anaesthetic agents have very low toxicity. Hypersensitivity is little more than a theoretical risk, and authenticated reports of such reactions are exceedingly few. Many so-called reactions to local anaesthetic agents are usually no more than coincidence.

In spite of the effectiveness of modern local anaesthetic preparations, a few practitioners are silly enough to use them in vast quantities and give five or ten cartridges in quick succession. Up to two cartridges, repeated if necessary after half-an-hour, provides more than adequate anaesthesia for the area which can be operated on within this space of time.

Lignocaine itself helps to stabilise cardiac rhythm, and after a myocardial infarct a standard procedure has been to give 100 mg of lignocaine rapidly intravenously. When given in this way there may sometimes be toxic effects including agitation, confusion, fits, sweating or drowsiness. Nevertheless these are not regarded as serious enough to contraindicate the use of lignocaine for these poor-risk patients. It can be seen therefore that toxic effects from lignocaine used in the normal manner and with reasonable restraint for dental purposes is unlikely to cause toxic effects.

The main toxic effect of prilocaine is to cause methaemoglobinaemia. This is rarely serious but life-threatening methaemoglobinaemia due to prilocaine has been reported in a previously healthy young patient.

Drug interactions

Anxiety continues to be expressed about interactions between vasoconstrictors and antidepressent drugs. There is, however, no clinical evidence of interactions between tricyclic antidepressants and local anaesthetics containing adrenaline or noradrenaline. A few patients, some of whom were taking tricyclic antidepressants, have had severe hypertensive responses to local anaesthetics containing *noradrenaline*. All of these patients had, however, been given noradrenaline in excessive amounts and those patients who were receiving tricyclic agents had no more severe reactions than those who were not.

In the case of adrenaline used in local anaesthetics for dental purposes *no clinical evidence has been found of acute hypertension or any other interaction with tricyclic antidepressants.*

At one time it was believed that adrenaline or noradrenaline could cause interactions with the monoamine oxidase inhibitor (MAOI) group of antidepressant agents. There is also no evidence that this is the case, and the idea probably arose as a result of misapprehensions about the pharmacology of these agents.

It must be appreciated that *tens of millions* of local anaesthetics are given each year and antidepressants are also used on a very wide scale. If, therefore, there were any serious risk of interactions, these would soon have made themselves only too evident. The fact that there is no clinical evidence of such reactions suggests that they are theoretical rather than practical problems.

Haemorrhagic disease

In haemophilia especially, a local anaesthetic needle can occasionally cause a small tear in the side of a vessel. This can be sufficient to cause severe deep, soft tissue bleeding. The risk is greatest with inferior dental blocks. From this site soft-tissue extravasation of blood can readily track down towards the glottis and cause respiratory obstruction. However, local infiltrations, even in mild haemophiliacs, can also cause alarming and possibly dangerous bleeding into the soft tissues. Such complications are uncommon but some haematologists will not allow a haemophiliac to have a local anaesthetic without protection with antihaemophilic factor.

Whether a dentist is prepared to accept the risk of giving a local anaesthetic to a haemophiliac without the protection of AHF depends on how enthusiastic a gambler he is. A possible alternative to giving AHF is to use the antifibrinolytic, tranexamic acid (Ch. 20).

Breaking the needle

Breaking a needle in the tissues should be a thing of the past now that disposable needles are (or should be) used for each patient and then discarded.

In the unlikely event of a needle having been broken in the tissues, the patient must be informed and reassured (broken needles have sometimes remained buried for years without complications) but referred for removal of the needle at open operation. No attempt should be made to remove the needle in the dental surgery unless part is protruding and can readily be grasped.

Injection of the wrong solution

Now that anaesthetic cartridges are so widely used this is a rare accident. In the past, serious injuries have been caused by the accidental injection of irritant chemicals.

Late complications

Some pain coming on as the anaesthetic wears off is not uncommon, especially after subperiosteal injections.

Pain may be due to (a) low-grade infection; (b) damage to the tissues if the needle is used clumsily or is blunt; or (c) to irritation by the solution injected. In this last respect the local anaesthetic may have an acid reaction, may not be isotonic with the body fluids or may contain an irritant antiseptic as a preservative. These objections have largely been overcome in present-day preparations.

Difficulty in opening the mouth

Transient difficulty in opening the mouth may occasionally accompany after-pain when inferior dental block injections have been given. This is due to inflammatory oedema.

Rarely, limitation of opening persists for several weeks after an inferior dental block and may have to be treated by manipulation under general anaesthesia. In some patients a programme of stretching exercises alone may be adequate, but up to 6 weeks may elapse before full opening is achieved.

The condition is painless and is the result of haematoma formation and fibrosis in the medial pterygoid region.

Infection at the site of injection

This may be carried by a dirty needle, by bacteria from the surface of the oral mucous membrane, or by injection of an infected solution. Infection is accompanied by the usual signs of acute inflammation, and its severity depends on the number and virulence of the organisms implanted. A severe infection involving the pterygomandibular and temporal fascial spaces may result from infection introduced with an inferior dental nerve injection.

Haematoma formation

This follows the tearing of the wall of a vein and leakage of blood into the tissues. If the bleeding is superficial it appears as a bruise under the skin. In patients with haemorrhagic disease, particularly haemophilia, haematoma formation is a serious hazard as mentioned earlier.

Ulceration of the lip

Severe superficial ulceration of the lower lip following an inferior dental block is an occasional complication. This is usually due to the patient's having bitten the lip and is especially likely to follow the use of lignocaine, which has a powerful and prolonged effect.

Other local complications

These include ulceration at or near the site of injection, prolonged anaesthesia and motor paralysis, but are all rare.

Hepatitis B

Hepatitis B can be transmitted from a carrier patient to another patient by an inadequately sterilised syringe or needle. The disease can also be transmitted from a reused anaesthetic cartridge, because blood leaks back into the cartridge at the end of the injection. An anaesthetic cartridge, even

if not visibly contaminated, should never be used up on another patient (see Ch. 20).

Intraligamentary injections

Using a special gun-like syringe with a very fine (30 gauge) needle, local analgesia can be obtained by direct injection into the periodontal ligament. Unexpectedly, this method is often considerably less painful than conventional injections and can achieve almost immediate abolition of sensation in a tooth with as little as 0.2% ml of local anaesthetic solution.

With upper anterior teeth where conventional injections tend to be particularly painful, intraligamentary injection seems to be considerably more pleasant for the patient.

In view of the small amount of local anaesthetic solution used, the rapid abolition of sensation and restriction of the effects to a single tooth, intraligamentary injection appears to have considerable potential advantages and is said to be greatly preferred by most patients, including children.

The disadvantages of intraligamentary injections are that *a.* they can sometimes cause persistent postoperative pain and *b.* overall, they are also less reliably effective than conventional injections.

A theoretical danger of intraligamentary injection is that it is likely to force bacteria of the periodontal plaque into the bloodstream. It may be advisable, therefore, as a precaution, to apply a potent antiseptic such as chlorhexidine or iodine in alcohol to the gingival sulcus just before injection.

Adverse effects of local anaesthetics—summary

Despite the possibility of several types of adverse effects from local anaesthetics such as lignocaine and adrenaline, the frequency of such mishaps must be viewed against the scale of use of these drugs. Lignocaine has been in use for over a quarter of a century, and the usage of dental local anaesthetics in Britain is estimated to be at least 40 *million* cartridges annually. In spite of this vast scale of use and in spite of the facts that incompetent practitioners may use these agents in recklessly large quantities and that a relatively high proportion of patients have unsuspected cardiovascular disease, significant adverse reactions are so rare as to make it almost impossible to collect meaningful statistics.

Patients with severe ischaemic heart disease are at greatest risk, but if these patients need dental treatment there is no safer way of doing it than under local anaesthesia. The only useful precautions that can be taken in such patients are to minimise anxiety (with, for example, diazepam) and to use no more of the local anaesthetic solution than necessary. There is no clinical evidence to suggest that in these circumstances prilocaine with or without felypressin is any safer, and it is probably less effective than lignocaine with adrenaline.

SEDATION

Sedation in the present context implies abolition of anxiety without complete loss of consciousness or loss of protective reflexes. By definition it should be possible to maintain communication with the patient, who should be responsive to commands throughout the procedure. The most satisfactory agents in current use are the intravenous benzodiazepines (diazepam and midazolam) and nitrous oxide with oxygen.

The intravenous benzodiazepines have no analgesic action, and though nitrous oxide is a potent analgesic for some types of pain it is not adequate for cavity preparation, though other procedures in the mouth become more comfortable for the patient. A local anaesthetic should therefore be given during sedation.

Intravenous barbiturates such as methohexitone are potent general anaesthetic agents and potent respiratory depressants. They are not suitable and too dangerous for dental sedation.

Oral sedation

Diazepam or, better, temazepam can be given by mouth. 5 mg of either, given the night before and again half an hour before treatment is frequently strikingly effective for abolishing anxiety. The chief disadvantage of oral sedation is that its effects are less predictable than intravenous sedation.

Intravenous sedation

Diazepam

Diazepam has a long record of safe and effective dental sedation, and the patient usually has complete amnesia for the operation.

Table 19.1   Advantages of intravenous diazepam

1. Effective and well tolerated by most adults
2. Requires no special equipment for administration
3. Amnesia for the period of sedation
4. Toxic effects (respiratory depression) insignificant in healthy patients (but see Table 19.2)
5. No major adverse cardiovascular effects
6. No unpleasant after-effects apart from drowsiness
7. Few significant interactions with other drugs (but see Table 19.2)

The usual procedure is to prepare the patient as for a general anaesthetic though fasting is unnecessary. Diazepam is injected (usually 10–15 mg) slowly while maintaining conversation until the patient's responses weaken or stop (though still rousable on command) or there is obvious ptosis with the eyelid drooping halfway across the pupil (Verrill's sign).

The airway should be protected with a sponge and a local anaesthetic given. If the latter is not given the patient may struggle or cry out during a painful procedure, though there will be no recollection of it afterwards.

With a single small dose, sedation is adequate for about 30 minutes but patients then remain drowsy and cooperative for a longer period and do not usually appear to be fully awake for at least an hour.

Adverse effects. Diazepam has proved to be remarkably safe and most complications have resulted from its misuse. However, it has the following toxic effects.

1. Respiratory depression. Diazepam causes a small but measurable degree of respiratory depression, and rapid injection can cause temporary apnoea. It should not be given to hypoxic patients, particularly those with chronic obstructive pulmonary disease. It should also not be given in combination with other drugs, such as opioids or barbiturates, which are more potent respiratory depressants, and deaths have resulted from use of such mixtures.

Table 19.2 Disadvantages and limitations of intravenous diazepam

1. Long-delayed recovery (metabolites also active and slowly excreted)
2. Irritant to blood vessels (vehicle rather than diazepam itself)
3. Respiratory depressant (dangerous in chronic obstructive pulmonary disease), especially if used with an opioid
4. Some patients 'resistant' or develop tolerance
5. Hypersensitivity (exceedingly rare)
6. Children may fail to respond or occasionally have paradoxical reactions
7. Not analgesic
8. Additive effect with other sedating drugs

However, for healthy patients, this degree of respiratory depression is not significant.

2. Hypotension. Diazepam can cause postural hypotension but the effect is not normally dangerous.

3. Delayed recovery. Diazepam has a half-life of 20–50 hours and persistently active metabolites. Even though the patient appears to be fully awake after treatment, consciousness is impaired. Diazepam also undergoes enterohepatic recirculation so that an apparently recovered patient can suddenly become drowsy hours after administration (second peak effect). All patients should therefore be forbidden to drive a motor vehicle for at least 12 hours after sedation and should be taken home by a responsible adult.

4. Vascular damage. Diazepam is not water soluble and is usually carried in propylene glycol (Valium injection). The latter is irritant to endothelium and can cause thrombophlebitis or, in the case of accidental intra-arterial injection, spasm and, rarely, gangrene of the fingers.

Diazemuls. This is diazepam in a non-irritant lipid emulsion, but this preparation is viscous and less convenient to use.

Recovery from diazepam. It is perhaps worth bearing in mind that though diazepam has a remarkable record for safety, its after-effects can be very dangerous in vehicle drivers, who are notorious for their failure to comply with instructions not to drive. Diazepam is particularly dangerous in this respect in that drowsiness often comes on after a variable period of apparent recovery (second peak effect) as a result of enterohepatic recirculation and active metabolites.

Midazolam

Midazolam has essentially similar properties to diazepam but has the following advantages.

1. It is water soluble and non-irritant to vessel walls.
2. It is more rapidly metabolised than diazepam and has no prolonged after-effects. However, the time to initial recovery is similar to that of diazepam.
3. It may give even more complete amnesia.

Adverse effects. These result from the facts that midazolam is approximately three times as potent as diazepam and susceptible patients can pass into a state of general anaesthesia. Overdose can result in dangerous respiratory depression, and a few patients, particularly the elderly, have died as a consequence. A factor which makes it easier to give an overdose is that sedation develops more rapidly than the clinical signs appear.

Because of these dangers, the General Dental Council have indicated that a dentist who administers sedation in the absence of a suitably trained assistant and proper resuscitative equipment 'would almost certainly be considered to have acted in a manner which constitutes serious professional misconduct'.

The current advice is to give no more than 5 mg of the dilute solution and then wait for signs of sedation to appear. A further dose can then be given if necessary.

However, if used with care to avoid the dangers indicated above and with particular care to limit dosage in the elderly, midazolam has, overall, considerable advantages over diazepam and to a great extent has replaced it.

Flumazenil

Flumazenil is a specific benzodiazepine antagonist which allows rapid arousal from diazepam or midazolam sedation. The main application of flumazenil is to counteract the effects of an accidental overdose. The half-life of flumazenil is considerably shorter than that of diazepam and recurrence of sedation is a possibility, though this suggestion has been contested.

Pulse oximetry

Pulse oximeters measure haemoglobin oxygen saturation by spectrophotometric analysis of the light passing through the tissues. The degree of arterial blood oxygenation is measured by a microprocessor which reads only the pulsatile component of the transmitted light.

A pulse oximeter can conveniently be attached to a finger and, within certain limitations, provides an indication of oxygen saturation throughout the body. They are an important safety measure which, though they have limitations, typically give a warning of dangerous falls in brain oxygen tension within 60 seconds of its onset.

Inhalational sedation with nitrous oxide—relative analgesia

Nitrous oxide is a potent anxiolytic. It is, unlike the benzodiazepines, a potent analgesic. However, this is of relative unimportance in sedation, as the analgesic effect is usually not sufficient to obtund the pain of cavity preparation and a local anaesthetic has usually to be given.

Relative analgesia can be used to induce in an anxious patient a state of tranquility during dental procedures without loss of consciousness or cooperation. However, individual requirements vary widely: the desired effect can often be achieved with a nitrous oxide concentration as low as 20%, but much higher concentrations may have sometimes to be used. In all cases nitrous oxide should be administered from apparatus specially designed to enable the nitrous oxide and oxygen concentrations to be controlled precisely and with a fail-safe device to prevent administration of not less than 30% of oxygen.

Indications for inhalation versus intravenous sedation

To a considerable extent these types of agent are interchangeable, and the operator's experience is a major determining factor. However, a survey in 1986 found that inhalation sedation was most widely used. Intravenous sedation has the obvious advantage that it requires no expensive equipment but, given a free choice of either method, the choice of relative analgesia depends on the following considerations:

1. *Patient preference.*
   a. Some prefer the drowsy, light-headed sensation that nitrous oxide induces.
   b. A few patients have needle phobia and refuse injections.
2. *Safety.* Nitrous oxide has negligible adverse cardiorespiratory effects and its excretion is not affected by liver or kidney disease.
3. *Difficult veins.* In a few patients, veins are so difficult to find that an intravenous agent is almost impracticable.

Table 19.3 Advantages of nitrous oxide/oxygen

1. Both analgesic and sedative
2. No respiratory depression
3. No adverse haemodynamic effects
4. No significant interactions with any other drugs
5. Patient remains cooperative, with consciousness only slightly impaired
6. Rapid recovery
7. Acceptable by, and effective for, children

4. *Rapid recovery.*
5. *Children.* Often more acceptable and easier to administer.

The limitations or disadvantages of relative analgesia include:

1. *Highly anxious patients.* Some cooperation is required from patients to administer relative analgesia satisfactorily, and this may be beyond the capabilities of a very anxious patient.
2. *Mask phobia.* Unpleasant anaesthetic experiences in the past may make a patient refuse an inhalational agent.
3. *Lack of amnesia.*
4. *Vomiting.* This is only an occasional complication.

Table 19.4 Disadvantages of nitrous oxide/oxygen

1. Rapid transition to anaesthesia in some patients
2. Fear of inhalational agents by some patients
3. Special equipment needed for administration (automatic cut-off essential if oxygen fails)
4. Risk of dependence with neurological complications
5. Pollution of surgery atmosphere

Nitrous oxide abuse

The properties of nitrous oxide which make it so valuable for sedation (relative analgesia) are those of drugs of dependence. There is the risk, therefore, of nitrous oxide abuse by anaesthetists and dentists, to whom it is readily available. A few reports of nitrous oxide addiction among dentists have appeared in the USA but, as with all types of drug abuse, the prevalence is inevitably greater than the number of reported cases. Prolonged use of nitrous oxide interferes with vitamin B12 metabolism, and some of these dentists have developed neurological complications as a consequence.

Xenon

Xenon (chemically a member of the noble gas group) has been used experimentally since 1951 for its anaesthetic properties. Recent reports indicate that it has advantages over nitrous oxide in having greater anaesthetic potency and stronger analgesic effects, and causing even less cardiovascular disturbance.

A current limitation of xenon is its cost, but this can be limited by use of a closed circuit system: this in turn reduces the possible hazard of operating room pollution. Also the anaesthetic apparatus has to be modified for xenon administration.

The value of xenon for sedation in dentistry has not as yet been reported.

GENERAL ANAESTHESIA

In the past, general anaesthesia was widely used for *brief* dental operations, particularly extractions. In these circumstances the risks are low, provided that the anaesthetist is competent and the patient is fit. Patients should be admitted to hospital for prolonged general anaesthetics, particularly for major oral surgery. Some anaesthetic agents, particularly the intravenous barbiturates, pose special problems because of their great potency and the ease with which dangerous complications can develop imperceptibly.

Since dental operations have to be carried out at the upper end of the airway the latter can only too readily become obstructed by a foreign body. The airway can only be fully protected by intubation and one of the dangers of general anaesthesia in the dental surgery is that intubation is not used. The use of general anaesthesia in dentistry therefore has important medicolegal implications.

The chief inhalational agents in use are nitrous oxide and oxygen, usually supplemented with halothane, enflurane, or isoflurane. The main intravenous agents are barbiturates, such as thiopentone or methohexitone.

Indications for general anaesthesia

With development of safe and satisfactory methods of conscious sedation there are few indications for general anaesthesia in dentistry. Its main uses are for:

1. major oral surgery
2. the severely physically or mentally handicapped
3. those for whom sedation is unacceptable or ineffective.

The General Dental Council has also indicated that general anaesthesia should only be given by or under the supervision of another dental or medical practitioner suitably trained in its use. It should be given only with suitable anaesthetic apparatus and with adequate resuscitative equipment being available. (See also Chapter 25.)

Contraindications to general anaesthesia

A general anaesthetic must not be given under the following circumstances.

1. A patient has had a recent meal (within the last 4 hours).
2. There is actual or potential respiratory obstruction, such as oedema of the neck.
3. No competent anaesthetist or adequate facilities are available.
4. The patient has systemic (particularly cardiovascular) disease.

Precautions and preparations for general anaesthesia

Before giving the anaesthetic:

1. The patient's fitness for anaesthesia should be assessed
2. The patient should have had nothing to eat or drink for 4 hours previously. It is also a good idea to make sure that the patient's bladder has been emptied

3. Another, competent person should be available to accompany the patient home afterwards.

For the administration of the anaesthetic the following are required.

1. A competent anaesthetist and nurse should be present
2. The anaesthetic equipment must be in full working order
3. Plenty of oxygen must be available, both in the anaesthetic apparatus and in reserve, together with means for providing positive pressure inflation of the lungs
4. Effective throat packs must be used to protect the airway
5. Efficient suction apparatus must be handy to keep the airway clear
6. Resuscitative equipment, including facilities for endotracheal intubation or tracheostomy, and appropriate drugs must be available.

After the operation the patient must be:

1. Put into a position where blood or saliva do not drain back into the pharynx
2. Kept under supervision until conscious
3. Allowed home only when fully recovered or it is reasonably certain that the accompanying adult can be responsible for the patient
4. Forbidden to drive a car or operate unguarded machinery until the following day at the earliest.

Premedication

If the patient is very nervous, premedication may be needed and this is usually given in hospital for anything more than the most minor operations. Premedication is not usually given in dental practice, partly because it is rarely necessary and partly because it tends to delay recovery. Diazepam 5 mg by mouth on the night before and, again, half an hour before the operation is often adequate.

Inhalation anaesthesia

Nitrous oxide and oxygen

Nitrous oxide is a pleasant non-irritant anaesthetic agent which is both analgesic and an effective sedating agent. It is the least toxic of all anaesthetic agents, has all the properties that can be desired, but is a weak anaesthetic. As a consequence anaesthesia often cannot be achieved if an adequate concentration of oxygen is given. The oxygen concentration should not be allowed to fall below 30%.

Recovery is rapid and occasionally accompanied by euphoria. There should be no significant after-effects, but there may occasionally be vomiting.

In cooperative patients nitrous oxide and oxygen alone can produce a light plane of surgical anaesthesia adequate for short operations such as dental extractions. The more resistant or uncooperative patients have a prolonged excitement stage, often with violent struggling. If oxygenation remains adequate, surgical anaesthesia is often unobtainable.

The chief limitation of nitrous oxide is that it is only a weak anaesthetic. Frequently therefore, it has to be supplemented with another agent such as halothane.

Halothane

Halothane is a potent non-irritating anaesthetic and is given with nitrous oxide and oxygen in concentrations of 2–3% for induction, then maintained at 0.5–2% for the remainder of the operation. For this purpose calibrated vaporisers have to be used to ensure accurate regulation of the concentration. Induction is smooth and relatively pleasant with minimal excitement. Surgical anaesthesia can be induced in 2–3 minutes. The halothane is usually stopped a few minutes before the operation is completed. Recovery is rapid (though less rapid than with nitrous oxide and oxygen alone) and there are usually no significant after-effects.

Halothane with nitrous oxide and oxygen can be used for brief dental operations, particularly on more difficult patients or for prolonged oral surgical operations in the operating theatre, and is the drug of choice for such purposes.

Toxic effects. The main toxic effects of halothane are (1) hepatitis and (2) induction of cardiac arrhythmias.

1. *Halothane hepatitis*. The mechanism of this reaction is unknown but it appears to be more

likely to follow repeated administration of halothane at intervals of less than 6 months. Otherwise, no other agent is known to be safer.

2. Cardiac arrhythmias. Halothane sensitises the heart to catecholamines such as adrenaline. Cardiac arrhythmias may therefore develop, especially if there is any respiratory depression and hypoxia.

Cardiac arrhythmias can be provoked by adrenaline, which is often given during oral surgery to give a bloodless field of operation. These effects of adrenaline can be counteracted by giving a beta-blocking drug if necessary.

Enflurane

Enflurane (Ethrane) is a newer halogenated ether inhalational agent which was introduced for clinical work in Britain in 1966. Enflurane has the advantages that it has a very rapid onset of action, allowing induction for simple extractions in about $1\frac{1}{2}$ minutes. Little enflurane (about 2.5%) is metabolised in the body and systemic effects seem to be minimal. Thus, cardiac rhythm is more stable than with halothane and there is less sensitisation of the myocardium to adrenaline injected to obtain a bloodless field. It is believed, on the basis of experimental work, that enflurane has no adverse effects on liver function and that even long exposure produces no persistent after-effects.

Recovery is more rapid than after halothane, for operations of equal duration.

The chief disadvantage of enflurane is that it depresses respiration more than halothane and appears to have epileptogenic potential. Nevertheless enflurane seems to have significant advantages over halothane.

Isoflurane

More recently still, isoflurane seems likely to replace enflurane (of which it is an isomer) in the USA. Isoflurane has the advantages of as rapid uptake and distribution as enflurane, lesser respiratory depression than enflurane (but greater than halothane), but considerably less adverse cardiovascular effects than either enflurane or halothane.

Unlike enflurane, isoflurane appears to have no epileptogenic action.

Overall, isoflurane appears to have significant advantages over halothane and enflurane. However, neither isoflurane nor enflurane are as pleasant to take as halothane, and they are considerably more expensive. Halothane, despite its possible dangers, is therefore still extensively used.

Intravenous anaesthesia

Intravenous anaesthetics are easy to administer, rapid in action and pleasant for the patient. The intravenous barbiturates in particular are powerful and dangerous. These agents should therefore be used only by experienced anaesthetists able to recognise complications and carry out resuscitative measures with speed and skill. Though several new agents have been introduced, the most frequently used intravenous anaesthetics are the barbiturates. Thiopentone (Pentothal) is widely used as an induction agent for general surgery, while in dentistry the more popular drug has been methohexitone (Brietal).

Thiopentone

Thiopentone is potent and rapid in action, giving a pleasant induction especially valued by patients who fear inhalation anaesthetics.

The usual method is (having made certain that the needle is in the vein) to give 2–3 ml of a 2.5% solution. After a pause of about a minute this is repeated until the necessary depth of anaesthesia is reached.

The dangers of thiopentone are essentially the same as those of methohexitone discussed below. However, thiopentone is somewhat more prone to cause spasm of the larynx and is also intensely irritant if injected outside a vein.

Local reactions to thiopentone can be particularly severe. If the drug is accidentally injected into the subcutaneous tissues there is severe irritation and the skin may slough. Injection close to a nerve may cause temporary or permanent paralysis. Intra-arterial injection is most dangerous. Arterial spasm is followed by thrombosis and sometimes by gangrene and loss of the arm.

Methohexitone

Methohexitone is more than twice as potent as thiopentone, but is generally preferred in dentistry, partly because the results of extravascular injections are less severe and partly because it has a shorter action. Subjectively at least, induction seems to be even more rapid than with thiopentone, and after a single injection the patient quickly recovers consciousness.

An important disadvantage of methohexitone is that it has no analgesic effect and may increase sensitivity to pain, and involuntary movements are common. As a consequence patients are restless in the light plane of anaesthesia desirable for dentistry.

Recovery after methohexitone. Methohexitone is rapidly distributed in the tissues but is also more rapidly metabolised than thiopentone. Nevertheless patients should be allowed at least an hour to recover, particularly if anaesthesia has been prolonged for more than a few minutes, and should be accompanied home by a responsible adult.

Complications

Both methohexitone and thiopentone are very potent drugs, and the patient passes through the stages of anaesthesia rapidly and almost imperceptibly. It is easy therefore to give an overdose.

Cardiovascular and respiratory effects. Methohexitone resembles thiopentone in causing significant respiratory depression and also some cardiovascular depression. Undetected hypoxia can cause further depression of the respiratory and cardiovascular centres to set up a vicious circle which may end fatally.

Though several deaths have been associated with methohexitone anaesthesia, the precise cause of some of them is not clear.

Excitatory phenomena. Hiccup and involuntary movements under light methohexitone anaesthesia are common, and it is regarded as being contra-indicated for epileptics.

Hypersensitivity reactions. The intravenous barbiturates can cause hypersensitivity reactions, probably by inducing mast cell degranulation. These reactions can result in bronchospasm or, rarely, fatal anaphylaxis.

The important conclusions to be drawn about intravenous anaesthetic agents, and barbiturates in particular, is that they are overall too dangerous for use by any except trained anaesthetists, and, even in their hands, there have occasionally been fatal accidents. In spite of statements to the contrary, intravenous barbiturates cannot be safely used for sedation.

Complications of general anaesthesia

These problems are discussed in text-books of anaesthesia, but they are of so serious a nature that they are also reviewed briefly in Chapter 21.

The main danger is obstruction of the airway. This is a hazard to which oral operations are especially prone.

SUGGESTED FURTHER READING

Brogden R N, Goa K L 1988 Flumazenil. A preliminary review of its benzodiazepine-antagonist properties, intrinsic activity and therapeutic use. Drugs 35: 448–467
Brown B R 1985 Halothane hepatitis revisited. New Engl J Med 312: 1347–1348
Committee on Safety of Medicines 1985 Midazolam (Hypnovel)—respiratory depression and hypotension. Current Problems No 14
Davies C A et al 1990 Reversal of midazolam with flumazenil following conservative dentistry. J Dent 18: 113–118
Ghonheim M M, Mewaldt S P 1990 Benzodiazepines and memory: a review. Anesthesiology 72: 926–938
Harris D, O'Boyle C, Barry H 1987 Oral sedation with temazepam: controlled comparison of a soft gelatin capsule formation with intravenous diazepam. Br Dent J 162: 297–301
Hosie H E, Brook I M, Holmes A 1987 Oral sedation with temazepam: a practical alternative for use in dentistry. Br Dent J 162: 190–193
Lachmann B, Armbruster S, Schairer W et al 1990 Safety and efficacy of xenon in routine use as an inhalational anaesthetic. Lancet 1: 1413–1415
Leading article 1988 Midazolam—is antagonism justified? Lancet 2: 140–142
Leading article 1988 Flumazenil. Lancet 2: 828–830
Lytle J J, Stamper E P 1990 The 1988 anaesthesia survey of the Southern California Society of Oral and Maxillofacial Surgeons. J Oral Maxillofacial Surg 47: 834–842
Neil H A W, Fairer J G, Coleman M P et al 1987 Mortality

among male anaesthetists in the United Kingdom 1957–73. Br Med J 295: 360–362

Nightingale J J, Norman J 1988 A comparison of midazolam with temazepam for premedication of day case patients. Anaesthesia 43: 111–113

Osborne-Smith C M D, Skelly A M 1987 The use of a benzodiazepine and an opioid for sedation for minor oral surgery under local analgesia. Proc Assoc Dent Anaesth 5: 1–2

Read Ward G 1990 Intravenous sedation in general dental practice—why pulse oximetry. Br Dent J 168: 368–369

Roberts G J 1990 Inhalation sedation (relative analgesia) with oxygen/nitrous oxide gas mixtures: 1. Principles. Dental Update 17: 139–147

Roberts G J 1990 Inhalation sedation (relative analgesia) with oxygen/nitrous oxide gas mixtures: 2. Practical techniques. Dental Update 17: 190–197

Shirlaw P J, Scully C, Griffiths M J et al 1986 General anaesthesia, parenteral sedation and emergency drugs and equipment in general dental practice. J Dent 14: 247–250

Simmons M, Miller C D, Cummings G C, Todd J G 1989 Outpatient dental anaesthesia. A comparison of halothane, enflurane and isoflurane. Anaesthesia 44: 735–738

Skelly A M, Boscoe M J, Dawling S, Adams A P 1984 A comparison of diazepam and midazolam as sedatives for minor oral surgery. Europ J Anaesthesiol 1: 253–267

Smallridge J A, Al Ghanim, Holt R D 1990 The use of general anaesthesia for tooth extraction for child out-patients at a London dental hospital. Br Dent J 168: 438–440

Spence A A 1990 Environmental pollution by inhalation anaesthetics. Br J Anaesth 59: 96–103

Whitwam J G 1990 The use of midazolam and flumazenil in diagnosis and short surgical procedures. Acta Anaesthesiol Scand 34 (Suppl 92): 16–20

20. Systemic disease and related problems affecting dentistry

Systemic disease can cause oral signs or symptoms which may be the earliest manifestation and therefore lead to the diagnosis. Alternatively disease may require dental treatment to be modified for the patient's safety. Drugs used in the treatment of systemic disease can also sometimes have effects on the mouth or also dictate modification of dental treatment. For example, a patient with systemic lupus erythematosus might have oral lesions caused by the disease or have a mucosal infection secondary to treatment with corticosteroids. In addition, the corticosteroid treatment would

441

mean that the patient was at risk from potentially lethal hypotensive circulatory collapse if subjected to surgery and anaesthesia without adequate preparation.

There are surprisingly few diseases, or their treatment, which do not have *some* relevance for dentistry, but in practical terms the problem is not often serious because routine dentistry under local anaesthesia can be tolerated (though not enjoyed) by most patients without any significant hazard.

While systemic diseases can affect the mouth in various ways, so, conversely, can systemic disease originate from the mouth. The main example is infective endocarditis, but oral microorganisms can cause a variety of metastatic or systemic infections (Ch. 8). Patients with immunodeficiency states are particularly at risk.

The relevance of systemic disease to dentistry can therefore be summarised as follows:

1. Systemic disease as a cause of oral lesions
2. Systemic disease that affects the dental management of patients
3. Drugs (used for the treatment of systemic disease) having either of these effects
4. Systemic disease originating from the mouth.

BLOOD DISEASES

Haematological disease is common and may be the cause of serious complications or oral symptoms, of which the main examples are:

1. Anaesthetic complications
2. Severe oral infections
3. Excessive bleeding
4. Mucosal lesions.

Haemoglobin estimation and routine indices are informative tests which should be carried out when any patient has abnormal signs in the mouth or is to undergo oral surgery.

Anaemia

Causes of anaemia

Causes of anaemia are shown in Table 20.1, but the following are particularly important.

Iron deficiency (microcytic) anaemia is the most common type and usually the result of chronic

Table 20.1   Important causes of anaemia

1. Iron deficiency	usually chronic blood loss
2. Folate deficiency	pregnancy, drug-associated malabsorption, dietary, alcoholism*
3. B12 deficiency	usually pernicious anaemia or malabsorption
4. Marrow disease	leukaemia and aplastic anaemia
5. Chronic inflammatory diseases	infections or the connective-tissue diseases
6. Haemolytic diseases	
7. Alcoholism*, liver disease, neoplasms and other causes	

* Alcoholism must always be excluded first in any patient with macrocytosis in the absence of anaemia—a characteristic early sign of alcoholism

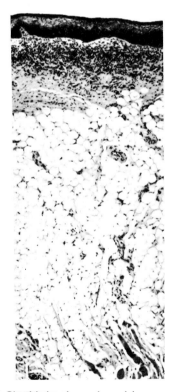

Fig. 20.1 Glossitis in advanced pernicious anaemia. The epithelium is thin and atrophic with inflammatory changes beneath. There is a striking loss of muscle tissue and replacement by fat. The muscle normally extends to immediately beneath the epithelium but here only a few degenerating fibres can be seen at the bottom of the picture (× 65).

blood loss. Women of child-bearing age or over, or men with peptic ulcer are mainly affected.

Pernicious anaemia chiefly affects women of middle age or over and, in them, is the main cause of macrocytic anaemia. Folate deficiency also causes a macrocytic anaemia, often in younger patients.

Leukaemia is an uncommon but frequently lethal cause of normocytic anaemia, but should be suspected in an anaemic child.

Sickle cell trait is most common in immigrants from the West Indies. Sickle cell anaemia is relatively rare. Thalassaemia is mainly seen in immigrants from the Mediterranean littoral.

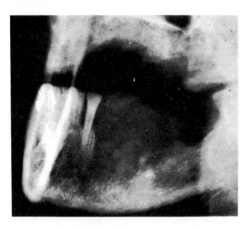

Fig. 20.2 Acute osteomyelitis in an anaemic patient. Acute osteomyelitis with widespread bone destruction followed straightforward extraction of the posterior teeth. The patient was found to have a haemoglobin level of 30%.

Clinical features

Apart from a few features distinguishing the individual diseases, anaemia, whatever the cause, produces essentially the same clinical features, as follows.

1. Pallor. The complexion is not a good guide. The conjunctiva of the lower eyelid, the nail beds, and sometimes the oral mucosa, give more reliable indications.
2. Glossitis and other mucosal diseases are discussed below.
3. General fatigue and lassitude.
4. Breathlessness on exertion.
5. Tachycardia and palpitations.

6. Oedema of the ankles. In severe cases cardiac failure can develop.

Features of anaemia important in dentistry

1. Mucosal disease. The main oral effects of anaemia or latent haematinic deficiencies include:

a. Glossitis
b. Angular stomatitis
c. Recurrent aphthae
d. Infection, particularly candidosis.

a. Glossitis. Anaemia is the most important, though not the most common cause of a sore tongue. Soreness of the tongue *can precede any fall in haemoglobin levels*, particularly as a result of deficiency of vitamin B12 or folate, and can be the first sign of such deficiencies. Later there may be overt inflammation and atrophy of the filiform papillae. However, the mechanism of these changes and the reason why such early manifestations are so localised is unknown.

The variants of sore tongue have been discussed in Chapter 15, but it is emphasised again that this symptom always requires adequate haematological investigation, initially by means of a haemoglobin level and routine indices. Even though the haemoglobin may be within normal limits, increase in erythrocyte size (mean corpuscular volume—MCV) is frequently indicative of pernicious anaemia.

If a deficiency state is found, the underlying cause such as gastrointestinal disease must be investigated.

b. Angular stomatitis. Inflamed cracks at the corners of the mouth constitute a classical sign, particularly of iron deficiency anaemia, but may be secondary to candidosis.

c. Recurrent aphthae. Aphthae are secondary to haematological deficiency, particularly of vitamin B12 or folate, in a minority of patients. This is typically in patients whose aphthae start or worsen late in life.

d. Candidosis. Iron deficiency, in particular, is a predisposing factor for candidosis as discussed in Chapter 15. Angular stomatitis is frequently associated.

2. Dangers of general anaesthesia. Further reduction of oxygenation of the tissues by a dental gas, for example, could precipitate irreparable brain damage or myocardial infarction. General anaesthesia should therefore be given in hospital with full oxygenation but preferably delayed until anaemia, if severe, has been treated. The dangers are particularly great in sickle cell disease, as discussed later.

3. Lowered resistance to infection. In addition to mucosal infection there may be more severe infection. In the past particularly, osteomyelitis could follow extractions in severe anaemia. Sickle cell disease in particular increases susceptibility to infection, as discussed below.

Sickle cell disease and sickle cell trait

Sickle cell anaemia mainly affects people of African, Afro-Caribbean, Indian, Mediterranean, or Middle Eastern origin. About 5000 persons in Britain are estimated to have sickle cell disease (homozygotes), but many more have sickle cell trait (heterozygotes).

The defect in sickle cell disease is an abnormal haemoglobin (HbS) with the risk of haemolysis, anaemia and other effects. In heterozygotes, sufficient normal haemoglobin (HbA) is formed to allow normal life with only rare complications.

Sickle cell disease

The complications arise from polymerisation of deoxygenated HbS which is less soluble than HbA. This forms long fibres which deform the red cells into sickle shapes and cause them to become readily haemolysed.

Chronic haemolysis causes chronic anaemia, but patients, under normal circumstances, typically feel well, as HbS more readily releases its oxygen content to the tissues than HbA.

Exacerbation of sickling causes increased blood viscosity and blocking of capillaries and sickling crises. Precipitating factors include (i) *hypoxia*, particularly from poorly conducted anaesthesia, (ii) *dehydration* and (iii) *infection* (including dental infections), acidosis and fever. These patients are also abnormally susceptible to infection, particularly pneumococcal or meningococcal, and osteomyelitis.

Sickle cell crises are of three main types, as follows.

Painful crises are caused by blockage of blood vessels and bone marrow infarcts. Painful crises can affect the jaws, particularly the mandible, and mimic acute osteomyelitis. The infarcted tissue forms a focus susceptible to infection, and Salmonella osteomyelitis is a recognised hazard.

Anaemic crises are due to marrow aplasia and require immediate transfusion.

Sequestration crises are probably the result of extensive sickling, particularly in the viscera. An acute chest syndrome, characterised by pain, fever and leucocytosis is the most common cause of death.

Dental aspects of sickle cell trait and disease

The sickling trait should be suspected, particularly in those of Afro-Caribbean origin, and investigated, if anaesthesia is anticipated. If the haemoglobin is less than 10 g/dl then it is probable that the patient is a homozygote with sickle cell disease and hospitalisation is necessary for anaesthesia.

In those with sickle cell trait the main precaution is that general anaesthesia, if unavoidable, should be carried out with full oxygenation.

In sickle cell disease the oral mucosa may be pale or yellowish due to haemolytic jaundice. Radiographic changes result from expansion of the haemopoietic marrow, causing thickening but osteoporosis of the bones of the skull. Infarcts in the jaws are painful and, with the radiographic changes can mimic osteomyelitis. Bone infarcts may appear relatively radiolucent at first, but become sclerotic, and opaque areas in the skull or jaws are left by earlier infarcts.

Occasionally, crises may be precipitated by dental infections such as acute pericoronitis. Regular dental care and prompt antibiotic treatment of infections is therefore important.

Painful bone infarcts should be treated with non-steroidal anti-inflammatory analgesics, and fluid intake should be increased. Admission to hospital is required for severe painful crises not responsive to analgesics.

Rigorous routine dental care is necessary because of the increased susceptibility to infection.

General anaesthesia, if utterly unavoidable, should be carried out in hospital.

The thalassaemias

The alpha-thalassaemias mainly affect Asians, Africans and Afro-Caribbeans, while the beta-thalassaemias mainly affect those from the Mediterranean littoral, such as Greeks (thalassaemia—literally, 'sea in the blood'). The thalassaemias result from decreased synthesis of the alpha or beta globin chains of haemoglobin. The imbalance between the production of the globin chains causes the normal chains to be present in the red cells in relative excess and to precipitate out. Haemolysis can therefore result.

The severity of the disease depends on the numbers of alpha or beta globin genes affected; in simplified terms the diseases are *thalassaemia minor* in heterozygotes and *thalassaemia major* in homozygotes.

Thalassaemia minor is characterised by mild but persistent microcytic anaemia but is otherwise asymptomatic apart sometimes from splenomegaly. Iron therapy is ineffective and can lead to iron deposition in the tissues.

Thalassaemia major (usually homozygous beta thalassaemia) is characterised by severe hypochromic, microcytic anaemia, great enlargement of liver and spleen and skeletal abnormalities due to extramedullary erythropoiesis. There is failure to thrive and early death if repeated transfusions are not given.

On radiographs the diploic spaces of the skull are enlarged and with a 'hair on end' appearance and a thin cortex. The maxillae may also be expanded causing severe malocclusion. The zygomatic bones are pushed outwards and the nasal bridge depressed in severe cases.

Regular transfusions are life-saving, prevent the development of bony deformities, but lead to increasing deposition of iron in the tissues. Haemosiderosis is the main cause of complications in survivors and leads to dysfunction of glands and other organs. Xerostomia can result from iron deposition in the salivary glands.

Desferrioxamine, a chelating agent, may reduce the effects of the iron overload, and folic acid treatment may ameliorate the haemolytic anaemia.

Polycythaemia vera

This is a rare disease in which the number of red cells is grossly increased. There may be cyanosis of the mucous membranes and skin, or bleeding from the gums.

Leukaemia

Increase in the number of white cells is the normal response to most acute infections but the most important cause of abnormal leucocytosis is leukaemia.

The effect of overproduction of white cells, the essential feature of leukaemia, is to suppress other cell lines of the marrow.

Leukaemia can affect virtually any of the white cell series (with some variation in its consequent manifestations) but the different types of acute leukaemia cannot be distinguished clinically.

Acute leukaemia

Acute lymphoblastic leukaemia is the most common leukaemia in children (usually between 3 and 5 years), while acute myeloblastic anaemia is the most common type in adults.

The consequences, particularly of acute leukaemia, are therefore:

1. *Anaemia* due to suppression of erythrocyte production
2. *Infections* due to deficiency or abnormalities of granulocytes particularly
3. *Bleeding* due to suppression of platelet production.

Splenomegaly or hepatomegaly or both are usually associated.

Mucosal pallor or abnormal gingival bleeding, particularly in a child, are strongly suggestive of acute leukaemia. Diagnosis depends on the peripheral blood picture and marrow biopsy

Oral and perioral aspects

Leukaemic manifestations include:

1. Gingival changes
2. Mucosal ulceration
3. Leukaemic deposits
4. Purpura

5. Anaemia
6 Cervical lymphadenopathy.

1. Gingival changes. As a result of low-grade infection at the gingival margins and lack of effective white cells, the gingival margins may become densely infiltrated and swollen with leukaemic cells. This is particularly characteristic of acute myelogenous leukaemias in adults. The gingivae are often purplish and may become necrotic and ulcerate. Also contributing to ulceration are immunodeficiency and the effects of cytotoxic drugs.

2. Mucosal ulceration. Ulceration is often a combined effect of immunodeficiency and cytotoxic drugs such as methotrexate. Herpetic infections and thrush are common, and ulceration may be caused by a variety of opportunistic microbes.

Also as a result of the immunodeficiency, the first sign of acute leukaemia may occasionally be an infection such as acute osteomyelitis following minor routine extractions.

3. Leukaemic deposits. Occasionally, tumour-like masses of leukaemic cells may form in the mouth or salivary glands.

4. Purpura. The haemorrhagic tendencies associated with leukaemia may appear as excessive gingival bleeding, purplish mucosal patches, blood blisters, or prolonged bleeding after surgery.

5. Anaemia. As mentioned earlier, mucosal pallor may be noticeable and is an important sign in children among whom anaemia is otherwise uncommon.

6. Cervical lymphadenopathy. This is particularly common in lymphocytic leukaemia but may be seen in other types, secondary to opportunistic infections in the mouth.

Ideally, patients with leukaemia or any others who are to be treated with cytoxic drugs should have the mouth brought to as healthy a state as possible to control the bacterial population, *before* complications develop.

Management of oral infections

Infections can sometimes be controlled by mouth rinses (0.2% chlorhexidine) and good oral hygiene. Oral hygiene together with antibiotic mouth rinses (with a tetracycline, amphotericin

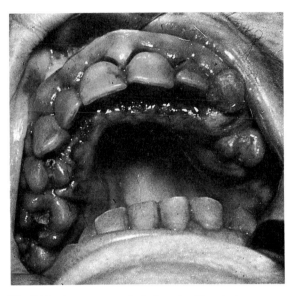

Fig. 20.3   Acute monocytic leukaemia. The gingivae are grossly swollen and purplish; in addition there is ulceration along the palatal aspect of the anterior teeth due to the poor resistance to infection (see also Ch. 6).

mixture) will often control severe gingival changes. Mucosal ulceration by Gram-negative bacilli or anaerobes may need specific antibiotic therapy which is also necessary to prevent systemic spread of infection.

Oral ulceration caused by methotrexate may be controlled by giving folinic acid.

Extractions should be avoided because of the risks of severe infections, bleeding, or anaemia. If unavoidable, blood transfusion and generous antibiotic cover are essential.

Chronic leukaemia

Chronic leukaemia is a slowly progressive disease of adults. Chronic lymphocytic leukaemia can be completely asymptomatic.

Oral manifestations are relatively uncommon or mild, but occasionally there is gingival or palatal swelling, oral purpura and other effects of defective haemostasis. Oral ulceration can result from infection or cytotoxic therapy.

If surgical treatment is unavoidable, similar precautions may need to be taken as with acute leukaemia if there is significant anaemia, bleeding tendencies, or susceptibility to infection.

Leucopenia and agranulocytosis

Leucopenia is a deficiency of white cells (fewer than $5000/mm^3$). It is a peripheral blood manifestation of actual or incipient immunodeficiency. Immunodeficiencies of which leucopenia may be a sign are discussed in Chapters 8 and 21. Important causes of leucopenia are as follows:

1. Leukaemia.
2. Aplastic anaemia
3. Drugs (see below)
4. Autoimmune
5. HIV infection.

Leucopenia can be a chance haematological finding. It does not cause symptoms until it becomes so severe as to impair defences against infection. Thus lymphopenia in an apparently healthy person may be a sign of HIV infection.

Drug-induced leucopenia

Important causes are as follows:

1. Analgesics, especially phenylbutazone
2. Antibacterial agents, especially chloramphenicol or co-trimoxazole
3. Phenothiazine antipsychotic drugs
4. Antithyroid agents such as thiouracil
5. Cytotoxic agents.

The treatment is to stop any drug which may be causative, to give antibiotics to control infections, and blood transfusions if necessary. Many cases of aplastic anaemia are nevertheless fatal but marrow transplantation has occasionally been successful.

Dental management comprises attention to oral hygiene and any other measures to control oral infections as described for acute leukaemia. Extractions or other surgical treatment should be avoided, but if essential and urgent, antibiotic cover must be given and transfusion may be necessary to combat any anaemia or haemorrhagic tendencies.

Agranulocytosis

This is a clinical syndrome of fever, prostration and mucosal ulceration, particularly of the gingivae and pharynx due to severe neutropenia which in some cases is drug-induced, and infections. In Britain the main cause of agranulocytosis, though usually reversible, has been co-trimoxazole—a reflection, in part, of its scale of use.

Aplastic anaemia

Aplastic anaemia is failure of production of all bone marrow cells (pancytopenia) with the result that there is loss of defence against infection and the systemic effects are not unlike those of acute leukaemia. Aplastic anaemia may be of unknown cause but probably autoimmune in nature. Otherwise drugs, such as cytotoxic agents, chloramphenicol and phenylbutazone are the main cause. The latter has caused many hundreds of deaths and its use is now severely restricted.

The oral effects—namely, opportunistic infections and anaemia—are generally similar to those of leukaemia.

The management is to stop any drugs that may be responsible and to give antibiotics and transfusions. Nevertheless approximately 50% of patients die within 6 months, usually from infection or haemorrhage. Dental management is as for acute leukaemia.

Cyclic neutropenia

This is characterised by a fall in the number of circulating neutrophils at regular intervals of 3 to 4 weeks. Oral ulceration secondary to cyclic neutropenia has been reported, but the disorder is so rare as to be little more than a pathological curiosity. One literature search in 1981 found only 40 reported cases since the disease was first described 70 years earlier.

THE HAEMORRHAGIC DISEASES

Disorders of the blood which cause abnormally prolonged bleeding are broadly divisible into purpura (platelet or, rarely, vascular defects) and clotting disorders.

Investigation of patients with a history of excessive bleeding

It is clearly impractical to put every patient through the rigours of full laboratory investigation before dental extractions and a careful history is all important.

The following are some of the questions that should be asked.

1. *Nature and results of previous dental operations.* A single episode of bleeding, particularly after a difficult extraction, is usually the result of local injury, but repeated episodes, particularly after simple extractions, suggest a haemorrhagic tendency.

2. *Duration of bleeding.* Bleeding for up to 24 hours after an extraction is usually due to local causes or to a minor defect of haemostasis which can be managed by local measures. Bleeding for longer periods is of serious significance. Even a *mild* haemophilic can bleed for several weeks after a simple extraction.

3. *Management of earlier haemorrhagic episodes.* Patients who have had to be admitted to hospital, and particularly those who have had to have blood transfusions, are likely to have haemorrhagic disease and should be referred to hospital for further investigation and management.

4. *Results of other operations or injuries.* Abnormally prolonged bleeding from any cause is an indication for investigation. Nevertheless it occasionally happens that a patient who bleeds persistently after dental extractions does not have any serious trouble from soft-tissue injuries. By contrast, it is certain that a patient who has had tonsillectomy without serious bleeding is not haemophilic.

5. *Family history.* Most of the severe haemorrhagic diseases such as haemophilia are hereditary. Information about other affected family members and their sex is therefore particularly important. However, in over 30% of haemophiliacs the family history is negative and the disease may only come to light after a dental operation.

6. *Drugs.* Anticoagulants are an obvious example, but several other drugs, including a few antibiotics, can cause haemorrhagic disease.

7. *Medical history.* Bleeding tendencies can be the result of other blood diseases, or liver or (occasionally) renal disease.

8. *Identity cards and hospital letters.* Patients with severe haemorrhagic diseases may carry a warning card, letter or identification tag and should be specifically asked whether they carry such warnings.

9. *Clinical examination.* Signs of anaemia and purpura should be looked for. A characteristic site of purpura is the palate where the posterior border of a denture presses into the mucous membrane.

Although the history is an essential aspect of the investigation of haemorrhagic diseases, it occasionally happens that they are first recognised as a result of prolonged bleeding after a dental extraction. Even haemophilia may not be diagnosed until after an injury such as this in an adult (see Fig. 21.7).

Examination of the mouth shows how the operation is to be planned. When many teeth are to be extracted they may have to be removed in small groups to allow the wound to be easily sutured or the sockets to be protected by an acrylic plate. A few extractions at a time are necessary only when the haemorrhagic condition cannot be rectified.

Radiographs should be taken to anticipate possible difficulties in the extractions.

In cases of doubt patients should be referred to hospital for physical and laboratory investigation.

Laboratory investigations

The details of these investigations should be left to the haematologist, but the nature of the problem must be made clear on the request form and should be expressed in some such terms as the following. 'This patient gives a history of prolonged bleeding after 2 previous dental extractions, but appears otherwise well. Would you please investigate this patient for possible haemorrhagic disease.'

Laboratory investigations usually include the following:

1. *Haemoglobin investigation and blood picture.* It is essential to look for anaemia because
   a. anaemia is an almost inevitable result of repeated bleeding
   b. any further bleeding as a result of surgery will worsen the anaemia
   c. anaemia increases the risks of general

anaesthesia and will need to be treated
before any surgery
  d. anaemia is also an essential feature of
     some haemorrhagic diseases, particularly
     acute leukaemia
2. *Tests of haemostatic function.* Essential tests
   include
  a. The bleeding time
  b. Prothrombin time, activated partial
     thromboplastin and thrombin times
  3. *Blood grouping and cross-matching.* These
     are necessary because transfusions may be
     needed before operation to improve
     haemostasis or afterwards if blood loss is
     severe.

The main types of haemorrhagic disease are

1. *Purpura* which is caused by deficiency or
   defects of platelets, or less commonly by
   vascular defects
2. *Clotting defects.* The most important is
   haemophilia.

Purpura

Purpura is the term given to bleeding into the skin
or mucous membranes, producing petechiae or ecchymoses. Excessive bleeding after injury or
surgery is associated. Unlike haemophilia, there is
no early arrest of haemorrhage, which starts immediately after the injury.

Purpura is typically the result of platelet disorders or is relatively rarely caused by vascular
defects. The bleeding time is prolonged but
clotting function is normal. An exception is von
Willebrand's disease, where there is an associated
deficiency of a clotting factor. Although platelets
are involved in the clotting process, even severe
depletion does not impair coagulation.

Table 20.2 Causes of purpura

I Platelet disorders
  1. Idiopathic thrombocytopenic purpura
  2. Connective-tissue diseases (especially SLE)
  3. Acute leukaemias
  4. Drug-associated

II Vascular disorders
  1. Von Willebrand's disease
  2. Corticosteroid treatment
  3. Ehlers Danlos syndrome
  4. Infective

General features of purpura

Purpura is characterised by superficial bleeding
('spontaneous bruising'). Penetrating injuries
cause prolonged bleeding. This tends to be less
prolonged than in the coagulation defects since the
blood ultimately clots normally.

Many women, if asked, say that they bruise
easily but this is no more than a self-flattering
belief that they have a 'delicate skin'—such
bruises are usually only a few millimetres in size.

Hess's test will detect formation of petechiae or
ecchymoses in the forearm after application of a
blood pressure cuff on the upper arm to obstruct
venous return. It is not particularly specific.

The most informative test of platelet function is
the *bleeding time* supplemented as necessary by
tests of platelet aggregation and adhesion.
Deficiency of platelets (fewer than 100 000 mm³),
is termed thrombocytopenia, but spontaneous
bleeding is uncommon until the count falls below
50 000 mm³.

Idiopathic thrombocytopenic purpura

The immediate cause of the thrombocytopenia is
IgG autoantibodies which bind to platelets. The
number of platelets in the peripheral blood is
greatly reduced.

The disease may affect children or young adult
women, and the first sign may be profuse gingival
bleeding or post-extraction haemorrhage. More
often there is spontaneous bleeding into the skin.

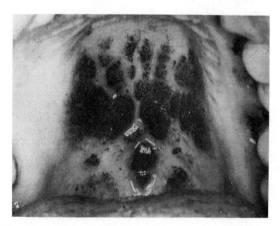

Fig. 20.4 Purpura. There is severe submucosal bleeding in
the palate, and blood can also be seen along the gingival
margins.

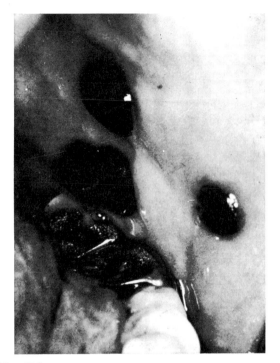

Fig. 20.5

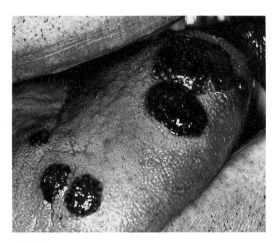

Fig. 20.6

Figs 20.5 and 20.6 Purpura. The 'blood blisters' are due to spontaneous submucosal bleeding. Operative treatment would clearly be hazardous for such a patient, and thorough haematological investigation is the first essential.

Management. Thrombocytopenic purpura frequently responds, at least in the short-term, to corticosteroids which can be used for urgently needed surgery. Long-term use of corticosteroids is associated with their usual hazards. Some cases resolve spontaneously but persistent cases may respond to splenectomy. However, 10% to 20% of cases are unresponsive to any form of treatment, and now that haemophilia is a manageable disease such cases have become one of the most troublesome of the haemorrhagic diseases. For operative treatment, transfusions of platelet concentrates can be given, but immunosuppressive drugs may have to be given at the same time to prevent destruction of the platelets by antibodies.

As with other platelet disorders, aspirin and other anti-inflammatory analgesics should be avoided.

AIDS-associated purpura

Autoimmune thrombocytopenia can complicate HIV infection and can be an early manifestation. Purpuric patches in the mouth, particularly in a young male, should suggest this possibility and also need to be distinguished from oral Kaposi's sarcoma.

Connective-tissue diseases

The main example is systemic lupus erythematosus, where there can be antiplatelet antibody formation and defective haemostasis as a result.

Acute leukaemia

Thrombocytopenia is a virtually invariable consequence of overgrowth of the white cells, and purpura can be an early sign, as discussed earlier.

Drug-associated purpura

Many drugs, particularly aspirin, interfere with platelet function, others act as haptens and cause immune destruction of platelets or suppress marrow function causing pancytopenia (aplastic anaemia) when purpura is frequently an early sign. The most frequent cause of aplastic anaemia in Britain has been phenylbutazone.

Important causes of drug-associated thrombocytopenia therefore include:

—Chloramphenicol
—Phenylbutazone

—Indomethacin
—Thiazide diuretics
—Quinine and quinidine.

If purpura develops, the drug should be stopped, but in the case of aplastic anaemia the process is sometimes irreversible and fatal.

Localised oral purpura

This is characterised by blood blisters forming in the oral mucosa as a result of minor or unnoticed trauma, but there is no abnormality of haemostasis. Occasionally such blisters form in the throat and cause a choking sensation ('angina bullosa haemorrhagica').

Systemic purpura can be firmly excluded by haematological examination, and the patient can be reassured.

Vascular purpura

Prolonged corticosteroid treatment, especially in the elderly, is probably the most common cause of vascular purpura.

Scurvy is now virtually only of historical interest, but severe purpura is a major feature and the cause of the swollen, engorged and bleeding gums seen in severe cases in the past.

Ehlers Danlos syndrome is discussed in Chapter 2.

Von Willebrand's disease

Von Willebrand's disease is characterised both by a prolonged bleeding time and deficiency of factor VIII. It is inherited as an autosomal dominant: both males and females are therefore affected.

The deficiency of factor VIII is usually mild in comparison with the platelet defect, so that bleeding into the skin or mucous membranes (purpura) is the more common manifestation of the disease. However, some patients have factor VIII levels low enough to cause a significant clotting defect.

The platelet defect is usually correctable with desmopressin, which may also be sufficient to correct any significant factor VIII deficiency. In unusually severe cases the deficiency of factor VIII is such that surgery has to be managed as for haemophilia A. However factor VIII remains active in the blood for a considerably longer period.

Clotting disorders

The main causes are as follows.

1. Heritable deficiencies of plasma factors. Haemophilia is by far the most important example. Only a minority of patients with von Willebrand's disease have a significant clotting defect.
2. Acquired clotting defects.

Haemophilia A

Haemophilia is the most common and severe clotting disorder. Haemophilia A (factor VIII deficiency) may affect approximately 6 per 100 000 of the population and is about 10 times as common as haemophilia B (Christmas disease, factor IX deficiency). In the past, extractions in haemophiliacs have been fatal, and extractions are still common emergencies or occasions when haemophiliacs need specific treatment.

Severe haemophilia typically causes effects in childhood, usually as a result of bleeding into muscles or joints after minor injuries. By contrast, mild haemophilia (factor VIII level over 25%) may cause no symptoms until an injury, surgery or a dental extraction causes prolonged bleeding. This may not happen until adult life.

Severe and prolonged bleeding deeply into the soft tissues can also follow local anaesthetic injections. Experiments with aspirating syringes suggest that in up to 10% of injections the needle damages or enters a vessel. A small laceration of a vessel wall caused in this way can leak copiously in a haemophiliac.

Inferior dental blocks are most dangerous both because of the rich plexus of veins in this area and because blood can leak down towards the glottis. Even a submucous infiltration can occasionally have severe consequences (Fig. 20.7), and a haematologist may require that anti-haemophilic factor be given whenever local anaesthetics are to be used.

General aspects of haemophilia. The characteristic feature is that bleeding typically starts after a short delay as a result of normal platelet and vascular responses which provide the initial phase of haemostasis. There is then persistent bleeding which, if untreated, can continue for weeks or until the patient dies. Pressure packs, suturing, or local application of haemostatics are ineffective.

In addition to the risk of haemarthroses, the most dangerous complication of uncontrolled haemophilia is intracranial haemorrhage. Deep tissue bleeding can also occasionally spread down from the neck and obstruct the airway.

Haemophiliacs are at risk from hepatitis as a result of repeated administration of untreated blood products. The majority of adult haemophiliacs have abnormal liver function tests as a consequence. Formation of antibodies to factor VIII is another complication.

A more recent hazard has been infection by HIV, before screening and heat-treated factor VIII were introduced. Many haemophiliacs have therefore developed AIDS or are carriers of the virus.

Dental management. The overall management of haemophiliacs depends on:

1. Recognition and assessment of patients
2. Decisions on treatment policy
3. Planning of essential extractions and other surgery
4. Preoperative preparation and replacement therapy
5. Choice of anaesthesia
6. Postoperative care.

1. *Recognition and assessment of patients.* The details of the history have been discussed earlier. The chief cause of confusion is von Willebrand's disease. The diagnosis and severity of haemophilia depend on the laboratory findings, which in typical cases are as follows:

a. Prolonged activated partial thromboplastin time
b. Normal prothrombin time
c. Normal bleeding time
d. Low factor VIII (or IX) levels on assay.

2. *Dental treatment policy.* Ideally, preventive dentistry and regular dental care should be such that extractions never become necessary. At the opposite extreme, when the dentition is already greatly damaged or neglect is irremediable, clearance may be the best policy in selected cases.

3. *Planning.* Radiographs should be taken to forestall any complications as a result of unsuspected disease and to help decide whether any additional extractions may need to be done. Arrangements must usually be made for admission to hospital.

The aim is to keep to a minimum the number of occasions when replacement therapy has to be given. When replacement therapy has been given, as much surgical work as possible should be done in that session. It is always wise to plan treatment with the possibility in mind that the next time the patient needs surgery, he may be in a place where

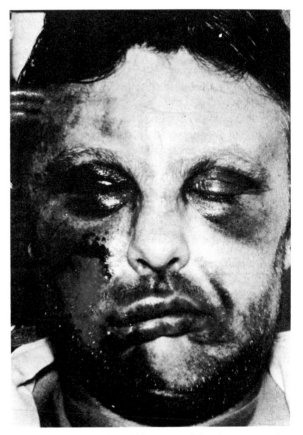

Fig. 20.7 Haemophilia. This was a mild and unsuspected haemophiliac who had never had any previous serious bleeding episodes. This enormous haematoma developed after a submucous injection for extirpation of an incisor pulp. (Reproduced by kind permission of Mr A. J. Bridge.)

replacement therapy is unobtainable or HIV or HBV are prevalent, or he may have developed antibodies to factor VIII.

4. *Preoperative preparation and replacement therapy*. A factor VIII level between 50% and 75% is necessary for dental extractions, and the amount of factor VIII to be given has to be estimated according to serum level and the expected severity of the surgical trauma.

Purified heat-treated factor VIII enables a known amount of factor VIII to be given in a very small volume. It is usual therefore also to give tranexamic acid or desmopressin to reduce the amount of factor VIII needed. Tranexamic acid or desmopressin alone can be used for other more minor dental procedures on haemophiliacs, as discussed later.

A typical sequence of events for dental extractions on a haemophiliac would therefore be to plan the operation for a morning and to give the calculated amount of factor VIII immediately before operation. Tranexamic acid is given 24 hours before operation and repeated 6 hourly by mouth for 7 to 10 days.

Surgery should be carried out with minimal trauma, and the soft tissues should be sutured to reduce the chances of disturbing or opening the wound during eating.

5. *Choice of anaesthesia*: If adequate replacement therapy has been given, either local or general anaesthesia (either intravenous or via an endotracheal tube) can be used. However, if an endotracheal tube is used it should be an oral cuffed latex tube to minimise abrasion of the trachea. If replacement therapy has not been given, an endotracheal tube can cause dangerous bleeding.

6. *Postoperative care*. It is usual to give an antibiotic such as oral penicillin (250 mg four times a day for 7 days) postoperatively to reduce the chance of infection of the wound and secondary haemorrhage.

Factor VIII is active for only about 12 hours and may have to be given postoperatively. The risks of bleeding are greatest on the day of operation and again from 4 to 10 days postoperatively. Factor VIII is sometimes therefore given prophylactically on the fourth or fifth day after operation, but this should be unnecessary if the initial dose has been adequate and the continued administration of tranexamic acid should provide adequate haemostasis.

If bleeding starts at any time after the operation, factor VIII must be given.

Analgesics and other drugs. In view of its tendency to enhance haemorrhagic tendencies and possibly to induce gastric bleeding, aspirin and other anti-inflammatory analgesics should be avoided in haemophiliacs. Paracetamol or propoxyphene are suitable alternatives.

Analgesics or other drugs should not be given to haemophiliacs by injection unless it is essential and factor VIII has been given within the previous 12 hours.

Other aspects of dental treatment. The risks from local anaesthetics should be borne in mind. Care should also be taken to avoid soft-tissue injuries. If minor bleeding starts it may be controllable with tranexamic acid or desmopressin.

Sedation. Relative analgesia is preferable, to avoid the risk from accidental damage to a vein.

Now that haemophiliacs have a personal stock of factor VIII for use in emergencies these problems have been greatly reduced. However, it may be necessary to check that the factor VIII has been taken.

Christmas disease (haemophilia B)

Christmas disease is inherited in the same way as, and is clinically identical to, haemophilia A. It has the advantage, however, that factor IX is more stable than factor VIII. The standard preparation for replacement therapy is NHS Three Factor Concentrate which contains factors IX, II and X.

Factor IX remains active in the blood for more than 2 days, so that replacement therapy can be given at longer intervals than for haemophilia A. All other aspects of the management of these patients are the same.

Acquired clotting defects

Overall these are more common than the inherited defects. The main causes include:

1. Vitamin K deficiency
2. Anticoagulant treatment
3. Liver disease.

Vitamin K deficiency

Causes of vitamin K deficiency include obstructive jaundice, or, less commonly, malabsorption. Important causes of obstructive jaundice are hepatitis, gall stones and carcinoma of the pancreas.

The underlying disease should if possible be dealt with and extractions or other surgery delayed until haemostasis returns to normal. In emergency, vitamin K can be given, preferably by mouth, and its effectiveness checked by the prothrombin time. If the latter does not return to normal within 48 hours there is probably parenchymal liver disease.

Anticoagulant treatment

Anticoagulants such as warfarin are used for thromboembolic disease, which can complicate atrial fibrillation or insertion of prosthetic heart valves, but is rarely given now after myocardial infarction.

The underlying disease may therefore influence dental management and is often more important than the anticoagulant treatment. The latter should be checked regularly using the prothrombin time, which should be kept at about 2 to $2\frac{1}{2}$ time the control level. Under such circumstances dental extractions can usually be carried out safely. However, as a precaution only a few teeth should be extracted at one session, trauma should be minimal, and the sockets can be sutured with a layer of oxidised cellulose enclosed. Anticoagulant treatment should not be stopped because of the risk of rebound thrombosis.

For more major surgery, anticoagulant treatment may have to be stopped, if the physician in charge agrees. If serious bleeding starts, tranexamic acid can be given, but, if otherwise uncontrollable, vitamin K may be needed.

Heparin anticoagulation. Short-term anticoagulation with heparin is given before renal dialysis sessions. Heparin is effective only for about 6 hours. Extractions or other surgery can therefore be delayed for 12–24 hours after the last dose of heparin, when the benefits of dialysis are also maximal.

Liver disease

Liver failure, from such causes as hepatitis or al-

coholism, causes failure of production of most clotting factors and inability to metabolise vitamin K. Haemorrhage can be severe and difficult to control. In mild cases vitamin K may be effective. In more severe cases, however, it is valueless, but tranexamic acid and fresh plasma infusion may control bleeding.

CARDIOVASCULAR DISEASE

Cardiovascular disease is common and is now the most frequent single cause of death in Britain. Heart disease is a problem of increasing magnitude and many of these patients need dental treatment. Though heart disease becomes more frequent and severe in later life, coronary disease is not uncommon in early middle age, while other types of heart disease affect children.

From the viewpoint of dental treatment, patients fall into two main groups. Young patients with valvular or other defects (either congenital or due to rheumatic fever) may be at risk from infective endocarditis. Severely affected patients may also be cyanotic and in cardiac failure. Older patients with ischaemic heart disease or in cardiac failure from any cause are particularly at risk from general anaesthesia and may be at even greater risk from endocarditis. There may be other complicating factors such as drug treatment as well.

Patients most at risk are therefore those who have or have had the following.

1. *Valvular or related defects* (either congenital or due to past rheumatic fever) or who have had a prosthetic valve inserted. These patients need prophylactic antibiotic cover, particularly before extractions (see Chapter 8 and Appendix I)
2. *Ischaemic heart disease* with or without severe hypertension. These patients need special protection to minimise the risk of dangerous arrhythmias. They are particularly at risk when given a general anaesthetic. Local anaesthetics have theoretical dangers, but at all events pain and anxiety must, as far as possible, be eliminated.
3. *Heart failure* from any cause. These patients are particularly at risk from general anaesthesia but in addition there may be the associated problems of the other two groups.

4. *Infective endocarditis.* Infective endocarditis has been discussed in Chapter 8.

Ischaemic heart disease

Patients are usually of middle age or over, though the disease is increasingly affecting younger people. The chief precautions are *first*, to minimise any stress upon the patient that dental treatment might entail as this might precipitate a heart attack in the dental surgery and *second*, to take account of some of the drugs these patients may be taking in order to avoid interactions or other complications. *Third*, general anaesthesia including so-called sedation with methohexitone should *not* be given in the dental surgery.

An association has been reported between poor dental health and myocardial infarction, but does not appear to have been confirmed. However, it has been found that patients who have silent (painless) myocardial infarcts have a high pain threshold, as indicated by pulp testing, while the opposite is the case in the larger group who have anginal pain.

General aspects of management

The patients chiefly at risk are severe hypertensives and those who have angina or have had a myocardial infarct. These patients have unstable heart rhythm, and anxiety or pain can cause outpouring of adrenaline which can both greatly increase the load on the heart and also precipitate dysrrhythmias.

To die of fright is not a figure of speech but is something which can happen as a result of dysrrhythmias. The first essential for these patients is therefore to ensure not merely painless dentistry but also to alleviate anxiety.

History. A careful history should be taken and the patient's current drug treatment noted. The patient should be asked about previous experiences of dental treatment and his attitude towards it. He should also be asked whether routine dental treatment under local anaesthesia is acceptable, and it should be explained that in any session of treatment as little or much will be done as the patient feels able to tolerate.

Sedation. Anxiety can be harmful to patients with cardiovascular disease. If therefore they are concerned about the prospect of dental treatment it may be adequate to give oral temazepam (5 mg on the preceding night and again half an hour before treatment).

If sedation is required, relative analgesia is safer because nitrous oxide has no cardiorespiratory depressant effects.

Local anaesthesia. The two essentials are that local anaesthesia should be acceptable to the patient and, second, that it should be completely painless. The most effective agent is 2% lignocaine with adrenaline and, after decades of use, no local anaesthetic has been shown to be safer. The injection should be given after effective surface anaesthesia and as slowly as possible to minimise pain.

General anaesthesia. Nitrous oxide sedation and local anaesthesia are usually adequate but if general anaesthesia is unavoidable (Ch. 19) it should be given by an expert anaesthetist in hospital, especially as some of the drugs used for cardiovascular disease increase the risks. Cardiovascular disease is the chief cause of sudden death under anaesthesia.

Cardiac failure

Failure is a relative term and treatment allows many patients to live almost normal lives. These patients as a consequence may seem well, but undue stress can prove dangerous. They should not therefore be given general anaesthesia in the dental surgery.

If in addition failure is secondary to severe congenital or rheumatic valvular disease, or to hypertension and ischaemic heart disease, then there are the associated problems (as described above) to be dealt with as well. Yet another problem is that of concurrent drug treatment.

Cardiac pacemakers

Pacemakers provide a stimulus to cardiac contraction when the normal rhythm is disturbed as a result of disease of the sinoatrial node or conducting tissues as a result, for example, of myocardial infarction.

Some ultrasonic scalers and some electrosurgical equipment can interfere with pacemaker function, they should generally be avoided. Other electromagnetic equipment such as pulp testers do not appear to confer a significant risk.

Infective endocarditis does not appear to be a particular risk for wearers of pacemakers, and antibiotic cover has not been recommended.

Aspects of drug treatment for heart disease

Some drugs used for cardiovascular disease, notably methyldopa, nifedipine and its analogues, and captopril can cause oral reactions (Ch. 15) but (despite ill-informed statements to the contrary), modern antihypertensive agents such as beta-blockers do not cause a dry mouth.

Other cardiovascular drugs may complicate dental management. Anticoagulants have been discussed earlier. Hypotensive agents are potentiated by general anaesthetics, and halothane in particular increases the risk of dysrrhythmias with digoxin.

Comment

Though patients with cardiovascular disease need to be treated with care, the risks of routine dental treatment under local anaesthesia (despite many statements to the contrary) and of adverse reactions appear to be very low. For example the Council of Community Health of the American Dental Association in a survey of the literature on the subject could apparently find only 6 relevant reports published between 1986 and 1988.

ENDOCRINE DISORDERS

With the exception of diabetes mellitus and thyroid disease, endocrine disorders are uncommon and rare causes of oral disease. Nevertheless, occasionally, oral changes can lead to the diagnosis of unsuspected endocrine disease. Patients with endocrine disorders such as Addison's disease, diabetes mellitus and thyrotoxicosis also need special care when having dental operations, and general anaesthetics should be avoided.

Pituitary hyperfunction—gigantism and acromegaly

Overactivity of acidophil cells of the anterior pituitary during the period of growth of the skeleton causes gigantism. After the epiphyses have fused, hyperfunction of these cells causes acromegaly.

Gigantism is characterised by overgrowth of the skeleton and soft tissues. The patient becomes a giant and in most cases acromegaly develops later.

Acromegaly is characterised by renewed growth of certain bones, notably the jaws, hands and feet, and overgrowth of some soft tissues. The condylar growth centre becomes active and the mandible becomes enlarged and protrusive. In radiographs the whole jaw can be seen to be lengthened and the obliquity of the angle is increased. The jaw and other bones are also increased in thickness due to subperiosteal deposition of bone. The teeth become spaced, or, if the patient is edentulous, the dentures cease to fit the growing jaw. Other changes are thickening and enlargement of the facial features, particularly the lips and nose, while the hands and feet become spade-like.

Headaches and visual disturbances due to the pituitary tumour are common. Later, weakness and, often, diabetes mellitus develop.

Irradiation or resection of the pituitary tumour may relieve the symptoms. Mandibular resection may be needed to reduce severe disfigurement.

Pituitary hypofunction—pituitary dwarfism

This rare disorder causes generally retarded growth and, as a result, well-proportioned dwarfism. Eruption of the teeth may be retarded.

Hyperthyroidism—thyrotoxicosis

Thyrotoxicosis is most common in young adults, particularly women.

The main features are irritability and anxiety, loss of weight, exophthalmos and tachycardia. Later, if the disease is untreated, cardiovascular disease or cardiac failure may develop, particularly in older patients.

The main dental importance of thyrotoxicosis is that patients may be difficult to manage because of nervousness and excitability. If these and other signs (such as exophthalmos) suggestive of thyrotoxicosis are apparent and the patient is not already under treatment referral to a physician is indicated. Patients with thyrotoxicosis of long

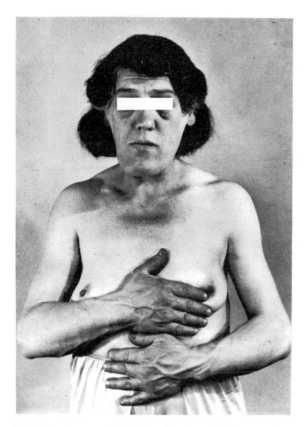

Fig. 20.8 Acromegaly. The jaw is enlarged and protrusive, the features thickened and the hands broad and spade-like.

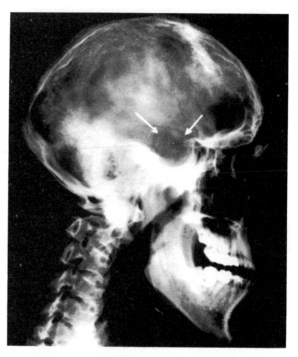

Fig. 20.9 Acromegaly. The mandible is enlarged with an elongated ramus and increased obliquity of the angle. The pituitary fossa is also enlarged due to the presence of the tumour causing the disease.

standing, and older patients with the disease, should not be given general anaesthesia, because of the risk of cardiac failure.

Severe thyrotoxicosis with excessive cardiac excitability is a theoretical contraindication to giving adrenaline with lignocaine. However, the risk appears to be largely theoretical, and no other local anaesthetics can be shown to be safer.

Treatment of hyperthyroidism is by surgical removal of part of the gland, or by means of drugs such as thiouracil, carbimazole or ^{131}I.

Hypothyroidism

Cretinism

Cretinism results from deficient thyroid activity at birth and causes retarded mental and physical development. Cretinism is most common in areas where simple goitre is found but is now rare since goitre has been effectively controlled with iodine.

A cretin is occasionally the offspring of a normal mother.

The main features are dwarfism and imbecility. Skeletal development and eruption of the teeth are much delayed. The face has a characteristic shape being excessively broad and rather flat; this is partly due to defective growth of the skull and facial bones. The tongue is large and usually protrudes. Other features are a dull facial expression, dry thick skin, short stocky build and, often, umbilical hernia.

Treatment with thyroid extract, if begun sufficiently early, leads to normal physical development and improvement in the mental defect.

Adult hypothyroidism

Hypothyroidism is frequently associated with autoantibodies or can follow removal of excessive thyroid tissue in the treatment of hyperthyroidism.

Hypothyroidism may cause weight gain, slowing of activity and thought, and a dry skin with loss

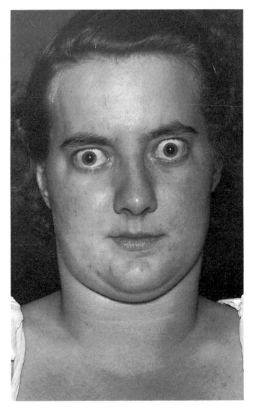

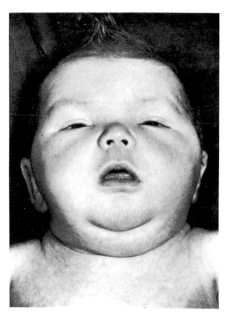

Fig. 20.11 Cretinism in a child of 2½. The facial expression, the excessive broadening of the features, and the protruding tongue are characteristic.

Fig. 20.10 Thyrotoxicosis. The exophthalmos is typical but the enlarged thyroid is not conspicuous. The patient had not then started to lose weight.

of hair. Ischaemic heart disease or cardiac failure are important complications.

In the dental management of hypothyroidism an important consideration is to avoid, or use in reduced doses, sedatives including diazepam, analgesics such as codeine, and general anaesthetics, as all of these may increase the risk of myxoedema coma. Anaemia or ischaemic heart disease may also necessitate modifications to dental treatment. Local anaesthesia is always preferable for these patients.

Very occasionally Sjögren's syndrome is associated with hypothyroidism.

Hyperparathyroidism

This uncommon disease is usually caused by an adenoma of the parathyroids. Increased parathyroid activity may cause decalcification of the skeleton and cyst-like areas of bone resorption

(osteitis fibrosa cystica—Ch. 12). Increased calcium excretion can lead to nephrocalcinosis and renal failure.

Hypoparathyroidism

Post-surgical hypoparathyroidism. The most common cause of hypoparathyroidism is thyroidectomy. The resulting hypocalcaemia causes increased neuromuscular excitability and tetany. These are controlled by giving the vitamin D analogue, 1,25 dihydrocholecalciferol (DHCC) orally. Later, any residual parathyroid tissue undergoes compensatory hyperplasia.

Idiopathic hypoparathyroidism. Early onset hypoparathyroidism is rare. In some cases it forms part of the polyendocrinopathy syndrome characterised by formation of autoantibodies to a variety of glandular tissues and deficiency states (particularly Addison's disease) and frequently mucocutaneous candidosis.

Idiopathic hypoparathyroidism is also characterised by enamel hypoplasia (Ch. 2). Otherwise the disease and its treatment are similar to post-surgical hypoparathyroidism.

Effects on calcified tissues

The main effects are retarded new bone formation and diminished resorption. Skeletal changes are rarely seen because these two factors seem usually to be in equilibrium.

In the rare early onset type of hypoparathyroidism there may be aplasia or hypoplasia of the developing enamel, which becomes deeply grooved. These changes are the result of ectodermal defects characteristic of the disease. The dentine may be incompletely mineralised but increased thickness of the lamina dura has also been described.

Tetany

In mild cases tetany is latent but can be elicited by tapping on the skin over the facial nerve; this causes the facial muscles to contract. In more severe cases there are muscle cramps and tonic contractions of the muscles which may go on to generalised convulsions. An early symptom of tetany is paraesthesiae of the lip and extremities.

Tetany more often results from overbreathing, often neurotic in origin (hyperventilation syndrome).

Adrenocortical insufficiency

Hypofunction of the adrenal cortices may rarely be primary (Addison's disease) or, far more frequently, secondary to corticosteroid therapy.

Addison's disease

Addison's disease is the result of atrophy of the adrenal cortices and failure of secretion of cortisol and aldosterone. In most cases it is autoimmune in nature with organ-specific circulating auto-antibodies. Tuberculosis and other infective causes of adrenal destruction are rare but can result from AIDS. The result is a severe disorder of electrolyte and fluid balance.

The clinical features of chronic adrenal insufficiency are lassitude, anorexia, weakness and fatigue, abnormal pigmentation, gastrointestinal disturbances, loss of weight and low blood pressure.

Pigmentation is often an early sign and, in the mouth, is patchily distributed on gingivae, buccal mucosa and lips; it is brown or almost black in colour. However, Addison's disease is a very rare cause of oral pigmentation.

The skin pigmentation looks similar to sun tan but with a sallow appearance due to underlying pallor. The exposed parts and normally pigmented areas are most severely affected.

Addison's disease may sometimes become apparent by development of an Addisonian crisis. This is characterised by a rapid fall in blood pressure, circulatory collapse (shock) and vomiting. These crises, which may be fatal, are often precipitated by such causes as infections, injuries, surgery or anaesthesia. Immediate treatment with intravenous hydrocortisone in large doses and fluid replacement is essential to save life.

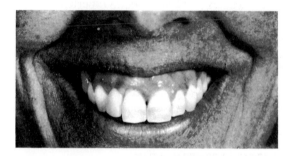

Fig. 20.12 Addison's disease. The patient, who normally has a fair complexion, shows the characteristic pigmentation of skin and gingivae. The teeth stand out in striking contrast to the darkening of the surrounding tissues.

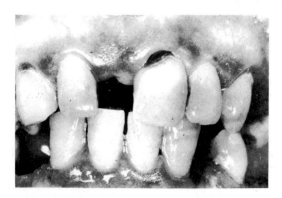

Fig. 20.13 Addison's disease. A close-up shows the characteristic distribution of pigment rather patchily along the attached gingiva. It is a brownish black in colour.

Though the disease is rare, a patient, other than a black, with pigmentation of the oral mucous membrane should be suspected of suffering from Addison's disease. A weak voice caused by general weakness and lassitude is also suggestive.

Long-term treatment of Addison's disease is usually by oral hydrocortisone which allows patients to live almost normal lives. Nevertheless these patients, like others receiving corticosteroids, have a low resistance to stress and injuries, and surgical treatment, particularly under general anaesthesia, may precipitate acute hypotension.

Corticosteroid treatment

Corticosteroids when given in sufficiently large doses have physiological effects resembling those of Cushing's disease. Thus there may be sodium and water retention, a raised blood sugar and impaired protein metabolism. Hypertension and diabetes are possible complications, and a characteristic moon-face appearance is produced.

Other important effects of corticosteroids include the following.

1. *Depression of adrenocortical function.*
   Long-term administration of corticosteroids leads to inability to respond to stress such as general anaesthesia, with the danger of a severe hypotensive crisis.
2. *Depression of inflammatory and immune responses*, and opportunistic infections.
3. *Depressed protein metabolism*, and, in particular, impaired wound healing.
4. *Masking serious disease.* This particularly dangerous effect can cause patients even with a lethal disease to appear, for a time at least, to be in perfect health with plump rosy cheeks and often a sense of well-being to match.

It cannot therefore be too strongly emphasised that, irrespective of how well a patient appears, the medical and drug history must be carefully evaluated. Thus, a young patient taking corticosteroids can look and feel well but be suffering from acute lymphocytic leukaemia. The dangers of dental treatment without due precautions on such a patient should be obvious.

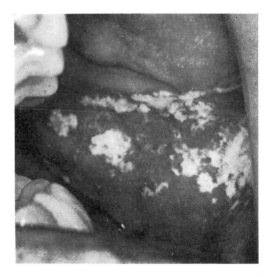

Fig. 20.14 Thrush in a patient on systemic corticosteroid treatment for pemphigus. Although the latter has been suppressed, the diminished resistance to infection has lead to persistent candidosis.

In summary, important complications of long-term corticosteroid treatment include:

1. Inability to withstand surgery and general anaesthesia
2. Reduced resistance to infection
3. Impaired healing
4. Concealment of serious disease.

The severity of these complications varies widely, but can be fatal.

The dental management of patients on systemic corticosteroid treatment is discussed in Chapter 21.

Diabetes mellitus

Diabetes mellitus is the most common endocrine disease and is the result of relative or absolute deficiency of insulin, causing a persistently raised blood glucose level. Approximately 2% of the population are affected but probably at least 50% of diabetics with mild or early disease pass unrecognised. There are two clinical types:

1. *Juvenile onset (insulin dependent) diabetes.*
   Symptoms typically become apparent before the age of 25 and the disease is usually severe with thirst, polyuria, hunger, loss of

weight and susceptibility to infection as early manifestations.

2. *Maturity onset diabetes.* Patients are typically over middle age and obese. The onset is insidious, often with deterioration of vision or pruritus or, sometimes, thirst, polyuria and fatigue. Many cases are asymptomatic, and the disease can be controlled by dietary restriction and, if necessary, oral hypoglycaemic agents.

The chief aspects of diabetes mellitus important in dentistry are as follows:

1. Diabetic emergencies, particularly hypoglycaemic coma (see Ch. 21)
2. Susceptibility to infection (mainly untreated or poorly controlled diabetics)
3. The management of diabetics during dentistry and anaesthesia
4. Complications of long-standing diabetes.

Susceptibility to infection. Rapidly destructive periodontal disease can be a feature of severe untreated diabetes mellitus but is unlikely to be seen now. However, even treated diabetic children have slightly poorer periodontal health than controls. As well as greater severity of gingivitis, diabetics also have higher DMFT levels (despite the sugar-free diet) and earlier loss of teeth than controls. Susceptibility to candidosis is also well-recognised. Occasionally in an unrecognised diabetic a dry mouth may be the main symptom of dehydration. Oral lichenoid reactions have also been reported as uncommon side effects of chlorpropamide and other hypoglycaemic agents.

The management of diabetics during dental operations

Local anaesthesia should be used for routine dentistry. The amount of adrenaline in the local anaesthetic solution is not significant in its effect on the blood sugar. Sedation can be given if required. Treatment should be so timed as not to interfere with the times of meals or of taking insulin or other hypoglycaemic agents—shortly after breakfast is therefore the ideal time.

General anaesthesia. Dental operations under general anaesthesia should be carried out in hospital under expert supervision.

Complications of long-standing diabetes

The chief complications are deterioration of sight (diabetic retinopathy), renal disease, peripheral arterial disease leading to gangrene of the feet and—of most importance in dentistry—ischaemic heart disease.

IMMUNOLOGICALLY MEDIATED DISEASE

Of the many diseases that are believed to be immunologically mediated, most have some dental relevance because of such considerations as the following:

1. Systemic effects that may affect dental management
2. Direct effects on the mouth or mucosal lesions (e.g. pemphigus or Sjögren's syndrome)
3. Treatment with drugs which can affect dental management (e.g. corticosteroids)
4. Abnormal reactions to drugs (e.g. penicillin anaphylaxis).

Immunologically mediated diseases fall into two main groups. By far the most common are atopic disease and contact dermatitis, which are abnormal reactions to exogenous antigens. The autoimmune diseases, by contrast, appear to be mediated by antibodies directed against host tissues. Intermediately, antibodies to exogenous antigens may cross-react with and possibly damage the tissues—the main example is cardiac damage in rheumatic fever, which may be mediated by anti-streptococcal antibodies.

Atopic disease

Atopic disease is the common type of allergy and affects approximately 10% of the population. Susceptibility to atopic disease is genetically determined and is mediated by IgE. There are no oral manifestations of atopic disease itself, and there is no oral counterpart to eczema. Acute angiooedema (as a reaction to a drug for example) can, however, indirectly involve the mouth if the acute oedema causes a swelling in the floor of the mouth. In such cases the important consideration is the threat to the airway.

Patients with atopic disease are said to be more susceptible to drug reactions, particularly acute anaphylaxis to such drugs as penicillin or intravenous anaesthetic agents, but this has not been confirmed. Drugs used in the treatment of atopic disease (particularly asthma) may complicate dental treatment. The main examples are as follows.

Antihistamines. Drowsiness, potentiation of sedatives and hypnotics, and dry mouth are the main relevant side-effects.

Corticosteroids. Systemic corticosteroids used particularly for severe asthma can increase susceptibility to infection, particularly oral candidosis, but, more important is the risk of severe hypotensive reactions (p. 460).

Corticosteroid sprays (such as Becotide and Bextasol) used to deliver minute doses directly to the airways do not apparently cause adrenocortical suppression but can promote oropharyngeal thrush in a few patients. Acute severe asthma is a potential cause of an emergency in the dental surgery (Ch. 21).

Contact dermatitis is a skin disease resembling eczema but is a cell-mediated (type 4) reaction. Again there is no convincing evidence of any oral counterpart to contact dermatitis, and patients who are sensitive to mercury, for example, can tolerate mercury-containing amalgams without ill-effect provided that the mercury does not come into contact with the skin. Contact dermatitis to materials used in dentistry is a hazard to dentists and especially to laboratory technicians. However, even though methyl methacrylate monomer in particular is known to be a sensitising agent, contact dermatitis is a surprisingly rare occupational hazard of dentistry.

Mercury allergy. See Chapter 25.

The autoimmune diseases

This blanket term is used for a great variety of diseases where there is defective modulation of immune responses and production of autoantibodies which can cause tissue damage by a variety of mechanisms, by no means all of which are clearly understood. The autoimmune diseases have a variety of features in common as summarised in Table 20.3, and all of those listed in Table 20.4 are likely to show these features. For example,

Sjögren's syndrome (Ch. 17) is approximately ten times as common in women as in men.

Table 20.3   Typical features of autoimmune disease

1. Significantly more common in women
2. Onset typically in middle age or older
3. Family history frequently positive
4. Usually increased levels of immunoglobulins (autoantibodies)
5. Circulating autoantibodies frequently also detectable in unaffected family members
6. Circulating autoantibodies to several tissues but not all attacked (e.g. antithyroid antibodies common in Sjögren's syndrome but thyroiditis is rare)
7. Often an increased risk of developing other autoimmune diseases (e.g. increased risk of patients with thyroiditis developing pernicious anaemia)
8. In some cases immunoglobulin and/or complement detectable at sites of tissue damage (e.g. pemphigus vulgaris)
9. Often associated with HLA B8 and DR3
10. Immunosuppressive treatment frequently limits tissue damage*

* Though immunosuppressive treatment will control most autoimmune processes it is not necessarily the most satisfactory form of treatment. At one extreme it is life-saving in pemphigus vulgaris, at the other extreme it will control joint destruction in rheumatoid arthritis but may lead to exacerbation of the disease when it is stopped. In other cases such as Sjögren's syndrome, symptoms result from extensive tissue destruction, and immunosuppressive treatment is too late.

By far the most common of these diseases is rheumatoid arthritis, and the main types of autoimmune diseases that can affect the oral or paraoral tissues are shown in Table 20.4.

The connective-tissue diseases. These diseases are characterised by a multiplicity of autoantibodies, none of which is specific to the tissues under attack and which frequently also are not specific to the disease either. Thus in rheumatoid arthritis the most constantly found autoantibody (rheumatoid factor) is not directed against the joint tissues but against an immunoglobulin. Moreover, rheumatoid factor is frequently detectable in other diseases of this group in the absence of arthritis. It is thought that the connective-tissue diseases are mediated by immune complex (type 3) reactions causing inflammation and tissue damage. However, apart from rheumatoid arthritis and systemic lupus erythematosus, the immunopathogenesis of many of these diseases is obscure.

Table 20.4 Some immunologically mediated diseases relevant to dentistry

Atopic disease and related allergies (type I)
  Asthma; eczema; hay fever; urticaria; food allergies
  Drug reactions
  Anaphylaxis and acute allergic angio-oedema

Autoimmune diseases
  The connective tissue diseases
    Rheumatoid arthritis
    Sjögren's and sicca syndromes★
    Lupus erythematosus★
    Systemic sclerosis★

Gastrointestinal disease
  Chronic atrophic gastritis and pernicious anaemia★
  Coeliac disease

Haematological disease
  Pernicious anaemia★
  Idiopathic and drug-associated thrombocytopenic purpura★
  Drug-associated leucopenia★
  Autoimmune haemolytic anaemia

Endocrine disease
  Addison's disease★
  Hypothyroidism (Hashimoto's thyroiditis)
  Hyperthyroidism
  Idiopathic hypoparathyroidism★

Mucocutaneous diseases
  Pemphigus vulgaris★
  Mucous membrane pemphigoid★

★ Diseases which can produce characteristic intraoral changes

Rheumatoid arthritis

Rheumatoid arthritis is by far the most common of the connective-tissue disorders and affects at least 3% of the whole population. Although it is a multisystem disease, arthritis (as might be expected) is the most prominent feature. The temporomandibular joints are frequently affected in the more severe cases, but the clinical effects are frequently insignificant (Ch. 14).

The chief importance of rheumatoid arthritis in dentistry is its association with Sjögren's syndrome. In addition, drugs used in the management of rheumatoid arthritis (particularly aspirin and other anti-inflammatory agents, corticosteroids, antimalarials, gold and penicillamine) can affect dental management or occasionally cause oral reactions. Many patients with rheumatoid arthritis are anaemic as a result of the disease itself, or alternatively or in addition as a result of gastric blood loss induced by aspirin and other analgesics.

Sjögren's and sicca syndromes

These have been discussed in Chapter 17.

Systemic lupus erythematosus

Systemic lupus erythematosus can have overt effects on almost any of the body systems, many of which may affect dental management, but oral mucosal lesions are seen in only about 20%.

SLE is characterised by a multiplicity of autoantibodies of which the most important are antinuclear factors, several of which are shared with other diseases in this group; only antibodies against double-stranded DNA (anti dsDNA) are peculiar to SLE.

Clinically the features vary according to the main organ systems affected. The so-called classical picture of a young woman with a butterfly rash across the mid-face is uncommon, and such rashes are not peculiar to SLE. The organs or tissues that can be affected are shown in Table 20.5: joint pains are the most common manifestation.

Corticosteroids and other immunosuppressives or antimalarials are the main forms of treatment.

Dental aspects. The oral lesions somewhat resemble lichen planus. However, they are very much more difficult to treat and may not respond to the doses of systemic corticosteroids which control more major manifestations of the disease.

Table 20.5 Organs and tissues affected in systemic lupus erythematosus

Joints	Joint pains and arthritis
Skin	Rashes
Mouth	Stomatitis, Sjögren's syndrome
Serous membranes	Pleurisy, pericarditis
Heart	Endocarditis, myocarditis
Lungs	Pneumonitis
Kidneys	Nephritic syndrome
Central nervous system	Neuroses and psychoses, strokes, cranial nerve palsies
Eyes	Conjunctivitis, retinal damage
Gastrointestinal tract	Hepatomegaly, pancreatitis
Blood	Anaemia, purpura

Antimalarials used in treatment can also produce oral lichen planus.

Otherwise dental management may be affected according to the pattern of systemic involvement, but in many cases the treatment is likely to affect dental management more than the disease itself. The chief dental considerations are therefore:

1. Corticosteroid and other immunosuppressive drugs
2. Painful oral lesions
3. Sjögren's syndrome
4. Bleeding tendencies (antiplatelet antibodies or anticoagulants)
5. Anaemia
6. Cardiac disease (rarely goes on to failure; infection of endocardial vegetations is possible).

Discoid lupus erythematosus

Discoid LE is characterised by mucocutaneous lesions essentially similar to those of SLE but without the latter's serological changes and systemic disorders.

Systemic sclerosis (scleroderma)

Systemic sclerosis is a rare disease characterised by subcutaneous and visceral fibrosis. It has a poor prognosis.

The pathogenesis of the progressive fibrosis and stiffening of the skin and often the gastrointestinal tract, lungs, heart and kidneys is unknown. Inflammatory changes are minimal. Circulating antinuclear antibodies are detectable in about 50% of patients but their role is also unknown.

Clinically the most common early sign is Raynaud's phenomenon and joint pains. Later the skin becomes thinned, stiff and pigmented and the facial features become smoothed-out and mask-like.

Fibrosis of viscera is liable to cause dysphagia, dyspnoea and pulmonary hypertension. Later there may be renal involvement, hypertension and cardiac failure.

Immunosuppressive drugs appear to be ineffective and the 5-year survival rate is only about 50%.

Intraoral changes tend to be slight, apart from the presence of Sjögren's syndrome in a minority, but opening of the mouth becomes limited by fibrosis.

A characteristic dental change is widening of the periodontal ligament shadow, but this is only seen in a few (7%) of cases. Gross resorption of the jaws has been reported. Firm whitish-yellow fibrotic plaques on the oral mucosa have been described but must be exceedingly rare.

Localised scleroderma (morphoea)

Morphoea is characterised by localised fibrosis resembling that of scleroderma but without the latter's systemic involvement of serological changes.

The face is frequently the chief site and the area of fibrosis resembles the scar from a sabre cut (coup de sabre). Childhood morphoea is a possible cause of facial hemiatrophy.

Wegener's granulomatosis

Wegener's granulomatosis is an uncommon disease causing inflammation of the upper airways, vasculitis and renal involvement which, in the absence of early treatment, is fatal. The pathogenesis is unknown. Anticytoplasmic autoantibodies have been reported and tissue damage is caused by vasculitis, but there appear to be no other associations with the connective tissue diseases with which it is frequently grouped.

Clinically involvement of the nasal tissues can result in destruction of, for example, the nasal septum and a saddle nose deformity.

In a minority of patients a characteristic form of gingivitis is the first sign. The gingivae typically undergo superficial proliferative changes initially resembling pregnancy gingivitis but becoming swollen with a granular surface and dusky or bright red in colour—an appearance described as 'strawberry gums'. The changes can be widespread or patchy. Mucosal ulceration may also develop.

Biopsy of affected gingivae typically shows a finely nodular surface, epithelial proliferation, a dense inflammatory infiltrate, collections of giant cells and, in the deeper tissues, vasculitis with destruction of small arteries.

Early recognition of these changes and biopsy confirmation is important, as early treatment at this stage may be life-saving.

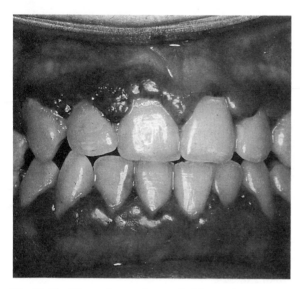

Fig. 20.15 Wegener's granulomatosis. The erythematous proliferative gingivitis ('strawberry gums') is readily mistaken for pregnancy gingivitis as it was in this young woman.

Midline granuloma syndromes

This group of diseases, in which Wegener's granulomatosis may be included, has acquired many names such as Lethal Midline Granuloma or Midfacial Granuloma. Their main features are variable degrees of destruction of the central facial tissues and a fatal outcome. These diseases, which are not necessarily clinically distinguishable, are now recognised in most cases to result from Wegener's granulomatosis or a peripheral T cell lymphoma.

Midfacial T cell lymphomas. These rare lymphomas can start in the nasal cavity and cause extensive destruction of the centre of the face. Nasal obstruction, discharge and crusting are typical early signs. Oral symptoms can result from extension through the palate to cause a small ulcer, and this may extend until the whole of the palate becomes necrotic.

Microscopic diagnosis is difficult as these lymphomas are pleomorphic and attack blood vessels, and thus simulate a vasculitis. Secondary inflammation may also obscure the lymphoma cells.

In the past, death could result from infection secondary to facial tissue necrosis. Usually now death results from dissemination of the lymphoma, but this may be delayed by radiotherapy.

Granulomatous diseases

Confusingly the term 'granuloma' is used *clinically* for lesions where there is proliferation of granulation tissue, as in apical granulomas. *Histologically* the term refers only to conditions where there is formation of tuberculosis-like follicles. These consist of rounded collections of large, pale histiocytes ('epithelioid cells') sometimes surrounded by lymphocytes, and often containing giant cells. Midline granulomas are *not* therefore granulomas microscopically.

There are very many causes of this type of reaction, the more important of which are shown below. All of them can affect mouth or cervical lymph nodes and most have been discussed in earlier chapters. Important examples of granulomatous diseases are:

* Infections
  — Tuberculosis and nontuberculous mycobacterioses
  — Leprosy
  — Syphilis
  — Deep mycoses, particularly histoplasmosis, cryptococcosis blastomycosis and coccidioidomycosis
  — Cat scratch disease
  — Toxoplasmosis
* Unknown causes
  — Sarcoidosis
  — Crohn's disease
* Reactive
  — Secondary to carcinoma or radiotherapy
* Foreign body reactions.

Sarcoidosis

Sarcoidosis is a chronic disease of unknown cause, in which granulomas form particularly in the lungs, lymph nodes (especially the hilar nodes), salivary glands and other sites such as the mouth.

Oral lesions, usually painless swellings, may be seen, and the most frequently affected sites are the gingivae, lips, palate and buccal mucosa. In over 50% of patients with bilateral hilar lymphadenopathy, biopsy of a labial salivary gland shows typical granulomas. Clinical involvement of the major salivary glands in uncommon but can cause tumour-like swelling.

Microscopically the granulomas are typically compact, non-caseating, contain multinucleated giant cells and are surrounded by lymphocytes.

Many minor abnormalities of immune responses such as anergy to some antigens such as tuberculin and, frequently, hypergammaglobulinaemia, are detectable, but patients are not unusually susceptible to infection.

Diagnosis depends on the combined clinical and laboratory findings and, in particular, pulmonary involvement, biopsy of affected tissue and a positive Kveim test. Granuloma formation in labial salivary glands may greatly facilitate diagnosis.

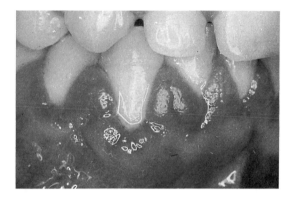

Fig. 20.17 Sarcoidosis. The gingival swelling is not clinically distinguishable from several other possible causes, but biopsy showed granuloma formation.

Treatment with systemic corticosteroids may be justified to control pulmonary fibrosis, cerebral lesions, or hypercalcaemia.

Crohn's disease

Crohn's disease is of unknown aetiology. It most frequently affects the ileocaecal region, causing thickening and ulceration. Effects include abdominal pain, variable constipation or diarrhoea and, sometimes, obstruction and malabsorption.

Orofacial involvement may occasionally precede abdominal changes. The main effects are diffuse soft or tense swelling of the lips, or mucosal thickening. A cobblestone-like thickening of the buccal mucosa, with fissuring and hyperplastic folds, is particularly characteristic. The gingivae may be erythematous and swollen. A minority of patients have painful mucosal ulcers. Glossitis due to iron, folate or vitamin B12 deficiency can result from malabsorption. Oral lesions, such as these, when associated with abdominal symptoms such as colicky pain, and alternating constipation and diarrhoea, are strongly suggestive of Crohn's disease.

Microscopically the granulomas are typically small, loose and with few multinucleate giant cells. They are often deep in the corium and may be difficult to find.

Oral symptoms may resolve when intestinal Crohn's disease is under control, or may respond to oral sulphasalazine or to intralesional injections of a corticosteroid.

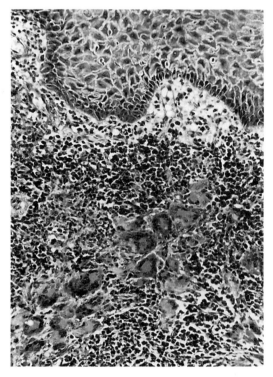

Fig. 20.16 Wegener's granulomatosis. Gingival biopsy from the patient shown in Fig. 20.15 showed the typical clusters of giant cells.

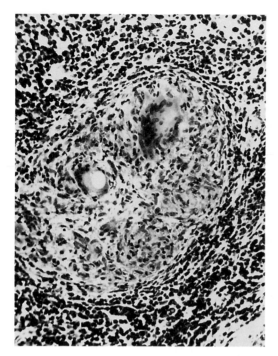

Fig. 20.18 Sarcoidosis. Microscopically the granulomas are compact with heavy peripheral lymphocytic infiltrate. However, they are not distinguishable by microscopy alone from other granulomatous diseases such as tuberculosis.

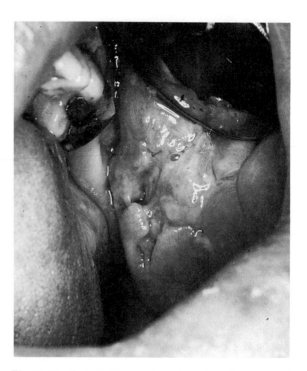

Fig. 20.19 Crohn's disease. Gross, irregular soft swelling of the buccal mucosa and ulceration, as here, is strongly suggestive of Crohn's disease, especially when associated with gastrointestinal symptoms.

Melkersson-Rosenthal syndrome

Melkersson-Rosenthal syndrome in its rare complete form comprises unilateral recurrent or fluctuating facial paralysis which may become permanent, labial or facial swelling and fissured tongue. The aetiology is unknown.

Recurrent, soft, painless facial swelling is most common, but may become persistent due to progressive fibrosis, and the buccal mucosa may have a cobblestone pattern like that in Crohn's disease. Facial palsy is troublesome and disfiguring.

Granulomatous reactions secondary to radiotherapy or chemotherapy

After treatment (usually radiotherapy) of oral carcinoma, a regional lymph node may become enlarged and firm, and tumour spread is suspected. However, such a node occasionally shows only a granulomatous reaction, probably in response to breakdown products from treatment of the tumour, and the patient can be reassured.

Foreign body reactions

Granulomas in response to implantation of foreign bodies are usually readily recognisable because of the clinical circumstances, most frequently implantation of amalgam or extrusion of root canal filling material. Such material is usually visible microscopically either directly or by polarised light. In starch granulomas (from glove powder), caseation can develop, but the granules should be recognisable by polarised light.

Zirconium (once used in dentifrices) can cause severe foreign body reactions.

Granulomatous reactions of unknown cause

The diagnosis of granulomatous reactions in oral tissues frequently depends on systemic investigation. However, a significant proportion of oral granulomatous reactions are unassociated with any detectable disease or local cause. In some, the patient may develop Crohn's disease or sarcoidosis

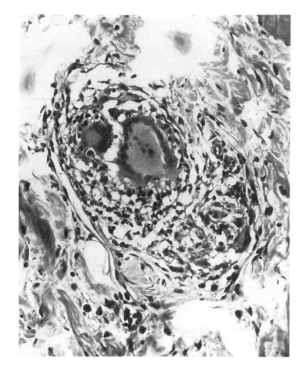

Fig. 20.20 Crohn's disease. The granulomas are frequently relatively deep in the mucosa, isolated and loose in texture with scanty peripheral lymphocytic infiltrate as here.

some time later, but many others remain healthy. In some of them the granulomatous reaction appears to result from common food additives such as cinnamon or tartrazine. Such causes can only be confirmed by an exclusion diet which, if faithfully maintained, may greatly lessen the swellings.

The term 'orofacial granulomatosis' has been introduced for this otherwise healthy group. However, this term is likely to cause confusion with midline facial granulomas which are lethal diseases.

When no cause can be found, regular follow-up should be maintained to ensure that systemic disease such as Crohn's disease or sarcoidosis is recognised at an early stage.

Immunodeficiency

Immune deficiencies can be primary or acquired (Table 20.6) and affect B to T lymphocytes, or both. However, the role of T lymphocytes in regulating B lymphocyte activity often means that a T cell defect affects antibody production. In addition there can be failures of production of individual antibodies such as IgA or of complement components.

Clinically, any patient who develops recurrent infections, and particularly if the infections respond poorly to treatment or are caused by otherwise harmless microbes (opportunistic infections), must be suspected of being immunodeficient.

Immunodeficiencies causing rapidly progressive periodontitis have been discussed in Chapter 6.

Table 20.6 Important causes of immunodeficiency

Primary (genetic)
—T or B lymphocyte defects (Swiss type agammaglobulinaemia, Di George's syndrome, etc.)
—IgA deficiency
—Complement component deficiencies
—Down's syndrome (multiple defects)

Secondary (acquired)
—Infections: AIDS, severe viral or bacterial infections, malaria, etc.
—Drug-induced: Immunosuppressive and anticancer treatment
—Malnutrition (worldwide a major cause)
—Cancer (particularly of lymphoreticular cells)
—Diabetes mellitus

The main causes of *severe* immunodeficiency are AIDS (Ch. 8) and immunosuppressive treatment for organ transplants or other purposes. Many cancer patients are also severely immunodeficient as a result both of the neoplasm and of the cytotoxic drugs used for its treatment.

The severe primary immunodeficiencies are rare and, unless a marrow transplant can be given, are usually fatal in childhood.

Oral manifestations of immunodeficiencies. The main effect, as mentioned earlier, is abnormal susceptibility to infections, particularly candidosis or viral infections such as herpes or deep infections such as osteomyelitis.

Selective IgA deficiency

Selective IgA deficiency is common and has potential relevance for the mouth. Selective IgA deficiency may affect about 1 in 600 of the general population and is associated with any of the following:

1. Normal health
2. Increased susceptibility especially to respiratory tract infections

3. Atopic disease
4. Connective-tissue disease, especially lupus erythematosus.

Susceptibility to infections. These infections mainly involve the respiratory tract and this may be due to an associated deficiency of IgG2.

The evidence regarding the effect of IgA deficiency on dental caries and periodontal disease is conflicting. There may also be compensatory secretion of other immunoglobulins into the mouth, and this may explain the variable findings. Both increased and decreased prevalence of dental caries have been reported. Gingivitis may be less than normal, but this may be the result of antibiotic treatment for respiratory infections.

There is no evidence of any significant association between oral mucosal infection and IgA deficiency.

Atopic disease. Asthma, eczema or any of the related diseases may be the presenting feature of IgA deficiency or the way by which the deficiency is discovered. The deficiency may allow increased absorption of allergens.

Graft-versus-host disease

Graft-versus-host disease is the result of an attack on an immunosuppressed host by transplanted immunocompetent cells. It is in effect a graft rejection reaction in reverse. It most frequently follows bone marrow transplantation both because of the deep immunosuppression necessary and because of the many immunologically active cells in the implanted marrow.

Oral manifestations of graft-versus-host disease are almost invariable. They comprise oral lichen planus and a Sjögren-like syndrome.

Hereditary angio-oedema

This disease is the result of a deficiency of C1 esterase inhibitor and, pedantically speaking, is an immunodeficiency disease. There is no neurotic component in the aetiology and the older term 'hereditary angioneurotic oedema' should be obsolete.

Since C1 esterase inhibitor is an inactivator of the first complement component, its absence leads to uncontrolled activation of the early components.

In the process C4 is consumed and its persistently low level in the serum provides confirmation of the diagnosis. As a result of stimuli such as minor trauma there are episodes of increased capillary permeability and gross but localised oedematous swelling.

Visceral angio-oedema can cause episodes of acute abdominal pain but, more important, oedema of the head and neck region can cause respiratory obstruction, and the disease has a significant mortality.

The most effective treatment and prophylactic agent is a synthetic androgen stanozolol which, if taken daily, maintains C1 esterase inhibitor at normal levels.

Hereditary angio-oedema must be distinguished from allergic angio-oedema (which can also threaten the airway) by the history of allergic disease in the latter and, usually, raised IgE levels.

LIVER DISEASE

Common types of liver disease are infections particularly viral hepatitis, obstructive jaundice, cirrhosis and tumours.

Rarely, liver disease can result from dental treatment when halothane has been given or as a result of transmission of hepatitis B.

As a broad generalisation the main effects of liver disease relevant to dentistry are:

1. Haemorrhagic tendencies
2. Impaired drug metabolism
3. Transmission, particularly of hepatitis B.

Haemorrhagic disease secondary to liver damage

Haemorrhagic tendencies can result either from obstructive jaundice (infective hepatitis also has an obstructive component) or from extensive liver damage. In obstructive jaundice vitamin K absorption may be severely impaired, while in liver failure vitamin K dependent clotting factors are not formed and severe bleeding tendencies result.

Impaired drug metabolism

Impaired drug metabolism results from severe parenchymal liver damage. There are few drugs which are not metabolised in the liver, and no drugs should be given to such patients without at least consulting the British National Formulary.

Causes of parenchymal liver disease and liver failure are shown in Table 20.7.

Most cases of cirrhosis are of unknown cause but cirrhosis is increasingly commonly the result of alcoholism. In Britain the incidence of alcoholic cirrhosis is as common in women as in men.

Halothane is a rare cause of severe liver damage but is important in relation to dentistry (Ch. 19).

Table 20.7 Important causes of parenchymal liver disease and liver failure

Idiopathic cirrhosis

Alcoholism

Viral hepatitis

Drugs, including halothane

Viral hepatitis

The main types are hepatitis A, B, D and non-A, non-B. Other viruses can also cause hepatitis but not as the primary manifestation of infection.

Hepatitis B and the associated delta agent (hepatitis D) are the chief risks to dental personnel but non-A, non-B hepatitis can also be transmitted during dentistry.

Hepatitis B

Hepatitis B can be readily transmitted during dentistry. Despite the outbreak of AIDS, hepatitis B is currently the greatest infective hazard to dental staff for the following reasons:

1. It is widespread
2. A chronic infective carrier state is common
3. Minute traces of body fluids can transmit infection
4. The virus survives well outside the body and is relatively resistant to disinfection
5. Infection can lead to chronic active hepatitis, cirrhosis and death from liver failure or liver cancer
6. There is no reliably effective treatment.

In addition, the hepatitis B virus may carry within it the delta agent which can cause a particularly virulent infection. However, active immunization is effective, safe and protects against both hepatitis B and delta infection.

The risk of transmission of hepatitis B by inoculation is emphasised by the fact that it was at one time termed 'syringe (or serum) jaundice' and, in the past particularly, countless cases were transmitted to patients via imperfectly sterilised syringes and needles.

Clinical aspects. The incubation period is long—at least 2 to 6 months. The majority of cases are subclinical (anicteric) but a minority develop acute hepatitis with loss of appetite, muscle pains, fever, jaundice and often a swollen, painful liver. The illness can be severe and debilitating but is usually followed by complete recovery and long-lasting immunity.

Nevertheless 5% to 10% of cases, particularly those who have had no overt illness, become persistent carriers and can transmit the infection.

The overall mortality rate is probably about 1% in those with clinical disease but occasionally has been as high as 30%, probably as a result of infection by the delta agent.

Biochemical markers of infection are the appearance of liver enzymes (transaminases, such as ALT, AST and GGT) in the serum, along with raised levels of bilirubin and often of alkaline phosphatase. However, confirmation of the diagnosis is by serology.

Serological markers of hepatitis B. The hepatitis B virus (HBV) is a DNA virus termed the Dane particle. The Dane particle consists of a central core and an outer shell. The core contains DNA, an enzyme (DNA polymerase: DNA-P) and the hepatitis B Core antigen (HBcAg). The protein shell forms the hepatitis B surface antigen (HBsAg).

1. The surface antigen (HBsAg). Particles of HBsAg are detectable in the late incubation period, and during acute and chronic infections.

Carriage of HBsAg indicates past infection, but unless HBeAg is also present, confers little risk of transmitting the infection.

2. Antibody to HB surface antigen (HBsAb). Antibody to the surface antigen begins to appear when recovery starts but HBsAg may briefly disappear before anti-HBs becomes detectable. Both serological tests then become negative.

During recovery, anti-HBs usually appears and

Table 20.8 Serological markers of hepatitis B immunity or carrier state

	HBsAg	Anti-HBsAg	HBeAg	Anti-HBeAg	Anti-HBcAg	DNA polymerase
Immunity	−	+	−	+	+	−
Carrier state*	+	−	+**	−	+	+**

★ Variable combinations of markers
★★ High infectively

rises in titre; its presence usually implies persistent immunity. Anti-HBs also appears after hepatitis B immunisation.

3. Hepatitis B core antigen (HBcAg). The core antigen is found only in liver cells, not the serum.

4. Antibody to HB core antigen (HBcAb). In contrast to the surface antibody, anti-HBc appears at the onset of disease. It quickly rises in titre, persists for many years and is one of the most sensitive indicators of past infection.

5. Hepatitis B e antigen (HBeAg). The e antigen is probably a breakdown product of the core antigen and an indicator of high infectivity. It appears in the serum simultaneously with HBsAg but disappears earlier if there is full recovery.

6. Antibody to e antigen (anti-HBe. HBeAb). The e antibody usually appears in the serum soon after the e antigen and heralds recovery. Failure of development of anti-HBe indicates high infectivity.

Carriers of both HBsAg and HBeAg but who lack anti-HBe are more likely to develop chronic active hepatitis and serious complications, and to transmit the infection.

7. DNA polymerase (DNA-P). DNA polymerase in the serum, like HBeAg, indicates high infectivity, since it is also part of the Dane particle.

The carrier state and complications. Most patients with acute hepatitis B recover completely within a few weeks, but approximately 4% to 5% fail to clear the virus within 6 to 9 months. The latter become chronic carriers with either of two main effects (sometimes with some overlap):

1. chronic carriage of HBsAg but not HBeAg and with a low risk from severe liver damage.
2. persistent carriage of both HBsAg and HBeAg and chronic active (aggressive) hepatitis. These patients have biochemical evidence of liver damage, are chronically ill, and at special risk from cirrhosis and, possibly, carcinoma of the liver.

The carrier state most frequently follows anicteric hepatitis and thus, since they have no history of jaundice, most carriers are unsuspected. Chronic active hepatitis with persistent malaise, and sometimes mild jaundice, is particularly likely to develop in the very young or old, and in those such as male homosexuals who are immunodeficient. Cirrhosis can result and lead to liver failure or hepatocellular carcinoma.

Risks to dental staff. The carriage rate of hepatitis B virus in the general population of Britain is 0.1–0.2%, but in hot climates such as Asia and Africa may be 5–40%, and dental staff there are at high risk. There are also high-risk groups (Table 20.9), and the hazard of infection is highest in inner urban areas and particularly for oral surgeons and periodontists.

In the USA, the carrier rate is 0.5–0.7% and rising, but nearly 30% of American dentists have serological evidence of previous infection and one of the highest infection rates of all health workers. In Danish dentists the prevalence of hepatitis B virus markers is double that of the general population but has remained stable over recent years; the risk to British dentists is probably of a similar order.

Transmission of HBV. Blood and blood products are most dangerous and can transmit infection in amounts of 0.0000001 ml particularly when the e antigen is present. Many cases have therefore followed needle stick injuries, injections and blood transfusions.

Saliva can also contain hepatitis B antigens and, experimentally, can transmit the virus. In addition, saliva is frequently contaminated with

Table 20.9 Patients with higher risk of being hepatitis B carriers

1. Promiscuous male homosexuals and STD (VD) clinic patients
2. Intravenous drug addicts
3. Patients and staff of dialysis and transplant units
4. Patients (especially with Down's syndrome) and staff of institutions for the handicapped
5. Immunosuppressed or immunodeficient patients
6. Patients receiving unscreened blood or blood products
7. Patients who have had acupuncture or tattooing, especially in tropical countries
8. Consorts of patients with hepatitis B or of any of the above
9. Certain associated diseases, particularly AIDS, some chronic liver diseases and polyarteritis nodosa
10. Temporary or permanent immigrants, or travellers returning from high-risk areas

NOTE: Hepatitis B is more common in the USA and tropical or subtropical countries. The carrier rate among Afro-Asians may be up to 40%.

blood, and saliva splashed on to the conjunctiva is a possible means of infection for dentists.

Hepatitis B can also be transmitted heterosexually, especially if promiscuous, but more readily by male homosexual activity. Promiscuous male homosexuals may carry the e antigen in high titre and are then potentially highly infective. This group, particularly in the USA are frequently also HIV positive, and in London 30% of male prostitutes (many of them teenagers) are estimated to be HBV carriers and 20% of them to be HIV positive.

As discussed earlier the risk of infection is related to the serological markers: HBeAg-positive patients are highly infectious but those who are HBeAg negative are of extremely low infectivity. Infective carriers can only be suspected if they have a history of jaundice or are in a high-risk group. Nevertheless it must be emphasised that only 1 in 4 patients with markers of HBV infection gives a positive medical history. In statistical terms, therefore, if a dentist treats 20 patients a day, one hepatitis B carrier will be encountered every 7 working days. Many infectious patients, as in the case of carriers of the AIDS virus, will therefore be treated unknowingly.

Dental staff who are carriers of or incubating hepatitis B can also transmit infection to patients, some of whom have died as a consequence.

The dangers to dentists have been emphasised by the death of an unvaccinated male nurse from hepatitis B, after being bitten by a mentally handicapped carrier patient.

The delta agent: hepatitis D virus (HDV)

The delta agent is a defective RNA virus that can only replicate in the presence of HBsAg. Delta infection is mainly transmitted by blood or blood products. It is widespread in intravenous drug abusers and in endemic areas such as the Mediterranean region. Delta infection causes acute hepatitis and, though this usually resolves, it can go on to fulminant liver disease.

Delta hepatitis, with occasional deaths, has been reported in dental patients.

Immunisation against hepatitis B also protects against the delta agent, and this strengthens the need for immunisation.

Non-A non-B hepatitis, including hepatitis C

Non-A non-B (NANB) hepatitis is so called because the infection resembles that caused by the other hepatitis viruses, but causative agents have not been identified until recently and others may as yet be uncharacterised. NANBH is the most common cause of post-transfusion hepatitis, and for this type of infection an RNA virus (hepatitis C virus) has been identified and appears to be the major cause of hepatitis after blood transfusions. Acute NANB hepatitis is similar in most respects to hepatitis B except that it is generally less severe but chronic liver disease is more common.

Worldwide, NANBH causes a high proportion of all cases of viral hepatitis and there are many carriers, especially among intravenous drug abusers, including over 50% of heroin addicts in London, and haemophiliacs. However, most have not yet been recognised because of the lack until recently of serological tests of NANBH infection, and diagnosis has had to depend principally on exclusion of other known agents.

More recently still, hepatitis E virus has been identified as a cause of another form of NANB hepatitis which resembles hepatitis A in its transmission and epidemiology.

Non-A non-B hepatitis as a hazard in dentistry. Since, NANBH, and particularly hepatitis C, can be transmitted in a similar way to hepatitis B and there are many carriers it must be considered as a risk in dentistry and there is some evidence that this is the case. The same care in cross-infection control should therefore be adopted as for hepatitis B. This is particularly important as there is no vaccine available as yet.

Control of transmission of viral hepatitis

Because of the ease of transmission of hepatitis the following basic precautions should always be taken (see also Appendix II).

1. All patients should be treated as infectious.
2. Gloves should be worn for all clinical dental work.
3. Special care should be taken to avoid needle-stick injuries.
4. Disposable instruments should be used and all others autoclaved.
5. *Clinical dental staff should be immunised against hepatitis B.*

The last is the single most important measure as it is virtually impossible completely to prevent transmission of this infection by other means. There is as yet no vaccine against hepatitis C and there are some strains of hepatitis B against which the current vaccine apparently confers no protection, but though the hazard from these is statistically small the risk from them emphasises the need to maintain rigorous cross-infection control.

Table 20.10 Sterilisation and disinfection for hepatitis B

Sterilisation
  Autoclaving at 134°C for 3 minutes OR
  Hot air at 160°C for 1 hour

Disinfectants
  Glutaraldehyde 2%
  Sodium hypochlorite 10% of stock solution
  (corrosive to metals)

As mentioned earlier, it is not merely for his own protection that the dentist should make sure that his cross-infection control procedures are up to standard, but it is also a legal obligation under the Health and Safety at Work Act.

It is worth emphasising again that gloves, masks and eye shields provide only partial protection. A single pair of gloves certainly does not provide an effective barrier, and double gloving is necessary for surgeons at high risk from acquiring or transmitting these infections. Active immunisation against hepatitis B is therefore essential for clinical dental staff. Three injections should be given at intervals into the deltoid muscle, but adequate protection may not develop until after 6 months. Side-effects are mild and rare, but a few (particularly the obese) do not produce adequate antibody levels after a normal course of vaccination and need it to be repeated. Booster doses are needed at 3- to 5-year intervals, or more frequently in some persons in whom the half-life of the vaccine is brief.

Those who have not been immunised, but are wounded while treating a high-risk patient or known carrier, should have immediate active immunisation. Passive immunisation with hepatitis B immune globulin as well has also been advised but there is now doubt as to its value.

Hepatitis A

Hepatitis A is the common form of infectious hepatitis. It is frequently acquired from contaminated food during a holiday abroad in the sun. There is little evidence that hepatitis A is transmitted during dentistry.

RENAL DISEASE

Renal disease has become more important in dentistry because of the increasing number of patients who, as a result of renal dialysis or transplantation, survive renal failure.

Renal dialysis patients. These patients, though dependent on regular dialysis, remain otherwise in reasonably good general health, though its level is related to the length of time since the last dialysis. About 70% can return to full-time work. However they are heparinised before dialysis and haemostasis is impaired for 6 to 12 hours. These patients are also at greater risk of having hepatitis B or becoming carriers.

In addition, these patients have a permanent venous fistula for the dialysis lines. This fistula is susceptible to infection, and antibiotic cover should be given for dental surgical procedures. Drugs, including sedation, should not be given intravenously, as the patency of the superficial veins which are the patient's lifelines must be preserved at all costs.

Dialysis patients also have an increased incidence of cardiovascular and cerebrovascular disease.

Renal osteodystrophy and secondary hyperparathyroidism. These can result from prolonged dialysis or renal failure and are now a more common cause than primary hyperparathyroidism of osteolytic giant-cell lesions which may first become apparent in the jaws (Ch. 12).

Renal transplant patients. Normal renal functions and health can be restored apart from the possible complications of prolonged immunosuppressive treatment. In addition these patients have often been on dialysis while awaiting a compatible donor. Hence they too may be hepatitis B carriers.

Nephrotic syndrome. These form a small group of patients who have a fairly good prognosis if given immunosuppressive treatment. The latter is the main factor affecting dental management, but these patients may also be susceptible to ischaemic heart disease as a result of accelerated atherosclerosis secondary to hypercholesterolaemia.

Chronic renal failure. Patients in chronic renal failure are a much smaller group than those already described. However, some patients are unsuitable for, or unable to obtain, dialysis.

Oral features of chronic renal failure. Any of the following may be seen:

— Mucosal pallor (anaemia)
— Xerostomia
— Purpura
— Ulceration
— Thrush or bacterial plaques
— White epithelial plaques
— Giant-cell lesions of the jaws (secondary hyperparathyroidism).

The white epithelial plaques may affect the floor of the mouth, edges of the tongue, or buccal mucosa and may resemble hairy leukoplakia. They regress when renal function is restored by dialysis or transplantation. Giant-cell lesions of the jaw can result from secondary hyperparathyroidism.

Dental management of these patients may be affected by any of the following:

1. Corticosteroid and other immunosuppressive treatment
2. Haemorrhagic tendencies
3. Anaemia
4. Impaired drug excretion
5. Hypertension
6. Hepatitis B carriage
7. Underlying cause of renal failure (e.g. diabetes mellitus, hypertension, or connective-tissue disease).

SYSTEMIC INFECTIONS

Systemic infections, particularly the childhood fevers and rarely syphilis or tuberculosis, can affect the mouth.

Other systemic infections such as infective endocarditis can be caused by oral bacteria (Ch. 8), while AIDS can affect dental management in other ways. One of the most important systemic infections relevant to dentistry—hepatitis B—has been discussed earlier.

Remote effects of dental infections

Bacteria grow in enormous numbers, particularly at the gingival margins and in periodontal pockets. These organisms are swallowed, may be inhaled, or may enter the bloodstream. On rare occasions, especially before the era of antibiotics, an acute oral infection such as osteomyelitis might spread to cause septicaemia. Under certain circumstances, bacteria from the mouth can reach distant parts of the body and may cause metastatic or systemic infections, particularly in immunodeficient patients. However, the main complication of this kind is infective endocarditis (Ch. 8).

NUTRITIONAL DEFICIENCIES

Patients with nutritional deficiencies are rarely seen in Britain. Those most liable to be affected are the elderly living on an inadequate diet, food cranks and severe alcoholics living on a grossly unbalanced diet, or patients with malabsorption syndromes. Several oral conditions of doubtful cause, such as periodontal disease or glossitis, have been ascribed to vitamin deficiencies though the patient is otherwise well and is living on an adequate diet. In these cases the giving of vitamin preparations brings no benefit. Vitamin deficiencies are not a contributory cause of dental caries.

Vitamin deficiency

Vitamin A deficiency

In rats, diet deficient in vitamin A causes severe effects on secretory epithelium; the columnar cells become squamous in type and keratinised. Ameloblasts fail to differentiate but form a layer of flattened cells; formation and mineralisation of enamel matrix are defective. Failure of organisation of enamel-forming epithelium removes the stimulus which normally causes odontoblasts to differentiate, and dentine formation is defective. The epithelial cells, having failed to differentiate, continue to proliferate and invade the underlying pulp where foci of amorphous dentine form. The secretory cells of salivary glands also become squamous and keratinised. However, there is no evidence that vitamin A deficiency causes dental hypoplasia in man.

In man, vitamin A deficiency causes night blindness and, later, xerophthalmia leading to infection and inflammation of the eye. Even in the presence of these signs, the teeth and mouth are unaffected, and, in a group of adults deprived of the vitamin for over a year, no dental disease could be found attributable to the deficiency.

Effective treatment of keratotic plaques (leukoplakias) with retinoids (vitamin A derivatives) has been reported but not confirmed, and the side-effects of these drugs are severe. Epidemiological investigations have reported an association between low vitamin A intake and oral and other cancers.

Retinoids may benefit a variety of skin diseases but, in addition to other toxic effects, are teratogenic.

Thiamin (B1) deficiency

In man, deficiency of thiamin and of other factors causes beriberi (neuritis and cardiac failure); the disease is mainly seen in rice-eating populations of the East. No oral changes are attributed to deficiency of thiamin.

Bizarrely, a case of beriberi due to malnutrition secondary to tooth decay has recently been reported in Britain.

Riboflavin (B2) deficiency

Riboflavin deficiency causes inflammatory and degenerative changes in the mucous membranes of the lips and tongue. The disease is rare in Britain but occasionally results from a malabsorption syndrome. By contrast, in the USA the disease remained endemic until the 1940s and the findings in many thousands of patients have been described. Angular stomatitis, consisting of red, painful fissures at the angles of the mouth, and shiny redness of the mucous membranes are characteristic. The tongue is commonly sore and red. A peculiar form of glossitis in which the tongue becomes magenta in colour and granular or pebbly in appearance, due to flattening and mushrooming of the papillae, has been described but is uncommon. The gingivae are not affected.

A greasy dermatitis round the alae nasi and eyes, and conjunctivitis are other features.

The disorder clears up in a matter of days when adequate doses of riboflavin (5 mg three times a day) are given. Riboflavin is usually ineffective in the treatment of the commonly seen cases of glossitis and angular stomatitis, which are rarely due to vitamin deficiency.

Nicotinamide deficiency (pellagra)

Pellagra affects the skin, gastrointestinal tract and nervous system. The disease is rare in Britain, but may very occasionally be seen as a result of a malabsorption syndrome or alcoholism. In the USA the disease was endemic until the 1940s.

The early symptoms are weakness, loss of appetite, and changes in mood or personality followed by glossitis or stomatitis and dermatitis.

Glossitis and stomatitis are sometimes early changes. The tip and lateral margins of the tongue become red, swollen and, in severe cases, deeply ulcerated. The dorsum of the tongue becomes coated with a thick, greyish fur which is often heavily infected. The gingival margins also become red, swollen and ulcerated, and generalised stomatitis may develop. Other changes in the gastrointestinal tract such as nausea and vomiting develop late; in acute cases diarrhoea may be a feature.

Dermatitis, when present, is characterised by its symmetrical distribution on the exposed parts of the skin and sites subject to irritation. The skin becomes red and, later, scaly, rough and pigmented.

Vitamin B12 deficiency—pernicious anaemia

This disease, unlike the others described in this section, is primarily a defect of absorption not a dietary deficiency. The characteristic features are chronic anaemia and disorders of the nervous system, as discussed earlier.

Folic acid deficiency

This can be the result of malnutrition but is more often seen in pregnancy, or as a result of malabsorption or drug treatment, particularly with phenytoin as discussed earlier.

Vitamin C deficiency—scurvy

This disease, once common among crews of sailing ships, is now exceedingly rare. In this country scurvy may very occasionally be seen among elderly people with an inadequate income, or in those devoted to eccentric diets. The main features of scurvy are dermatitis and purpura, while anaemia, delayed healing of wounds and, in advanced cases, swollen bleeding gums may also develop. In children bone formation may be disturbed (Ch. 12).

There is no evidence that deficiency of vitamin C plays any part in periodontal disease except in frank scurvy, and there is no correlation between low plasma ascorbic acid levels and gingivitis in patients. There is no reason for giving ascorbic acid to healthy patients with periodontal disease.

Vitamin D deficiency

Vitamin D plays an essential role in the absorption of calcium and phosphorus from the gut, and in their metabolism. Deficiency of this vitamin, during the period of bone development causes rickets (Ch. 12).

The main source of vitamin D is fish liver oils, but small amounts are also present in eggs and butter. In strong sunlight vitamin D can by synthesised in the skin. In Britain margarine is fortified with vitamins A and D. The requirements are, however, small except during periods of bone growth and pregnancy.

There is no basis for the idea that dental caries is due to poor calcification of the teeth resulting from vitamin D deficiency, and the giving of vitamin D and calcium for the prevention or reduction of dental caries is valueless. There are also dangers associated with increasing children's intake of vitamin D. Some children are sensitive to the action of this potent drug; hypervitaminosis D causes hypercalcaemia and renal calcinosis.

The teeth. Dental defects (hypocalcification) are a feature only of exceptionally severe rickets (Chs 2 and 12).

Pregnancy

Pregnancy may have effects on the mouth and has implications affecting dental management.

The chief oral effects are aggravation of gingivitis and possible development of a pregnancy epulis (pyogenic granuloma—Ch. 16). Occasionally, recurrent aphthae remit during pregnancy.

As to dental management, a minority of women in late pregnancy become hypotensive when laid supine, as a result of the swollen uterus impeding venous return; they should be treated in a sitting position. Alternatively hypertension or eclampsia may complicate management. Iron or folate deficiency anaemia, with possible oral or other manifestations, are other possible hazards.

Respiratory reserve is decreased and there is a risk of fetal hypoxia. Neonatal respiration is further depressed by drugs such as general anaesthetics, especially with barbiturates, diazepam and opioids all of which cross the placenta. Another risk is that of vomiting if general anaesthesia is given. If sedation is necessary, relative analgesia is preferable. Though there is a theoretical risk of fetal effects from depression of vitamin B12 metabolism by nitrous oxide, this does not appear to be significant after brief exposure.

With regard to local anaesthesia, prilocaine can rarely cause methaemoglobinaemia and, possibly, fetal hypoxia. It has also been suggested, but not substantiated, that felypressin, being related to oxytocin, might cause premature uterine contractions. However, local anaesthesia is generally safe during pregnancy.

The main risks of fetal abnormalities are from drugs and radiation: the hazard is greatest during organogenesis in the first trimester. Few drugs are known to be teratogenic for humans, and in many cases the risk is no more than theoretical or results from prolonged high dosage. For example any teratogenic risk of metronidazole for humans has never been substantiated. Non-steroidal anti-inflammatory agents in high dosage may cause premature closure of the ductus arteriosus and fetal pulmonary hypertension. Aspirin may also increase the risk of neonatal haemorrhage. Paracetamol is therefore the preferred analgesic.

Systemic corticosteroids can cause fetal adrenosuppression, and there is a possible teratogenic risk from sulphonamides. However, the only drugs known to be teratogenic (in the present context) are thalidomide (used experimentally for major aphthae), etretinate (used experimentally for leukoplakia) and possibly azathioprine (used experimentally for Behçet's syndrome and sometimes for connective-tissue diseases). In addition tetracyclines can cause irreversible discolouration of the teeth and in high doses can cause maternal hepatoxicity. (For further details of drug usage in pregnancy, see the current British National Formulary.)

The risks from dental radiography are small but only essential radiographs should be taken, the minimal radiation exposure should be given, and a lead apron should be worn by the patient as discussed in Chapter 22.

COMPLICATIONS OF SYSTEMIC DRUG TREATMENT

Problems that may result from systemic diseases have been indicated, but it may be worth emphasising again that drugs given for these conditions can also complicate dental treatment.

In some cases it may be difficult to decide whether the underlying disease or the drug is likely to cause the most serious difficulties. It is estimated that about 10% of ambulant outpatients are having some form of drug treatment but, though the problem is not yet at least a common source of difficulties in dentistry, it must always be borne in mind. Complications, when they happen, can sometimes be catastrophic.

Systemically administered drugs can have the following effects relevant to dental treatment:

1. Drugs may complicate dental treatment itself; anticoagulants, for example, may cause prolonged bleeding after dental extractions.
2. Drugs may react with or potentiate drugs given for dental purposes; hypotensive agents, for example, can cause a severe fall in blood pressure during general anaesthesia.
3. Drugs may cause stomatitis or have other oral effects, as discussed in Chapter 15.

The main groups of commonly used drugs which can cause complications during dental treatment include the following.

Antibiotics. These may cause superinfection, particularly candidosis, due to interference with the normal oral flora. Patients who have previously received antibiotics may occasionally become hypersensitised unknowingly, particularly to penicillin, and react acutely to further antibiotic treatment.

Anticoagulants. If anticoagulants are being given under adequate haematological supervision, extractions can usually be carried out without excessive bleeding. Any underlying heart disease may be a more serious problem of management.

Cardiovascular drugs. There is a great variety of agents used for treating hypertension, itself a common disease. The main hazards are during general anaesthesia, when there may be a dangerous fall in blood pressure unresponsive to normal methods of treatment.

Nifedipine and its analogues as well as anti-arrhythmic agents such as diltiazem can cause gingival hyperplasia.

Anticonvulsants. Gingival hyperplasia is a well-known effect of phenytoin; less common is lymphadenopathy. Because of the many adverse effects of phenytoin it is being displaced, for major epilepsy, by carbamazepine. The latter has rarely been reported to cause marrow depression.

Analgesics. Aspirin is generally safe but can dangerously potentiate haemorrhagic tendencies from any cause and should also not be given to patients with peptic ulceration or to children. Torrential haematemesis is a rare but recognised complication that occasionally results even from small doses of aspirin.

Hypnotics, sedatives and tranquillisers. There is a great variety of these drugs; many of them potentiate each other, general anaesthetic agents and hypotensive agents. Barbiturates, especially phenobarbitone, have rarely been reported as causing Stevens–Johnson syndrome (bullous erythema multiforme).

Neuroleptics ('major tranquillisers'), particularly the phenothiazines, cause troublesome dry mouth. Other adverse effects of phenothiazines and related antipsychotic agents include tardive dyskinesia (uncontrollable facial movements) which may make dental treatment difficult, parkinsonian tremor, postural hypotension and pigmentation of the oral mucosa. Metoclopramide also has phenothiazine-like activity and causes clenching of the jaw muscles.

Benzodiazepines ('minor tranquillisers') by contrast have few adverse effects apart from sedation (which is additive with other CNS depressants) and slight respiratory depression which is not significant in normal persons.

Antidepressant agents. Tricyclic antidepressants have an anticholinergic action and cause an unpleasantly dry mouth. They are *not* a cause of important interactions with adrenaline in local anaesthetics. Monoamine oxidase inhibitors can cause dangerous interactions with narcotic analgesics, particularly pethidine, which is often given postoperatively.

Antihistamines. These commonly used drugs often cause drowsiness, potentiate sedatives and cause dry mouth.

Insulin. Patients may lose consciousness (hypoglycaemic coma) if, after taking their insulin, they are prevented by dental treatment from taking food at the normal time. The consequences are more serious if this happens during general anaesthesia.

Corticosteroids. Systemic therapy causes suppression of normal adrenal function with the risk of circulatory failure, particularly during surgery under general anaesthesia. Corticosteroids, particularly in heavy dosage, also reduce resistance to infection; thrush is a well-recognised manifestation. These drugs are also dangerous because of the misleading appearance of good health that they can give to seriously ill patients.

Precautions

Cytotoxic and immunosuppressive drugs

Several of these, but particularly methotrexate, cause severe oral ulceration. In addition they promote opportunistic infections, which can cause or worsen existing ulceration.

The anticancer drug cisplatin can cause greyish gingival pigmentation.

Cyclosporin has less tendency to promote opportunistic infections but can cause gingival hyperplasia.

Though these problems are no more than an occasional cause of difficulties, patients must always be asked whether they are under medical treatment. In such enquiries the word 'drugs' should be avoided as inevitably leading to misinterpretation. Patients should be asked whether they are taking 'medicines, tablets, injections, or any sort of medical treatment for *any* purpose' or have received any of these recently, or whether they have been given any sort of hospital card.

Drug dependence

Drug dependence, particularly addiction to intravenous drugs, is an increasingly frequent phenomenon, particularly in the larger cities. However, alcohol remains the most widely abused drug.

There are few direct effects of drug dependence, and difficulties in management are more common. These include the following.

1. Stealing prescription pads or attempting to manipulate the dentist into prescribing drugs, particularly opioids, for example by complaining of pain. However, multiple drug abuse is common, and attempts may be made to obtain any drugs such as

benzodiazepines or antihistamines which have mood altering or sedative properties.

2. Carriage of hepatitis or HIV by intravenous addicts.
3. Maxillofacial injuries, particularly among alcoholics.
4. Impaired liver function secondary to alcoholism or hepatitis, and consequently impaired drug metabolism.
5. Lymphadenopathy secondary to drug injection in unusual sites.
6. Infective endocarditis. This is secondary to dirty injections, but, once the heart has been damaged, the risk of endocarditis after extractions or periodontal treatment is considerably increased.
7. Severe infections such as osteomyelitis, particularly among alcoholics.
8. Increased risks from general anaesthesia as a result of liver damage, respiratory disease, or covert use of the drug of abuse preoperatively.
9. Gross oral neglect and sometimes increased sensitivity to or fear of pain.
10. Rarely, ulceration of the palate secondary to cocaine-induced ischaemia of the nasal cavity.

CHANGES IN THE MOUTH CAUSED BY SYSTEMIC DISEASE—SUMMARY

Changes in the mouth and jaws caused by systemic disease have been discussed in this and other chapters. These disorders are often serious and may sometimes be lethal; oral changes may be of diagnostic importance. They are reviewed briefly here to serve as a reminder of the variety of changes that may be seen.

The teeth. Changes in the teeth due to systemic disease are rarely of general diagnostic importance except as indications of disease during the developmental period. In a few cases, the disease process is still active.

Abnormal colour. Causes include:

1. Tetracycline (yellow to brown or grey)
2. Fluorosis (opaque white or brown patches)
3. Severe jaundice (yellow or greenish)
4. Porphyria, a rare hereditary disorder of haemoglobin metabolism (purplish red)

5. Dentinogenesis and osteogenesis imperfecta (purplish or brownish but increased translucency).

Hypoplasia. Causes include:

1. Congenital syphilis. The characteristic deformity is notched and peg-shaped permanent incisors; the molars may also be deformed. This is exceedingly rare.
2. Severe childhood fevers. Horizontal grooves or pits particularly of the incisors may rarely be seen.
3. Severe fluorosis. Rough pitting in addition to white and brown opacities is seen in very high fluoride areas.
4. Severe rickets. Grooving or pitting of the enamel have rarely been described.
5. Hypoparathyroidism. Grooving or pitting of the enamel is caused by the associated ectodermal defects.

It should be emphasised that all these abnormalities are rare and cause defects only if active during dental development.

The oral mucous membrane. The main signs of systemic disease in the oral mucous membrane may be summarised as follows.

Abnormal colour.

1. Pallor due to anaemia
2. A yellowish tint due to jaundice
3. Brown pigmentation (in white people) may be due to Addison's disease.

Gingival or mucosal bleeding.

1. Purpura. This includes many diseases, such as acute leukaemia and AIDS. Purpura may be seen both subcutaneously and submucosally, and excessive gingival bleeding may be a feature.
2. Disorders of clotting. Excessive gingival bleeding may be a feature but purpura is not present. Haemophilia is the most important cause.

Acute gingivitis.

1. Acute leukaemia, immunodeficiencies, AIDS, agranulocytosis and uncontrolled diabetes mellitus are the main causes.

2. Vitamin deficiencies. Scurvy and pellagra are exceedingly rare causes.

Stomatitis.

1. Systemic infections. The most important are measles (in the prodromal stage), chickenpox and secondary syphilis.
2. Diseases affecting skin and mucous membranes. Pemphigus, mucous membrane pemphigoid and erythema multiforme have the most serious effects, but lichen planus is much more common.
3. Iron, vitamin B12, or folic acid deficiency can cause or contribute to aphthous stomatitis.
4. Drug therapy. Barbiturates, gold, sulphonamides, cytotoxic agents and many others are occasional causes.
5. Other causes. In the later stages of uraemia there may be ulceration of the mouth and of other parts of the gastrointestinal tract.

Keratoses.

White patches can result from AIDS, renal failure, or tertiary syphilis.

Glossitis.

1. Anaemia. This is the most common identifiable cause and is most frequently due to iron deficiency. Latent deficiencies are also important.
2. Vitamin deficiencies. Riboflavin deficiency and pellagra are rare causes of glossitis in this country, but, in malabsorption syndrome, vitamin deficiencies may cause glossitis and other effects.

Multiple effects. The great variety of effects of AIDS, but in particular opportunistic infections such as thrush, and tumours, are discussed in Chapter 8.

Changes in the jaws. Areas of resorption or patchy resorption and sclerosis in the jaws are sometimes caused by widespread skeletal diseases and associated with changes in the blood chemistry. The main causes are:

1. Paget's disease
2. Widespread metastases of carcinoma, or multifocal neoplasms
3. Hyperparathyroidism (primary or secondary).

The cervical lymph nodes. Oral sepsis is so common a cause of enlargement of the cervical lymph nodes that it is easy to forget that they become involved in serious diseases of the reticuloendothelial system of which they may be the first sign. Important systemic causes of generalised enlargement of lymph nodes are as follows:

1. Glandular fever
2. Hodgkin's disease
3. Non-Hodgkin lymphoma
4. Lymphocytic leukaemia
5. AIDS and its prodromes.

These and other causes of cervical lymphadenopathy have been discussed in Chapters 8 and 16.

SUGGESTED FURTHER READING

Albrecht M, Banoczy J, Tamas G 1988 Dental and oral symptoms of diabetes mellitus. Community Dent Oral Epidemiol 16: 378–380
Aledort L M 1989 New approaches to bleeding disorders. Hospital Practice February: 207–225
Amerena V, Andrew J H 1987 Hepatitis B virus: the risk to Australian dentists and dental health care workers. Aust Dent J 32: 183–189
Anon 1989 Sickle cell disease and the non-specialist. Drug and Therapeutics Bulletin 27: 9–12
Badenoch J 1988 Legionnaires' disease. Med Int 52:
Barrett A P 1987 Clinical characteristics and mechanisms involved in chemotherapy-induced oral ulceration. Oral Surg, Oral Med, Oral Pathol 63: 424–428
Bolewska J, Holmstrup P, Moller-Madsen B, Kenrad B et al 1990 Amalgam-associated mercury accumulations in normal oral mucosa, oral lesions of lichen planus and contact lesions associated with amalgam. J Oral Pathol Med 19: 39–42
Boucek C D 1988 Blood in the mouth. New Engl J Med 319: 1607
Burge S M, Frith P A, Millard P R, Wojnarowska F 1989 The Lupus band test in oral mucosa, conjunctiva and skin. Br J Dermatol 121: 743–752
Cannell H 1988 The development of oral and facial signs in B-thalassaemia major. Br Dent J 164: 50–53
Carlsson E B, Chewning L C 1989 Polycythemia vera in an oral surgical patient. Oral Surg, Oral Med, Oral Pathol 67: 673–675
Cawson R A 1965 Gingival changes in Wegener's granulomatosis. Br Dent J 118: 30–32
Centers for Disease Control 1987 Outbreak of hepatitis B

associated with an oral surgeon—New Hampshire. Morbid Mortal Week Rep 36: 132–133

Centers for Disease Control 1988 Update: Universal precautions for prevention of transmission of human immunodeficiency virus, hepatitis B and other bloodborne pathogens in health-care settings. J Am Med Assoc 260: 462–465

Chan J K C, Ng C S, Lau W H, Lo S T H 1987 Most nasal/nasopharyngeal lymphomas are peripheral T cell neoplasms. Am J Surg Pathol 116: 418–429

Chott A, Rappersberger K, Schlossarek W, Radaszkiewicz T 1988 Peripheral T cell lymphoma presenting primarily as a lethal midline granuloma. Hum Pathol 19: 1093–1101

Colten H R 1987 Hereditary angioneurotic edema 1887–1987. New Engl J Med 317: 43–45

Communicable Disease Report 1990 Kawasaki disease (KD) surveillance. CDR 90/08: 1

Cottone J A 1986 Delta hepatitis: another concern for dentistry. J Am Med Assoc 112: 47–49

Cross C E, Lillington G A 1989 Serodiagnosis of Wegener's granulomatosis: pathobiologic and clinical implications. Mayo Clin Proc 64: 119–122

Davis L G, Weber D J, Lemon S M 1989 Horizontal transmission of hepatitis B virus. Lancet 1: 889–893

Dreizen S, McCredie K B, Bodey G P, Keating M J 1986 Quantitative analysis of the oral complications of antileukemia chemotherapy. Oral Surg, Oral Med, Oral Pathol 62: 650–653

Eddleston A 1990 Modern vaccines: hepatitis. Lancet 1: 1142–1145

Fagan E A, Partridge M, Sowray J H, Williams R 1988 Review of hepatitis non-A, non-B: The potential hazards in dental care. Oral Surg, Oral Med, Oral Pathol 65: 167–171

Fagan E, Vergani D, Williams R 1987 Delta hepatitis. Lancet 332: 1322–1323

Falcone C, Sconocchia R, Guasti L et al 1988 Dental pain threshold and angina pectoris in patients with coronary artery disease. J Am Coll Cardiol 12: 348–352

Falk H, Hugoson A, Thorstensson H 1989 Number of teeth, prevalence of caries and periapical lesions in insulin-dependent diabetics. Scand J Dent Res 97: 198–206

Field E A, Tyldesley W R 1989 Oral Crohn's disease revisited—a 10-year-review. Br J Oral Maxillofac Surg 27: 114–123

Fiese R, Herzog S 1988 Issues in dental and surgical management of the pregnant patient. Oral Surg, Oral Med, Oral Pathol 65: 292–297

Foley F F, Gutheim R N 1956 Serum hepatitis following dental procedures: a presentation of 15 cases including 3 fatalities. Ann Intern Med 45: 469–470

Fotos P G, Westfall H N, Snyder I S et al 1985 Prevalence of Legionella-specific IgG and IgM antibody in a dental clinic population. J Dent Res 64: 1382–1385

Friedlander A H, Runyon C 1990 Polymyalgia rheumatica and temporal arteritis. Oral Surg, Oral Med, Oral Pathol 69: 317–321

Friedlander A H, Yoshikawa T T 1990 Pathogenesis, management and prevention of infective endocarditis in the elderly. Oral Surg, Oral Med, Oral Pathol 69: 177–181

Geppert T 1990 Southwestern internal medicine conference: Clinical features, pathogenic mechanisms and new developments in the treatment of systemic sclerosis. Am J Med Sci 299: 193–206

Hall S M Communicable disease report. British paediatric surveillance unit/CDSC Reye syndrome surveillance scheme. CDR 89/38: 3

Handlers J P, Waterman J, Abrams A M, Melrose R J 1985 Oral features of Wegener's granulomatosis. Arch Otolaryngol 111: 267–270

Hardman P K, Gier R E, Tegtmeier G 1990 The incidence and prevalence of hepatitis B surface antigen in a dental school population. Oral Surg, Oral Med, Oral Pathol 69: 399–402

Herrin R A, Boyd J F 1988 Desmopressin acetate prophylaxis in a patient with hemophilia A: report of a case. J Am Dent Assoc 117: 593–595

Israelson H, Binnie W H, Hurt W C 1981 The hyperplastic gingivitis of Wegener's granulomatosis. J Periodontol 52: 81–87

Jenison S A, Lemon S M, Baker L N, Newbold J E 1987 Quantitative analysis of hepatitis B virus DNA in saliva and semen of chronically infected homosexual men. J Infect Dis 156: 299–307

Kolbinson D A, Schubert M M, Flournoy N, Truelove E L 1988 Early oral changes following bone marrow transplantation. Oral Surg, Oral Med, Oral Pathol 66: 130–138

Lamey P J, Taylor J A, Devine J 1988 Giant cell arteritis. A forgotten diagnosis? Br Dent J 164: 48–50

Laurell L, Hugoson A, Hadansson J et al 1989 General oral status in adults with rheumatoid arthritis. Community Dent Oral Epidemiol 17: 230–233

Lettau L A, Smith J D, Williams D et al 1986 Transmission of hepatitis B with resultant restriction of surgical practice. J Am Med Assoc 255: 934–937

Mazze R I 1986 Nitrous oxide during pregnancy. Anaesthesia 41: 897–899

Melmed S 1990 Acromegaly. New Engl J Med 322: 966–976

Minor M W, Fox R W, Bukantz S C, Lockey R F 1987 Melkersson–Rosenthal syndrome. J Allergy Clin Immunol 80: 64–67

Mitchell K, Ferguson M M, Lucie N P, MacDonald D G 1986 Epithelial dysplasia in the oral mucosa associated with pernicious anaemia. Br Dent J 161: 259–260

Mori M 1984 Status of viral hepatitis in the world community; its incidence in dentists and other dental personnel. Int Dent J 34: 115–121

Murray-Lyon I M 1989 Strategies for preventing hepatitis B. Q J Med 71: 277–278

Platt J C, Tomich C E, Campbell S 1989 Malignant lymphoma presenting as a midline lethal granuloma. J Oral Maxillofac Surg 47: 511–513

Pogrel M A 1988 Unilateral osteolysis of the mandibular angle and coronoid process in scleroderma. Int J Oral Maxillofac Surg 17: 155–156

Porter S R, Scully C 1990 Non-A, non-B hepatitis and dentistry. Br Dent J 168: 257–259

Probert C S J 1989 Beriberi secondary to tooth decay. Lancet 335: 51–52

Pye M 1988 Lingual and scalp infarction as a manifestation of giant cell arteritis: delay in diagnosis leading to blindness. J Rheumatol 15: 1597–1598

Raustia A M, Autio-Hramainen H I, Knuutila M L E, Raustia J M 1985 Ultrastructural findings and clinical follow-up of 'strawberry gums' in Wegener's granulomatosis. J Oral Pathol 14: 581–587

Reingold A L, Kane V A, Hightower A W 1988 Failure of gloves and other protective devices to prevent transmission of hepatitis B to oral surgeons. J Am Med Assoc 259: 2558–2560

Rogers S N 1989 A study of the dental health of patients undergoing heart valve surgery. Postgrad Med J 65: 453–455

Royer J E, Bates W S 1988 Management of von Willebrand's disease with desmopressin. J Oral Maxillofac Surg 48: 313–314

Sanholm L, Swanljung O, Rytomaa et al 1989 Periodontal status of Finnish adolescents with insulin dependent diabetes mellitus. J Clin Periodontol 16: 617–620

Scheutz F, Melbye M, Esteban J I et al 1988 Hepatitis B virus infection in Danish dentists: a case-control and follow-up study. Am J Epidemiol 128: 190–196

Scully C 1989 Orofacial manifestations of the rheumatic diseases. Dental Update July/August: 240–246

Scully C, Cawson R A 1991 Medical problems in dentistry, 3rd edn. Wright, Bristol

Shaw F E, Barrett C L, Hamm R et al 1986 Lethal outbreak of hepatitis B in a dental practice. J Am Med Assoc 255: 3260–3264

Shopper T P, Boozer H B 1987 Serum chemistries for dentists. JADA 114: 197–200

Siew C, Gruninger S E, Hojvat S A 1988 Screening dentists for HIV and hepatitis B. New Engl J Med 318: 1400–1401

Sjostrom L, Laurell A, Hugoson A, Hakannson J P 1989 Periodontal conditions in adults with rheumatoid arthritis. Community Dent Oral Epidemiol 17: 234–236

Smith H M, Alexander G J M, Birnbaum W, Williams R 1987 Does screening high risk dental patients for hepatitis B virus protect dentists? Br Med J 295: 309–310

Stevens C E, Taylor P E, Pindyck J et al 1990 Epidemiology of hepatitis C virus. J Am Med Assoc 263: 49–53

Sullivan L W 1987 The risks of sickle-cell trait. Caution and common sense. New Engl J Med 317: 830–831

Theaker J M, Porter S R, Fleming K A 1989 Oral epithelial dysplasia in vitamin B12 deficiency. Oral Surg, Oral Med, Oral Pathol 67: 81–83

Wahlen Y B, Matsson L 1988 Oral mucosal lesions in patients with acute leukaemia and related disorders during cytotoxic therapy. Scand J Dent Res 96: 128–136

Weel F, Jackson I T, Crookendale W A, McMichan J 1987 A case of thalassaemia major with gross dental and jaw deformities. Br J Oral Maxillofac Surg 25: 348–352

Weiner A J, Kuo G, Bradley D W et al 1990 Detection of hepatitis C viral sequences in non-A, non-B hepatitis. Lancet 335: 1–3

Whittaker S, Foroni L, Luzzato L et al 1988 Q J Med 65: 645–655

Wood R E, Lee P 1988 Analysis of the oral manifestations of systemic sclerosis (scleroderma). Oral Surg, Oral Med, Oral Pathol 65: 172–178

21. Sudden loss of consciousness and other emergencies in dental practice

Fainting
Cardiac emergencies
Angina
Myocardial infarction
Cardiac arrest and cardiopulmonary resuscitation (CPR)
Anaphylaxis
Asthma and status asthmaticus
Circulatory collapse associated with corticosteroid therapy
Convulsions

Acute hypoglycaemia
Prolonged haemorrhage
Strokes
Severe maxillofacial injuries
Drug reactions
Anaesthetic and sedation accidents
Hyperventilation syndrome
The emergency drug kit
Disturbed behaviour

Fortunately, serious emergencies are uncommon in dental practice, but when they happen the dentist's skill and prompt response can sometimes be life-saving. The main problems that may have to be faced have been listed above.

FAINTING

Fainting is the most common cause of sudden loss of consciousness in the dental surgery. It is due to a transient fall in blood pressure and cerebral ischaemia. It is usually emotional in origin.

Very nervous patients may be helped by being given premedication with, for example, temazepam 10 mg an hour before treatment.

Predisposing factors

Anxiety, pain, hunger and a hot humid atmosphere. Some patients have a tendency to faint readily in response to particular stimuli, such as injections or the sight of blood. Typical signs are:

—Confusion, dizziness or complaint of feeling faint
—Pallor and sweating
—Nausea; sometimes vomiting
—Dilated pupils
—Slow pulse
—Rarely, a minor fit or incontinence.

Management

- Lay the patient flat.
- Raise the legs above the level of the head.

Smelling salts and similar old fashioned 'stimulants' are of no value but a sweet drink after recovery is helpful.

If response to laying the patient flat is not rapid and the pulse does not recover its normal strength and rhythm, consider the possibility of other causes such as (according to circumstances) anaphylaxis, a heart attack, or acute hypoglycaemia.

CARDIAC EMERGENCIES

Anginal

Anginal attacks must be distinguished from myocardial infarcts. There have usually been previous attacks and the chest pain is usually recognised by the patient as anginal.

In such cases give the patient's usual medication (nitrates) by the usual route (under the tongue). Pain uncontrollable in this way suggests a myocardial infarct.

Myocardial infarction

There is sometimes a history of angina or the patient may be known to be a severe hypertensive.

Signs are variable but typically include:

— Severe, crushing chest pain
— Pain may radiate to the left shoulder, arm or jaw
— Nausea and vomiting
— Shallow breathing
— Weak, rapid, often irregular pulse
— Increasing pallor and sweating.

Management

The essential initial measures are:

1. To make sure the patient can breathe
2. To relieve pain
3. To relieve anxiety.

- Put the patient in a comfortable position where breathing is easiest (usually sitting back). Laying the patient flat may make breathing difficult.
- Reassure the patient.
- Give nitrous oxide and oxygen 50/50 (or intravenous morphine 10 mg at 2 mg/min).
- Call an ambulance.
- If there is no improvement, consciousness is lost and pulse becomes impalpable, there may be cardiac arrest, and standard cardiopulmonary resuscitation may be needed.

Cardiac arrest and cardiopulmonary resuscitation (CPR)

Treatment must be immediate and efficient if life is to be saved. The chances of survival and of avoiding brain damage are heavily dependent on the duration of the circulatory failure. Death is likely within 4 minutes of cessation of cardiac contraction. The chief considerations are therefore;

1. To be alert to the possibility of cardiac arrest

2. To be aware of possible predisposing causes
3. To be able to recognise arrest
4. To have a trained dental team ready
5. To start resuscitation as soon as arrest is recognised.

Dental staff in any practice therefore should be trained in CPR to enable them to act as an efficient team.

Cardiac arrest can be a totally unpredictable event in an apparently healthy person, but precipitating events include myocardial infarction, anaphylaxis, anaesthetic accidents (overdose or severe hypoxia), or a severe hypotensive reaction in a patient on corticosteroids.

Signs of arrest include:

— Sudden, complete loss of consciousness
— Absence of any pulse (best felt at the carotid artery just in front of the sternomastoid muscle)
— Pallor or ashen grey colour and cold clammy skin

To wait for later signs such as cyanosis or pupillary dilatation and loss of reaction to light, is likely to be fatal or the patient may survive with irreversible brain damage.

Management

In essence this comprises the ABC of,

Airway
Breathing (mouth to mouth)
Circulation (chest compression)

The following are the main measures.

- Put the patient on a *firm* flat surface—keep in the chair, if of a suitable type. Otherwise put on the floor, but this can be difficult with a heavy patient and may delay the start of treatment.
- Call for help—the dental team in the first instance. One of them should telephone for an ambulance.
- Clear the airway and keep the jaw forward and the neck extended.
- Start chest compression at 60 per minute, with one hand over the other on the lower

sternum. The arms should be stiffly extended and the full upper body weight (40–50 kg) used. The risk of breaking a rib should be ignored.

- Inflate the lungs vigorously (mouth-to-mouth or preferably using a mask and oxygen via a respirator bag with a plastic airway in the patient's mouth) between each five compressions of the sternum. The chest should be seen to be inflated. Do not otherwise interrupt chest compression for more than 10 seconds.
- Continue until there are signs of recovery or expert help arrives. If there is no sign of recovery after 15 minutes the attempt has usually failed.

A trained dental team is needed to carry out these different tasks. There should be two operators to carry out the resuscitation itself—one compressing the chest, the other inflating the lungs then changing over as the first tires. Number 2 should monitor the pulse between lung inflations.

Clinically, ventricular fibrillation cannot be distinguished from arrest, and sometimes ventricular fibrillation can be stopped by giving a heavy blow on the sternum. However, some authorities advise against it because it may, in other cases, precipitate fibrillation.

Signs of recovery include:

—Return of colour and pulse
—Blinking
—Lightening of consciousness
—Spontaneous movements—not mere twitching.

After recovery the patient should be admitted to hospital for any ancillary treatment and investigation. Some patients who collapse unexpectedly and are revived by CPR show no evidence of myocardial infarction, and may survive for years without another attack.

Effectiveness of cardiopulmonary resuscitation. Increasingly, commercial organisations are encouraging their staff to take courses in cardiopulmonary resuscitation. Even when imperfectly performed by lay persons in the street, CPR has been life-saving on many occasions. Modern city traffic is such that lives are frequently lost because of the time lost before an ambulance reaches the victim.

Causes of failure

The most common mistakes are:

1. Giving external cardiac compression without artificial ventilation
2. Giving artificial ventilation without external cardiac compression
3. Failing to clear the airway and to ensure that it remains open by hyperextending the head adequately
4. Failing to close the nose during mouth-to-mouth respiration
5. Failure to get a close fit with the mask when using a bag respirator
6. Failing to make sure that ventilation is adequate, as indicated by the movement of the chest
7. Timidity in applying external cardiac compression and insufficient force to squeeze the heart
8. Failing to release pressure on the chest completely between compressions and thereby preventing cardiac filling
9. Compressing the chest too rapidly to allow the heart to fill between compressions
10. Putting the hands in the incorrect position on the sternum
11. Failing to act sufficiently quickly and fretting about minutiae rather than getting on with external cardiac compression and artificial ventilation.

ANAPHYLAXIS

Anaphylactic reactions are usually to injected drugs (particularly penicillins and some intravenous barbiturate anaesthetics) and very rarely to drugs by mouth. The main effect is acute, severe hypotension.

Typical signs are:

—Onset one to several minutes after an injection
—Initial paraesthesia, flushing and oedema of face
—Itching, sometimes with visible urticaria

—Wheezing (bronchospasm)
—Weak, rapid or impalpable pulse
—Loss of consciousness unresponsive to laying flat
—Increasing pallor or cyanosis; cold, clammy skin.

Management

- Lay the patient flat and raise the legs.
- Give intramuscular adrenaline (1:1000, 0.5–1 ml). Repeat after 10 minutes if necessary.
- Adjunctive treatment:
  —Intravenous hydrocortisone 100–300 mg to prevent further deterioration in severe reactions.
  —Intravenous antihistamine such as chlorpheniramine 10–20 mg, well diluted with blood and given *slowly* (over 1 minute) may help restore the blood pressure.
- Telephone for an ambulance.

ASTHMA AND STATUS ASTHMATICUS

Asthma is a state of reversible airways obstruction. It can be an allergic reaction (type 1) or non-allergic. Attacks can therefore be precipitated by specific allergens such as a drug, or other stimuli such as anxiety. Asthma is a serious disease and, though treatable, causes between 2000 and 2500 deaths a year in Britain.

An attack is characterised by:
—Noisy wheezing
—Difficulty in breathing
—Hyperinflation of the chest.

Management. An attack usually responds to quick use of the medication such as a salbutamol inhaler which asthmatics normally carry with them. If the attack is severe, oxygen should also be given. The patient should not be laid flat.

Status asthmaticus

This is a potentially fatal emergency characterised by:

—Lack of response to routine medication

—Persistent and increasing difficulty in breathing
—Involvement of accessory muscles of respiration
—Cyanosis.

Status asthmaticus can also result if the patient cannot find his/her normal medication.

If intravenous salbutamol or comparable drugs are not available the management is to:

- Give adrenaline 0.5–1 ml subcutaneously.
- Call an ambulance.
- Give oxygen.
- Give intravenous hydrocortisone succinate 200 mg.

CIRCULATORY COLLAPSE IN PATIENTS ON CORTICOSTEROID TREATMENT

The response of patients on long-term corticosteroid treatment to surgery is unpredictable. Near fatal circulatory collapse has been seen after dental extractions in a patient taking only 5 mg of prednisone a day. Since large doses of corticosteroids given for a short period are safe—and for these patients may be life-saving—the policy should be to be, if anything, overprotective. Prevention is all-important, since circulatory collapse is sometimes unresponsive to treatment. All patients therefore who are having systemic corticosteroids, and even those who have had these drugs in the past, are at risk; it has been suggested that cortical function may take up to 2 years to recover. Corticosteroid ointments used lavishly, particularly for widespread eczema, also have systemic effects and have been known to cause severe reactions.

Types of dental treatment hazardous for these patients are surgical treatment of any type including extractions, especially under anaesthesia or so-called sedation with methohexitone. Local anaesthesia is considerably safer.

The following principles are a general guide for the management of patients under systemic corticosteroid treatment.

1. Major oral surgery must be carried out in hospital.
2. Minor operations including extractions should preferably be carried out under local anaesthesia,

but an intravenous corticosteroid should be given prophylactically.

3. If even a brief general anaesthetic is unavoidable, then a corticosteroid must be given prophylactically. *At least* 100 mg of hydrocortisone succinate should be given intravenously just before the operation and the patient's condition carefully watched throughout. At the least sign of a falling blood pressure (pallor with a rapid but weak pulse) immediate corticosteroid supplementation (100 to 500 mg intravenously) must be given.

4. For extractions under local anaesthesia 100 mg of hydrocortisone should be given intravenously and repeated if there is the least doubt as to the patient's condition.

5. These patients should be kept under observation for at least an hour after operation.

6. Restorative dentistry under local anaesthesia is probably not dangerous. There is probably no need for corticosteroid supplementation but there should, on the other hand, be no hesitation in giving large amounts intravenously if circulatory collapse seems imminent.

The suggestion of doubling the patient's normal dose of corticosteroid the day before and the day of treatment is probably ineffective, as relatively enormous doses (that is hundreds of milligrams) are needed to prevent or manage circulatory collapse.

Management of hypotensive collapse. If inadequate corticosteroid cover has been given and the patient shows signs of circulatory failure (pallor, rapid weak or impalpable pulse, falling blood pressure and loss of consciousness) the following are the essential measures:

1. Lay the patient flat and *raise the legs*
2. Give *at least* 200 mg of hydrocortisone sodium succinate intravenously. Repeat as necessary if response not obvious
3. Give oxygen and apply cardiopulmonary resuscitation if necessary
4. Call an ambulance.

CONVULSIONS

Epilepsy. In most cases fits are the result of tonic-clonic (grand mal) epilepsy in a known epileptic. The fit may be precipitated by such factors as hunger, fatigue, stopping or changing medication, or flickering tube lights. The manifestations are:

—Instantaneous loss of consciousness sometimes preceded by a cry
—Violent generalised muscular contraction
—Cyanosis
—Tonic (jerking) muscular contractions follow
—Slow recovery but often persistent drowsiness.

All that can be done is to protect patients from injuring themselves or breaking equipment during an attack. Insertion of a mouth prop is often recommended but is difficult to do quickly enough.

Patients are typically drowsy after an attack and, after resting, should be accompanied home. Treatment of complications such as lacerations of the tongue, fractures or displacement of teeth, or subluxation of the jaw may be necessary.

Rarely, as mentioned earlier, a minor fit can result from deep loss of consciousness in a faint, particularly if the patient is not laid flat. They are also a possible complication of a large intravenous bolus of lignocaine (for control of dysrrhythmias after myocardial infarction) but only a *theoretical* possibility as a result of overdose of lignocaine as a local anaesthetic. Lignocaine has also been recommended as a *treatment* for epilepsy.

Status epilepticus in which fits follow one another without recovery of consciousness is a life-threatening emergency. Treatment is with intravenous diazepam 10 mg and repeated after 10 minutes if necessary.

ACUTE HYPOGLYCAEMIA

The patient may be aware of what is happening and (if sensible) will warn the dentist before losing consciousness. The attack resembles a faint in some respects, but the features are:

—Anxiety or irritability*
—Pallor and sweating
—Rapid pulse
—Loss of consciousness
—Failure to respond to laying flat.

---

* Signs of failing consciousness are highly variable and can include paraesthesiae, tremor, truculence, disorientation, blurred vision, slurred speech or fits.

Management. Before consciousness is lost, give sugar, at least 4 heaped teaspoonfuls in water, by mouth.

If consciousness is lost:

- Lay the patient flat and raise the legs.
- Give intravenous sterile 50% glucose solution (up to 50 ml) *OR* intramuscular glucagon 1 mg followed by oral sugar when consciousness is regained.

If none of the latter are available and the patient appears to be lapsing into coma, intramuscular adrenaline 0.5–1 ml can be given but must be followed by oral sugar as soon as consciousness returns.

PROLONGED HAEMORRHAGE

Though bleeding may be occasionally alarming for dentist and patient alike a major vessel is unlikely to be damaged as a result of dental surgery, and hence the patient is unlikely to lose any dangerous quantity of blood if promptly dealt with.

The most severe bleeding is likely to come from an unrecognised haemophiliac. This can only be controlled by giving anti-haemophilic factor. It is necessary therefore to control the bleeding as well as possible by means of a pressure pad and supporting the patient's jaw with a firm barrel bandage, and to get the patient admitted to hospital as quickly as possible where appropriate treatment can be given.

Continued bleeding due to local causes is much more common and is really only an emergency in the sense that the dentist may be woken up at 3 o'clock in the morning to deal with it. The simplest and most effective treatment (Ch. 9) is to give a local anaesthetic, to tidy up the socket and to suture it.

STROKES

Cerebral haemorrhage or thrombosis is a common complication of hypertension in the elderly. In younger patients, rupture of a berry aneurysm of the circle of Willis causes subarachnoid haemorrhage which has been known to follow acute hypertension caused by noradrenaline in a dental local anaesthetic.

Typical features of cerebrovascular accidents include:

—Sudden loss of consciousness
—Weakness or paralysis of one side of the body (hemiplegia) and sometimes drooping of one side of the face.

In many cases consciousness is not recovered but goes on to fatal coma.

Little can be done for such patients, and the main measures are to protect the airway and call for an ambulance.

SEVERE MAXILLOFACIAL INJURIES

These have only to be faced by the dentist in general practice if he happens by mischance to be on the scene at the time of the accident or (even less likely) the accident is nearby and the patient is brought to him.

The most important aspect, as explained in Chapter 13, is to ensure that the airway is clear. The injuries to the facial skeleton themselves, though alarming in appearance, do not endanger life unless they affect the airway. There may, however, be loss of consciousness due to head injury. Signs of shock are indications of severe damage to other parts of the body, such as internal bleeding, for which emergency treatment in hospital is needed.

DRUG REACTIONS

There are very few that can endanger life but these include the following.

Noradrenaline when used as a vasoconstrictor in excessive concentration (1:20 000) can occasionally cause acute hypertension which may result in cerebral haemorrhage or even death.

Quite apart from its dangers, noradrenaline has no advantages and should not be used in local anaesthetic solutions.

Monoamine oxidase inhibitors can cause severe reactions with narcotic analgesics *particularly pethidine*. The reaction can be very sudden. Monoamine oxidase inhibitors also interact with indirectly acting sympathomimetic agents (such as ephedrine used as a nasal decongestant), but *not* adrenaline or noradrenaline, to cause acute severe hypertension.

General anaesthetic agents are one of the chief causes of fatal accidents in the dental surgery as described earlier.

Corticosteroids given systemically for any disease can lead to circulatory collapse which in several cases has been fatal when patients are subjected to stress, as described earlier.

ANAESTHETIC AND SEDATION ACCIDENTS

Deaths as a result of anaesthetic accidents, particularly with intravenous methohexitone, have given rise to considerable adverse publicity for the dental profession and caused the General Dental Council to publish a Notice for the Guidance of Dentists who practice anaesthesia or sedation (see Ch. 19).

The main dangers are:

— Respiratory obstruction
— Respiratory failure
— Overdose of the anaesthetic agent
— Cardiac arrest (often secondary to hypoxia)
— Anaphylactoid reactions to intravenous anaesthetic agents
— Circulatory collapse of patients on long-term corticosteroids.

Intravenous sedation. Deaths have followed the use of diazepam with pentazocine, and midazolam alone. The cause in such cases is respiratory failure. In the case of midazolam this can follow over-rapid injection, particularly in an elderly person.

In such cases immediate resuscitation (positive-pressure ventilation with oxygen) must be given, and it is a requirement of the General Dental Council that resuscitative equipment should be available wherever sedation is practised.

HYPERVENTILATION SYNDROME

Hyperventilation can be due to organic causes or caused by anxiety. In the latter case it can cause alarming symptoms such as:

— Rapid breathing
— Shortness of breath or a sense of suffocation
— Numbness of the extremities
— Tightness of, or pain in the chest
— Faintness or blurring of vision
— Palpitations
— Tetany due to carbon dioxide washout.

Management. Frequently the patient is unaware of overbreathing, and the main measures are:

• Reassurance
• Persuade the patient to breathe deeply and slowly.

If this fails, the patient should be persuaded to rebreathe the expired air from a plastic bag, for example, if nothing else is available.

THE EMERGENCY DRUG KIT

A variety of kits have been suggested or are available commercially. The latter are expensive but, whether the drugs are bought as a kit or individually, they are likely to be rarely used. Their expiry dates must therefore be noted and replacements obtained as necessary. The following are suggested:

1. Adrenaline Injection, 1 in 1000. 1 ml ampoules
2. Chlorpheniramine (maleate) Injection, 10 mg/ml, 1 ml amps.
3. Diazepam Injection, 5 mg/ml, 2 ml amps.
4. Sugar, glucose tablets or sweet drinks
5. Glucagon Injection, 1-unit vials with solvent.
6. Glucose Injection, 50%, 50 ml amps.
7. Hydrocortisone sodium succinate 100 mg with solvent
8. Oxygen
9. Nitrous oxide OR Entonox (N_2O/O_2, 50/50).

In addition there should be sterile, disposable syringes and needles, apparatus for administering oxygen and nitrous oxide, an oral airway and a powerful aspirator.

DISTURBED BEHAVIOUR

Neurotic patients may behave in a tiresomely abnormal fashion under the emotional stress of having dental treatment or in almost any other circumstances. There may be spectacular convulsions and the attack mistaken for epilepsy. The patient nevertheless usually manages to avoid injury. There is also no incontinence but consciousness may appear to be disturbed for a long period.

It is often difficult to be sure that these reactions are neurotic in nature though there may be a strong suspicion that this is the case. There is also the possibility that there is some underlying organic disorder such as atypical epilepsy. In any case further dental treatment is impossible for the time being, and the attack has usually to be allowed to take its course.

The patient's doctor should be consulted before any further dental treatment is undertaken.

SUGGESTED FURTHER READING

Auster K F 1974 Systemic anaphylaxis in the human being. New Engl J Med 291: 661–664

Baskett P J F, Bennett J A 1971 Pain relief in hospital: the more widespread use of nitrous oxide. Br Med J 2: 509–511

British Medical Journal 1976 First aid in acute myocardial infarction. 1: 356–357

Cawson R A, James J 1973 Adrenal crisis in a dental patient having systemic corticosteroids. Br J Oral Surg 10: 305–309

Dental Clinics of North America 1982 Medical emergencies in the dental office. Saunders, Philadelphia

Drug and Therapeutics Bulletin 1975 Penicillin allergy 13: 9–11

Edmondson H D, Frame J W 1986 Medical emergencies in dental practice. Dental Update 11: 263–273

Freeman N S et al 1977 Office emergencies: an outline of causes, symptoms, and treatment. JADA 94: 91–96

Gray H H 1989 Cardiopulmonary resuscitation. Med Int 71: 2968–2974

Kerr F, Brown M G, Ludwig J B 1975 A double-blind trial of patient-controlled nitrous oxide/oxygen analgesia in myocardial infarctions. Lancet 1: 1397–1400

Marsden K 1989 Guidelines for cardiopulmonary resuscitation. Basic life support. Br Med J 299: 442–447

Pantridge J F, Geddes J S 1976 Management of acute myocardial infarction. Br Med J 2: 168–170

Plumpton F S, Besser G M, Cole P V 1969 Corticosteroid treatment and surgery. 1. An investigation of the indications for steroid cover. 2. The management of steroid cover. Anaesthesia 24: 3–18

Rowlands D J 1976 Cardiac arrest. Br J Hospital Med 16: 310–319

Scully C, Cawson R A 1991 Medical problems in dentistry, 3rd edn. Wright, Bristol

22. Effects of radiation on the mouth and jaws and radiation protection in dentistry

The effects of radiation of special importance to the dental surgeon are the dangers to the patient and operator during diagnostic dental radiography, and the complications arising from radiotherapy of cancer of the mouth.

Types and nature of radiation

Biological effects of irradiation depend on its power of ionisation. An atom is normally electrically neutral and consists of a positively charged nucleus and negatively charged satellite electrons. Loss of an electron leaves a positively charged atom; the addition of an electron produces a negatively charged atom. These positively and negatively charged atoms are ions and the process is known as ionisation.

X-rays and gamma rays strike electrons from atoms in their path. Each electron attaches itself to another atom which thereby becomes negatively charged. One of the pairs of ions thus formed has gained, and the other lost, an electron.

Different types of radiation vary in their ability to penetrate the tissues and in the number of ion pairs they produce in a given distance of travel. Thus an α-particle causes dense ionisation of superficial tissues but is unable to penetrate further; γ-rays, on the other hand, cause a lower ion density but penetrate tissues deeply and may do more harm to body cells as a result.

Units

Radiation dosage is expressed in terms of joules (energy) per kilogram of absorbing tissue, and 1 J/kg is termed 1 gray (1 Gy = 100 cGy). However, the radiation dose equivalent depends on the biological effectiveness of a particular form of radiation and is expressed in sieverts (1 Sv = 1000 mSv). For X rays, the dose equivalent in sieverts is equal to the absorbed dose in grays, and sometimes these terms are used indifferently. An indication of the scale of these units is that exposure of the whole body to 10 Sv is lethal within about 30 days, while exposure to 100 Sv is lethal within hours. For localised therapeutic radiation, a tumour of the head and neck region would require about 50 Sv to kill all the tumour cells. By contrast, natural background radiation in most areas of Britain accounts for less than 2 mSv a year.

Sources of radiation

Sources of radiation are natural or artificial. Everyone is submitted to natural and inescapable sources of radiation. Some artificial sources such as 'fallout' contribute to general background radiation, while others such as X-rays affect individuals only occasionally.

Natural sources. Natural rock and soil formations are radioactive to varying degrees. Cosmic radiation reaches the earth from outer space and is so penetrating that protection is virtually impossible. Food and water may contain traces of radioactive isotopes.

Other sources are:

1. Diagnostic and therapeutic X-rays
2. Radioactive substances handled in various occupations
3. Atomic explosions and fall-out from these explosions
4. Radioactive waste from atomic reactors and industry
5. Radon emitted from rock formations, particularly granite.

HARMFUL EFFECTS OF RADIATION

The harmful effects of ionising radiation can be on the recipients or on their offspring and can be summarised as follows:

1. Direct effects on the tissues
   a. Cellular damage
   b. Systemic effects
       i. Radiation sickness
      ii. Central nervous system syndrome
     iii. Gastrointestinal syndrome
      iv. Haemopoietic syndrome
   c. Carcinogenesis
2. Secondary effects (tissue damage secondary to radiation-induced ischaemia)
3. Genetic effects.

Though the different types of cells of the body respond in a similar way to irradiation, the effect on a particular tissue or organ depends on the interplay of many factors such as the sensitivity of the tissue to radiation, its importance to the body as a whole and its anatomical site. The immediate and delayed effects of radiation on the cells are as follows.

Mechanisms of cell injury by ionising radiation

Though the exact mechanisms are not all clear, it is generally believed that ionising radiation damages tissues in the following ways.

Direct effects. These result from damage, mainly to DNA, by the high energy of radiation. This can cause changes in DNA structure resulting in *point mutations* or *chromosomal breaks*.

In cellular terms the effects may be

1. arrest of mitotic division
2. cell death by apoptosis (energy-dependent nuclear compaction, and nuclear and cellular fragmentation)

Indirect effects. In cellular terms these result from ionisation of water and formation of toxic, free radicals. Endothelial cells are not merely more vulnerable, but obstruction of the vessels they line has far-reaching effects on the tissues supplied. The endothelial cells swell or die and thrombosis follows. The small lumens of capillaries and small arteries are readily obstructed in this way.

Systemic effects (acute radiation syndromes)

Acute radiation syndrome (radiation shock) is the term given to the effects of massive doses of radiation to a localised area or of lesser doses to the whole body. They result from such causes as atomic bombing or severe radiation accidents, as at Chernobyl. After whole body exposure to 2–5 Sv, survival is possible with adequate treatment, but exposure to 5–20 Sv is usually rapidly lethal. Exposure to 50 Sv or more is lethal within 24 hours from damage to the brain (CNS syndrome). Also vulnerable are the gastrointestinal tract and the bone marrow.

In Hiroshima and Nagasaki acute radiation syndromes caused tens of thousands of deaths within hours or days, as well as consequences such as leukaemia, which are still developing almost half a century later.

Radiation sickness is the term given to the effects on several body systems of doses of more than 5 Sv or heavier doses to part of the body, particularly the upper trunk. It is therefore a possible consequence of irradiation for cancer of the breast or lung.

Symptoms can start within hours and include headache, debility, nausea and vomiting, or diarrhoea and often anxiety and insomnia. Heavier doses can cause dysrhythmias and hypotension.

After these prodromal symptoms, if the dosage has been sufficiently great, more severe effects can follow after variable latent periods. These effects depend on the total dose and nature of the ionising radiation and, to some extent, on the part of the body exposed.

Neoplastic change

This phenomenon is of a different type from those just described; it is uncommon and characterised by a long latent interval, usually several years, between the first exposure to irradiation and appearance of the lesion. Malignant change usually affects those who have received large doses of irradiation such as those given for the treatment of cancer, or many smaller doses repeated over a long period. Examples of neoplastic change caused by irradiation include the following:

1. *Cancer of the skin* sometimes develops in persons, particularly radiologists, who have repeatedly

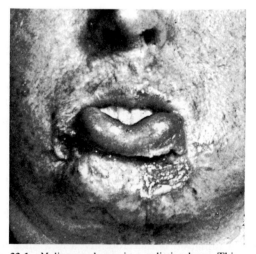

Fig. 22.1 Malignant change in a radiation burn. This patient, a woman of 55, had been given irradiation for lupus, some years previously. There is a chronic radiation burn of the skin with scarring around the periphery, and a carcinoma has developed in the ulcerated area.

allowed their hands to get in the path of the rays. This has been known to happen to a dentist who was used to holding intraoral films in place with his fingers. Carcinoma of the skin may also affect patients who have received radiotherapy for a neoplasm, or for superficial conditions such as tuberculosis (lupus) of the skin, or even unwanted hair.

2. *Bone sarcomas* were a complication of the ingestion of radioactive paints. This is now rare, but the dangers of Strontium 90 in fall-out, in this connection, cannot yet be assessed.

3. *Leukaemia* is one of the most common complications of radiation. Radiologists and survivors from atomic explosions have shown a high incidence of this disease, which may sometimes also follow therapeutic radiation of the spine for rheumatic disease.

4. *The salivary glands.* A disproportionate increase in salivary gland cancer developed after the atomic explosions at Hiroshima and Nagasaki. Salivary gland cancer has also been noted as a complication of therapeutic irradiation of the head and neck area. In a case/control study an increased incidence of salivary gland neoplasms, particularly malignant tumours, has been reported to be related to dental diagnostic radiography.

5. *Sarcoma of the tongue, jaw or other parts of the mouth* has, on a few occasions, followed irradiation of oral cancer.

Overall, however, the tissues most susceptible to radiation-associated carcinoma are the bone marrow, breast, lung and thyroid. In the region of the mouth the parotid glands appear to be most susceptible.

The mechanisms of neoplastic change following irradiation are probably the result of damage to nuclear DNA. Though it is uncommon, it is a serious and often lethal complication that forbids the use of irradiation for anything but the treatment of malignant disease.

Genetic effects of radiation

The effects of radiation just described are upon the person receiving it; genetic effects are upon subsequent generations.

Small doses of radiation, much less than the amount necessary to damage cells or to produce detectable signs of injury, affect the genes. Mutation of genes takes place normally and is one of the factors in the process of evolution; the effect of radiation is to increase the rate of mutations. When radiation reaches the gonads the patient's offspring may suffer from congenital disorders produced by such a mutation. Apart from increasing the number of mutations, there is no evidence that irradiation can cause any special abnormalities. Nevertheless, it is believed that these mutations will be generally harmful.

The increased risk of neoplasia and the possibility of harmful genetic effects is the main basis of the current concern about radiation and has been the stimulus for the introduction of legislation to limit radiation for medical purposes—*including dental radiography*—as discussed later.

Importance of the various sources of irradiation

The danger to the population in peacetime from various sources of radiation may be considered under three main headings, as follows.

1. Background radiation

This is radiation to which the general population is exposed and cannot escape. It emanates from natural sources, from the escape of radioactive material from atomic explosions (fall-out) and from atomic power plants.

The amount of background radiation received by an individual is small when compared (for example) with a course of deep X-ray therapy, but is not insignificant. The effect of background radiation is admittedly unknown but it is potentially dangerous because of effects on the genes and because, by its cumulative effects, it may increase the incidence of neoplasms such as leukaemia.

A danger of atomic fall-out is the dissemination of Strontium 90. This isotope is taken up by bones and developing teeth and, in sufficient dosage, is known to cause development of bone sarcomas. The effects on the population of the ingestion of this substance are unknown but the hazard is obvious.

Domestic radon exposure. More than a century ago, miners in central Europe (Schneeburg and Joachimsthal) developed a then-unidentifiable but fatal lung disease. This was later recognised as lung cancer resulting from the inhalation of the radioactive gas radon 222 from the surrounding rocks. More recently it has become appreciated that radon in significant amounts is emitted from rocky strata, particularly granite, underlying many residential areas such as Cornwall and other parts of the West Country, Aberdeen, Cumbria and elsewhere.

In the USA the levels of radon 222 and its decay products in some homes is over 200 times what is regarded as a 'safe' level. It has been estimated that 5000 to 20 000 cases of lung cancer may be at least partly due to domestic radon inhalation.

In view of the possible dangers of radiation in relatively low dosage, every precaution must be taken to minimise an individual's total dose. Particular care should therefore be taken during the use of radiographic apparatus.

2. Special occupational hazards

These are faced by radiologists and radiographers, and by workers with radioactive isotopes in research and industry. The effect from these hazards is reduced by appropriate methods of protection and care on the part of the workers. Even under these circumstances there is a substantial increase in the total amount of radiation received by the individual. Greater amounts of radiation received in these occupations are known to cause cancer of the skin or leukaemia. Accidents with highly radioactive isotopes can be fatal or cause serious injuries or cancer later.

3. Hazards of radiotherapy

Irradiation is widely used for the treatment of malignant disease. The aim is to give a dose of radiation lethal to the tumour but, as far as possible, restricted in its effects to the growth. A heavy dose of radiation is therefore given to a small area of the body. If an overdose is given, tissues other than the tumour are damaged or destroyed and a radiation burn results. Even when the dose is carefully regulated, tissues in the neighbourhood of the tumour may suffer the indirect effects of radiation. Damage to the blood supply caused in this way makes the tissues vulnerable to injury and infection for years afterwards. In the case of the jaw, radiation-osteomyelitis may be the result.

Neoplastic change in the tissues near the site of irradiation is another, though uncommon, complication of therapeutic radiation.

EFFECTS OF RADIOTHERAPY ON THE MOUTH AND JAWS

The mouth and jaws may suffer immediate damage from the direct effects of radiation on the cells, or delayed effects from injuries to the blood supply.

Direct damage to adjacent tissues such as radiation mucositis is an unavoidable complication of therapeutic radiation but is generally mild and temporary. Indirect damage with its virtually permanent effect on the blood supply and persistently impaired local response to injury and infection is usually a much more serious problem.

Gross overdose causes a radiation burn; this is rarely seen nowadays. The tissues are made more susceptible to damage of this sort by sepsis, a poor blood supply or by repeated courses of radiation.

A radiation burn is heralded by pain and swelling developing near the end of a course of treatment. The necrotic tissues break down, forming an ulcer with a thickened edge, surrounded by erythema and oedema. Damage to the blood vessels delays healing of the burn, which may persist for a year or more.

The main measures are to control infection with antibiotics and, if possible, to excise the dead area and graft fresh tissue to healthy surroundings.

The following may be affected.

The skin

The weak penetrating powers of the radiation given by older types of therapeutic X-ray apparatus entailed that irradiation of a deeply situated tumour often led to damage to more superficial tissues.

Ultra-high-voltage equipment, linear accelerators, or radioactive isotopes of cobalt give deeply-penetrating radiation. Superficial damage is also minimised by irradiating a deeply placed growth from several points at different angles. Each dose of radiation passes through a different area of the superficial tissues, each of which receives a relatively low dose of radiation. Another method is to centre the rays on the tumour and to rotate the apparatus round the patient.

Radiation damage to the skin resembles in some ways a simple burn, but the effects go more deeply and the amount of damage to underlying tissues is disproportionate to the superficial injury.

The first change is erythema, appearing 6 to 48 hours after exposure; the subcutaneous tissues become oedematous and swollen. With mild overdosage the erythema and oedema resolve and the skin returns to normal. With severe overdose, damage to the epithelium and its appendages, to underlying connective tissue and to blood vessels, leads to permanent scarring. Hair follicles and sweat glands are destroyed. Coarse bundles of connective tissue are laid down, and the poor blood supply prevents full recovery of the epithelium, which remains thin and flattened.

Clinically the scarred area of skin appears tense, shiny, dry and atrophic; it becomes patchily pigmented and marked with telangiectases.

Malignant change may later develop in this scar and must be distinguished from recurrence of the original neoplasm.

Mucous membranes

The changes are essentially the same as those in the skin. The initial inflammatory reaction is seen as an area of erythema. After about a week, superficial cells which have been killed appear as a yellowish white membrane over the surface. This is usually shed after a further week, and the mucosa recovers its normal appearance. Minor salivary glands in the immediate area of irradiation are damaged or destroyed. These changes are known as *radiation mucositis*.

Heavier exposure causes loss of the full thickness of epithelium, leaving raw areas. Gross overdosage may cause mucous membrane and connective tissue to slough away entirely, exposing the bone. The rate and degree of healing then depend on the severity of damage to the blood vessels but may take years. In addition to the visible changes,

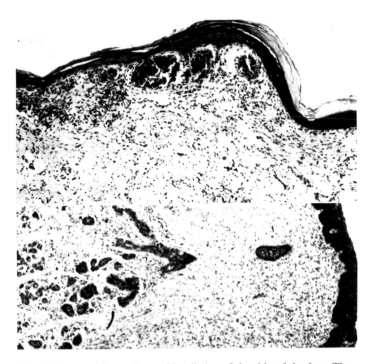

Fig. 22.2 (*upper*) Late effects of irradiation of the skin of the face. The epithelium is thin and atrophic. The skin appendages (hair follicles and sweat glands) have been destroyed; abnormal, thin-walled blood vessels (telangiectases) have formed just under the epithelium in the otherwise almost avascular dermis, and there are groups of chronic inflammatory cells (× 40).

Fig. 22.3 (*lower*) Late effects of irradiation of the mouth. Section of part of the tongue of a patient who had been irradiated about eighteen months previously. The mucous membrane is thin and there is an infiltration of chronic inflammatory cells. The mucous gland to the left has been largely destroyed, but some duct tissue remains (× 40).

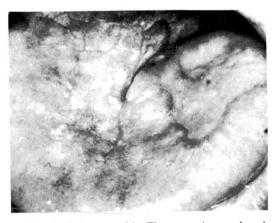

Fig. 22.4 Radiation mucositis. The tongue is smooth and covered by a whitish film due to death of superficial epithelial cells. On the right the full thickness of epithelium has been destroyed, leaving a raw area covered with fibrin.

the earliest effect noticed by the patient is loss or disturbance of taste sensation.

Salivary glands

Secretory tissue is sensitive to irradiation, and minor damage with temporary drying of the mouth is an almost unavoidable complication of irradiation of an oral tumour. More severe damage causes permanent reduction of secretion. The viscosity of the saliva changes and its lubricating power is lost. The mouth may feel uncomfortable even though it appears moist. More severe damage still is characterised by death of all secretory cells in the affected area, followed by fibrosis.

In cases where salivary secretion is reduced or

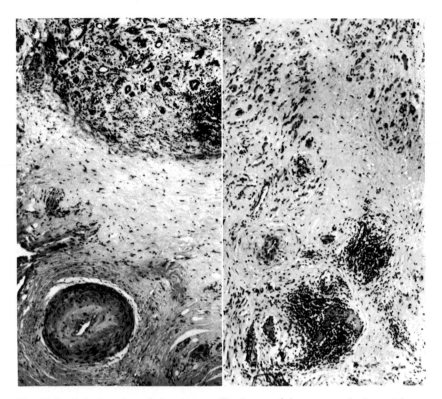

Fig. 22.5 (*left*) Chronic radiation damage. The lumen of the artery at the lower left has been almost obliterated by thickening of the intima. To the right there is an atrophic salivary gland of which only duct tissue remains in a fibrous mass infiltrated by chroinic inflammatory cells (× 40).

Fig. 22.6 (*right*) Chronic radiation damage to the tongue. Chronic inflammatory cells surround fragments of necrotic debris; nearby is an obliterated blood vessel. The rest of the tissue consists of coarse bundles of collagen among which can be seen shrunken muscle fibres in cross section (× 40).

affected in quality, patients may be helped by the use of artificial saliva, either flavoured methyl cellulose 2% (Hypromellose) or lemon-flavoured glycerine mouth-rinses.

An increased incidence of salivary gland cancer followed the atomic explosions at Hiroshima and Nagasaki and has been noted as a complication of therapeutic irradiation of the head and neck area. In a case/control study an increased incidence of salivary gland neoplasms, particularly malignant tumours, has also been reported to be related to dental diagnostic radiography, and another study by the same workers reported a significant association between intracranial meningiomas and full mouth dental radiography before the age of 20.

However, there findings have not as yet been confirmed.

Fibrosis and ankylosis of the temporomandibular joint

Modern sources of radiation are deeply penetrating. Degenerative changes in tissues through which radiation has passed are followed by fibrosis. This effect is most troublesome when the dose of radiation has been heavy and when the path of the rays is in the neighbourhood of the temporomandibular joint or masticatory muscles. In severe cases the skin, subcutaneous tissues and fascia covering the muscles become bound together and an area of muscle is replaced by fibrous tissue forming a boardlike layer. There may be limitation of movement of the temporomandibular joint or complete ankylosis. Treatment is difficult. Exercises to maintain movement of the joint and prevent contraction of the fibrous tissue should be instituted before limitation of movement becomes permanent. Later it may be necessary to separate muscle attachments by such operations as coronoidectomy on the affected side. In the most severe cases section of the angle or body of the mandible may have to be carried out to create a false joint.

The teeth and bone

The pulps may be killed by radiation; the teeth become brittle, and a well-recognised complication is rapid caries due mainly to the reduced flow of saliva. These effects on the teeth emphasise the importance of clearing the mouth before irradiation is begun unless the teeth and supporting tissues are exceptionally healthy and well cared for.

Growing bone and cartilage are sensitive to irradiation, which may stop development.

Heavy doses of radiation to bone can kill the osteocytes, producing aseptic necrosis. The bone becomes chalky and brittle but remains attached

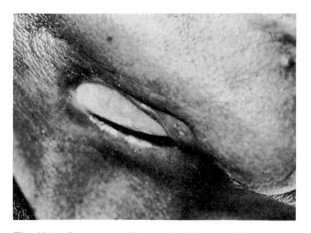

Fig. 22.8 Gross osteoradionecrosis of the mandible. The whole of the right mandible was non-vital but remained attached. Most of the upper border was exposed in the mouth while part of the lower border can be seen here protruding through the skin.

to adjacent healthy bone, from which there is no sharp line of demarcation. Inflammatory changes are slight provided that there is no secondary infection. The periosteum may lay down a thin layer of poorly formed bone to surround the dead tissue. The damaged tissue with its poor blood supply, and the mass of necrotic bone, are highly susceptible to infection. If infection can be avoided the necrotic bone may cause no symptoms but appears more radiopaque.

Irradiation-induced osteomyelitis

Osteomyelitis follows infection which reaches bone killed by the direct action of irradiation; this may occasionally happen soon after treatment. More often osteomyelitis is a late complication as a result of the damage to blood vessels by radiation. This causes ischaemia of the tissues, upon which infection becomes superimposed. Widespread infection and necrosis is the result of these combined effects.

The usual precipitating cause is infection around the teeth or, more often, extractions, and tissues remain vulnerable for years afterwards. A denture can also ulcerate the mucosa, precipitating osteomyelitis, and some regard heavy irradiation of the mouth as a contraindication to the fitting of dentures.

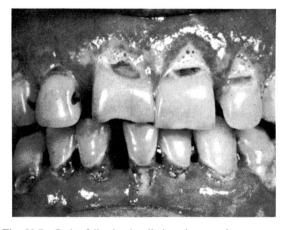

Fig. 22.7 Caries following irradiation. Acute caries particularly affects the necks of the teeth. The normal glistening film of saliva on the enamel is absent but bubbles of frothy fluid surround the gingival margins.

DENTAL MANAGEMENT OF PATIENTS RECEIVING RADIOTHERAPY

Pre-irradiation management

Many patients who receive radiotherapy for cancer of the head and neck are of middle age or over, are often edentulous or, if dentate, the teeth are unhealthy. These deteriorate rapidly after irradiation, with attendant complications, and they should be removed before treatment.

In patients with well-cared-for mouths, particularly the small number of young patients with malignant tumours, extensive extractions are probably not essential.

The procedure before irradiation should therefore be as follows:

1. *Assessment of the patient.* Preservation of the teeth (with its attendant hazards) can only be allowed if they are healthy and if the patient both wants to preserve them and will take the necessary care.

   The level of caries activity and the state of the periodontal tissues must be carefully evaluated. The soft tissues should also be examined for any other lesions which may complicate treatment.
2. *Radiographic examination.* A panoramic radiograph, supplemented as necessary with periapical and occlusal films, should be carried out to detect unsuspected disease.
3. *Extractions.* Unhealthy teeth should be extracted and any other lesions, such as a cyst of the jaw, should be dealt with.
4. *Periodontal treatment.* Thorough dental prophylaxis should be carried out and the periodontal state improved as far as possible.

During the course of radiotherapy oral hygiene procedures should be carried out weekly, preferably with a fluoridated polishing paste. Any infection, such as candidosis, developing as a complication of radiotherapy, should be treated with antifungal agents.

Post-irradiation management

The mouth and neck should be examined for recurrent disease or development of new lesions.

Regular dental prophylaxis should be carried out and preventive measures should be reinforced as follows.

1. *Oral hygiene.*
2. *Flouride rinses.*
3. *Dietary advice.* The patient should be *forbidden* to eat sweets and candy bars, and a non-cariogenic diet should be organised.

   Restorative dentistry should be carried out as necessary.
4. *Post-irradiation xerostomia.* Dryness of the mouth is troublesome and promotes infection. Xerostomia is managed as well as possible by the use of frequent sips of fluid and some form of artificial saliva, as described earlier (Ch. 17). Post-irradiation xerostomia is particularly difficult to ameliorate, possibly because of altered mucosal sensation.
5. *Diagnostic radiography. Essential* dental radiography is permissible. The dose from routine dental diagnostic radiographs is insignificant in comparison with the dose that has been given for therapeutic purposes.

Treatment of complications

When the dose of radiation has been heavy, osteomyelitis can develop after extractions in spite of all precautions and sometimes even many years after therapy. The best that can be done may be simply to retain the teeth but control the local infection by use of antibiotics. In more favourable cases extractions may be considered under protection of adequate antibiotic cover. A single, simple extraction may be done first as a trial; an adequate dose of an antibiotic should be given before operation, the tooth removed with the minimum of trauma, and antibiotic therapy continued until healing is established. A dry socket may be an inevitable result but, provided that infection localised to this extent, further extractions can be carried out with similar precautions.

Even in the edentulous patient, lower dentures can traumatise the underlying tissues, causing ulceration and sometimes deep extension of infection. If may be inadvisable therefore to allow irradiated patients to wear a lower denture.

COMPLICATIONS OF IRRADIATION—SUMMARY

Radiation causes direct damage by killing cells but often a secondary effect, namely tissue ischaemia caused by obliterative endarteritis, is more troublesome. This change in bone leaves it persistently vulnerable to infection following minor injury or extractions.

Heavy doses of radiation may cause a radiation burn or necrosis of bone and destroy salivary glands.

Therapeutic radiation of oral tumours of moderate radiosensitivity should cause little more than temporary discomfort. The mouth may be dry for a time; there is soreness as superficial epithelium is shed, and the sense of taste is impaired. With heavier dosage salivary secretion is permanently reduced. However slight the symptoms, any remaining teeth are more susceptible to caries; regular dental care, avoidance of sweet-eating, and use of fluorides are essential. In addition, the bone of the jaw has a reduced blood supply and is prone to infection; prophylactic clearance of the teeth before radiation is essential in patients with neglected mouths.

HAZARDS OF DENTAL RADIOGRAPHY

The output of radiant energy from dental X-ray apparatus is small and the radiation is not normally directed towards any particularly vulnerable sites. Nevertheless, there is always some scattered radiation reaching other parts of the patient and the operator. This minute amount of energy adds to the level of background radiation and to its dangers. The operator is exposed to this stray radiation for the greater part of his working life and its total effect may not be negligible.

The scatter of X-rays is due to their having some of the properties of light; within the tissues the rays scatter in all directions in much the same way as light is scattered by fog. The main dangers from this scattered (secondary) radiation is to the gonads of the patient and of the operator. In addition, because of the operator's frequent exposure, the cumulative effect of the radiation may be enough to damage the bone marrow and induce leukaemia. The high incidence of leukaemia among medical radiologists before safety measures were rigorously observed shows the reality of this danger.

Reduction of radiation hazards

The widespread concern about radiation hazards, particularly their potential cancer-inducing and genetic effects, has led to the formation of an International Commission on Radiological Protection (ICRP). The aim is to reduce radiation dosage to the absolute minimum.

The doses of radiation for diagnostic radiographs are small but not negligible. In the past, dentists have lost fingers or developed cancer as a result of holding films in patients' mouths. One dentist, at least, is known to have died from radiation exposure, and there was a significantly increased incidence of leukaemia among medical radiologists before the risks were appreciated.

The cancer risk from radiotherapy is well recognised but the cancer risk from diagnostic radiography is uncertain. However, a recent report concluded that there was a significant association between dental radiography and cancers of the parotid glands. Since the only known cause of salivary gland cancers is ionising radiation, this report, though unconfirmed, can hardly be ignored. Another study reported a significant association between intracranial meningiomas and full mouth dental radiography before the age of 20.

It should also be noted that dental radiography is not merely a greater consumer of X-ray film than medical radiography, but also the number of dental radiographs (unlike medical radiographs) has increased dramatically over the years. The situation has been encapsulated in a *Lancet* Editorial entitled 'Dental X-rays for caries or cash?'.

There appears to be no threshold dose for radiation to contribute to cancer risks. Nevertheless the greater the individual or cumulative dose the greater the risk. As a result, the cumulative exposure of staff to X-rays in a busy practice can be significant.

ALARA (As Low As Reasonably Achievable) is the acronym defining the essential principle underlying the reduction of radiation risks.

Moreover the recommendations regarding radiation dose reduction are enforceable by law in Britain through regulations made under the Health and Safety at Work Act.

The Department of Health booklet *Radiation Protection in Dental Practice* is essential reading for all dentists taking radiographs. They must be fully familiar with its contents and implement its recommendations. Further advice can be obtained from the National Radiation Protection Board (NRPB). However, the employer (such as the principal of a large practice), even if he himself takes no radiographs, still has the ultimate responsibility for compliance with the regulations.

All dentists who use radiographs must therefore possess the Core of Knowledge (Appendix III) required for radiation safety. Failure to implement the Approved Code of Practice may bring action from the Health and Safety Inspectorate. This could lead to an embargo on all radiography until the situation is remedied. During such a period, a practice would be greatly limited in the work that could be done. It is also conceivable that such neglect might also be regarded as a breach of National Health Service conditions of service and lead to difficulties with the local Dental Services Committee (Ch. 25).

If the dentist continued to take radiographs after being found to fail to take the required precautions he might render himself liable to prosecution under the Health and Safety at Work Acts.

It should also be noted that dentists must be fully aware of correct radiographic techniques and processing procedures, since dose limitation is highly dependent on taking good-quality radiographs and avoiding re-takes.

The basic precautions therefore include the following.

1. Take radiographs only when absolutely necessary.
2. Define a Controlled Area round the X-ray set, and exclude all persons from it, other than the patient, during radiography.
3. Use equipment of adequate power (preferably 70 kVp) that does not emit stray soft X-rays.
4. Collimate the beam to the minimum area necessary. For intraoral films the field should not be more than 6 cm in diameter.
5. Use a filter (not less than 1.5 mm aluminium for tube voltages up to 70 kV) to block soft X-rays.
6. Limit the area exposed. For intraoral films for example, a field-defining spacer cone should be used to maintain a minimal focal-spot-to-skin distance of not less than 20 cm for voltages over 60 kV.
7. *Make sure that the films are of the optimal quality to avoid re-takes*, by precautions which include the following:
   a. Use the fastest film (D or E speed) possible compatible with image quality, and use intensifying screens when appropriate
   b. Place the patient and film correctly for the view required
   c. Give the correct exposure
   d. Process the film for the recommended period at the correct temperature in fresh developer (replaced fortnightly)
   e. Make sure that the film is fully fixed and washed to avoid degradation of the image by stains
   f. Review all procedures if image quality starts to deteriorate.
8. Never hold the film in the patient's mouth.*
9. Stand at least 2 m from the tube and patient, outside the Controlled Area and the line of the beam.
10. Monitor staff if the workload exceeds 150 intraoral or 50 panoramic films a week. A film monitor may be worn and a lead protective apron may be required.**
11. Provide a lead apron protection for the patient's body and particularly for women who are of childbearing age or are pregnant.

---

*If this is done, the hand is exposed to approximately 4000 times the dose that would have been received if the operator were standing 2 m away. The remainder of the body would also receive a correspondingly increased dose. Overall, one of the best protections from radiation is distance, since the intensity falls off according to the inverse square law.
**The current dose limit for exposure for radiation workers is 50 mSv/year, though this may be reduced, if a recent recommendation is implemented, to 15 mSv/year.

12. The X-ray equipment should be of such a nature that

   a. radiation ceases immediately pressure on the switch is released even when a timer is fitted

   b. the emission warning light operates synchronously with emission of X-rays. The apparatus must also be fully assessed by a competent authority such as the National Radiation Protection Board, to check on these points as well as radiation dosage, emission of stray X-rays and authentication of regular maintenance checks at not more than 3-year intervals.

Special precautions have to be taken in large practices with a heavy workload (more than 300 intraoral or 50 panoramic films a week). In these circumstances a separate X-ray room has to be provided and must be large enough to allow the operator to keep 2 m away from the apparatus and patient. The walls should be dense enough (brick or its equivalent), or covered with lead ply, to shield adjacent working areas.

Panoramic radiography

Radiation dosage can sometimes be reduced by using panoramic films which, by replacing multiple intraoral films, can reduce overall dosage. Unsuspected disease in the jaws may also be revealed. Panoramic films are particularly useful for such indications as fractures of the jaws. However, for routine dentistry, detail is generally less good than in intraoral films. Doses for individual dental films are as follows:

   1 intraoral = 10 μSv
   1 extraoral = 15 μSv
   1 panoramic = 80 μSv

Intraoral panoramic units give unnecessarily high exposure to tissues, such as the tongue, outside the field being examined. Such units should be replaced or, if still being used, tongue protection should be provided.

SUGGESTED FURTHER READING

Berger R P, Symington J M 1990 Long-term clinical manifestation of osteoradionecrosis of the mandible. J Oral Maxillofac Surg 48: 82–84

Council of Scientific Affairs 1989 Harmful effects of ultraviolet radiation. J Am Med Assoc 262: 380–384

Editorial 1983 Dental X-rays for caries or cash? Lancet 2: 609

Epstein J B, Wong F L S, Stevenson-Moore P 1987 Osteoradionecrosis: clinical experience and a proposal for classification. J Oral Maxillofac Surg 45: 104–110

Evans J H 1990 Leukaemia and radiation. Nature 354: 16–17

Gratt B M, White S C, Halse A 1988 Clinical recommendations for the use of D-speed film, E-speed film and xeroradiography. J Am Dent Assoc 117: 609–614

Henshaw D L, Eatough J P, Richardson R B 1990 Radon as a causative factor of myeloid leukaemia and other cancers. Lancet 335: 1008–1012

Hutchison I L, Cope M, Delpe D T et al 1990 The investigation of osteoradionecrosis of the mandible by near infra-red spectroscopy. J Oral Maxillofac Surg 28: 150–154

Hutchison I L, Cullum I D, Langford J A et al 1990 The investigation of osteoradionecrosis of the mandible by 99m TC methylene disphosphonate radionuclide bone scans. J Oral Maxillofac Surg 28: 143–149

Keene H J, Fleming T J 1987 Prevalence of caries-associated microflora after radiotherapy in patients with cancer of the head and neck. Oral Surg, Oral Med, Oral Pathol 64: 421–426

Marciani R D, Ownby H E 1986 Osteoradionecrosis of the jaws. J Oral Maxillofac Surg 44: 218–223

Morton M E 1986 Osteoradionecrosis: a study of the incidence in the Northwest of England. Br J Oral Maxillofac Surg 24: 323–331

Morton M E, Simpson W 1986 The management of osteoradionecrosis of the jaws. Br J Oral Maxillofac Surg 24: 332–341

Standing Dental Advisory Committee (undated) Radiation protection in dental practice. Department of Health, London

The Ionising Radiations Regulations 1988 Guidance notes for the protection of persons from ionising radiation in medical and dental use. Department of Health, HMSO, London

Whaites E 1991 The essentials of dental radiography and radiology. Churchill Livingstone, Edinburgh

Widmark G, Sagne S, Heikel P 1989 Osteoradionecrosis of the jaws. Int J Oral Maxillofac Surg 18: 302–306

23. Oral disease in the child

Dentistry in the child should logically start with teething, but it is usually the family doctor who has to deal with this largely mythical disorder.

The chief problem is that of dental caries, though it has shown a great decline in recent years. Childhood caries differs from that in the adult in respect of its great rapidity of development; reactionary dentine often cannot form fast enough to protect the pulp. The deciduous teeth can sometimes decay down to the gum level in a quite remarkably short space of time.

Gingivitis is also common but destructive periodontal disease (juvenile periodontitis) is a rarity.

Establishment of good oral hygiene habits during childhood is of the utmost importance and, ideally, children's dentistry should be synonymous with preventive dentistry.

Dentistry in children, partly because of its involvement with orthodontics, has become a specialty of its own and will not therefore be discussed in detail here.

Teething

Teething is the term given to the supposed troubles associated with the eruption of deciduous teeth. In the past, teething has been thought, quite irrationally, to be a cause of serious illness, and the enormously high infant mortality of the 18th century was often ascribed to it at the time. Arbuthnot in 1732 wrote that 'Above one-tenth part of all children die in teething (some of them from gangrene)'.

Eruption starts with movement of the tooth from within the alveolar process and continues until the tooth is in occlusion. During this process the crown passes through the gingiva to appear in the oral cavity; this stage is supposed to be the source of all the trouble. The crown of the unerupted tooth is, however, covered by enamel epithelium which, as it nears the surface, fuses with the gingival epithelium. Breakdown of epithelial cells at the centre of this point of union exposes the tip of the crown to the oral cavity.

Thus there is no rupture of the mucosa and no wound to bleed or become infected.

There are *no systemic complications of teething*. During this period the child is susceptible to many infections, since protection conferred by passive transfer of maternal antibodies has been lost and the infant's defence mechanisms are poorly developed. Purely coincidental systemic infections are the reason why teething has been blamed for diseases ranging from gastroenteritis to convulsions.

A carefully conducted study on teething carried out on 126 normal infants in an institution in Finland has clearly showed that eruption of a tooth bore no relation to the incidence of infection, diarrhoea, bronchitis, fever, rashes or convulsions.

The danger inherent in the belief that teething can cause systemic upsets is that early signs of serious infections, such as otitis media, tonsillitis, meningitis, gastroenteritis, pneumonia or pyelitis may be dismissed as 'teething', and the child given a 'teething powder' or a purgative. Whenever a child becomes unwell during teething, a cause outside the mouth must therefore be looked for.

In the past, teething powders containing mercury were given but caused pink disease (acrodynia). There is also, of course, no justification for the giving of purgatives or any other drugs.

Oral infections that may coincide with teething.

Stomatitis is *not* caused by teething but may happen to *coincide* with it.

There are two main causes:

1. *Thrush* usually precedes teething and can develop at any time in the neonatal period.

2. *Herpes simplex*. Primary herpetic stomatitis (Ch. 15) is the main cause of a sore mouth at the time of teething but is common in this age group only in poor and underdeveloped communities.

The initiation of dental care

A few infants are brought by zealous parents for advice about care of the teeth almost as soon as they have erupted. Most children are brought at the age of 2 or 3, when caries may have started. This, however, is an ideal time to put the patient's and parents' feet on the road to preventive care. In fact the main emphasis in dentistry for children must be on prevention.

There are few conditions of the mouth peculiar to children, who share most of the common oral diseases with adults. The principles of management of these common diseases are also the same for both, though there are differences in detail.

The features of dentistry special to childhood can be summarised as follows:

1. The problems of managing children
2. Teaching the principles of preventive dental care
3. Orthodontic care if necessary
4. Oral diseases special to children
5. Management of the handicapped child.

Dental disease

Both caries and gingivitis start early but childhood is the time when caries is most active, as the teeth are more vulnerable and sweet-eating or the use of syrup-soaked comforters accelerate the process. The management of caries and its sequels or—preferably—its prevention forms the vast bulk of dental treatment for children. At this stage gingivitis is reversible or entirely preventable if the teeth are brushed effectively.

Interacting with both these diseases in many children is the need for orthodontic treatment. Irregularities of the teeth can create additional stagnation areas and make plaque control more difficult. Conversely, early loss of teeth (usually as a consequence of decay) can create a need for orthodontic treatment to enable the permanent successors to erupt into the arch. However, orthodontic appliances themselves enhance stagnation so that plaque control is more difficult.

Premature loss of deciduous teeth can leave too little space for the permanent successors, which can become malpositioned as a consequence. To maintain an intact arch for as long as necessary various types of pulp treatment are often used in children, in whom a less long-lasting effect is needed than in the adult.

Orthodox endodontic treatment of deciduous

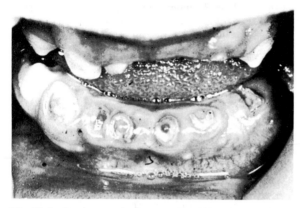

Fig. 23.1 Rampant caries in a young child. The anterior teeth are destroyed down to gum level leaving the pulp exposed but vital. Severe caries affecting the anterior teeth is a characteristic effect of allowing the child to suck a syrup-soaked comforter.

molars is technically difficult because of the narrow and often curved root canals and limited access. In any case, such efforts are rarely justified when the aim is to retain the tooth only for a limited period. Neglected caries and periapical infection of a deciduous tooth can also damage the underlying successor, but this is rare.

Injuries to the teeth

Injuries to the anterior teeth are particularly common in children. Trauma or caries exposing the pulp of the permanent incisors brings with it the problems of root canal treatment of a tooth with an open apex, as discussed in Chapter 5.

Analgesic choice in childhood—Reye's syndrome

This syndrome of rapidly developing liver failure with encephalopathy typically, but rarely, follows childhood viral infections such as chickenpox. Increasing drowsiness is followed by death in approximately 30% of cases.

Aspirin appears to increase the risk of Reye's syndrome, particularly if given to a young febrile child, and the number of reported cases in Britain had declined to 29 in 1988/89 following warnings against its use. Aspirin is therefore contraindicated

for dental pain in children under 12, and it is replaced with paracetamol.

ORAL DISEASES OF CHILDREN

As mentioned earlier, caries, though its prevalence has greatly declined, is the chief dental disease of children in terms of frequency and destructiveness of the dentition.

It might be expected that developmental defects would be conspicuous in childhood, but surprisingly often no complaint is made until adult life. Developmental defects have been considered earlier in Chapter 2, but it may be useful to be reminded of them and other diseases particularly likely to be seen in children:

1. *Defects of the teeth*
   Hereditary amelogenesis imperfecta
   a. Hypoplastic type
   b. Hypocalcified type
   Dentinogenesis imperfecta
   Tetracycline pigmentation
   Fluorosis
   Other developmental defects
2. *Periodontal disease*
   Hereditary gingival fibromatosis
   Juvenile periodontitis
   Syndromes associated with juvenile periodontitis
3. *Mucosal disease*
   Herpetic stomatitis
   Hand, foot and mouth disease
   Candidosis (particularly thrush)
   White sponge naevus
   Aphthous stomatitis
   Geographical tongue
4. *Tumours and tumour-like lesions*
   Congenital epulis
   Progonoma (pigmented neuro-ectodermal tumour)
   Cherubism
5. *Temporomandibular joint disease*
   Juvenile chronic arthritis

Dental defects

The chief need is to disguise them to produce a more attractive appearance. They do not in general increase—and fluorosis actually decreases—susceptibility to caries.

Periodontal disease

The main consideration is the control of gingivitis by effective toothbrushing. In adolescence gingivitis often shows prominent inflammatory oedema (so-called hyperplastic gingivitis) but its control is by orthodox means.

Hereditary gingival fibromatosis and juvenile periodontitis are discussed in Chapter 6.

Stomatitis

Infections. Thrush in infancy and herpetic stomatitis or hand, foot and mouth disease at any time in childhood are the only types of infective stomatitis likely to be seen (Ch. 15).

White lesions. Virtually the only white lesion likely to be seen in a child is the white sponge naevus (Ch. 16).

Chronic mucocutaneous candidosis can also produce leukoplakia-like lesions in children but is rare.

Aphthous stomatitis. Aphthae can start at any time after infancy. The features and management are the same as when the disease starts in adolescence or early adult life (Ch. 15). In children, particularly, aphthae have to be distinguished from herpetic stomatitis.

Geographical tongue shows hereditary tendencies and probably remains unnoticed in many infants. In others the appearance causes anxiety or the child may complain of sensitivity to salty or spicy foods. Reassurance is all that can be given, but this is often all that is needed.

Kawasaki's disease (mucocutaneous lymph node syndrome)

This childhood disease is of unknown cause and though considerably more common in Japan, accounts for more than 100 cases a year in Britain and causes approximately twice as many deaths here as Reye's syndrome.

Kawasaki's disease is characterised by fever, a rash, conjunctivitis, redness and oedema of the oral mucosa with swelling of the lingual papillae (strawberry tongue), as well as cervical lymphadenopathy. The chief cause of death is myocardial infarction or myocarditis. Vasculitis is a prominent feature of the pathology.

Tumours and tumour-like lesions

Congenital epulis is a rare lesion present at birth, usually on the anterior maxillary gum. Females are most often affected. The swelling is rounded and up to 2 cm in diameter or, occasionally, even larger. Histologically there are large, pale close-packed granular cells similar to those of the granular cell myoblastoma.

The condition is benign, responds to excision and is so uncommon as to be of little practical importance.

Pigmented neuroectodermal tumour is a rare tumour of the anterior maxilla usually detected in the first year of life (see Ch. 11).

Other tumours of childhood. Malignant neoplasms are rare in childhood. Nevertheless, they are the single largest cause of death (excluding accidents) between the ages of 1 and 15 years. Acute leukaemia accounts for a high proportion, but leukaemic oral changes apart from anaemia or bleeding are uncommon in children.

Swellings of the jaws

Cysts of the jaws are uncommon in children. Developmental cysts, including dentigerous but not—surprisingly—primordial cysts, may occasionally be seen (Ch. 10).

Cherubism sometimes causes bilateral swellings, especially in the region of the angles of the jaws (Ch. 12).

Juvenile chronic arthritis

There are some tens of thousands of children with juvenile arthritis. One type resembles rheumatoid arthritis, while another has features in common with ankylosing spondylitis. The most severe type (Still's disease) causes polyarticular joint destruction, fever and a rash; lymphadenopathy and cardiac disease may be associated. Destruction of the temporomandibular joint can lead to ankylosis and deformity.

THE HANDICAPPED CHILD

The prevalence of major handicaps is surprisingly high and is estimated very approximately as being between 1.5 and 2 per 1000 live births. Of these, mental handicaps account for approximately 0.9 per 1000 and major physical handicaps for the remainder. The management of dental care for these patients varies not merely with the type of handicap but also according to parents' attitudes. Mental or physical handicap does not necessarily mean, however, that any compromise may have to be made with standards of dental care, though in many cases this is inevitable.

The ways in which dental care may have to be modified vary according to the underlying disorder, but the difficulties fall into the following categories:

1. Inability of the child to cooperate during normal dental treatment. This usually means that the patient is also unable to undertake routine home oral care and hygiene.
2. Ability to accept normal dental treatment but inability to carry out normal home oral care and hygiene.
3. Ability to cooperate for normal dental treatment and carry out normal oral hygiene at home, but for whom dental treatment may have to be modified in some way.

The major mental and physical handicaps are summarised below, and this provides an indication of the scale of the problem. One other difficulty that may be met is that occasionally some parents may be reluctant to subject their handicapped children to dental treatment. Others, while wishing for the best for their children, may nevertheless indulge them excessively in sweets to comfort or reward them or as an attempt to compensate for their own delusions of guilt about their child's defects.

Major mental and physical handicaps

Those of particular relevance to dentistry are as follows:

1. *Mental handicaps*
   a. Psychiatric disorders
   b. Subnormality (including Down's syndrome)

2. *Physical disorders*
   a. Cerebral palsy
   b. Epilepsy
   c. Cleft palate
   d. Severe defects of the hands or arms
   e. Heart disease
   f. Haemorrhagic disease (particularly haemophilia)
   g. Diabetes mellitus
   h. Long-term corticosteroid treatment.

Physical and mental defects are frequently combined, as in Down's syndrome and some cases of cerebral palsy.

There are many other types of mental and physical handicap but these are some of the most important in relation to dentistry. As can be seen from their very varied nature, they can affect dental management in several ways.

Mental retardation (often associated with physical disabilities) is by far the largest group of handicapped children needing dental care. All patients with Down's syndrome, many spastics and some epileptics are also mentally retarded. Other handicapping conditions are few compared with these four groups which account for approximately 70–75% of handicapped children.

With patience and sympathy the great majority—perhaps 90% of handicapped children can be satisfactorily treated by conventional means, and general anaesthesia is needed for only a minority.

Psychiatric disorders

This covers a wide range of disorders from emotional disorders to psychotic personalities. At one extreme it may be impossible to communicate with, or manage, autistic children, for example, without heavy sedation or general anaesthesia. At the other, kindness and patience may achieve all that is needed. Those with personality defects can sometimes be exceedingly difficult, in that they may be totally uncooperative in the conscious state in the dental chair and may be equally uncooperative about oral hygiene at home. Like the severely mentally retarded, the best that can be hoped for in such cases may merely be to repair severe dental disease under general anaesthesia.

Mental retardation

Retardation may be unassociated with any physical disorder, or physical defects may be severe, as in some cases of cerebral palsy.

Mentally retarded children do not present any specific dental disorders, but oral hygiene is usually poor; gross accumulation of plaque and gingivitis or destructive periodontal disease are therefore common. Caries is less often severe unless they are fed too many sweets.

The level of dental care and health depends to a large extent therefore on the degree of subnormality. Mildly retarded children can usually be coaxed into accepting regular treatment and (if the parents are adequate) to maintain acceptable standards of oral hygiene. At the other extreme all that may be possible, particularly for the child with continuous uncontrollable muscular activity such as clenching of the jaws, is first aid dentistry under general anaesthesia. All intermediate grades exist but the level of dental health that can be achieved depends greatly upon the level of the dentist's skill and devotion to the task.

Management

The child's ability to cooperate and respond to dental treatment must be assessed. The parent's attitude and intelligence must also be considered.

Most handicapped children are nervous at the prospect of the incomprehensible unknown that dentistry represents, but with gentle sympathetic handling, can come not merely to accept but positively to enjoy dental treatment.

The mildly retarded can with understanding and patience, be managed with no more difficulty than a normal 8- to 10-year-old child. If the child is *unable* to cooperate in the conscious state, then general anaesthesia or sedation may have to be used.

With patience, too, some of these children can eventually be taught how to brush their teeth, but this depends very much on the parents or nurses and on the severity of the mental defect.

Little more than dental first aid can therefore be provided for the severely retarded. Many of these, of course, are institutionalised and there is little hope of their maintaining any oral hygiene.

Heavy sedation may make the problem even worse. The best that can be done is often merely to patch up the teeth as necessary under general anaesthesia to avoid pain and prevent loss of teeth for as long as possible.

Vaccination against hepatitis B is essential for the dentist working with the mentally handicapped, particularly Down's syndrome children in institutions where the carriage rate may be high.

Down's syndrome

Down's syndrome is the most common clinically recognisable type of mental subnormality. The incidence is estimated to be 1 in 700 live births.

Down's syndrome is the result of a chromosomal abnormality, and not usually an hereditary disease. The total chromosome complement is 47 instead of the normal 46. In most cases this is the result of three chromosomes 21 (trisomy 21) instead of the usual two.

General features

Down's children have a characteristic 'mongoloid' facial appearance, abnormalities of the skull and frequently of the dentition, increased susceptibility to infection (particularly viral) due to immune defects and, in up to 50% of cases, congenital cardiovascular disease. Once seen, Down's syndrome is readily recognised but the facial appearance is easier to illustrate than to describe adequately.

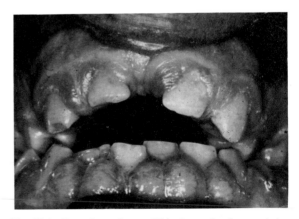

Fig. 23.2 Down's syndrome. This shows the characteristic anterior open bite together with gross gingival hyperplasia caused by phenytoin treatment for concomitant epilepsy.

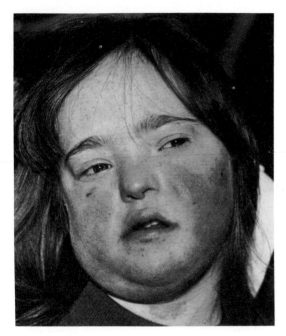

Fig. 23.3 Down's syndrome. This shows both the characteristic facial appearance and a cyanotic flush caused by associated congenital heart disease.

The prominent medial epicanthic skin fold gives the eyes their well-known appearance.

There is hypoplasia of the mid-face, associated with poorly developed paranasal sinuses and a malformed upper respiratory tract. Upper respiratory tract infections are common, and snorting breathing is often a feature.

The underdevelopment of the maxillae is usually associated with a protrusive mandible and a Class III malocclusion, with anterior open bite. Other types of malocclusion are also common.

The tongue is often protrusive and the dorsum is typically very deeply fissured or scrotal. The lips are often everted, thick, dry and crusted. Eruption of the teeth is often delayed, while hypodontia and morphological or hypoplastic defects of the teeth are common. The teeth most commonly absent are (as in normal people) the third molars and maxillary lateral incisors but other teeth are frequently also absent.

Dental disease

This has an unusual pattern; caries activity tends to be low but periodontal disease is common and often rapidly progressive and severe. The low caries activity has been ascribed to the form and spacing of the teeth and to the characteristics of the saliva. This has a high bicarbonate content and pH.

Poor oral hygiene, due to the patient's disabilities and made worse by mouth breathing, contribute to the early onset of periodontal disease. This is otherwise similar in pattern and distribution to that in normal patients, with heavy accumulations of plaque on the teeth. Acute ulcerative gingivitis is common and often recurs.

Rapid progress of periodontal disease with destruction of bone leads to early loss of teeth, particularly the lower anteriors.

These patterns of dental disease associated with the immunodeficiencies characteristic of Down's syndrome present an interesting paradox to those who accept some of the current ideas about the role of immunological mechanisms in caries and periodontal disease.

Associated abnormalities. The high incidence of congenital cardiac defects causes a high mortality during early infancy, and those that survive may be susceptible to bacterial endocarditis.

Susceptibility to infection is increased as there are often defects or deficiencies of some of the white cell series, impaired cell-mediated immunity and, often, abnormal immunoglobulin patterns. Gastrointestinal, respiratory and dermal infections are common, while viral hepatitis B is frequent especially in those in institutions.

Dental management

Management depends upon three factors: the level of oral health and hygiene, the severity of mental defect and the associated abnormalities, particularly cardiovascular disease.

The mental defect varies widely and, although all Down's children are subnormal, some are less severely affected and are trainable to some degree. A mitigating factor is that most of them (though there are exceptions) are good-natured, cooperative within their ability, and affectionate. As a result many parents become devoted to these children. The success of dental treatment is mainly dependent on the level of care provided. The more intelligent ones can be treated normally in the dental chair, while the lowest grades, who are usually institutionalised, must be treated like any other severely retarded child. General anaesthesia may therefore be unavoidable.

In those with congenital heart disease appropriate antibiotic cover must be given, particularly before extractions, to prevent infective endocarditis.

The main difficulty is that of the periodontal state. The more intelligent Down's children may manage a moderate standard of home care, but in many cases extractions may become unavoidable. Treatment of the periodontal state is otherwise by orthodox means. Nevertheless it is preferable to try to retain the teeth as long as possible. Dentures are usually poorly tolerated because of the mental condition, the occlusal abnormalities, the large tongue and poor muscle tone which make retention difficult. Orthodontic treatment is rarely feasible.

Cerebral palsy

These children, often loosely referred to as spastics, suffer various types of neuromuscular dysfunction. Cerebral palsy is common and is one of the most severe handicaps. The neuromuscular dysfunction can be so severe as to make speech impossible (dysarthria) and cause the child to appear mentally defective. As a consequence it has become recognised only in recent years that intelligent children with cerebral palsy have been confined for life to institutions for the mentally retarded. Oddly, the unintelligible noises that a person with cerebral palsy makes in the attempt to communicate may be understandable only by another person with cerebral palsy. Although many spastics are of low intelligence, this is not necessarily the case, and the mental abilities of such children can now be reasonably accurately assessed. The dentist should therefore make sure he knows the child's capabilities.

The three main types of neuromuscular dysfunction due to cerebral palsy are as follows.

Spasticity affects approximately 50% and is characterised by fixed contraction of the affected muscles and general stiffness. This may be so great that it may not even be possible to move an affected limb passively.

Hemiplegia is the most common type of spasticity, and in such cases mental retardation is uncommon but other neurological disorders, such as epilepsy, are frequent. At the other extreme, quadriplegics are frequently mentally retarded but less often epileptic.

Athetosis is characterised by involuntary jerking movements, often of a wriggling character and sometimes accompanied by grimacing. Athetosis is slightly more common than spasticity and probably accounts for about 45% of affected children.

Ataxia is characterised by lack of balance, an unsteady gait and poor control over voluntary muscular movements. It is relatively uncommon and affects about 5–10%.

In addition to variants of these three main types of disease, different parts of the body may be affected to a greater extent than others.

Dental management

Obviously enough, the dental management of these children is difficult, however willing they may be. Many have severe caries and often periodontal disease due to inability to maintain oral hygiene. Considerable skill and experience may therefore be needed to modify treatment procedures to cater for the physical and mental condition of the patient.

The first consideration is adequate assessment of the patient's capabilities, with the help of the physician looking after the child. The dentist can then assess the child's ability to deal with dental disease. If at this stage it is obvious that the child is uncontrollably anxious, then premedication or sedation may be given before treatment.

Provided that the disabilities are not too severe, many of these children can be treated satisfactorily in the dental chair. The chief difficulty with athetotic children is the irregular movements. These may make it impossible to carry out good restorative work and also make it easy for the child to be injured with sharp dental instruments. These children should not be physically restrained but may need general anaesthesia if the movements are too great to make routine dentistry possible. One necessary precaution with conscious athetotic patients is always to use a mouth prop, as the jaws may suddenly clench. The prop should not be kept in the mouth for too long without pauses for rest.

These problems require time, experience and skill to overcome. As a consequence, it is of the utmost importance that the highest standards of preventive dentistry be practised to reduce the amount of time in the dental chair. Time must therefore be spent with both child and parent demonstrating toothbrushing and oral hygiene procedures, and making sure that these are faithfully carried out, if at all possible. An electric toothbrush is usually a great help. The parents must also be made to understand that the more sweets the child eats the more time he will have to spend having dental treatment.

The use of fluoride gels in special trays may be a useful measure which these patients can easily tolerate. It may be possible also for the child to take fluoride tablets regularly.

There are no specific dental defects associated with cerebral palsy but malocclusion (possibly as a result of the abnormal muscle behaviour) is common.

Epilepsy

Minor or even major epilepsy should, with modern methods of treatment, present no special difficulties, unless associated with other handicaps. It is important, however, to minimise the development of fibrous gingival hyperplasia in those on long-term phenytoin by high standards of oral hygiene.

It is also important to be able to recognise and manage a grand mal attack (Ch. 21) should it happen in the dental surgery.

Cleft lip and palate

Cleft defects are present in 2 to 3 per 1000 live births. Cleft lip alone is more common in males and is usually repaired at about 3 months.

Cleft palate is more common in females and is associated in up to 20% with other congenital abnormalities, some of which, such as cardiac defects, may not be obvious but are a potential cause of complications. Clefts are characteristic of many developmental craniofacial syndromes and sometimes associated with mental defect. For example, clefts are present in about 0.5% of cases of Down's syndrome, but in the less common trisomy 13 (Patau's syndrome) mental defect is associated with clefts in 75%, and cardiac defects in 80%.

The surgical repair of cleft palate is typically carried out at about 15 months but dental aspects of management of these patients can include:

1. The making of a plate to facilitate feeding and to prevent collapse of the maxilla
2. Care of the teeth in contact with a plate or simple obdurator
3. Replacement of congenitally missing teeth
4. Treatment of hypoplastic defects of the teeth by crowning or other means
5. Orthodontic treatment
6. Antibiotic cover for extractions when there are cardiovascular defects.

Spina bifida

Spina bifida is the name given to failure of fusion of the vertebral arches. In its mildest form (spina bifida occulta) the defect is common but no more than a radiographic finding, sometimes with a tuft of hair overlying the defect. In its severe forms (spina bifida cystica) there is a gross defect in the lower vertebral canal, through which the meninges and often also nerve tissue protrude as a sac which may be covered by skin. The consequences are paralysis and deformities of the lower limbs with loss of sensation and reflexes, incontinence and other complications. Meningitis is an obvious hazard and epilepsy is frequently associated.

Since the upper part of the body is normal, the main difficulty in dental management is getting the child into the chair. Associated epilepsy may also affect dental management.

Hydrocephalus

Hydrocephalus may be seen in isolation or be associated with spina bifida. Compression of the cerebral tissue can cause severe mental defect, but the intracranial pressure may be relieved by insertion of a catheter to shunt the cerebrospinal fluid directly into the right atrium or sometimes the peritoneal cavity. This shunt is susceptible to infection, and, for dental operations likely to cause bacteraemia, prophylactic antibiotics should be given as for infective endocarditis.

In addition to the disabilities already mentioned, severe hydrocephalus can cause the skull to be so distended and heavy that the head has to be supported during treatment.

Severe defects of the limbs

These are rare but have been brought to public notice by the thalidomide tragedy. One of the striking effects of this drug is phocomelia, that is absence of the proximal part of a limb. Thus the hands, often also defective, are attached close to the shoulder.

These children can receive normal dental chair care, but are totally dependent on parents for toothbrushing. Again, preventive measures to reduce caries activity are important.

Heart disease

Congenital is now more common than rheumatic heart disease in children. Congenital heart disease may be associated with virtually any of the developmental disorders mentioned earlier and should always be suspected in any child with a congenital defect such as a cleft palate.

Management of children with cardiac disease is therefore that of prophylaxis against infective endocarditis (Ch. 8) together with dealing with any other congenital disorder that may be associated. Again, high standards of oral hygiene and preventive dentistry are particularly important to minimise gingival sepsis and to avoid, as far as possible, extraction of teeth.

Haemorrhagic disease

Haemophilia is both the most common and severe haemorrhagic disease (Ch. 20). Two aspects are particularly important in childhood:

1. Deciduous teeth must be allowed to be shed spontaneously. Minor bleeding that may result from exfoliation should be controllable with a plasminogen inhibitor (tranexamic acid) but, if more severe, anti-haemophilic factor may have to be given.

2. Establishment of good habits of oral health care is essential to reduce the risk of extractions later—at one time this could have meant the difference between survival and early death.

Diabetes mellitus

Childhood diabetes is usually the most severe form of the disease. Despite the reduced sucrose intake, caries rates appear to be higher than in controls. Periodontal disease is also more active, despite diabetic control, with the result that teeth are typically lost earlier. Dental infections can also occasionally impair diabetic control. For all these reasons a high standard of regular dental care is particularly important for these children. However, most diabetic children, as a result of the disciplined life that they have to lead, are particularly cooperative patients.

The muscular dystrophies

Muscular dystrophies, of which the Duchenne type is the most common (approximately 1 in 5000 male births), are the main crippling diseases of childhood. Weakness of the muscles leads to progressively severe disability and is frequently associated with cardiomyopathy and respiratory impairment.

There appear to be no specific dental problems apart from that of propping up a severely affected child in the chair. General anaesthesia is dangerous in the presence of cardiovascular disease.

Dental care for the handicapped—summary

In summary, handicapped children present a wide variety of problems of dental management, but probably up to 90% of them can be managed by conventional means without the help of general anaesthesia.

Nevertheless, handicapped children, especially those in institutions, are a dentally neglected group, even though in recent years valiant attempts have been made to overcome this deficiency. Understandably enough, the average person is unlikely to be attracted to the care of what they expect to be drooling and grimacing mental defectives. Surprisingly therefore, those who manage handicapped children say that the work is considerably more rewarding than the dental care of normal children. Such is the hideous emptiness of these children's lives, particularly when institutionalised, that dental treatment, which involves both relatively prolonged personal attention and a change from other endless dreary days, can be a pleasure for them. One Down's syndrome child, for instance, though well looked after by affectionate parents, was in a state of mysteriously eager expectation for days at the prospect (it was later found) of having a chest X-ray. Dental treatment may therefore be a real source of pleasure for those so deprived.

It is noticeable that there is a welcome concern about the dental care of handicapped *children*. It seems almost to be forgotten that handicaps persist for the rest of life and little is heard about the less emotive subject of the care of the handicapped adult.

SEDATION AND ANAESTHESIA FOR CHILDREN

Oral sedation. Some children respond well to oral temazepam, usually not less than 5 mg on the night before and again about half an hour before treatment. Oral sedation is often worth a trial as being the safest and simplest means of controlling anxiety.

Intravenous sedation. The main limitations are that venepuncture may be difficult and that some children fail to respond or occasionally react paradoxically and become hyperactive.

Nitrous oxide analgesia. Relative analgesia is relatively safe and effective, but patience may be needed in getting the child to accept the nose mask.

General anaesthesia. General anaesthesia should be avoided as it has a small but unavoidable morbidity and should be reserved for the following situations.

1. Where a child is totally unable to cooperate and all other measures have failed
2. The severely mentally retarded child, where communication is impossible
3. Central nervous system disorders with severe involuntary movements
4. Difficult or prolonged dental operations

All these categories of patient should be treated in hospital.

SUGGESTED FURTHER READING

Adams M M et al 1981 Down's syndrome: recent trends in the United States. J Am Med Assoc 246: 758–760

April M M, Burns J C, Newburger J W, Healy G B 1989 Kawasaki disease and cervical lymphadenopathy. Arch Otolaryngol Head Neck Surg 115: 512–514

Bissenden J G, Hall S 1990 Kawasaki syndrome: lessons for Britain. Br Med J 300: 1025–1026

British Medical Journal 1975 Teething myths 4: 604

Communicable Disease Report 1990 Kawasaki disease (KD) surveillance. CDR 90/08: 1

Drug and Therapeutics Bulletin 1969 Helping parents with the handicapped child. 7: 49–51

Enwonwu C O 1985 Infectious oral necrosis (cancrum oris) in Nigerian children. Community Dent Oral Epidemiol 13: 190–194

Goldberg M P 1978 The oral mucosa in childhood. Pediatric Clinics of North America 25: 239–262

Gratrix D, Taylor G O, Lennon M A 1990 Mothers' dental attendance patterns and their children's dental attendance and dental health. Br Dent J 168: 441–444

Hardman P K, Gier R E, Tegtmeier G 1990 The incidence and prevalence of hepatitis B surface antigen in a dental school population. Oral Surg, Oral Med, Oral Pathol 69: 399–402

Libman R H, Coke J M, Cohen L 1979 Complications related to the administration of general anaesthesia in 600 developmentally disabled dental patients. JADA 99: 190–193

Manford L M, Roberts G J 1980 Dental treatment in young handicapped patients. Anaesthesia 35: 1157–1168

Melville M R B et al 1981 A dental service for handicapped children. Br Dent J October: 259–261

Moller P 1973 Treatment of the handicapped child. In: Finn S B, Clinical pedodontics, 4th edn. Saunders, Philadelphia

Office of Population Censuses and Surveys 1985 Children's Dental Health in the United Kingdom 1983. HMSO, London

Ord R A, El-Attar 1987 Osteomyelitis in children—clinical presentations and review of management. Br J Oral Maxillofac Surg 25: 204–217

Pearson P A 1973 Dental treatment for the handicapped patient. Dental Update 1: 135–139

Pool D 1981 Dental care for the handicapped. Br Dent J
October: 267–270

Scully C 1976 Down's syndrome and dentistry. Dental
Update 3: 193–196

Scully C 1976 Dentistry for the handicapped in general
practice, Part 1. Dental Practice, November: 6–8

Scully C 1976 Dentistry for the handicapped in general
practice, Part 2. Dental Practice, December: 7–9

Scully C, Cawson R A 1991 Medical problems in dentistry,
3rd edn. Wright, Bristol

Seward M H E 1976 A survey and statistical evaluation of
the complications attributed to the eruption of the
primary dentition. Br Dent J 141: 370

Todd J E, Walker A M 1985 Children's dental health in the
United Kingdom 1983. HMSO, London

24. Oral disease in the elderly

The dental problems of the older patient are the consequence of the interaction of the following factors:

1. Age changes in the tissues
2. The advance of periodontal disease
3. Difficulties with dentures
4. Oral diseases peculiar to or more common in the elderly
5. Systemic diseases associated with advancing age.

Though all of these are important in varying degree the main dental need of most elderly patients is the provision of effective and comfortable dentures. Elderly patients tend to become even more infrequent visitors to the dentist than they once were, especially when dentures have been provided. As a consequence, cancer of the mouth, which both becomes more common as age advances and is insidious in development, is particularly likely to be missed in its earlier stages. The majority of cases of cancer of the mouth are at an advanced stage by the time they come for treatment.

Though the major part of treatment of the elderly is prosthetic dentistry, it is easy to become so involved in the technical problems as to lose sight of any other disabilities the patient may have.

It is important to take a somewhat less restricted view.

AGE CHANGES IN THE MOUTH AND JAWS

The changes seen in the mouth as age advances are partly the consequences of age itself, partly the result of wear and tear on the tissues, and partly the consequences of the fact that certain diseases become more common as age advances. These changes include the following.

The teeth

The teeth can undergo attrition, abrasion, hypercalcification and frequently, continued destruction by caries.

Attrition

Severe attrition is rarely seen in the indigenous population of Britain, partly because the diet is so soft and partly because the majority of people have lost their teeth by middle age.

Attrition is the wearing down of the occlusal surfaces of the teeth by mastication and is severe in those living on a coarse, gritty diet. Attrition may occasionally also be produced by nervous habits, particularly grinding the teeth at times of stress or during sleep. Chewing a pipe stem can cause localised attrition.

In advanced attrition the incisal edges and cusps of the teeth are worn away until the teeth become peg-shaped with a flat or hollowed occlusal surface, sharp margins and wide exposure of the dentine.

Since the process is slow, attrition leads to progressive reactionary dentine formation. This is made visible when wear advances so far as to show the original position of the pulp.

Attrition is usually incompatible with active caries or periodontal disease as these cause destruction, mobility, or loss of teeth before attrition can develop. Partly also the kind of diet that produces attrition also has a low sugar content. Attrition is, however, associated with periodontal disease in India, for example, where the diet is often abrasive and periodontal disease starts early.

A special form of attrition is characteristic of dentinogenesis imperfecta where the enamel splits off, exposing the dentine which rapidly wears down until level with the gums as described in Chapter 2. This is the only type of attrition seen in children.

Abrasion

Abrasion is the wearing away of tooth tissue, usually by overvigorous toothbrushing. The areas most severely affected are the labial or buccal surfaces of the necks of the teeth. In a right-handed person the left canine and pre-molar teeth are usually most severely damaged. The main contributory factors are the vigorous use of a hard toothbrush with a horizontal sawing action and, sometimes, abrasive tooth powders.

Cementum and then dentine become exposed, and eventually grooves are worn into the necks of the teeth. At first, the exposed tissue at the neck of the teeth may be abnormally sensitive, causing discomfort or pain during eating. In other cases there are no symptoms and, with reactionary dentine formation, deep notches may be formed, with exposure of the pulp. Occasionally the damage is so severe that the crown of the tooth snaps off.

Simultaneously with the abrasion of tooth substance the gingival margin wears away,

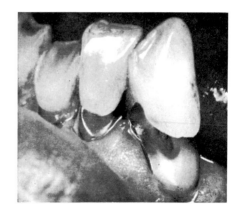

Fig. 24.1 Abrasion and attrition. This elderly patient has worn deep grooves into the teeth by vigorous toothbrushing for many years. The pulps have retreated behind successive layers of reactionary dentine. The incisal edges also show attrition; irregular facets have been worn by the opposing teeth, exposing the dentine.

progressively exposing the roots. Recession is often severe but usually combatible with healthy gingivae because the vigorous toothbrushing effectively removes plaque and leaves the gingivae pale, firm and tightly attached.

The combination of deeply abraded teeth with firm healthy gingivae indicates the great resistance of the gingival margins to mechanical injury.

Hypercalcification

The roots of the teeth gradually become hypercalcified by progressive obliteration of the dentinal tubules. The roots may as a consequence become completely calcified and virtually transparent (Ch. 9), but the main clinical consequence is that they become progressively more brittle and liable to fracture during extraction.

The periodontal tissues and jaws

Osteoporosis is the loss of bone tissue which takes place progressively with ageing, particularly in women. Though there is a constant turnover of bone, bone loss exceeds bone deposition after the age of about 35. The whole skeleton is affected but there is very wide individual variation.

The extent to which osteoporosis contributes to bone loss in periodontal disease is unknown. It seems likely that the jaws escape the effect of osteoporosis. Though there is little evidence of any significant association, it is noteworthy that women, who as a group suffer more severe osteoporosis, consistently lose their teeth earlier than men despite evidence of better dental care (Ch. 26).

In the dentate elderly, therefore, the alveolar bone usually shows the long-term effects of periodontal disease, with severe alveolar bone loss.

The majority of elderly patients are edentulous and show progressive alveolar bone loss. Gross alveolar bone loss in the edentulous jaw is often said to have been the result of delay in extracting the teeth until periodontal disease is far advanced.

Progressive loss of denture-bearing bone brings with it the well-known prosthetic difficulties, particularly with retention and stabilisation of dentures. Later, as excessive amounts of bone become resorbed, pain can be caused by the dentures pressing upon anatomical structures, such as the mylohyoid ridge or genial tubercles, which become prominent after loss of overlying bone.

The temporomandibular joints

Osteoarthritis of the weight-bearing joints is a common and often disabling disease as age advances. By contrast osteoarthritis of the temporomandibular joints is not a significant problem. The condition is uncommon and, if found, it is likely to have been an incidental finding in radiographs. Even when present, in sharp contrast to its effects on weight-bearing joints, osteoarthritis of the temporomandibular joint rarely causes pain.

Pain or other symptoms from the temporomandibular joint in the elderly are remarkably uncommon.

The mucous membrane

Changes in the oral mucous membrane seen as the patient ages are partly the result of age changes; others are pathological changes which cannot be said to be a direct consequence of ageing.

Fodyce's granules. These sebaceous glands in the oral mucosa, particularly in the buccal regions, become more numerous and larger with age. In some patients the soft, yellowish gland acini seen immediately beneath the buccal mucous membrane are very numerous and cover a wide area. They must be distinguished from the more superficial white thickening of the mucosal epithelium seen in keratotic lesions.

Lingual varicosities. The veins in the underside of the tongue become larger, more prominent and, possibly, more numerous.

Foliate papillae. This normal lymphoid tissue, sometimes known as the lingual tonsil, is seen on each side of the lateral border of the tongue at the junction of the anterior two-thirds and the posterior third. These papillae become enlarged and red in elderly people and are sometimes mistaken for neoplasms.

Age-changes in the mucosa. It is sometimes suggested that, with age the oral mucosa becomes thin or atrophic.

One feature of senility is loss of dermal collagen; heavily stressed areas, particularly the denture-bearing areas, may therefore be affected since the denture-bearing mucosa is mucoperiosteum. Weakening of the collagen support of this area of tissue could have the effect of making the mucous membrane less resistant to trauma.

Salivary function

It is often stated that salivary secretion diminishes with age, but this has not been confirmed in large-scale studies. However, depressed salivary flow is overall more common in the elderly as a result of such causes as Sjögren's syndrome and the use of drugs with anticholinergic activity for a variety of conditions (Ch. 17).

Elderly patients who have a dry mouth must therefore be investigated accordingly.

DISEASES AFFECTING THE EDENTULOUS MOUTH

Between the ages of 55 and 64, the proportion of the population who are edentulous in the UK as a whole is 37%, but 53% in Northern England, and higher still in the lower socioeconomic groups.

Though mastication with dentures is less efficient than with healthy teeth, this seems to matter little, and most denture wearers suffer no more than discomfort or social embarrassment from time to time from these repulsive appliances.

Other troubles affecting the denture wearer may come from a variety of causes. The denture can for example damage the underlying tissues or promote infection beneath it. Alternatively, the fit of the denture can be affected by changes in the underlying tissues which distort the denture-bearing area. In addition, mucosal lesions can develop under or at the margins of dentures to cause severe discomfort or pain. Some of these mucosal lesions, particularly cancer, become increasingly common as age advances and tend to be seen more often in denture wearers. Troubles affecting the denture wearer may therefore fall into the following categories:

1. Lesions caused directly or indirectly by dentures
2. Lesions which may affect the fit of the denture
3. Lesions of the oral mucous membrane coincidentally affecting the denture-bearing area.

In the first two categories the primary complaint is usually of discomfort from the denture. In the first group the denture needs to be modified. In the second group the denture is not at fault but the underlying cause must be dealt with. The primary complaint of the third group may not be related to the denture, but includes oral diseases seen more often in this older age group, such as sore tongue or carcinoma. However, even these may be blamed on the denture.

Lesions directly or indirectly due to dentures

Traumatic ulcers

These are usually seen when the denture is new, and are the result of overextension or rough spots on the fitting surface. The usual sites are in the sulcus on the labial or lingual frena. The cause of these ulcers is usually obvious from their history and clinical features, but the diagnostic criterion is that the ulcer heals within a few days when the denture is removed or adequately relieved.

Continued resorption of supporting bone can cause traumatic ulcers later or (as described earlier) can cause pain when the denture presses on

such structures as the genial tubercles or mylohyoid ridge. When this happens the denture has usually to be remade.

Denture hyperplasia (Denture granuloma)

These lumps usually form at the margin of the denture as a result of overextension. Long-standing low grade irritation leads to fibrous proliferation.

Histologically these lumps are formed of fibrous connective tissue with a covering of stratified squamous epithelium. There is little or no infiltration with inflammatory cells unless the surface is ulcerated.

Clinically the lesion forms a rubbery mass with a smooth or slightly lobulated surface. An essentially similar type of fibrous overgrowth may form in the vault of the palate but becomes flattened and leaf-like (leaf-fibroma or leaf-granuloma). These fibrous nodules should be excised and the diagnosis confirmed by histopathology.

Denture stomatitis

This form of candidosis is caused by occlusion of the mucous surface by an upper denture, producing, in susceptible patients, favourable conditions for the proliferation of the fungus. The proliferation of *Candida albicans* in the interface between denture and mucosa causes chronic inflammation of the denture-bearing mucosa. Angular stomatitis frequently accompanies these changes (Ch. 15).

Prosthetists have been strangely anxious to prove that denture stomatitis is traumatic in origin; there is no evidence to support this idea, and the condition responds to antifungal drugs.

Papillary hyperplasia of the palate

Papillary hyperplasia is not itself caused by dentures and is seen in dentate mouths where no dentures are worn. It is, however, made worse when associated with denture stomatitis or when mechanically irritated by a denture. There is no evidence that papillary hyperplasia is premalignant—the vault of the palate is hardly ever affected by cancer.

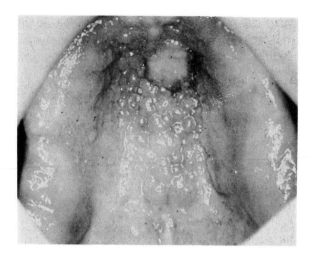

Fig. 24.2 Papillary hyperplasia of the palate. The absence of inflammation is noticeable.

Changes at the angles of the mouth

As a result of loss of elasticity and atrophy of the supporting muscles, the skin of the face sags. Furrows usually therefore form at the angles of the mouth in the elderly, irrespective of whether they are wearing dentures or not.

Furrows at the angles of the mouth are made deeper by (a) loss of vertical dimension and (b) by loss of support to the upper lip by resorption of the underlying bone. Though establishment of correct vertical dimension and increasing the thickness of the labial flange of the upper denture can slightly lessen these furrows at the angles of the mouth, they cannot usually be eliminated in this way. Plastic surgery is required when patients are anxious to have signs of age removed.

Furrows can become inflamed as a result of infection by *Candida albicans* or *Staphylococcus aureus* (Ch. 15). Angular stomatitis is also a well-recognised feature of iron deficiency, and may then be mediated by increased susceptibility to infection, particularly by *Candida albicans*.

Frictional keratosis and other hyperkeratotic lesions

Keratosis may be seen particularly under the lower denture and, though uncommon, is seen more often as age advances. It is probable that friction plays a part in the development of these patches,

but it is rarely possible to get rid of them by any modification of the denture. The only certain test is to take the denture away from the patient for two or more weeks to see whether the area reverts to normal.

Other hyperkeratotic lesions (leukoplakias) also increase in frequency as age advances and are often unrelated to a denture. The older the patient and the longer a leukoplakic lesion has been present the greater the chance of malignant change (Ch. 16).

Lesions which may affect the fit of dentures

The main examples of lesions that can affect the denture-bearing area are:

a. Buried teeth, roots, or (rarely) odontomas
b. Cysts. Residual and, less often, keratocysts are the main types affecting edentulous patients
c. Tumours. Carcinoma is the most important superficial neoplasm. Among tumours of the jaws ameloblastomas are uncommon in the over 50s, while secondary carcinomas are increasingly frequent
d. Osteodystrophies. Paget's disease or, less often, acromegaly or hyperparathyroidism can affect this age group
e. Fractures of the jaws.

The effect of all these lesions, as far as the dentures are concerned, is that they impair the fit or cause discomfort or pain. These are usually therefore the first symptoms.

Buried teeth or roots cause increasing discomfort as they erupt: first as the mucosa becomes crushed between the tooth and denture base then later as the denture rides on the protuberance.

Swellings of the jaw, either localised as in the case of cysts and tumours, or a general change in the form of the jaw (as in Paget's disease or acromegaly) produce characteristic clinical features.

Carcinoma, the most lethal disease of the mouth, can develop in the denture bearing area. In the early stages the tumour is usually painless and can grow to 2 or 3 cm in diameter with no other complaint than that the denture no longer fits. Later, pain and ulceration develop but these too may be blamed on the denture. Biopsy is of course essential.

Fractures of the jaw are less common among older, edentulous patients but can be secondary to gross resorption or be pathological if a tumour develops. Increasingly also, elderly people have become the victims of violence. If the dentures are available and unbroken, they can be used as a temporary splint. If there is malunion it interferes with the fit of the denture and causes pain. The denture should be remade.

It must be emphasised therefore that the cause of progressive deterioration of the fit of dentures must be looked for and not simply evaded by repeated 'eases'.

Lesions of the mucous membrane which can affect the denture-bearing area

Some mucosal diseases become more common as age advances and so are more likely to be seen in denture wearers. Others become less common but may occasionally nevertheless present problems. These disorders, which are described more fully in Chapter 15, can affect various sites but may impinge on the denture bearing area. These diseases, most of which cause soreness of the mouth, include the following:

1. Aphthous stomatitis
2. Lichen planus
3. Mucous membrane pemphigoid
4. Pemphigus vulgaris
5. Herpes zoster
6. Glossitis
7. Carcinoma.

Aphthous stomatitis

Aphthae are remarkably uncommon among edentulous patients. This is partly an age-related phenomenon, as these ulcers reach their peak frequency much earlier in life.

If recurrent aphthae start or become worse after middle age an underlying systemic cause should be looked for. A deficiency state, particularly vitamin B12 deficiency, is a strong possibility at this age.

Rarely, aphthae form in the sulcus under the edge of the denture and are aggravated by trauma.

As a consequence healing can be delayed and proliferative changes can develop. The lesion can then simulate a tumour and biopsy becomes necessary.

Aphthae do not affect the main denture-bearing mucoperiosteum.

Lichen planus

Lichen planus is common in people of middle age or over but only rarely extends so far into the lower buccal sulcus as to be traumatised by the denture flange. The atrophic or erosive lesions of the lichen planus are painful irrespective of whether a denture is worn or not.

Mucous membrane pemphigoid

This disease increases in frequency with age. Large shallow ulcers (erosions) may occasionally form under a denture and may make a lower denture unwearable. Erosions may be tolerated under the more stable upper denture. Biopsy is necessary, particularly to exclude the pemphigus vulgaris.

Pemphigus vulgaris

This is a vesiculo-bullous disease mainly of the middle aged but may affect the elderly. It tends not to affect the denture-bearing area itself, but, like mucous membrane pemphigoid, can cause intense soreness of the mouth. Biopsy is essential.

Herpes zoster

Zoster causes a vesiculating stomatitis and facial rash together with intense aching pain. It is considerably more common after middle age. The whole of the denture-bearing area of one side can be affected.

In elderly patients especially, post-herpetic neuralgia, resembling trigeminal neuralgia, can be a particularly troublesome sequel.

In up to 10% of patients there may be an underlying lymphoma.

Carcinoma and leukoplakia

Cancer and leukoplakia become increasingly common as age advances and coincidentally therefore are more common in denture wearers.

There is no reason to believe that denture irritation can cause malignant change, but it is easy for the patient (or clinician) to mistake the early signs for denture trauma. Moreover, once edentulous, patients rarely attend a dentist. Early asymptomatic lesions can thus be missed.

Cancer is the most lethal disease of the mouth affecting edentulous (and for that matter dentate) patients. It is essential therefore to be certain of the diagnosis of minor lesions that develop in relation to dentures. They must not be dismissed as traumatic unless they heal completely within a few days of easing or removing the denture (Ch. 16).

Radiation injury

Radiotherapy to tumours of the mouth, or nearby, tends to cause varying degrees of damage to the bone of the jaw. A major factor is the development of obliterative endarteritis and ischaemic changes. The tissues are, as a consequence, susceptible to minor trauma which can lead to severe and almost intractable osteomyelitis. Denture trauma can have this effect, and experts in this field may not permit patients to wear lower dentures after radiotherapy (Ch. 22).

Glossitis

Soreness of the tongue is a common complaint among older patients. Though it may be blamed on the denture ('lack of tongue space') there is no evidence that a denture can cause diffuse soreness of the tongue. It is important to exclude systemic disease, particularly iron deficiency or pernicious anaemia. The latter increases in frequency as age advances. Depression is also common in the elderly (Ch. 15).

Dry mouth

The complaint of dry mouth becomes more common as age advances. The main causes (apart from those who have had radiotherapy to the mouth or jaws) are drugs and Sjögren's syndrome (Ch. 17).

IMPLANTS

As mentioned earlier, a major requirement of the elderly is the provision of stable and effective dentures. For this purpose, conventional prosthetic techniques may be inadequate, as shown by the frequency of claims for compensation for unsatisfactory dentures. As a consequence, methods of implanting denture attachments into the bone have been the subject of experimentation for many years. However, there are two important difficulties. First, the material of the implant must not merely be tolerated by the tissues but must become integrated with the bone to become firmly stable. Second, there is the risk of infection tracking into the bone where the implant penetrates the mucosa.

With earlier blade implants, results were unpredictable, and, though bone sometimes grew into the interstices of the implant, the latter was usually separated from the bone by a layer of collagen which could develop similar changes to chronic periodontitis with slow or rapid loosening.

The principles of *osseointegration* depend on the finding, first, that in the preparation of the implant site, heating the bone, by rapid cutting, above the critical temperature of 47°C for more than 1 minute interferes with healing. Second, pure titanium (as shown by experience since 1965) is completely biocompatible and bonds to bone (osseointegration) via the oxide film that forms on its surface. Scanning electron microscopy has shown that osteoclasts will grow on the surface of pure titanium. Titanium is also strong enough to form a satisfactory implant. Third, provided that the implant is fully osseointegrated and immobile, there is little downgrowth of epithelium but it forms an apparently permanent, weak attachment to the implant. However, strict oral hygiene must be maintained after the prosthesis has been inserted.

Following development of the original Brånemark osseointegrated implant, others using similar principles have been introduced.

An alternative to titanium in the Tubingen implant is ceramic (polycrystaline aluminium oxide) which is biocompatible and inert. It is claimed that this presents an electrically charged surface to the tissues and that this attracts macromolecules from tissue fluid to form a monomolecular layer on the ceramic, and that plaque forms less readily on it than on natural teeth. Microporosity, grooves and lacunae in the ceramic aid retention. However, the ceramic is weaker than titanium.

The practical considerations with Brånemark implants are as follows.

1. Selection of the patient. The patient must have mandibular bone of sufficient volume to hold an implant and must also be able to tolerate an initial operation lasting up to 2 hours. However, this can frequently be carried out under local anaesthesia with sedation.
2. After raising the mucoperiosteal flap great care has to be taken to avoid heat trauma to

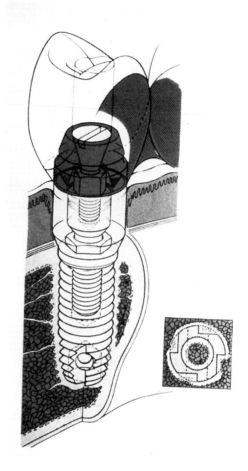

Fig. 24.4 The Brånemark implant. Diagram showing the essential features of the implant threaded into the bone and the method of attaching an abutment to it. At lower right is a section of the special bur used for threading the bone cavity. (By kind permission of Nobelpharma).

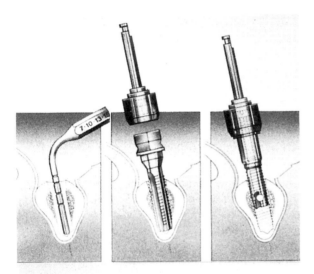

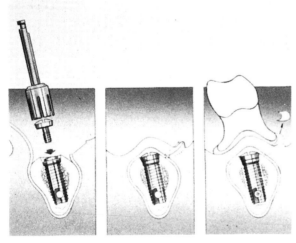

Fig. 24.3 Diagram of the stages of preparation for insertion of a Brånemark osseointegrated implant. The last picture shows a temporary denture with soft lining, worn while osseointegration develops. (By kind permission of Nobelpharma).

the bone by use of an ultra-low-speed handpiece. The cavity has also to be cut very precisely with specially made drills to fit the implant, and strict asepsis must be maintained. The number of implants inserted is governed by the amount and quality of bone which has to support the load of mastication.

3. The titanium implant is firmly inserted into its site and the incision is closed. It is then left unloaded for 3 to 6 months to allow osseointegration to develop.
4. After osseointegration is complete, the implant is exposed at a second operation and

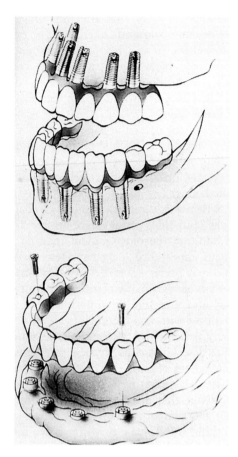

Fig. 24.5 Diagrams showing the attachment of full dentures to a series of Brånemark implants. Space allowed between the denture base and the mucosa allows cleaning between them. (By kind permission of Nobelpharma).

tested for immobility. If satisfactory, the abutments to attach the denture are fixed to the implants and the wound sutured.

5. After healing of the second operation wound the prosthesis can be fitted to its abutments.

In essence the Brånemark implant consists of a hollow titanium screw onto which a gold cylinder is fitted with a gold screw. By this means it extends through the mucosa and abutments are attached.

The advantage of correctly fitted, implant-supported prostheses include: (1) their stability, (2) the lack of functional stress imposed on the underlying mucosa, and (3) the transmission of functional stress directly to the bone allowing greater masticatory force.

Regular radiographic and clinical monitoring should be carried out to confirm the retention of the implants and the health of the tissues around them.

Failure of implant-supported prostheses may result from such factors as: (1) too few implants to support the imposed loads, in relation to the amount and quality of the supporting bone; (2) poor design or technique allowing excessive stress to be imposed on one implant; (3) poor oral hygiene.

Although implants are mentioned here because of the frequent difficulties in making satisfactory dentures for the elderly, implants can be used where necessary in younger persons, for example to replace a single missing incisor. Though the cost of osseointegrated implants is considerable, it must be set against that of multiple replacements of conventional dentures and the long functional life (10 or more years) of at least 75% of implants.

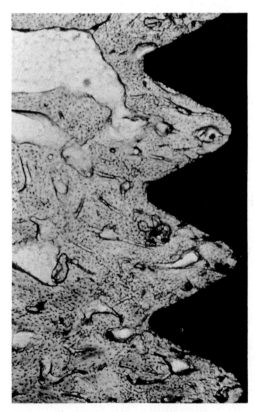

Fig. 24.6 Section showing integration of the bone with the Branemark implant and total lack of inflammatory reaction. (By kind permission of Nobelpharma).

SYSTEMIC DISEASE IN THE ELDERLY

Systemic diseases which particularly affect the elderly are shown in Table 24.1.

Table 24.1   Diseases more common in the elderly

1. Diseases of the nervous system
    Mental deterioration and psychiatric disorders
        Depression
        Dementia (particularly Alzheimer's disease)
        Confusional states
        Paranoia
        Dependence on hypnotics
    Parkinson's disease
    Strokes
    Ataxia

2. Cardiovascular disease
    Hypertension and ischaemic heart disease (Ch. 20)
    Cardiac failure (any cause) (Ch. 20)
    Giant-cell (temporal) arteritis and polymyalgia rheumatica (Ch. 18)

3. Respiratory disease
    Chronic bronchitis
    Pneumonia

4. Musculoskeletal
    Osteoarthritis (Ch. 14)
    Paget's disease (Ch. 12)

5. Haematological
    Anaemia (especially pernicious anaemia) (Ch. 20)
    Chronic leukaemia (Ch. 20)
    Myeloma (Ch. 11)

6. Oral or predominantly oral
    Lichen planus
    Mucous membrane pemphigoid
    Trigeminal herpes zoster
    Carcinoma, premalignant and other white lesions
    Sore tongue
    Sjögren's syndrome
    Candidosis (denture stomatitis)

7. Miscellaneous
    Cancer of most kinds
    Nutritional deficiencies
    Deterioration of vision and hearing

Diseases of the nervous system

Deterioration of mental function

This deterioration (an almost inevitable consequence of ageing) affects all aspects of mental activity, such as intelligence, memory, emotional state and personality. These different functions tend to be affected to a variable and unpredictable extent. Thus the patient may seem bright enough but may immediately forget instructions given, for example about how to look after dentures. Other patients become confused, querulous, or even aggressive, behave in an irresponsible fashion, have delusions of persecution and are generally 'difficult'. Alzheimer's disease, the most common cause of dementia after middle age, can present in any of these ways.

In general, the older the patient, the less adaptable he is likely to be. While preservation of teeth for as long as possible may be desirable, it may create greater problems if extractions have to be postponed until late in life. The wearing of full dentures demands a remarkable feat of adaptation at any age, and older patients face greater difficulties. In addition the older patient may no longer care about appearance, may have few social contacts and may prefer a soft diet. Motivation, which plays so large a part in adaptation to denture wearing, may also therefore be diminished.

Difficulties with and complaints about dentures by elderly patients may therefore be as much due to mental deterioration as physical problems. Poor communication, often due to deafness, makes matters worse. Exasperating though such complaints may become, they must be treated with understanding and sympathy. This mental deterioration is something we all have to suffer if we live long enough; in the words of a physician 'insightless atrophy and ultimate obliteration of normal mental life . . . is a remorseless enemy of the natural dignity of man'.

Parkinson's disease

This common disease is characterised by rigidity often most obvious as a mask-like fixity of facial expression, tremor sometimes affecting the lower jaw, and often dribbling as a result of impaired neuromuscular function.

The disease, which affects the basal ganglia, may be associated (because of the age of affected patients) with mental deterioration. The appearance, particularly the poverty of facial expression, which is easily mistaken for incomprehension, and the defective speech also unjustly suggest impaired mental function. It is important to take care therefore not to offend a patient with Parkinson's disease by making such an assumption.

Parkinson's disease can cause difficulty with the management of dentures because of the loss of fine control of muscular movement. If there is also mental deterioration the difficulties are proportionately increased.

The effects of Parkinson's disease can be diminished by giving anticholinergic drugs such as benzohexol (Artane), which tend to cause a dry mouth. But more effective are dopaminic agents such as levodopa.

Trigeminal neuralgia

This disease, which causes intense lightning pains in the trigeminal area, is particularly a disease of those past middle age. It is described in Chapter 18 together with post-herpetic neuralgia, for which it can be mistaken.

Cardiovascular disease

Cardiovascular disease, particularly hypertension and ischaemic heart disease, are the commonest causes of death in the Western world. All diseases of the cardiovascular system worsen as age advances. In the edentulous patient this may cause no special difficulties; in general the greatest problems are likely to arise if a general anaesthetic is needed (Ch. 19). A myocardial infarct may happen during dental treatment in a patient with ischaemic heart disease. The event may be precipitated by acute anxiety, and possible causes might include a sense of suffocation if excess impression material slips towards the pharynx (Ch. 20).

A variety of drugs used for cardiovascular disease can also cause oral reactions (Ch. 15). As noted earlier, the elderly with heart lesions are at the highest risk for infective endocarditis and form the peak age group for this disease.

Nutritional disorders

These are particularly likely to affect the elderly. Poverty, reduced mobility (which interferes with both cooking and shopping), and mental deterioration are some of the contributory factors. Poorly functioning dentures and impairment of taste sensation may make matters worse.

However, deficiency states, particularly scurvy and vitamin B group deficiencies, are remarkably rare nowadays even in old age. It is important nevertheless that denture function should be the best possible in order not to worsen nutritional problems in older patients.

Anaemia

Pernicious anaemia due to impaired absorption of vitamin B12 is mainly seen after middle age. Iron deficiency often persists into later life or may be made worse by defects of absorption.

These conditions can cause oral signs and symptoms, particularly sore tongue (Ch. 20). Sore tongue or signs of atrophy of the mucosa should be investigated by haematological examination.

Factors affecting dental care of the elderly

Many factors limit the mobility of elderly patients who are frequently arthritic, may be unsteady on their feet, unwell for a variety of reasons or simply be unable to afford the cost of dental care or transportation. Domiciliary care of the elderly is lamentably inadequate, however.

SUGGESTED FURTHER READING

Brånemark P-I, Adell R, Albrektsson T et al 1982 Osseointegrated titanium implants in the rehabilitation of the edentulous patient. In: Lee A J C, Albrektsson T, Brånemark P-J (eds) Clinical applications of biomaterials. John Wiley, New York

Brånemark P-I, Breine U, Adell R et al 1969 Intraosseous anchorage of dental prostheses. 1. Experimental studies. Scand J Past Reconstr Surg 3: 81–100

Cumming C G, Wight C, Blackwell C L, Wray D 1990 Denture stomatitis in the elderly. Oral Microbiol Immunol 5: 82–85

Flint S, Scully C 1988 Orofacial age changes and related disease. Dental Update 15: 337–341

Ibbetson R J, Setchell D J 1989 Treatment of the worn dentition: 1 & 2. Dental Update 16: 247–252, 300–304

Johns R 1990 The role of osseointegrated dental implants in the treatment of elderly people. Dental Update 17: 19–23

Quayle A A, Cawood J, Howell R A et al 1989 The immediate or delayed replacement of teeth by permucosal intra-osseous implants: the Tubingen implant system. 1.

Implant design, rationale for use and pre-operative assessment. Br Dent J 166: 365

Quayle A A, Cawood J, Howell R A et al 1989 The immediate or delayed replacement of teeth by permucosal intra-osseous implants: the Tubingen implant system. 2. Surgical and restorative techniques. Br Dent J 166: 403

Sheiham A 1990 Dentistry for an ageing population: responsibilities and future trends. Dental Update 17: 70–75

Smith D G, Seymour R A 1988 Periodontal disease and treatment in the elderly. Dental update 15: 18–22

Walls A W G, Barnes I E 1988 Gerodontology: the problem? Dental Update 15: 186–190

Walls A W G, Barnes I E 1989 Treatment planning for the ageing patient. Dental Update 14: 438–443

Ward-Booth P 1988 Oral surgery for the older patient. Dental Update 15: 410–414

Watson R M, Forman G H, Davis D M 1989 Osseointegrated implants—Principles and practice: 1. Osseointegration and surgical techniques with the Nobelpharma implant system. Dental Update 16: 327–344

Watson R M, Forman G H, Davis D M 1989 Osseointegrated implants—Principles and practice: 2. Prosthetic rehabilitation with osseointegrated implants. Dental Update 16: 374–381

25. Occupational hazards to dental staff and patients

Innumerable *possible* hazards related to the practice of dentistry can be imagined. Though there are relatively few which are either frequent or have severe consequences, some remarkable accidents in the dental surgery are on record and there have been occasional deaths of both dental staff and patients. No more than a few examples can be offered here, and reference should be made to specialised texts and to the many publications of official bodies, such as the medical protection organisations, the Health and Safety Executive and the General Dental Council, which publish guidelines or regulations.

HAZARDS TO DENTAL STAFF

The chief hazards to dental staff include the following:

1. Infections, particularly hepatitis B
2. Accidents, including burns or eye injuries
3. Radiation injuries
4. Adverse effects of chemicals or drugs
5. Drug dependence
6. Involvement in medicolegal problems
7. Stress and difficulties with hostile patients
8. Postural disorders.

Infections

The possibilities of acquiring potentially-fatal infections have been discussed in Chapters 8 and 20. However, there are many other infections of varying degrees of seriousness that may be acquired in dental practice. These include the following:

—Hepatitis (Ch. 20)
—AIDS (Ch. 8)
—Herpetic infections (Ch. 15)
—Hand, foot and mouth disease (Ch. 15)
—The common cold and other respiratory viral infections
—Tuberculosis (Ch. 15)
—Syphilis (Ch. 15)
—Legionellosis.

The level of hazard that these diseases represent varies widely. Among them, some such as hand, foot and mouth disease are highly infectious but mild, others such as influenza are readily acquired and usually only incapacitating for a time, while the hepatitis B virus is widespread, highly contagious and potentially lethal but preventable by immunisation.

In addition to considering the hazards to the dentist from these various infections from the illness itself, it should be borne in mind that they also cause loss of working time and income. Further, there is the possibility of transmitting infections such as herpes simplex or hepatitis B to patients, as discussed below. Claims for compensation in such cases have been successful.

As mentioned in earlier chapters, the main measures are to maintain a high standard of cross-infection control: to wear protective clothing, to take great care in the use and disposal particularly of local anaesthetic needles, to maintain a high standard of asepsis and antisepsis. These measures alone should provide adequate protection against herpetic infection (herpetic whitlow or possibly keratitis) and the more remote possibility of occupationally acquired syphilis. In addition and more important is immunisation against hepatitis B and possibly tuberculosis, though the risk from the latter is small. The concern about AIDS is understandable, but as described in Chapter 8, only a single dentist is yet known to have acquired occupationally-acquired AIDS even though he worked in an exceptionally high-risk area (New York) and had many minor occupational injuries.

During surgical procedures, droplets of blood can be splashed into the eyes and can cause either eye infections or enter the body by this route to cause systemic infection. Ordinary glasses do not provide adequate protection and plastic protective spectacles should therefore be worn. These will block contaminated blood splashes and also injuries to the eye from particles projected from a fast-rotating bur or of calculus during scaling.

Cross-infection control is discussed in Chapter 20 and the main measures are summarised in Appendix II. However, it should be noted that adequate cross-infection control is not merely for the protection of the dentist, but it is also a legal obligation under the Health and Safety at Work Acts to protect staff and patients.

Legionellosis

In addition to infections discussed in earlier chapters, legionellosis is a potential hazard in the dental surgery. Various legionellae (usually *L. pneumophila*) can cause fatal pneumonia, particularly in elderly persons, and also a non-pneumonic illness (Pontiac fever). Most of these infections have been spread by aerosols from contaminated air-conditioning systems, but legionellae can also be harboured in stagnant water in dental units, and there is an increased prevalence of antibody carriage among dental personnel. There is therefore the possibility that patients or dental staff could be infected from dental water sprays.

Units which stand idle for long periods, as in hospital dental departments, are particularly likely to contain legionellae, and some have had to be closed to enable disinfection to be carried out.

Though the risk of spreading Legionnaires' disease from a dental unit appears to be small, it is probably prudent to flush through all water sprays after idle periods such as weekends. If infection of a unit is confirmed, it should be disinfected, preferably with hypochlorite.

Accidents

Obvious examples are penetrating wounds from sharp instruments or from a rotating bur, burns from recently autoclaved instruments or, as mentioned above, eye injuries. Eye injuries are of major importance and can result from fragments projected from a rotating bur, chemical or blood splashes, or other causes. The free end of a wire being cut is sharp and can be projected like a missile. Rarely, dentists have lost the sight of an eye from such causes.

However, the majority of accidents in the dental surgery are the result of tripping over some unnoticed obstruction. As a result, sharp or hot instruments that are being carried can be projected through the air. Alternatively, injuries may result from falling onto dental equipment or any other hard object.

Another possible danger is that of electric shock from faulty equipment, and dental staff may be at greater risk because their hands are often wet.

The dental surgeon as an employer has a duty to protect staff under the Health and Safety at Work Acts. As a consequence he may face litigation if an accident results from, for example, a poorly maintained autoclave. Patients may also claim compensation for such injuries.

Radiation

X-rays are the chief cause of anxiety, both because of the known dangers of ionising radiation (as well as public alarmism about the subject) and because of the enormous numbers of diagnostic radiographs taken in dentistry. Though the contribution of dental radiographs to the total radiation load on any individual is small, it may nevertheless be significant. Dental staff taking many radiographs, day after day, can be at risk, and adequate precautions must be taken (Ch. 22).

A more recent consideration is that, since June 1990, all dentists are required to have the Core of Knowledge regarding radiation protection and to implement their related statutory responsibilities. The possibility therefore exists that those who lack this degree of training or fail to fulfil the legal requirements may no longer be allowed to take radiographs.

Other sources of radiation that can be injurious are lasers and ultraviolet light. The latter has been used for the curing of plastic restorations but has been largely or entirely replaced by blue light.

Lasers may be used in surgery and can cause burns of tissues accidentally exposed and blindness if directed towards the retina.

Chemicals or drugs

Either of these groups of substances can have direct toxic effects or cause hypersensitivity reactions such as dermatitis. Toxic effects of drugs are discussed in Chapter 21 and are more frequently hazards to patients than staff. However, pollution of the surgery atmosphere with anaesthetic agents may possibly be a hazard to dental staff, as are hypersensitisation or direct toxic effects of mercury as discussed below. Methyl methacrylate monomer, as another example, is both irritant, particularly if splashed into the eye, and also a

sensitising agent. However methylmethacrylate allergy, even among dental laboratory staff who are habitually handling it, is remarkably uncommon.

Mercury toxicity and allergy

The dangers of mercury are either from systemic absorption, particularly of organic mercury compounds such as methyl mercury, or from the development of hypersensitivity (contact dermatitis).

Hypersensitivity to mercury or its salts causes an inflammatory and sometimes vesiculating reaction of exposed skin. This can readily be confirmed by patch testing, but even those who have objectively confirmed sensitivity to mercury can tolerate mercury amalgams in the mouth.

Despite almost constant exposure to mercury, contact sensitivity to it is remarkably rare among dental staff. In the unlikely event that it develops, adequate protection should be provided by the wearing of gloves and covering the arms (as required anyway for adequate cross-infection control) during preparation and insertion of amalgams.

Systemic mercury toxicity is a possible occupational hazard of dentistry. Mercury and particularly methyl mercury are neurotoxic, but it is not clear to what extent the metal is converted to organic compounds in the body. Thus many dentists have had decades of exposure to mercury and inevitably absorbed some of it, but this mercury burden has not been shown to cause clinically significant effects. Sensitive neurological testing may, however, show some slight deficit by retirement age.

Care should therefore be taken in handling mercury and preventing it from being spilt or scattered in fine particles during amalgam mixing. Spilt mercury can be picked up with a plastic pipette or adsorbed onto waste amalgam. Drilling out old amalgams also gives off traces of mercury vapour if the bur is inadequately cooled. Serious difficulties arise from spilling a substantial quantity of mercury, particularly onto carpeted wooden flooring. Decontamination can then present an almost insuperable problem. Even worse is when (as has happened) a DSA spills mercury behind an autoclave and is then too ignorant or nervous to speak of the accident. Mercury absorption by the dental staff can, as a result of the rapid evaporation, then rise to alarming levels.

Atmospheric pollution by anaesthetic agents

Traces of volatile or gaseous anaesthetics contaminate the atmosphere of some dental surgeries. There are known toxic effects of halothane (liver damage particularly after repeated exposure) and of nitrous oxide (depression of vitamin B12 metabolism after prolonged exposure) and some studies have suggested that, for example, female operating theatre staff have an increased rate of abortions or of fetal abnormalities. It has also been claimed that anaesthetists have increased risk of cancer or hepatic or renal disease. However, none of these findings has been substantiated.

Dental surgeries, particularly if small and ill-ventilated, may allow much higher concentrations of atmospheric nitrous oxide to accumulate than in operating theatres. Levels more than 200-fold the recommended maximum level of 25 ppm have been recorded in some dental theatres. Scavenging, particularly of patients' expired air during relative analgesia, should therefore be provided if N_2O is frequently used.

Dental staff may be exposed in the surgery or laboratory to many other potentially toxic drugs or chemicals, but it must be emphasised that in practical terms the risks from many of these are very small if reasonable precautions are taken.

Respiratory risks from dusts

Dental laboratory staff are at risk from a variety of dusts, and pneumoconioses can result from inhalation of silica or metals from various dental materials. Rarely, asthma can result from inhalation of methylmethacrylate or cyanacrylate vapours. Other vapours such as formaldehyde, or dusts such as nickel or chromium, are potential carcinogens.

Adequate face masks should therefore be worn, and equipment such as grinders or polishing lathes should be enclosed and locally ventilated.

However, the greatest respiratory risk in laboratories is smoking.

Drug dependence

Partly because of ready access to drugs, doctors and dentists are at greater risk of becoming drug-dependent than their lay peers. In addition dentists can (and some do) become alcohol-dependent, and this poses a greater threat to their careers than it does to non-professional persons. In the USA, N_2O-dependent dentists, with consequent neurological damage, have been reported. Nitrous oxide abuse is probably a greater hazard than opioids or cocaine, which are little used and less readily available in dentistry.

A drug-dependent dentist may injure a patient, and as consequence be subjected to claims for compensation or face criminal charges. However, even if there is no such accident, the dentist may be regarded as unfit to practice and as a consequence lose (or have restricted) this right and his livelihood, if the General Dental Council so decides.

Medicolegal problems

Involvement with legal complications is a significant occupational hazard in dentistry. They may not appear at first sight to be a threat to the dentist's health but can result in as much loss of working time as physical illnesses and even greater anxiety. It may also result in the loss of his right to practice. The first and most important precaution is to maintain a subscription with a professional protection organisation. However, even these organisations cannot provide a shield against all eventualities.

The main causes of trouble are likely to be the following:

1. Professional negligence
2. Professional misconduct
3. Breaches of the NHS terms of service
4. Failure to comply with the Health and Safety at Work Acts and other legislation.

Though offences under these headings are obvious causes for complaints, trouble is most likely to result from provoking patients by rudeness or by a casual, impatient, or patronising manner. Many more cases are brought as a result of patients being angered by dentists' or doctors' offhand or bad manners than by incompetence. It cannot be emphasised too strongly therefore that it is essential to maintain (difficult though it may be) a courteous, considerate and caring manner and to obtain consent for any work that has to be done. It is also essential to keep full and adequate records for reference, in case claims are made later.

Consent

An operation on a patient, such as extraction of a tooth, without consent is, legally speaking, an assault. Consent also has to be *informed*: that is, reasonable explanation of the need for and the nature of an operation and its possible complications (within reason) should be given and phrased in a way that the patient can understand.

Consent can be verbal or even implied by, for instance, the mere fact of a patient with toothache coming to dentist, but it is preferable to obtain written consent, particularly for the more hazardous procedures. This documentary evidence may be valuable if claims for compensation are made some time later.

Consent is not of course required for *essential*, life-saving measures such as provision of an airway, in an emergency.

Professional negligence

This term implies that the work carried out falls below a standard judged to be reasonable for the practitioner's training and experience. It would, for example, be regarded as negligent if a dentist failed to diagnose and offer to treat periodontal disease or if he precipitated a medical emergency or serious illness as a result of failing to take an adequate medical history. Successful claims have been on just such grounds.

Many claims have been made because of unsatisfactory dentures and for the complications of extractions, particularly third molars. As mentioned earlier (Ch. 9) it is important not to attempt to extract misplaced third molars unless there is a clear indication for so doing. It is also essential for the dentist to know the current recommendations for the prophylaxis of infective endocarditis, as failure to comply with them has also lead to successful claims.

General anaesthesia and sedation

General anaesthesia is potentially the most dangerous procedure used in dentistry. Death of a patient under anaesthesia may result in a charge of manslaughter, criminal proceedings and erasure from the Dentists Register. This is most likely to happen when the dentist tries to act as both operator and anaesthetist. An illustration of the hazards of such practices, to both patient and dentist, is the case of a dentist in California who used a cocktail of methohexitone and other drugs, and was responsible for the death of three patients. As a consequence, he was found guilty of second-degree murder and given a 15-year prison sentence.

Intravenous sedation with diazepam or midazolam are far safer. However, diazepam given with an opioid such as pentazocine, or sedation with midazolam alone, have caused some deaths.

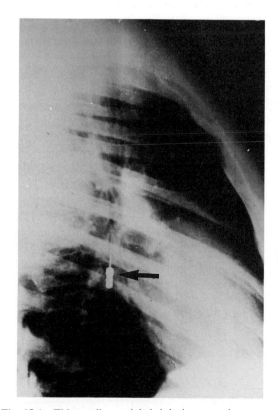

Fig. 25.1 This needle was inhaled during general anaesthesia as a result of absence of a throat pack. Such an accident could lead to claims for compensation and probably a charge of professional negligence.

The General Dental Council has therefore laid down guidelines for the conduct of these procedures. The main requirements are that (a) the dentist must be assisted by another person adequately trained to monitor the patient's vital signs and able to assist in resuscitation, (b) emergency procedures should be laid down and regularly rehearsed by all staff and (c) adequate and effective resuscitative equipment should be immediately to hand when required. The essential points in the GDC guidelines have been mentioned in Chapter 19 and are set out in detail in the Dentists Register, and must be closely adhered to.

A recent source of claims has resulted from patients experiencing fantasies of sexual assault during benzodiazepine sedation. It is essential therefore to have a witness such as the dental nurse present to guard against any such unjustified assertions.

Professional misconduct

Professional misconduct includes unprofessional behaviour (such as sexual or non-sexual assault) towards patients as well as criminal offences, whether or not they are related to dental practice. Examples of the latter include defraudment of the Dental Estimates Board or conviction for drunk driving. Criminal convictions, apart from minor motor offences, are automatically reported to the GDC and are likely to lead to disciplinary procedures.

Perhaps more alarmingly, failure (even if completely accidental) to pay the General Dental Council's annual Registration fee will result in erasure from the Dentists Register. The absence of such registration is no mere formality but can lead to a charge of unlawful dental practice in a Magistrate's Court, with a consequent fine (currently not more than £1000) and the prosecution's costs.

Breaches of National Health Service terms of service

Dental surgeons working within the National Health Service are under contract to their Family Practitioner Committee (FPC) and are required (among other considerations) to employ an appropriate degree of skill in their work and provide treatment necessary to achieve dental fitness. In addition, of course, claims for reimbursement should be made only for work that has been done, and only for work included within the provisions of the Scale of Fees.

Complaints about poor quality of dental treatment or overtreatment may come from patients or from the Dental Estimates Board and are normally dealt with by a Dental Service Committee (DSC) which has both dental and lay members.

If a formal investigation is justified, an oral hearing is usually held for both the complainant and the dental surgeon to present their cases. If the complaint is found to have been justified, the Dental Service Committee can recommend to the FPC one of several possible alternatives:

1. To warn the dentist to comply more closely with the Terms of Service
2. To deduct a sum, from the dentist's remuneration, sufficient to cover any reasonable expenses incurred by anyone as a result of the breach of Terms of Service
3. To withold a further sum from the dentist's remuneration
4. To set a period during which all procedures, except examinations or emergency treatment, must be submitted for prior approval by the DEB
5. To consider, via the National Health Service Tribunal, whether the dentist should remain on the Dental List.

Complaints to the FPC must not therefore be taken lightly. Moreover, if the case is regarded as sufficiently serious and results in the witholding of at least £750, the case may also be referred to the General Dental Council to consider whether the dentist may have been guilty of professional misconduct. If so, the consequences can be even worse.

At the time of writing, a preliminary scheme of inspection of practices by Dental Practice Advisers (DPAs) is being tested in several areas. The purpose is to examine such matters as radiation protection, cross-infection control and any other matters which may affect the quality of treatment provided.

The Health and Safety at Work Acts and other legislation

A dentist as an employer or as the occupier of the premises in which he practises is under legal obligations to ensure that working conditions are healthy and that all reasonable precautions are taken to protect both staff and visitors against accidents. Contravention of any of the requirements of the Act can result in a fine of £1000 or more. An employer also needs to insure against any employee's civil claims for injuries or illnesses and to display the certificate of insurance. In addition he has to formulate and display a Safety Policy for the practice and to make sure that all employees are aware of its provisions.

Health and Safety Inspectors can visit a practice at any time (though normally by appointment) to assess the level of safety, particularly of X-ray and general anaesthetic equipment, autoclaves, cross-infection precautions, safety training and the storage and handling of flammable or explosive materials. If the Inspector finds that a statutory provision is contravened, he can serve an Improvement Notice. Further, if the Inspector feels that the conditions present a serious threat to health then he can serve a Prohibition Notice which may oblige cessation of dental practice until remedial measures have been taken. In extreme cases, contravention of the Act can result, on conviction in a Crown Court, in a fine of unlimited amount or imprisonment for up to 2 years or both. The injured person can also sue their employer for negligence in a civil action.

In addition to safety measures related to the practice of dentistry, the premises themselves must be safe under the requirements of the Occupiers' Liability Act as discussed below.

The Employment Protection Act

An employer is obliged to adhere to the conditions of the Employment Protection Act to avoid charges of unfair dismissal or of discrimination against employees on the grounds of their race or sex, or because of disablement. It may be worth noting that claims by dental staff of unfair dismissal or harassment are increasing and can be a considerable source of trouble to the dentist. Practitioner employers should have a copy of, and be familiar with, the ACAS (Arbitration and Conciliation Advisory Service) Code of Practice. They should also make sure that applicants for posts should have a clear job description and preferably also a detailed contract of service. Dismissal of an unsatisfactory employee can be difficult if the nature of the work they are required to do has not been made absolutely clear.

Stress

The apprehension experienced by very many patients before a dental appointment, and anxiety-induced 'difficult' behaviour during treatment, can transmit themselves to the dentist and put a considerable strain on his emotional resources. For those who find the management of anxious patients difficult, use of sedation will usually make the task easier and also more pleasant for the patient.

Dentists' anxiety can be further heightened by trying to keep to a tight timetable of appointments and by irritating delays when anything goes wrong. Unrealistic ideas of the desired income, and taking on an excessive workload to achieve it, can be a major factor. How to cope with such problems is a matter for each individual, and expert counselling may sometimes be needed. At all costs, however, sympathetic and considerate relationships with patients must always be maintained and will make things easier and lessen tension. However, if this cannot be achieved and relationships with patients become strained, work may become an unbearable burden and be poorly carried out. Medicolegal complaints can follow as discussed earlier.

Assaults by patients are an uncommon hazard of dentistry. Sympathy and reassurance may prevent such situations from getting out of hand but violent psychotic patients may be controllable only by parenteral sedation (*not* diazepam), and the police should be called before anyone is injured or too much damage has been done.

Postural complaints

Dentistry carried out over long periods in the traditional standing posture can lead to disabling back pain in susceptible persons and be a significant occupational hazard. Seated dentistry can lessen but may not abolish this problem. Obvious precautions are to discover the most comfortable working position that can be sustained and to take up leisure activities that strengthen the back muscles.

HAZARDS TO PATIENTS

The main hazards to patients result from:

1. Ill-judged or incompetent treatment
2. General anaesthesia or sedation
3. Infections
4. Toxic effects of other drugs or chemicals
5. Accidents, including physical injuries or chemical burns
6. Radiation
7. Complications arising from underlying systemic disease.

Ill-judged or incompetent treatment

One of the more common causes for claims is for mistaken or incompetent treatment, such as removing the wrong tooth. A major cause of trouble is extraction of misplaced or asymptomatic wisdom teeth in adults, as discussed earlier. There is usually no justification for so doing and there is a significant risk of a fracture or severe infection as a consequence. A claim for assault may also result if informed consent has not been given, particularly when there have been complications such as these.

General anaesthesia and sedation

Some of the physical hazards to patients have been mentioned earlier. In addition, patients may claim that they have been assaulted while consciousness was impaired. Alternatively they may injure themselves during a violent induction or recovery phase. One patient even managed to sever his Achilles tendon in these circumstances.

Anaesthesia and possibly sedation should be avoided during pregnancy. If a stillbirth or production of a defective fetus ultimately follows, it may be difficult to convince a patient that this is mere coincidence. There is a theoretical hazard from nitrous oxide, which, by interfering with vitamin B12 metabolism, can affect DNA production. Though there is no firm evidence that brief exposure during dental sedation could affect a fetus in this way, it may be preferable to avoid its use, particularly during the first trimester.

Infections

Just as the dentist may acquire an infection from a patient so too can patients acquire infection from dental personnel. With good cross infection control this risk is generally small but there have been outbreaks particularly of hepatitis B and of herpes simplex infections (from herpetic whitlow) transmitted to patients by dental staff.

Other drugs and chemicals

Some of the dangers of general anaesthetic agents have already been mentioned, but most anaesthetic accidents are the result of mismanagement rather than toxic effects of the anaesthetic agents themselves. The toxic effects of other drugs are discussed in Chapter 20.

Mercury

Though mercury and particularly its organic compounds are undoubtedly toxic, as discussed earlier, public anxiety about mercury poisoning or allergy allegedly caused by dental amalgams has been fanned by unscrupulous practitioners, scaremongers and others. It was noteworthy, for example, that the alleged dangers of mercury toxicity achieved sudden publicity at the same time as a new and expensive composite restorative material was introduced.

No convincing evidence has been produced to establish that dental amalgams are toxic to patients or are the cause of vague symptoms such as poor memory, lassitude and depression from which pretty well everyone seems to suffer, most of the time. It has been shown that patients who complain of vague symptoms from 'mercury allergy' tend also to suffer from a variety of complaints (such as irritable bowel syndrome) which have no clear organic basis. In a group of 20 patients com-

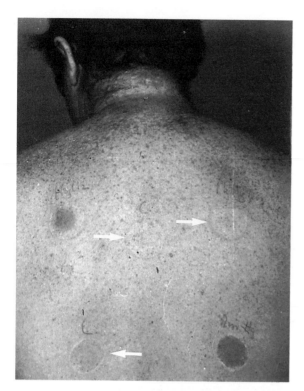

Fig. 25.2 Mercury allergy (delayed hypersensitivity). The reaction to a mercury salt (top right and bottom left) can be contrasted with the lack of reaction to control substances (arrowed). Despite being sensitive to mercury this patient was able to tolerate insertion of amalgam fillings without reaction.

plaining of amalgam-related symptoms, recently investigated, none was found to be hypersensitive to mercury. It also, incidentally, cannot be shown that alternative materials such as composites, of which there is much less experience, are necessarily safer. Some of these, for example, give off traces of formaldehyde, which is suspected of being carcinogenic.

A *few* patients are genuinely sensitive to mercury but, even in these, amalgam restorations can safely be inserted, provided that no amalgam touches the patient's skin. Nevertheless, in these patients, it is usually simpler to use composite materials to obviate the precautions necessary to ensure that no mercury comes into contact with their skin.

Though it can be shown that minute traces of mercury can be absorbed through the oral mucosa from amalgams there is no evidence that they have any clinical effects. In the words of the Council on Dental Therapeutics of the American Dental Association, 'there is insufficient evidence to justify claims that mercury from amalgam restorations has an adverse effect on the health of the patients'.

Accidents

Precautions must obviously be taken against possible accidents during dental practice, such as wounds from a bur, burns from recently autoclaved instruments, or chemical burns from corrosive substances such as phenol. Whenever there is any risk of eye injuries, eye protection should be provided.

In addition, patients may have accidents as a result, for example, of tripping on an ill-lit step or faulty flooring. These too can lead to claims under the Occupiers' Liability Act and for which adequate insurance should be held.

Accidents may lead to allegations of professional negligence and claims for compensation. In the event of an accident, the patient should be given whatever treatment is appropriate. Careful notes should be taken of the event, and the medical protection organisation should be informed. It is important to mollify the patient's feelings but not to admit direct liability.

Radiation

Some of the main considerations have been discussed earlier, and the subject is dealt with in more detail in Chapter 22.

Complications from underlying systemic disease

The more important emergencies due to underlying disease are discussed in Chapter 21.

SUMMARY

Avoidance of all accidents is of course impossible, but important precautions against possible trouble include the following.

1. Practice dentistry to the highest possible clinical and ethical standards and do not perform overambitious procedures beyond your competence.

2. Take and record careful histories and keep good records of all treatments and any that has been refused.

3. Ensure that patients give fully informed consent to all procedures.

4. Avoid at all costs discourtesy and offending patients by an indifferent or abrupt manner.

5. Maintain membership of a Protection Society to make sure of regular payment both of this and of the General Dental Council's registration fee, and take out adequate insurance against possible claims by staff or patients.

6. Keep abreast of current clinical knowledge, especially about such matters as antibiotic

prophylaxis, and make sure that the rest of the dental team are adequately trained in all the work, such as radiography and cross-infection control, they are required to perform.

7. Avoid the use of general anaesthesia and, if practising sedation, make sure that the Notices for the Guidance of Dentists, in the Dentists Register, are scrupulously followed.

8. Keep informed of current legislation applicable to dental practice such as the Health and Safety at Work Acts and the Employers' Liability Act, and of any Notices for the Guidance of Dentists, published by the General Dental Council.

SUGGESTED FURTHER READING

Basu M K, Browne R M, Potts A J 1988 A survey of aerosol-related symptoms in dental hygienists. J Soc Occup Med 38: 23–25

Belfrage S, Ahlgren I, Axelson S 1966 Halothane hepatitis in an anaesthetist. Lancet 2: 1466–1467

Bleicher J N, Blinn D L, Massop D 1987 Hand infections in dental personnel. Plast Reconstruct Surg 80: 420–422

Burge E S 1989 Occupational risks of glutaraldehyde. Br Med J 299: 342

Cavanagh J B 1988 Long term persistence of mercury in the brain. Br J Indust Med 45: 649–651

Cohen E N, Brown B W, Wu M L, Whitcher C E, Brodsky J B 1980 Occupational disease in dentistry and chronic exposure to traces of anaesthetic gases. JADA 101: 21–31

Cook T A, Yates P O 1969 Fatal mercury intoxication in a dental surgery assistant. Br Dent J 127: 553

Council on Dental Materials and Dental Therapeutics 1989 Safety of amalgam—an update. JADA 119: 204–205

Council on Dental Practice 1987 Chemical dependency and dental practice. J Am Dent Assoc 114: 509–518

Eley B M, Cox S W 1987 Mercury from dental amalgam fillings in patients. Br Dent J 163: 221–226

Ericson A, Kallen B 1989 Pregnancy outcome in women working as dentists, dental assistants or dental technicians. Int Arch Occup Env Health 61: 329–333

Franz G 1982 The frequency of allergy to dental materials. J Dent Assoc South Afr 37: 805

Glotry R R, Ayer W A 1986 Head neck & oral abnormalities in dentists participating in the health assessment program. JADA 112: 338–341

Gutman L, Johnsen D 1981 Nitrous oxide-induced myeloneuropathy: report of cases. J Am Dent Assoc 103: 239–241

Harley J L 1978 Eye and facial injuries resulting from dental practice. Dent Clin North Am 22: 505–515

Herber R F M, de Gee A J, Wibowo A A E 1988 Exposure of dentists and assistants to mercury: mercury levels in urine and hair related to conditions of practice. Community Dent Oral Epidemiol 16: 153–158

Langan D C, Fan P L, Hoos A A 1987 The use of mercury

in dentistry: a critical review. J Am Dent Assoc 115: 867–879

Leading article 1985 Lung disease in dental technicians. Lancet 1: 1200–1201

Martin M V 1987 The significance of the bacterial contamination of dental water system. Br Dent J 163: 152–154

Merfield D P, Taylor A, Gemmell D M, Parrish J A 1979 Mercury intoxication in a dental surgery following unreported spillage. Br Dent J 141: 179

Meurman J H, Porko C, Murtomaa H 1990 Patients complaining about amalgam-related symptoms suffer more often from illnesses and chronic craniofacial pain than their controls. Scand J Dent Res 98: 167–172

Moller-Madsen B, Hansen J C, Kragstrup J 1988 Mercury concentrations in blood from Danish dentists. Scand J Dent Res 96: 56–59

Naleway C, Sakaguchi R, Mitchell E et al Urinary mercury levels in US dentists, 1975–1983: review of health assessment program. JADA 111: 37–42

Nilsson B, Nilsson B 1986 Mercury in the dental practice. I. The working environment of dental personnel and their exposure to mercury vapor. Swed Dent J 10: 1–14

Peterson R L, Avery J K 1988 The alcohol-impaired dentist: an educational challenge. J Am Dent Assoc 117: 743–748

Richards J M, Warren P J 1985 Mercury vapour released during the removal of old amalgam restorations. Br Dent J 161: 231–233

Scully C, Cawson R A 1987 Medical problems in dentistry, 2nd edn. Wright, Bristol

Scully C, Cawson R A, Griffiths M 1990 Occupational hazards to dental staff. The British Dental Association, London

Shapiro I M, Sumner A J, Spitz L K et al Neurophysiological and neuropsychological function in mercury-exposed dentists. Lancet 1: 1147–1150

Spence A A 1987 Environmental pollution by anaesthetic gases. Br J Anaesth 59: 96–103

Verschoor M A, Herber R F M, Zielhuis R L 1988 Urinary mercury levels and early changes in kidney function in dentists and dental assistants. Community Dent Oral Epidemiol 16: 148–152

Wilson S J, Wilson H J 1985 Mercury vapour levels in a dental hospital environment. Brit Dent J 161: 233–234

26. Epidemiological aspects of oral disease and community dentistry

Community dentistry aims to investigate the need and demand for dental care in a population, and to determine how to provide for optimal dental health of a community.

The provision and use of dental care by the community is largely dependent (as discussed later) on epidemiological studies. Those who feel that this subject is remote from pathology should remember that epidemiology is an important method of investigating the aetiology and control of disease. The role of fluorides in reducing dental caries, and the value of fluoridation of water supplies (for example), have been determined by epidemiological studies. Knowledge of the causes and mechanisms of oral disease is also of no real value unless it is used for providing means of prevention or treatment, ensuring that the public uses these facilities. One purpose of community dentistry is to determine the extent to which these happen.

The concept of community dentistry is perhaps a little difficult to comprehend, in that dental treatment is provided in an individual, person to person fashion. It is relevant therefore to consider the parent subject of community medicine to identify common features between community medicine and community dentistry.

Community medicine

Community medicine is mainly concerned with two basic concepts. The first is the maintenance or improvement of the general health of the community. This, in principle at least, is achieved by epidemiological studies to determine the needs, then by the application of public health measures to deal with the problem. The second objective is that of relating medical care more closely to the needs of the community and keeping medical care as closely as possible within the community.

Though the expression 'community medicine' may be relatively new, the concept is old. The Romans had effective public health measures, while detailed epidemiological studies and preventive measures for specific diseases go back to the early 18th century.

Public health measures affect the community profoundly, whether or not they are aware of it. These measures range from the provision of a safe water supply to vaccination programmes. The establishment of effective sewerage systems in particular, by preventing faecal contamination of drinking water, has caused water-borne diseases such as typhoid, cholera and dysenteries to disappear from cities where once they accounted for hundreds of thousands of deaths a year. Vaccination combined with rigorous supervision of immigrants has abolished smallpox throughout the world.

Preventive medicine has achieved such successes as to have had a vast impact on the health, welfare and size of the population of the world. By such standards the achievement of more or less complete dental health on a nationwide scale might seem a modest task. But, alas, it is questionable whether there is the general will or even methods available to achieve this objective within the foreseeable future.

Social aspects of disease

The second objective of community medicine is concerned predominantly with the social aspects of disease. The most obvious example is that major threats to health in many countries are the interrelated social problems of the spread of AIDS and of drug dependence. Limiting the spread of AIDS is dependent on health education and persuading all concerned to adopt less risky habits. In the USA, this has resulted in a relative decline in the incidence of AIDS among male homosexuals but a corresponding increase among the many drug abusers and prostitutes, particularly from the poor, uneducated minority groups who are least accessible to health education. Since AIDS is as yet untreatable or preventable by immunisation, its control is essentially a social problem.

In relation to dentistry, a striking example of the gulf between hospital medicine and social problems, which are so often ignored, is illustrated by the problem of mouth cancer. Very often these patients receive highly skilled treatment provided by the coordinated efforts of many experts using sophisticated equipment. Impressive though these efforts genuinely are, the fact is that many patients return home to linger in misery, sometimes because they are too poor or ignorant to know how to look after themselves. Often, no-one tells them how to manage their diet. Some, ashamed by what they regard as obvious stigmata of cancer, become isolated and lack even their neighbours' help or company.

Health economics

Somewhat less obviously, community medicine is concerned with politico-economic problems. First, medical care has to be paid for, and if this care is to be community-based then it must be paid for by the state—more precisely, the taxpayer. Hence, the allocation of resources and the priorities given to different aspects of medical care present a touchy problem affected by a wide variety of influences. Second, a huge amount of illness can perhaps only be controlled by political means. Examples are the effects of cigarette smoking and of motor vehicle accidents, which together cause tens of thousands of deaths a year and countless cases of disability. Both *in theory* could be controlled completely, but only with the loss of enormous tax revenue from cigarettes, by throwing hundreds of thousands of people out of work, and by making decisions which would probably overthrow any government.

Community medicine is therefore a complicated subject. It is in some respects a medical discipline but in other ways a social movement and has, as a consequence, produced its own jargon. First, of course, such phrases as 'community health measures' sound more attractive and are more emotive than the actuality, which might merely be the provision of a new main drain. Second, the prefix 'community' is liberally applied to any medical or paramedical workers, irrespective of what it implies. Thus, in the present Health Service there are Community *Health* doctors and Community *Medicine* doctors who—if it can be believed—do different jobs and receive different salaries.

One may perhaps therefore ask in what way a community dentist might differ from any other.

Community dentistry

Generally speaking, the attitudes and problems underlying community medicine have remarkably little in common with any concepts of community dentistry. Dental disease in no way isolates the patient from the community. Moreover there is, so far, only *one* public health measure—fluoridation of water—which can even partially affect dental disease. The rest depends almost entirely on treatment or instruction given by individual dentists to individual patients. The level of dental health in the community therefore depends on the extent to which people seek dental care and apply preventive measures. These in turn depend on the individual's attitude towards dental health and whether a natural dentition is valued more highly than artificial dentures.

It is therefore a facile oversimplification to assume that, since dental disease is largely preventable, all that is needed is sufficient money (provided by the taxpayer) to apply these measures on a national scale to accomplish a dental utopia.

While few would dispute the desirability of improving the dental health of the community, some sense of proportion is needed to consider how few preventive measures are available and to assess how effective they are likely to be in relation to the scale and nature of the problem.

To a great extent, dental disease is in effect self-inflicted or the result of neglect. Self-inflicted diseases are some of the most difficult to control, as mentioned earlier. Drug dependence and alcoholism can hardly be said to have declined in response to an enormous amount of well-intentioned effort and expense.

The content of community dentistry

Community dentistry, like community medicine, comprises both investigation—epidemiology in all its aspects—and action, namely public health measures. The investigational aspect of community dentistry forms the major component of the subject at the moment.

The main areas of investigation relevant to community dentistry are therefore:

1. The prevalence of dental disease and the need for treatment
2. Factors affecting the prevalence and distribution of dental disease
3. The demand for dental treatment and factors affecting demand for treatment and attitudes towards dental health
4. Factors affecting types of treatment given by dentists
5. Evaluation of means of improving dental

health in the community, including health education
6. Assessment of manpower needs to accomplish these aims and of optimal means of deployment and distribution of dental manpower
7. Establishment of the optimal composition of the dental team in terms of dentists and ancillaries of various kinds
8. Assessment of the training implications of these decisions and evaluation of dental education in relation to the needs of the community
9. Determination of the feasibility of dental health care measures in relation to finances available, and relating the priorities for dental public health measures to those for other services
10. Monitoring the effectiveness of dental health care measures that have been implemented, and modifying these measures in the light of the findings.

It is not feasible to try to discuss all these matters here, especially as some, such as the problems of finance and the 'cost-effectiveness' of various methods of dental health care, involve too many imponderables.

The question of the prevalence of dental disease, the demand for dental treatment and related problems are the field of *epidemiology*, which forms the groundwork for all community dental care programmes. The problem of how the dental health of the community could then be improved involves many more conjectural aspects which can be solved only by experimental studies monitored in turn by further epidemiological studies.

EPIDEMIOLOGICAL ASPECTS OF ORAL AND DENTAL DISEASE

Epidemiology can be defined as the study of the distribution of, and determinants affecting, disease in human populations. In other words, findings from epidemiological studies may suggest possible causes and factors affecting the distribution or spread of disease.

Epidemiology originated (not surprisingly) in the study of epidemics, but started even before the cause of infections was known. In spite of this lack of knowledge, remarkable progress was made.

The work of John Snow in the early 19th century exemplifies well not merely the nature of epidemiological studies and their purpose, but also what could be achieved. John Snow is best known for his remarkable work in 1824 when he followed the spread of a cholera epidemic in such detail as to be able to trace the source to a single well in Broad Street, Soho. From this finding he deduced the then unknown fact that the infection was water-borne. Snow was able both to stop further spread of the infection and also to confirm his theories as to its origin by a single simple action. The measure was so surprising in its simplicity and so completely effective as to demonstrate a touch of genius. The epidemic was in fact stopped simply by removing the handle of the pump.

Sadly, no-one has thought of a comparably simple and effective preventive measure for dental disease.

The purposes of epidemiology

Epidemiological studies are applied to many conditions other than infections and to many different aspects of disease. It is so well known that dental disease is virtually universal in Westernised countries that merely to accumulate data on the prevalence of dental disease can be of little value. Though often done to provide material for publications, it serves little other purpose if the information is not put to practical use.

The ultimate purposes of epidemiological studies must in the main be:

1. To seek factors relating to the causes of disease
2. To assist in prevention
3. To assess the needs and demand for treatment
4. To evaluate treatment or preventive measures
5. To provide a basis for the allocation of financial resources.

Sources of information

Data on some diseases are collected as a statutory requirement. Causes of death have been registered in Britain since 1836. Though much of the data from death certificates is inaccurate, it is informative in the case of mouth cancer. The notification of infectious diseases such as diphtheria has also been compulsory since the 19th century but, though such data are relatively reliable, they can only record cases which have been severe enough to have come to a doctor, and they also depend on the accuracy of the diagnosis.

Cancer of all types is registrable and, since it is likely that every patient with cancer will sooner or later seek treatment and often die from the disease, a much fuller picture is available for this disease than for any other. These data are brought together by the Office of Population Censuses and Surveys (OPCS). Though inaccuracies can obviously be found as a result, for instance, of uncertainties about precise diagnosis of certain tumours, Britain has the largest source of data on incidence of, duration of survival, and mortality from malignant disease of all types anywhere in the world.

In the case of cancer of the mouth these data are particularly valuable and accurate since the disease can be recognised with reasonable certainty, at least in its later stages, by clinical examination alone. Histological confirmation is also straightforward. Mortality from cancer in specific sites has been continually recorded since 1897 by the Registrar General and has also been calculated from death certificates as far back as 1868. In view of the unusual degree of certainty of recognition of oral cancer compared with other sites, these data offer a unique historical perspective of the trends in this disease. These trends in turn provide a basis for hypotheses as to possible causative factors.

Probably more is known about the general epidemiological aspects of mouth cancer than any other disease of the mouth, and some of these data are discussed in Chapter 16.

A glance at the OPCS medical statistics for any year is, incidentally, well worthwhile to get an idea of the vast amount of data that have been accumulated about virtually every disease.

No comparable amount of information is available concerning dental disease; the only statistics regularly accumulated are those of items of treatment approved by the Dental Estimates Board. Obviously this covers only a selected sample:

namely, those who choose to ask for dental treatment through the National Health Service. Very many, however, do not bother with regular dental treatment and are therefore not represented except as casual extractions and, ultimately, dentures. A small minority have dental treatment at their own expense, so there are no data about these either. Nevertheless these statistics provide some indication of the extent to which people seek dental treatment and also of the relative frequency with which different kinds of treatment are provided by the Health Service.

Surveys are an important means of accumulating data about dental disease but also have limitations, in that examination of patients is time-consuming and expensive; a significant number of patients may also refuse examination. Some surveys can be carried out by means of interviews; this too is time-consuming, is affected by the subjective nature of the patient's answers and, again, those least interested in dental health are the least likely to participate.

Any decision to carry out a survey creates in turn a series of other needs if any useful information is ultimately to be produced.

Types of epidemiological studies

The aims of epidemiology can be achieved by different types of study. These are generally categorised as:

1. *Descriptive*
2. *Analytical*
3. *Experimental.*

1. *Descriptive studies* accumulate data about the incidence or prevalence of a disease and its distribution. Such studies provide data on the level of need for treatment but can do no more than suggest factors which may be related to the frequency or severity of disease. Examples of descriptive epidemiology are the studies carried out on the prevalence of caries in different areas of Britain or in different age groups. Unfortunately, many studies in dental epidemiology never get beyond this stage.

2. *Analytical studies* seek to identify variables which might be determinants of the disease in question. An example is the investigation of the relationship between the fluoride content of drinking water and mottling of the enamel. An analytical study such as this can be carried out in either of two ways. A group of patients with mottled teeth and a group of controls (an otherwise comparable group with normal teeth) can be collected and the difference in exposure to fluoride between the two groups compared. Alternatively what is known as a *cohort** study could be carried out. A cohort is a group sharing a common experience—in this case exposure to fluoride. To carry out such a study a particular population (a cohort) that had been exposed to high-fluoride drinking water is compared with a control group that has not been exposed; the difference in the frequency and severity of mottling in the two groups could then be compared.

Generally speaking case/control studies are easier to carry out than cohort studies. If the aim was, for instance, to examine the association between drinking habits and mouth cancer it would be easier to find patients with mouth cancer and look into their drinking habits. The alternative would be to assess the incidence of mouth cancer among a group (cohort) of chronic alcoholics. This would be difficult because the incidence of cancer is so low that many thousands of alcoholics would have to be found and examined before any significant number of cases was found.

Studies can also differ in another respect: they may be *cross-sectional*, that is to say looking at a group of patients at a particular point of time. *Longitudinal* studies, by contrast, follow a group of patients over a period to observe the changes that develop. In the investigation of periodontal disease in particular, longitudinal studies are of the greatest value in showing the progress of the disease in relation to such variables as the level of oral hygiene or specific forms of treatment. Unfortunately it is exceedingly difficult to follow a group of patients for an adequate length of time.

3. *Experimental studies.* The earlier reference to John Snow's removal of the handle of the pump which supplied infected water is an example of an experimental preventive measure. Snow had no

---

* Cohort—literally one of the 10 companies in a Roman legion and therefore consisting of 300 to 600 men. One wonders how such a unit got into epidemiological terminology.

way of knowing the cause of the infection but his experimental measure was remarkably successful.

Closer to home have been the experiments on fluoridation of water supplies followed by epidemiological evidence that confirmed conclusively its value and safety as a preventive measure.

Practical aspects of epidemiological studies

Accuracy of observations

The standard and consistency of diagnosis obviously affects the accuracy of observations. In the case of periodontal disease, this is particularly difficult. Decisions that have to be made before a survey is carried out therefore include the following.

1. *The observation to be made.* In most cross-sectional studies of dental caries, for example, the observation made is usually that of the number of decayed, missing and filled teeth. More precise studies might require different kinds of observation such as the rate of development of cavities. This in turn would bring increased difficulties because of the problems of assessing the size of carious cavities.
2. *The choice of technique.* The requirement of an ideal technique are considered below, but in the case of dental caries it might involve examination merely with mirror or probe or might use radiographs in addition. Though this brings greater accuracy it is also more time-consuming and costly.
3. *The training of personnel.* Errors enter in because of variations in the standards and skill of different observers and because of variations, by each observer, in the quality of his observations. These difficulties are particularly great in studies on periodontal disease where assessments are necessarily subjective.

   The performance of observers has therefore to be calibrated by training them to examine for the chosen variable on the same group of patients repeatedly until their results are consistent both within the group and by the same person on each occasion.

4. *Testing the technique.* Pilot studies on a small test group are necessary to test whether the observational technique works under field conditions and whether the observers are performing to an adequate standard.

Quality of observational techniques

For epidemiological studies to be useful the techniques used must be:

1. *Valid.* The observation should be both sensitive and specific. For detection of early occlusal caries a sticky fissure has been shown to fulfil these criteria. By contrast, DMF measurements provide no information about the reason why teeth have been lost nor about the rate of development of dental caries, and much has to be derived from such observations by inference only. The problems of measuring periodontal disease are particularly great, as discussed below.
2. *Practical.* The detection of early dental caries involves both probe and mirror examination and the use of radiographs for interstitial caries. In a large survey it may be impractical to attempt to use radiology because it is time-consuming and the facilities may be difficult to obtain. There is also a general need to minimise radiation exposure.
3. *Accurate.* Periodontal disease is very difficult to quantify, and there are no precise objective methods of assessing its severity. These problems are made worse by the variation in the severity of the disease in different parts of the mouth and even at different points round the circumference of a single tooth.
4. *Under standardised conditions.* The conditions under which the observations are to be made must be carefully specified and standardised throughout the survey. In the case of dental caries in particular it is important to standardise such things as the type and quality of lighting and the type of probes used. If radiographs are also to be taken, then the many variables such as tube distance, angulation, exposure and type of film have also to be carefully standardised.

Quantification of disease

The most basic observation is that of the number of cases. Though this is a crude observation, it may itself be of value in that it provides some indication of the amount of treatment needed. Such information must also be related to the size of the population at risk. Such rates are subject to many variables, in that some diseases affect only children, others affect only women, while yet others affect any member of the whole population. Many figures quoted may therefore be misleading unless the size and composition of the population at risk is known. The number of affected patients in relation to the population at risk is described as a *disease rate*.

A *disease rate* may be defined as the number of persons with a disease in relation to the population at risk (the sum of those affected and those unaffected) at any given point of time.

Rates express either *morbidity* (the frequency of an illness) or *mortality* (the frequency of deaths). In the case of dental disease, morbidity is obviously the chief concern, but in the case of cancer, mortality is important.

Incidence and prevalence rates

Incidence rates can be defined as the number of cases of a disease which develop in a measurable population during a specified period of time. Calculations of incidence rates depend on the disease having a definable starting point. Infectious diseases, for example, have a clearly definable onset so that the incidence (sometimes called the *attack rate*) can be defined in terms of the ratio of the number of persons starting the illness (new cases) to the size of a population or, more usually, per 100 000 of a population in a given week, month, or year. Similarly, for most patients cancer is a single disease from which they survive or die. The incidence of new cases of oral cancer in a year is therefore also readily definable.

Prevalence rates define the proportion of a population affected by a disease at a particular time. The prevalence rate is affected both by the *incidence* and by the *duration* of the disease. Dental disease in particular rarely has a detectable starting point and is a more or less continuous process. Figures for DMF in a given population are there-fore an indication of the prevalence of caries rather than of its incidence.

Population and samples. While cancer, especially, is no respecter of persons, most diseases are affected by the make-up of the population at risk. This in turn is affected by a wide variety of attributes and variables; these include such factors as age, sex, marital state, occupation, socio-economic status, ethnic group, or environment. Broadly speaking, the level of dental health varies with age, sex, socio-economic status and geographical situation of the sample.

It must be emphasised that in studies of dental disease, as of any other, the controls must be carefully matched with the population under examination, as most of these variables affect the severity and extent of dental disease and the type of treatment sought.

Indices of dental disease

These are needed (i) to carry out prevalence studies for epidemiological purposes, (ii) for clinical trials, to test the response to treatment.

Indices provide a measure of the severity of the diseases investigated. They are also needed to standardise as far as possible the observations made. This in turn allows, in theory at least, comparisons to be made between studies carried out at different times or in different places.

Indices of dental caries

The main examples are:

1. *Decayed, missing and filled teeth DMF* is probably the most widely used method. However, in young children, shedding of deciduous teeth increases the number of missing teeth, while in adults an increasing number of teeth are lost due to periodontal disease. In addition, once a tooth has been attacked by caries, further attacks by the disease on other surfaces of the tooth are not measured.

2. *DMF surfaces (DMFS)* is a more sensitive and accurate measure of dental caries but depends on radiographs to detect interstitial caries, as well as probe and mirror examination to detect occlusal lesions. Surface counts have the advantage that new

points of attack on the same tooth can be detected, and this gives an index of the activity of the disease, particularly in mouths where caries is already severe.

Indices of periodontal disease

Several variables can be measured such as

1. Amount of plaque
2. Extent of gingivitis (colour or bleeding)
3. Extent or depth of pocketing
4. Amount of alveolar bone loss.

All of these methods are essentially subjective. There is wide variation between different observers, and the same observer rarely produces completely consistent results. The figures obtained for these assessments of gingivitis must also not be regarded as being in any way quantitative. It is a spurious way of recording judgements to use digits to represent (for instance) 'Good', 'Moderate', 'Bad', or 'Very Bad'. These scores cannot or *must not* therefore be manipulated mathematically.

Assessment of plaque

A disclosing agent must be used and the extent of plaque or debris (they are indistinguishable) is assessed by methods such as the following.

The Plaque Index.

0 No plaque in the gingival area

1 Plaque adhering to the gingival margin and adjacent tooth surface
2 Moderate accumulation of plaque within the gingival pocket, on the gingival margin and/or adjacent tooth.
3 Abundant plaque within the gingival pocket and/or gingival margin and adjacent tooth.

The Oral Hygiene Index (simplified). For this index six tooth surfaces are usually chosen (buccal surfaces of upper first molars; lingual surfaces of lower first molars; labial surfaces of upper right and lower left central incisors). Each surface is scored for plaque and calculus separately as follows:

- *Plaque*
  0 None present

1 Plaque covering not more than one-third of the tooth
2 Plaque covering more than one-third but less than two-thirds of the tooth
3 Plaque covering more than two-thirds of the tooth.

- *Calculus*
  0 None present
  1 Supragingival calculus covering not more than one-third of the tooth
  2 Supragingival calculus covering more than one-third but not more than two-thirds of the tooth or flecks of subgingival calculus round the neck of the teeth or both
  3 Supragingival calculus covering more than two-thirds of the tooth or a continuous heavy band of subgingival calculus round the neck of the tooth or both.

The mean plaque score and the mean calculus score are (unjustifiably) added to give the Oral Hygiene Index.

To add to the confusion, a high Oral Hygiene score does *not* mean good oral hygiene but indicates severe oral neglect.

The Gingival Index. For this assessment the circumference of the gingival margin is divided into four (mesial, distal, buccal and lingual) and each is scored as follows:

0 Normal gingiva
1 Mild inflammation; slight change in colour, slight oedema and no bleeding on probing
2 Moderate inflammation; redness, oedema and glazing; bleeding on probing
3 Severe inflammation, severe redness and oedema; ulceration; spontaneous bleeding.

The score for each area is totalled and the sum divided by 4 to provide the Gingival Index for the whole mouth.

It will be obvious that this assessment is even more subjective than the plaque measurements. By how much, for instance, does 'Mild' differ from 'Moderately' and how firmly must the probe be used to elicit bleeding? Unfortunately, no better methods have been devised.

The Periodontal Index. This is similar in essence to the Gingival Index but is widely used to assess more severe degrees of tissue destruction in addition to gingivitis. The gingivae and supporting tissues of each tooth are assessed as follows:

0   Neither overt inflammation nor loss of function due to destruction of supporting tissues
1   Mild gingivitis. Inflammation of the gingival margin but this does not surround the tooth
2   Gingivitis. Inflammation surrounds the tooth but there is no detectable break in the epithelial attachment
6   Gingivitis with pocket formation. There is true pocketing but no mobility nor migration and no interference with function
8   Advanced destruction with loss of masticatory function. The tooth may be loose, have drifted or may be depressible in its socket and may sound dull on percussion.

The Periodontal Index is the sum of the scores for the individual teeth divided by the number of teeth examined.

The Community Periodontal Index of Treatment Needs (CPITN). The CPITN method of scoring was proposed by the World Health Organization. A special periodontal probe which has a 0.5 mm ball end, and is colour coded between 3.5 and 5.5 mm from its tip, must be used. Probing force should not exceed 20–25 g. In adults, a single score for each sextant with two or more functioning teeth is recorded in a simple box chart as follows:

Code 4:   6 mm or deeper pathological pocket
Code 3:   5–5 mm pathological pocketing
Code 2:   Supra or subgingival calculus or defective margin or filling or crown
Code 1:   Bleeding after gentle probing
Code 0:   Healthy periodontal tissues.

Only one code—the *highest*, corresponding to the *worst* condition observed—is recorded for each segment.

In children and young persons under 20, when a designated tooth is absent, the sextant is recorded as missing. Between the ages of 7 and 11 it is suggested that only bleeding, calculus, or defective restorations are recorded.

Treatment needs. The suggested management is related to the disease scores as follows:

Code 0:   No need for periodontal treatment
Code 1:   Oral hygiene instruction (OHI) needed
Codes 2   Scaling and root planing (Sc+RP)
  & 3:   needed in addition to OHI
Code 4:   Complex treatment as well as OHI+Sc+RP.

These recorded figures in turn suggest the amount of time needed for treating each patient.

Needless to say, this scoring system has been criticised on various grounds but is intended only as a screening procedure to suggest (as its name implies) the treatment needs of a community.

ADULT DENTAL HEALTH IN BRITAIN

The first surveys on a national scale, by means of dental examinations and interviews, were carried out in 1968 in England and Wales and in 1972 in Scotland. Further surveys have been carried out in the whole of Britain in 1978 (with samples of over 3000 persons examined and nearly 20 000 interviewed) and in 1988 on a smaller scale, and only limited data from it were available at the time of writing.

Annual surveys by means of interviews on approximately 10 000 households have also been carried out annually by the Office of Population Censuses and Surveys (OPCS), and the 1987 data are available.

These different surveys do not all provide the same type of information, but some indices (particularly loss of teeth) make clear a slow but steady improvement in dental health of the population. The earlier surveys are also still informative in terms of trends in dental health and of a population's ideas about how better dental health could be achieved.

A noticeable feature of these surveys is the lower state of dental health in the north compared with the south, in professional classes compared with manual and, particularly, unskilled workers. These differences are illustrated by, for example, the proportions of these different groups who have become edentulous and in their patterns of dental attendance as discussed below.

In the following summaries the latest available data are quoted.

Total loss of teeth

No more than some sample figures can be given, but between 1968 and 1988 the proportion of edentulous persons (all ages) fell from 37% to 20% in England and Wales. In Scotland these figures fell from 44% to 26% between 1972 and 1988.

Tooth loss is of course related to age. In 1968, 1% between ages 16 and 24 were found to be edentulous but none in this group in the later surveys, except in Scotland in 1988 where 1% of these young people had lost all teeth. At the opposite end of the age scale, 80% of those over 75 were edentulous in 1988 in England and Wales.

The disparities in the size of the edentulous population in the different areas is further indicated by the fact that it constituted 27% of the population in the north of England and only 16% in the south in 1988.

Despite the fact that women consistently report that they more regularly attend for check-ups, a significantly higher proportion of them have been found to be edentulous in all the surveys, in all regions and at all ages. For example, in England and Wales 24% of women, but only 17% of men overall, and in Scotland 34% of women and 23% of men, were edentulous in 1987.

In terms of the disparities in dental health between the different socio-economic groups, the proportion edentulous in 1983, for example, was only 8% among professionals but 44% among manual workers.

In summary, therefore, in the 20 years between 1968 and 1988 the proportion of edentulous persons (aged 16 or over) in England and Wales had fallen from 37% to 20%. All surveys also consistently showed larger edentulous populations in northern Britain compared with the south, among unskilled compared with professional workers, and among women compared with men.

The condition of the teeth

Between 1968 and 1978 the proportion of adults with some decay fell from 64% to 59%. Overall, there was an average of 2 decayed teeth per mouth

in 1978 and this had fallen to 1 by 1988. In this decade the number of sound, untreated teeth had risen corresponding from 13 to 15. In this last survey the numbers of missing and filled teeth were on average 7.6 and 8.1, respectively, and just under 15 sound and untreated in the arch. This represented a slight improvement on the findings of the 1978 survey but the disparities between different areas remained virtually unchanged.

Periodontal disease

The proportion having some debris on the teeth was 65% for the UK as a whole: this ranged from 64% for ages 16–24 to 70% for age 55 and over. 58% of these claimed to have regular dental check-ups.

Calculus was found in 72% of persons in the UK as a whole and increasingly frequently with age. Thus it was found in 54% for ages 16–24 and in 83% for those over 45 and in 64% of those claiming to have regular check-ups.

Some gingivitis was present in 83%. It was present in 77% of those aged 16–24 and in 87% of those over 45. Gingivitis was found even in 78% who had regular check-ups.

Periodontitis was found in 27% overall and ranged from 3% of those aged 16–24 to 64% of those over 55.

In total, therefore, plaque and/or calculus and gingivitis and/or periodontitis were found in 91% of the adult population.

In all areas fewer women showed these components of periodontal disease, except for gingivitis which was equally common in both sexes.

Even taking into account the possibility of variations in diagnostic criteria the findings for periodontal disease show no improvement over those made 10 years earlier and patients were equally unaware of their periodontal state.

These data are from the 1978 survey, but no more recent information on this scale is yet available.

Patterns of dental attendance

These figures had changed little by 1987, when 46% (women 56%, men 41%) in England and

Wales and 41% in Scotland (women 55%, men 35%) stated that they had regular check-ups. As noted earlier, despite the persistently higher rate of dental attendance by women, an appreciably higher proportion of them lost all their teeth than men, in all age groups. In effect therefore women tended to lose all their teeth earlier than men.

Attitudes towards total tooth loss

Nearly 70% of edentulous persons stated that they were glad to have got rid of, or were not worried about, having lost their teeth in 1978. With regard to dentate patients, only 53% expressed themselves as being very upset at the idea of losing their teeth.

CHILD DENTAL HEALTH 1973 TO 1983

Only illustrative samples of the main findings in these 2 studies can be presented.

The state of the childrens' health was assessed by examination, but background information was gathered by postal questionnaires. This is in contrast to the 1973 study, when the parents were interviewed.

Caries prevalence

The number of 5-year-olds with decayed or filled deciduous teeth fell from 71% in 1973 to 48% in 1983. The average number of deciduous teeth with signs of decay fell from 3.4 to 1.7. As before, there were sharp differences between south and north, with the average number of decayed deciduous teeth at 5 years being 1.1 in England, 2.6 in Scotland and 3.0 in Northern Ireland.

There was an increase in decay among older children when compared with 1973, but this was because improved dental care had allowed filled deciduous teeth to be retained longer.

Loss of permanent teeth due to decay

In the UK overall, tooth loss from decay was very small and by age 15 accounted for only an average of 0.6 teeth.

Dental attendance

Regular dental attendance in 1973 was recorded as 39% for 5-year-olds and 53% for 12-year-olds. By 1983, these figures had risen to 57% and 64% but the figure was only 59% for 15-year-olds. Similarly, attendance only for trouble, which was 53% and 32% for 5- and 12-year-olds respectively in 1973, had fallen to 24% and 22%.

In 1987, 72% of 5-year-olds and 79% of 15-year-olds had attended for a check-up or 'to get used to the dentist'.

Ideas about causes and prevention of decay

In 1973 approximately 80% of mothers stated that sweet things were the main cause, and in 1983 between 68% and 78% (according to their children's ages) of mothers still thought so. Only a minority in 1973 thought that decay could be prevented by avoiding sweets, and by 1983 between 37% and 48% of mothers still thought the same, and 71% to 75% of them thought that cleaning the teeth was the most important preventive measure. Over 25% thought that a balanced diet (whatever that may be) was a useful preventive measure. Little credit was given to dentists and only 3% to 4% thought that their preventive treatment was of value.

As to fluorides, fewer than 6% of mothers in 1973 thought that fluorides were of any benefit and this had not significantly changed by 1983. By this time less than 3% overall thought that fluoride in drinking water might prevent decay, and only slightly more (between 5% and 8%) thought that use of fluoride toothpastes was of value.

Approximately half the mothers stated that their children brushed their teeth twice a day and the number had not changed significantly by 1983.

Gingivitis, plaque, calculus and pocketing

There was depressingly little change between 1973 and 1983. In 1983 gingivitis present in 5-, 10- and 15-year-olds was 18%, 50% and 49% respectively. The figures for 1973 were 26%, 56% and 51% and showed no apparent improvement. Calculus was found in 3%, 16% and 33% of 5-, 10- and 15-year-olds in 1983, while in 1973 it was found in 5%, 16% and 34% at the same ages. 'Debris' was found on the teeth of 19%, 56% and 47% of 5-, 10- and 15-year-olds in 1983, while in 1973 it was found in 39%, 65% and 51% respectively. It was therefore concluded that the teeth were slightly cleaner than their counterparts 10 years earlier.

Pocketing was only assessed in 15-year-olds and was present in 9% (the UK as a whole). However, pocketing and gingivitis were associated in only 7%, so that it appeared that in 2% pocketing had developed in the absence of gingivitis.

In conclusion it is apparent that there has been a great improvement in the level of child dental health, as suggested by smaller local surveys, but it seems that the decline in caries prevalence has not continued further. However, the findings of the 1988 national survey on child dental health were not available at the time of writing.

SUMMARY

1. The dental health of the community is gradually improving. The main index is that, overall, the proportion of edentulous persons (all ages) has fallen from 37% in 1988 to 20% in 1988 in England and Wales. Among dentate patients the average number of sound, untreated teeth per mouth has risen from 13 in 1978 to 15 in 1988.

2. Despite evidence of more regular dental check-ups, 24% of women had become edentulous as compared with 17% of men. Total tooth loss is higher among women than men at all ages and in all areas.

3. Dental health is considerably better among professional classes than among unskilled workers. Of these 8% and 44% respectively were edentulous in a recent survey.

4. A depressingly high proportion of the population still seem relatively undismayed at the prospect of having their teeth replaced by dentures.

5. Among children, the number of 5-year-olds with decayed or filled deciduous teeth fell from 71% in 1973 to 48% in 1983, and the average number of deciduous teeth with signs of decay fell from 3.4 to 1.7.

6. As with adults there remain wide differences between south and north with, for example, the average number of decayed deciduous teeth at 5

years being 1.1 in England, 2.6 in Scotland and 3.0 in Northern Ireland.

7. There appears to be little improvement in periodontal health over a decade in either children or adults.

8. Dental health education seems to have had little impact on mothers' ideas about achieving dental health for their children. Remarkably few, for example, believe use of fluorides to be important in preventing decay. The persistently high expenditure on confectionery and soft drinks (over £5 600 000 000 in 1988) also suggests that few are aware of, or concerned about, the effects of sugar on the teeth.

9. Few mothers also seem to think that dentists contribute appreciably to improving dental health.

10. Fluoridation of water supplies remains the only widely applicable dental health measure, but its value is decreasing in many areas such as southern England and many parts of the USA, probably as a result of the widespread use of fluoride toothpastes.

THE EUROPEAN ECONOMIC COMMUNITY (EEC)

One of the effects of the so-called Common Market is that dental training has had to be harmonised to enable dentists to practice in any of the constituent countries. In particular, Italy and, more recently, Spain have had radically to change their dental curricula to something similar to that in Britain, and even this textbook is published in Italian and Spanish. In Spain there is currently so great a demand for places in dental schools (there are many unemployed or underemployed doctors) that the educational standards for entry are the highest for any university subject.

However, there is as yet no sign that the UK is being overwhelmed by foreign dentists hoping to make a better living here, or that British dentists are migrating to other countries for the same reason.

Another consideration is that the member countries provide widely differing standards of public health care and methods of remunerating doctors and dentists. Inevitably, governments look at such provisions in other countries to see whether health care can be delivered more efficiently and economically by emulating them, and ultimately this might have an effect on the British National Health Service.

CURRENT PROBLEMS AFFECTING THE DENTAL PROFESSION, AND THEIR POSSIBLE EFFECTS ON DENTAL HEALTH

The image of the dental profession in the eyes of the public, and its own ideas of itself, need to be considered. In addition the changes in the dental needs of the population as shown by the dental health surveys inevitably affect various aspects of dental practice. The greatest problem is that improvement of dental health, and in particular periodontal disease, depends almost entirely upon the individual efforts of practitioners. There are no public health measures that can deal with this aspect of health. Though industry and advertising appeared to have convinced a high proportion of the population of the value of toothbrushing this does not as yet appear to have had any significant effect on the prevalence or severity of periodontal diseases.

Some of these problems that need to be considered are therefore as follows.

1. The greatly decreased prevalence of dental caries in children, and the scanty evidence of improved periodontal health, imply that the emphasis on restorative dentistry is decreasingly justified.

2. Whether or not more widespread fluoridation of water supplies is possible or even necessary in many areas such as the south-east of England has to be considered.

3. The findings of national surveys do not suggest that the contribution of the dental profession to dental health education and prevention of dental disease is very great, but the current system of remuneration within the NHS provides little financial incentive for such effort.

4. The increasing costs particularly of dentures which are unremunerative and as a consequence are increasingly difficult to obtain in the NHS by the large numbers of edentulous persons present in all areas, especially in northern Britain.

5. The increasing NHS fees for most forms of dental treatment and anxieties about pricing dentistry out of the NHS. This also particularly affects the north, where incomes are generally lower.

6. Difficulties in recruiting dentists to practices in many areas, especially the north where dental health is poorest.

7. Overprescribing of the more remunerative dental procedures—namely, restorative and orthodontic treatment—that has been confirmed in surveys reflects poorly on the dental profession and has given rise to adverse publicity.

8. The scant evidence of increasing rates of regular dental attendance or of expressed confidence in the contribution of dentists to improving dental health is a possible cause for concern.

9. Anxiety about cuts in financial support for the NHS and about future forms of remuneration within the NHS such as the possibility of remuneration by capitation fee and whether any such changes will, on the one hand, reduce dentists' incomes or, on the other, benefit patients.

10. Doubts about the extent or value of dental health education, especially on the lower socio-economic groups, as shown by, for example, expressed ideas about how best to achieve dental health or about total tooth loss, despite high levels of regular dental attendance.

11. Difficulties in recruiting suitable candidates for dental training, partly because of doubts about the future of the dental profession and competition from more remunerative occupations.

12. Low morale among NHS and university dental staff, particularly concerning the future of both, especially as a result of increasing cuts in financial support for both.

SUGGESTED FURTHER READING

Anon 1986 The 1983 Update on adult dental health from OPCS. Br Dent J 162: 246–253

Anon 1988 Adult dental health. Br Dent J 166: 279–281

Anon 1990 The Annual Report of the Chief Medical Officer of Health: Dental health. Br Dent J 168: 119–120

Ciancio S G 1986 Current status of indices of periodontitis. J Clin Periodontal 13: 375–378

Dennis G (ed) 1990 Annual Abstract of Statistics No 126 (1990). HMSO, London

Fischman S L 1986 Current indices of plaque. J Clin Periodontal 13: 371–374

Gratrix D, Taylor G O, Lennon M A 1990 Mothers' dental attendance patterns and their children's dental attendance and dental health. Br Dent J 168: 441–444

Greene J C, Louie R, Wycoff S J 1990 Preventive dentistry II. Periodontal diseases, malocclusion, trauma and oral cancer. J Am Dent Assoc 263: 421–425

Holloway P J, Lennon M A, Mellor A C et al 1990 The captitation study. 1 Does captitation encourage 'Supervised neglect?' Br Dent J 1990 166: 119–121

Office of Population Censuses and Surveys 1985 Children's dental health in the United Kingdom 1983. HMSO, London

Office of Population Censuses and Surveys 1989 General Household Survey 1987. HMSO, London

Pilot T, Barmes D E 1987 An update on periodontal conditions in adults, measured by CPITN. Int Dent J 37: 169–172

Renson C E 1989 Global changes in caries prevalence and dental manpower requirements: 1. Assembling and analysing the data. Dental Update 16: 287–299

Renson C E 1989 Global changes in caries prevalence and dental manpower requirements: 2. The reasons underlying the changes in prevalence. Dental Update 16: 345–352

Renson C E 1989 Global changes in caries prevalence and dental manpower requirements: 3. The effects on manpower needs. Dental Update 16: 382–390

Todd J E, Walker A M 1985 Children's dental health in the United Kingdom 1983. HMSO, London

Appendix I The prophylaxis of infective endocarditis

The recommendations of the British Society for Antimicrobial Chemotherapy for the antibiotic prophylaxis of infective endocarditis are based on the most recent information available and give special consideration to the problems of general dental practice.* The recommendations are as follows.

Patients who require antibiotic cover

Patients at risk are those with acquired cardiac valve disease, with congenital valve or other endocardial defects, with prosthetic valves or with a history of previous attacks of infective endocarditis. The last are a special, high risk group who should be referred to hospital.

Operations for which cover should be given

Cover should be given for extractions, scaling and surgery involving the periodontal tissues. Other procedures, though capable of causing bacteraemias, do not offer a significant threat.

Recommended antibiotic regimens are as follows.

RECOMMENDATIONS FOR ENDOCARDITIS PROPHYLAXIS (1990)

Dental extractions, scaling, or periodontal surgery under local or no anaesthesia

(a) For patients not allergic to penicillin and not prescribed a penicillin more than once in the previous month:

Amoxycillin
Adults: 3 g single oral dose taken under supervision 1 hour before dental procedure
Children under 10: half adult dose
Children under 5: quarter adult dose

(b) For patients allergic to penicillin:

Erythromycin stearate
Adults: 1.5 g orally taken under supervision 1–2 hours before dental procedure plus 0.5 g 6 hours later
Children under 10: half adult dose
Children under 5: quarter adult dose

or

Clindamycin*
Adults: 600 mg single oral dose taken under supervision 1 hour before dental procedure
Children under 10: 6 mg/kg body weight single oral dose taken under supervision 1 hour before dental procedure

---

* Simmons N A, Cawson R A, Clarke C A et al 1990 Prophylaxis of infective endocarditis. Lancet 1: 88–89
See also Cawson R A, 1983, British Dental Journal 154: 183–4, for additional notes.

---

* Note: Clindamycin, *as a single oral dose*, is suggested for patients allergic to penicillin as an alternative to erythromycin. In comparison with erythromycin, clindamycin is considerably better and more reliably absorbed (hence the need for only a single dose) and is also less likely to cause nausea or vomiting. As to toxicity the Committee on Safety of Medicines have received only 10 reports of adverse effects from 1970 to the time of publication of the current recommendations. Of these, there was only a single case of diarrhoea, all the rest were of a minor nature or not an effect of the drug itself, and there was no report of pseudomembranous colitis. However, it is important to note that the risk of pseudomembranous colitis is considerably increased if repeated doses are given.

Under general anaesthesia

(c) For patients not allergic to penicillin and not given penicillin more than once in the previous month:

Amoxycillin intramuscularly

Adults: 1 g in 2.5 ml 1% lignocaine hydrochloride just before induction plus 0.5 by mouth 6 hours later
Children under 10: half adult dose

or

Amoxycillin orally

Adults 3 g oral dose 4 hours before anaesthesia followed by a further 3 g by mouth as soon as possible after operation
Children under 10: half adult dose
Children under 5: quarter adult dose

or

Amoxycillin and probenecid orally

Adults: amoxycillin 3 g together with probenecid 1 g orally 4 hours before operation

Special risk patients who should be referred to hospital:

(i) Patients with prosthetic valves who are to have a general anaesthetic
(ii) Patients who are to have a general anaesthetic *and* who are allergic to penicillin or have had a penicillin more than once in the previous month
(iii) Patients who have had a previous attack of endocarditis
Recommendations for these patients are:

(d) For patients not allergic to penicillin and who have not had penicillin more than once in the previous month:

Adults: 1 g amoxycillin intramuscularly in 2.5 ml 1% lignocaine hydrochloride *plus*

120 mg gentamicin intramuscularly just before induction: then 0.5 g amoxycillin orally 6 h later
Children under 10: amoxycillin, half adult dose; gentamicin 2 mg/kg body weight

(e) For patients allergic to penicillin or who have had penicillin more than once in the previous month.

Adults: vancomycin 1 g by slow intravenous infusion over 60 min followed by gentamicin 120 mg intravenously just before induction or 15 min before the surgical procedure
Children under 10: vancomycin 20 mg/kg intravenously, gentamicin 2 mg/kg intravenously

Additional measures

1. Application of an antiseptic such as 0.5% chlorhexidine to the gingival margins before the dental procedure should reduce the severity of any resulting bacteraemia and may usefully supplement antibiotic prophylaxis in those at risk.

2. Regular dental care for the maintenance of optimal dental health is important for those at risk. Good dental health should reduce both the frequency and severity of any bacteraemias and also the need for extractions.

3. It is essential that, even when antibiotic cover has been given, patients at risk should be instructed to report any unexplained illness. Infective endocarditis is typically exceedingly insidious in origin and can develop 2 or more months after the operation. Late diagnosis considerably increases the mortality or disability among survivors.

4. Patients at risk should carry a warning card to be shown at each dental visit to indicate the risk of infective endocarditis and the need for antibiotic prophylaxis.

Appendix II Cross-infection control—summary

These principles are based on the fact that (i) the great majority of carriers of hepatitis viruses, or HIV, or both cannot be recognised clinically, (ii) contamination of instruments and hands is inevitable and (iii) imperceptibly small traces of blood can transmit hepatitis B and the virus is difficult to kill. ALL PATIENTS MUST THEREFORE BE REGARDED AS POTENTIALLY INFECTIOUS.

MAJOR MEASURES TO MINIMISE CROSS-INFECTION

1. Have immunisation against hepatitis B.
2. Take extreme care with needles or other sharp instruments and discard disposables safely into appropriate impervious bins.
3. Make sure of effective sterilisation (autoclaving) of instruments and disinfection of working areas.
4. Wear gloves, mask, protective goggles,* or face shields* and clean clinical garments in the surgery.
5. Maintain meticulous personal hygiene.
6. Give patients a 0.2% chlorhexidine mouth rinse preoperatively to reduce the number of oral microbes.
7. Use rubber dam (wherever feasible) and high-speed evacuation
8. Try to avoid causing bleeding.
9. Keep working area to a minimum; use tray system or cover surfaces with disposable material. Uncovered surfaces and equipment should be cleaned and disinfected after treatment of each patient.

10. Take a careful medical history and take particular care in observing these precautions with high-risk patients.**

CARE OF EQUIPMENT AND WORKING AREAS

1. Heavy duty rubber gloves should be worn for all cleaning and disinfection.
2. Clean all blood and debris from instruments before sterilisation.
3. Autoclave all possible equipment, unwrapped, usually at 134°C for 3 minutes.
4. Discard all disposables and waste into an impervious bin for incineration.
5. Handpieces and other non-autoclaveable equipment may have to be sterilised in a hot-air oven or chemically, after thorough cleaning.
6. Disinfect working surfaces with 1% hypochlorite, change any disposable covering material and disinfect impressions.

---

* Eye protection is important not merely to protect against infection but also against injuries.

** It may seem contradictory to recommend that full cross-infection control measures should be taken with all patients but also to advise *extra* care with high-risk patients. Most cannot be identified, but a patient with visible signs of AIDS or its prodromes, for example, has a significantly higher level of viraemia and is potentially more liable to transmit the infection than a recently infected, asymptomatic person (Ch. 8).

However, *IF* a high risk patient can be identified, it is important to make absolutely certain that all infection control measures are being strictly observed. Extra precautions such as double-gloving may be taken, and referral to a specialist unit may be required.

Table AII.1 High-risk groups for AIDS and hepatitis

1. Promiscuous male homosexuals and bisexuals
2. Intravenous drug abusers
3. Haemophiliacs and others who have received untreated blood products or unscreened blood
4. Sexual contacts of any of the above
5. Visitors from high-risk areas*

* Some surveys have shown that this group have the highest frequency of hepatitis B carriage.

Appendix III The core of knowledge relating to radiation protection of patients

(Summarised from the Schedule to the Ionising Radiation (Protection of Persons Undergoing Medical Examination or Treatment) Regulations 5 and 6 1988 (SI 1988 No. 778).

The person physically directing medical exposures (taking radiographs) is expected to know:

1. The nature of ionising radiation and its interactions with the tissues
2. The genetic and somatic effects of ionising radiation and how to assess these risks
3. The ranges of radiation dose that are given to a patient for a particular procedure and the principal factors which affect the dose and how to measure it
4. The principles of quality assurance and quality control as applied to both equipment and techniques
5. The principles of dose limitation and the various means of dose reduction to the patient, including protection of the gonads
6. The specific requirements of women who are or may be pregnant, and of children
7. If necessary, the precautions necessary for handling sealed and unsealed sources of radiation
8. The organisational arrangements for advice on radiation protection and how to deal with suspected cases of overexposure
9. The statutory responsibilities (see below).

   For those making clinical requests for radiographs ('clinically directing medical exposure') the following additional knowledge should be acquired:

10. The clinical value of the individual diagnostic and therapeutic procedures which the person expects to use, as compared with other techniques used for the same or similar purpose
11. The importance of using existing information (previous radiographs or reports or both) about the patient.

THE STATUTORY RESPONSIBILITIES. TO MEET PRESENT LEGISLATIVE REQUIREMENTS IT IS ESSENTIAL TO:

1. Notify the *Health and Safety Executive* of the use of X-ray equipment
2. Appoint a suitably qualified and trained person within the practice as a *Radiation Protection Supervisor* (RPS)
3. Ensure that equipment meets all *appropriate standards* in respect of radiation safety and is regularly *checked and maintained*
4. Provide and display *Local Rules*, which must include the name of the RPS, description of the Controlled Area, and any special local provisions
5. Provide adequate *information, instruction and training* for all staff
6. Ensure that staff *are not exposed* to an instantaneous dose rate exceeding 7.7 μSv h
7. Provide a *contingency plan* to specify actions to be followed in the event of an equipment malfunction
8. Appoint a *Radiation Protection Advisor*, if any staff are likely to be exposed to an instantaneous dose more than 7.5 μSv h or if any person other than the patient is to be in the Controlled Area during X-ray emission.

Index